THIRD EDITION

Measuring Occupational Performance

Supporting Best Practice in Occupational Therapy

THIRD EDITION

Measuring Occupational Performance

Supporting Best Practice in Occupational Therapy

Edited by

MARY LAW, PHD, FCAOT
McMaster University
Hamilton, Ontario, Canada

CAROLYN BAUM, PHD, OTR/L, FAOTA
Professor, Occupational Therapy, Neurology and Social Work
Elias Michael Director, Program in Occupational Therapy
Washington University School of Medicine
St. Louis, Missouri

WINNIE DUNN, PHD, OTR, FAOTA
Professor
Department of Occupational Therapy Education
University of Kansas
Kansas City, Kansas

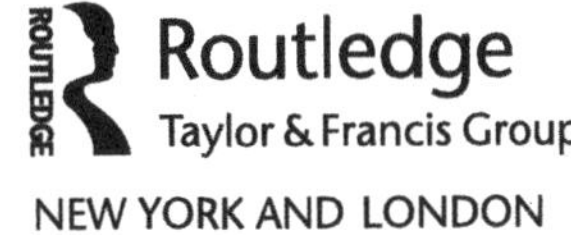

NEW YORK AND LONDON

Instructors: *Measuring Occupational Performance: Supporting Best Practice in Occupational Therapy, Third Edition Instructor's Manual* is also available. Don't miss this important companion to *Measuring Occupational Performance: Supporting Best Practice in Occupational Therapy, Third Edition*. To obtain the Instructor's Manual, please visit http://www.routledge.com/9781630910266

First published in 2017 by SLACK Incorporated

Published 2024 by Routledge
605 Third Avenue, New York, NY 10017
4 Park Square, Milton Park, Abingdon, Oxon OX14 4RN

Routledge is an imprint of the Taylor & Francis Group, an informa business

Library of Congress Cataloging-in-Publication Data

Names: Law, Mary C., editor. | Baum, Carolyn Manville, editor. | Dunn, Winnie, editor.
Title: Measuring occupational performance : supporting best practice in occupational therapy / [edited by] Mary Law, Carolyn Baum, Winnie Dunn.
Description: Third edition. | Thorofare, NJ : SLACK Incorporated, [2017] | Includes bibliographical references and index.
Identifiers: LCCN 2016046083 (print) | ISBN 9781630910266 (hardcover : alk. paper) |
Subjects: | MESH: Occupational Therapy--standards | Outcome Assessment (Health Care) | Practice Guidelines as Topic | Evidence-Based Medicine
Classification: LCC RM735 (print) | NLM WB 555 | DDC 615.8/515--dc23
LC record available at https://lccn.loc.gov/2016046083

ISBN: 9781630910266 (hbk)
ISBN: 9781003525042 (ebk)

DOI:10.4324/9781003525042

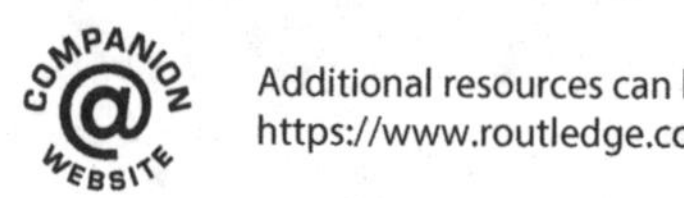

Additional resources can be found at
https://www.routledge.com/9781630910266

Dedication

To our colleagues who have collectively dedicated themselves to making the most effective, creative, and relevant measurement possible. Your efforts are reflected in this book and serve to contribute to both the growth of evidence for the profession of Occupational Therapy and the improvement of people's quality of life.

Contents

Instructors: *Measuring Occupational Performance: Supporting Best Practice in Occupational Therapy, Third Edition Instructor's Manual* is also available. Don't miss this important companion to *Measuring Occupational Performance: Supporting Best Practice in Occupational Therapy, Third Edition*. To obtain the Instructor's Manual, please visit http://www.routledge.com/9781630910266

Acknowledgments

We are very grateful to all of the authors who have shared their knowledge in the chapters of this book. Their ability to analyze measures and to synthesize that information in easy-to-use tables is outstanding. Thanks also to our colleagues at McMaster University, Washington University in St. Louis, and the University of Kansas Medical Center for your continuing support of our work.

Mary wishes to acknowledge the ongoing support that she receives from her family—thanks to Brian, Mike, Geoff, Andy, Jenna, Rebecca, and Laura. She wishes to thank her friends and colleagues from CanChild Centre for Childhood Disability Research at McMaster University for being the best support network ever!

Carolyn would like to acknowledge the colleagues and participants who have fostered her interest in measurement, and particularly Mary Law, Joy Hammel, Dorothy Edwards, Julie Bass, and Allen Heinemann who unselfishly share their knowledge and support.

Winnie would like to acknowledge Anna Wallisch, Mark Burghart, and Benjamin Evans for their work preparing references and obtaining background material.

About the Editors

Mary Law, PhD, FCAOT is Professor Emeritus, School of Rehabilitation Science and CanChild Centre for Childhood Disability Research at McMaster University in Hamilton, Canada.

Carolyn Baum, PhD, OTR/L, FAOTA is the Elias Michael Director and Professor of Occupational Therapy, Neurology and Social Work at Washington University School of Medicine in St. Louis, MO.

Winnie Dunn, PhD, OTR, FAOTA is Professor and Chair of the Department of Occupational Therapy Education in the School of Health Professions at the University of Kansas, Kansas University Medical Center in Kansas City, KS.

Contributing Authors

Catherine Backman, PhD, OT(C), FCAOT (Chapter 15)
Professor, The University of British Columbia
Senior Scientist, Arthritis Research Canada
Affiliated Investigator, Vancouver Coastal Health
British Columbia, Canada

Julie D. Bass, PhD, OTR/L, FAOTA (Chapter 17)
St. Catherine University
Minneapolis, Minnesota

Jackie Bosch, PhD, OT Reg. (Ont.) (Chapter 13)
Associate Professor, School of Rehabilitation Science
Investigator, Population Health Research Institute
McMaster University
Hamilton, Ontario, Canada

Mark Burghart, MOT (Chapter 3)
Doctoral Student
Department of Occupational Therapy Education
University of Kansas
Lawrence, Kansas

Mary A. Corcoran, PhD, OTR/L, FAOTA (Chapter 6)
Associate Dean, Faculty Development for Health Sciences
Professor, Clinical Research and Leadership
School of Medicine and Health Sciences
The George Washington University
Washington, DC

Oana Craciunoiu, MScOT, OT(C) (Chapter 16)
Department of Occupational Science and Occupational Therapy
University of British Columbia
Child and Family Research Institute
Vancouver, British Columbia, Canada

Mary Forhan, PhD, OT(C) (Chapter 15)
Assistant Professor
University of Alberta
Edmonton, Alberta, Canada

Lauren Foster, OTD, OTR/L (Chapter 12)
Adjunct Assistant Professor
University of Kansas Medical Center
Kansas City, Kansas

Apeksha Gohil, BOT (Chapter 3)
Candidate for Post-Professional Clinical Doctorate in Occupational Therapy
Department of Occupational Therapy
University of Illinois at Chicago
Chicago, Illinois

Meredith P. Gronski, OTD, OTR/L (Chapter 5)
Methodist University
Fayetteville, North Carolina

Joy Hammel, PhD, OTR/L, FAOTA (Chapter 8)
University of Illinois at Chicago
Chicago, Illinois

Kathryn M. B. Haugen, REHS/RS (Chapter 17)
U.S. Centers for Disease Control and Prevention
Minnesota Department of Health
St. Paul, Minnesota

Jenna Heffron, PhD, OTR/L (Chapter 8)
Ithaca College
Ithaca, New York

Margo B. Holm, PhD, OTR/L, FAOTA, ABDA (Chapter 14)
Professor Emerita
Department of Occupational Therapy
School of Health and Rehabilitation Sciences
University of Pittsburgh
Pittsburgh, Pennsylvania

Vicki Kaskutas, OTD, OTR/L, FAOTA (Chapter 11)
Associate Professor
Washington University School of Medicine
Program in Occupational Therapy
St. Louis, Missouri

Danbi Lee, PhD, OTD, OTR/L (Chapter 8)
Northwestern University
Evanston, Illinois

Lori Letts, PhD, OT Reg. (Ont.) (Chapters 13, 16)
Assistant Dean, Occupational Therapy Program
Professor, School of Rehabilitation Science
McMaster University
Hamilton, Ontario, Canada

Joy MacDermid, BScPT, PhD (Chapter 4)
Professor
School of Rehabilitation Science
McMaster University
Hamilton, Ontario, Canada

Susan Magasi, PhD (Chapter 3)
Assistant Professor
Department of Occupational Therapy
University of Illinois at Chicago
Chicago, Illinois

Mary Ann McColl, PhD, MTS (Chapter 7)
Queen's University
Kingston, Ontario, Canada

Kira Meskin, OTD, OTR/L (Chapter 8)
Northern Suburban Special Education District
Highland Park, Illinois

Laura Miller, PhD, BSc(OT)(Hons), MHSM (Chapter 10)
Senior Lecturer
School of Allied Health
Australian Catholic University
Virginia, Queensland, Australia

Becky Nicholson, OTD, OTR/L (Chapter 12)
Clinical Assistant Professor
Department of Occupational Therapy Education
University of Kansas
Kansas City, Kansas

Monica S. Perlmutter, OTD, OTR/L, SCLV, FAOTA (Chapter 5)
Program in Occupational Therapy
Washington University
St. Louis, Missouri

Nancy Pollock, MSc, OT Reg. (Ont.) (Chapter 7)
School of Rehabilitation Science
McMaster University
Hamilton, Ontario, Canada

Anne A. Poulsen, PhD, BOccThy (Hons) (Chapter 10)
Senior Researcher
School of Health and Rehabilitation Sciences
The University of Queensland
St Lucia, Queensland, Australia
Honorary Senior Research Fellow
Mater Medical Research Institute (MMRI)
South Brisbane, Queensland, Australia

Patricia Rigby, PhD, OT Reg. (Ont.) (Chapter 16)
Associate Professor, Department of Occupational Science and Occupational Therapy
Rehabilitation Sciences Institute
University of Toronto
Toronto, Ontario, Canada

Joan C. Rogers, PhD, OTR/L, FAOTA (Chapter 14)
Professor Emeritus
Department of Occupational Therapy
School of Health and Rehabilitation Sciences
University of Pittsburgh
Pittsburgh, Pennsylvania

Jill Stier, MA, OT Reg. (Ont.) (Chapter 16)
Department of Occupational Science and Occupational Therapy
University of Toronto
Toronto, Ontario, Canada

Anna Wallisch, MOT (Chapter 3)
Doctoral Student
Department of Occupational Therapy Education
University of Kansas Medical Center
Kansas City, Kansas

Jenny Ziviani, PhD, BAppSc(OT), BA, MEd (Chapter 10)
Professor
Children's Allied Health Research
School of Health and Rehabilitation Sciences
The University of Queensland
St Lucia, Queensland, Australia

PREFACE

The journey from the conceptualization of an idea for a book to its completion is often a long, meandering pathway. That is the case with this text. We initially conceived the idea for this book in conversations during the Can-Am Occupational Therapy Conference in Boston in 1994. All of us were enthusiastic about the idea of assembling knowledge about the measurement of occupational performance in occupational therapy practice. As you can imagine, the tasks of identifying the focus and content of the book and appropriate authors and writing have taken longer than expected. However, there has been a benefit from the time taken. Measurement in occupational therapy has become more sophisticated, and this is reflected in many assessments reviewed in this book.

It has been exciting and rewarding to work together on this text. There is no doubt that this book has been enriched from the collaboration between the three of us. From the many faxes and emails to the time that we spent together at conferences, on teleconference meetings, and over 2 days in St. Louis, our interactions have been stimulating and fun. This time to work together has been a wonderful opportunity for growth and professional collaboration.

This edition marks a new era in occupational therapy measurement. We have more validated instruments than ever before. Our interprofessional collaborations have illuminated other measures that are useful to certain areas in occupational therapy. Our colleagues in practice are more sophisticated consumers and so have a more discerning eye for quality methods to support their evidence-based practices. Collectively, we understand the many ways to document participation so our work is convincing to others.

It is our hope that student occupational therapists, occupational therapy practitioners, and occupational therapy educators will find the material in this book useful in their daily studies and practice. We welcome your comments and thoughts about the content and layout of the book. Faculty can access the *Instructor's Manual* to support their work as well.

Mary Law, Carolyn Baum, and Winnie Dunn

Foreword

In my Foreword for the first edition of this book, I stated that global health care trends were becoming congruent with the core values and beliefs of occupational therapy. I am happy to report that now, several years later, these trends continue as health care policy and the prevalent health paradigm increasingly supports our values and beliefs. Among these values and beliefs are that health is greater than or even different from the sum of the intact anatomical, physiological, and behavioral components of individuals; that client-centered experience of well-being is essential to health; and that health is inseparable from the social and physical environment of daily living.

These trends have been fueled by globalization, research findings, and evidence-based practice. As different cultures have come together and exchanged knowledge, practices, and artifacts of living, it has become clear that the traditional Western view of health as the absence of bodily pathology is only partially true, and therefore, only a partially effective model for improving health. A more bio-psycho-social-cultural view is required. Research findings generally have supported the need for a model of health in which mind, body, action, and situation are interactive and transactive. The rise of evidence-based practice has encouraged critical scholarship and the testing of deeply held assumptions by the various health care disciplines, creating and supporting the climate of change that underlies the emerging trends.

Although the trends in health care are promising, they have far to go. The new policies are not yet backed uniformly or consistently by economic and management systems that provide the infrastructure for the practices needed to implement these trends. Practitioners continue to hold disparate and nonconvergent models of health, either because of lack of training relevant to the new trends or inability to accommodate to these trends because of the poor infrastructure. There is a need for leadership on how to do the health care represented in these trends: specifically, a need for the clear explication of healthy living, for the development of interventions to promote it, for the valid and trustworthy assessment of its achievement, and for the dissemination of this body of knowledge to clients, health care providers, managers, and policy makers.

Now, more than ever, occupational therapy has much to contribute to the path of health care. We are trained in mind-body health and its relationship with the meaning and importance of the routines of daily living; we are experts in the content, rhythms, and situations of living; and we have a philosophy of optimism and pragmatism that girds our intervention—a seeing of possibilities, and the roll-up-your-sleeves, hands-on doing of what needs to be done. Most importantly, we aim to see clients' lives through their eyes, to understand what is important from their point of view. Having this aim, even if its achievement is difficult, is essential to effective cross-ethnicity and cross-cultural therapeutic relationships, as well as to the development of high-quality and globally relevant assessments, interventions, practice theory, and research.

However, in fulfilling our potential as leaders in health care, we occupational therapists also have much to learn. Only now are we recognizing that our "commonsense" approach to daily living is our primary strength; that, indeed, it is worthy of the intense critical scholarship, research, and theory development that we saw previously as secondary to the doing of our work with clients, or as reserved for the more "basic science" disciplines. The editors of this text, Mary Law, Carolyn Baum, and Winnie Dunn, have been instrumental in naming the strengths of an occupational paradigm and giving a voice to the meaning of health from an occupational perspective. Among their many works, they have brought together the esteemed contributors to this book to explain how our core values and beliefs can be put into everyday practice in this changing environment.

My statement in the Foreword to the first edition bears repeating because it continues to be true in this second edition. The contributors to this book show how the manifestation of our values and beliefs in practice creates the best practice for our clients and supports the continued integration of these values and beliefs into the larger health care system. Their guidance is based specifically on current research evidence about the importance and validity of measuring occupational performance. They summarize the measurement tools needed to assess client occupational performance, to provide the best intervention, and to document the effectiveness of that intervention. The tools are not merely a compilation of all that are available for measurement relevant to occupational therapy; rather, they are an elite group of tools carefully selected by the contributors through a process of rigorous theoretical, clinical, and scientific reasoning. As a result, the book is an essential reference manual for the evidence-based practitioner, the occupational performance researcher, and the health care policy consultant.

Although occupational therapy continues to develop as a profession, it has recently achieved a new level of rigor and expertise in its scholarship and research-based knowledge. Now, several years after the printing of the first edition, I believe that occupational therapists are ready to play major roles in defining the multi- and interdisciplinary approach to health. The assessments in this book address health concepts and constructs that are at the intersections of the various disciplines, and they bridge the dichotomies that often differentiate the disciplines. These assessments connect mind to body, action to environment, and individual to community. They do so because this is how occupational therapists view health. Occupational therapists are ready to lead the way to a new and collaborative health care paradigm, using the voice of connection that exists within the assessment procedures of this book.

Linda Tickle-Degnen, PhD, OTR/L, FAOTA
Tufts University
Medford, Massachusetts

Introduction

Foundations of Occupational Therapy Measurement Practice

Occupational therapists serve persons, groups, and organizations that want support to participate in occupations (ie, self-care, work, voluntary activities, play, leisure) that facilitate their quality of life. The World Health Organization (WHO) has recognized the importance of participation in occupations and its influence on health and well-being in their widely adopted *International Classification of Functioning, Disability and Health* (ICF).[1] This book provides the student and the clinician with the focus and tools to measure occupational performance and support best practice in occupational therapy.

What challenges do occupational therapists face as they pursue the measurement of occupational performance? Let's illustrate a few of them:

- "I want to evaluate the occupational performance outcomes of my clients, but the team I work with expects me to provide information about range of movement, strength, and endurance. They also want numbers."
- "It would be easier to justify reimbursement for services if we used outcomes measures that provided evidence about the changes that we see in clients' day-to-day activities. It's so hard to know where to start in using outcomes measures. How do we decide what it is we want to measure, and what are the best assessments to use?"
- "I know that I should encourage my clients to identify the occupational performance issues for which they need occupational therapy services, but I just don't have enough time to allow them to do that. It's so much easier just to do our standard assessment of performance components (eg, cognitive status, balance) and start therapy right away."

In writing this book, we hope to address these issues and eliminate concerns that limit measurement practices in occupational therapy. We have identified 5 fundamental objectives for the book.

Mine the Gold

There is a wealth of information in the occupational therapy literature and the broad health and social sciences literature that supports occupational therapy measurement practices. Using such information will enable occupational therapists to support their clinical observations and will lend credibility to their day-to-day clinical observations. Occupations are complex, individualized, and essential for health and well-being. We enhance evaluation of occupational performance—the outcomes of doing occupation—when we develop a broad measurement perspective. As a result, others will recognize the unique contribution of occupational therapy to their teams.

Become Systematic

Occupational therapists can use the information in this text to develop a consistent approach to measuring the outcomes of their practice. We provide a systematic guide to make decisions about measurement of occupational performance. This guide enables therapists and clients to knowledgeably identify outcomes of interest and select the most reliable and valid methods to assess these desired outcomes. We provide resources for the selection of the best assessments to support therapists for their practice or research situations. We index measures by assessment area, chapter, and title for ease of identification.

Use Evidence in Practice

Occupational therapists strive to practice effectively and efficiently. One of the most important underpinnings of an evidence-based occupational therapy practice is the consistent use of outcomes measures to evaluate occupational therapy service. Information from the application of outcomes measurement enables therapists to make decisions about which programs are most effective, thus building evidence to support occupational therapy intervention. In this text, we provide information about the selection and application of outcomes measurement to support an evidence-based occupational therapy practice.

Make Occupational Therapy Contribution Explicit

Occupational therapy makes a unique contribution to health, education, and community care through our focus on the occupations of everyday life. Through ongoing analysis of persons doing the occupations of their choice within different environments, occupational therapists identify factors that support or hinder performance and intervene to support optimal performance. Mattingly and Fleming, in a study of the occupational therapy clinical reasoning process, stated that "what occupational therapists do looks simple; what they know is quite complex."[2(p 24)] When occupational therapists consistently use measurement tools to identify the unambiguous outcomes of effective occupational therapy services, we clarify our contribution to the participation, health, and well-being of persons needing our services.

Engage in Occupation-Based, Client-Centered Practice

There is substantial research evidence to support the relationship between engagement in occupation and positive outcomes for a person's health and well-being.[3-6] Therapy that supports persons to do the occupations of their choice is most effective when delivered using a client-centered service delivery model.[7] Information in this text focuses on measurement of occupational performance from a client-centered perspective, and supports an occupation-based, client-centered practice.

This book is organized to be a tool for the student occupational therapist and the practicing therapist as they strive to organize and classify their occupational therapy experiences to best serve their clients. Section I of this text addresses the foundations of occupational therapy measurement practices. In Chapter 1, we outline the theoretical foundations for an occupation-based, client-centered practice. Chapter 2 focuses on central concepts to understand regarding measurement, including the importance of considering the context of measurement, and Chapter 3 discusses measure development and the properties that must be considered when evaluating a measure. In Chapter 4, we present a decision-making framework to guide occupational therapists in the identification, selection, and use of best measurement practices.

In Section II, we introduce topics that influence our understanding of assessment data (Chapter 5), including qualitative methods (Chapter 6), the need for client-centered care (Chapter 7) and self-management (Chapter 8). Finally, in Section III, we organize the occupational performance measurement areas into separate chapters for your use. Each chapter covers a critical area for your consideration.

References

1. World Health Organization. *International Classification of Functioning, Disability, and Health (ICF)*. Geneva, Switzerland: WHO; 2001.
2. Mattingly C, Fleming M. *Clinical Reasoning: Forms of Inquiry in a Therapeutic Practice*. Philadelphia: F.A. Davis; 1994.
3. Clark CA, Corcoran M, Gitlin LN. An exploratory study of how occupational therapists develop therapeutic relationships with family caregivers. *Am J Occup Ther.* 1995;49(7):587-594.
4. Law M, Steinwender S, LeClair L. Occupation, health and well-being. *Can J Occup Ther.* 1998;65(2):81-91.
5. Stav WB, Hallenen T, Lane J, Arbesman, M. Systematic review of occupational engagement and health outcomes among community-dwelling older adults. *Am J Occup Ther.* 2012;66:301-310.
6. Wilcock A. *An Occupational Perspective of Health*. Thorofare, NJ: SLACK Incorporated; 1998.
7. Law M. *Client-Centered Occupational Therapy*. Thorofare, NJ: SLACK Incorporated; 1998.

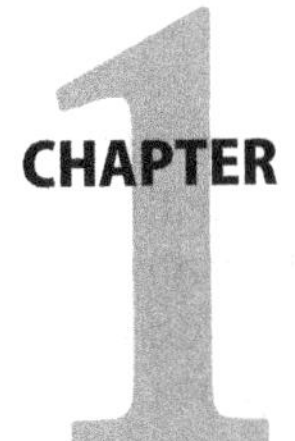

CHAPTER

Measurement in Occupational Therapy

Mary Law, PhD, FCAOT and Carolyn Baum, PhD, OTR/L, FAOTA

Our conception of man is that of an organism that maintains and balances itself in the world of reality and actuality by being in active life and active use.[1]

Occupational therapists support individuals, groups, and organizations to participate in the occupations of everyday life. The goal for occupational therapy services is to enhance occupational performance (ie, the doing and experience of occupation to satisfy life needs). Occupational therapists' unique contribution to society, therefore, is to enable clients to achieve their goals by helping them recognize what might limit their occupational performance.[2] To achieve this goal, our discipline must learn about the clients' physical, cognitive, neurobehavioral, and psychological capacities; their culture; their physical, social, and institutional environments; and the activities, tasks, and roles that the clients define as important. The process of providing occupational therapy is complex.

Within the health, education, and community care, each discipline has a developed area of focus. For example, physicians center on patients' impairments, medical history, and physical exam; physical therapists focus on movement; dietitians consider nutrition; and occupational therapists emphasize occupational performance. Rogers[3] describes medicine's efforts to limit the impact of disease as a contrast to occupational therapy's efforts in enabling the performance of work, play, or self-care "occupations." A critical point of Rogers is that there are individuals who experience occupational performance problems that are not accompanied by disease (ie, joblessness, behavior disorders, teen mothers, and people living in times of war, among others). The broad focus of occupational therapy on the "occupations of everyday life" makes it necessary to use measurement methods that are not dependent on a medical condition to determine the extent of the occupational performance dysfunction. Rogers argues convincingly that, through the emphasis on disease and functional deficit, rather than occupational performance and competence, the biomedical influences on traditional health care have been a limiting factor in the development of occupational therapy (and its measurement methods).

There is a sizable population of persons with disabilities in the world. For example, about 45 million Americans, or 1 in 6,[4] and 1 of 7 Canadians over the age of 15 years, about 3.4 million people,[5] have an impairment that limits their daily activities. Approximately one-third of these disabilities are severe enough that they limit participation in work and/or community life.[5] Disability is a public health problem—it affects not only individuals with a disability and their immediate families, but also society.[6] There are even more persons who are experiencing limitations in occupational performance for other reasons such as poverty, social crises, or war. Measurement of the outcomes of occupational therapy practice in all of these situations improves our ability to work together with clients, their families, and other groups in a client-centered occupational therapy practice.

In this chapter, we will discuss the foundations of occupational therapy measurement practices, including the philosophical influences, sociocultural factors, central concepts for contemporary practice, interdisciplinary models that are consistent with our philosophy, and models for considering occupational performance in a best practice measurement process.

Philosophical Influences on Occupational Therapy

The values, beliefs, and principles of a discipline have a major influence on its identity and development, and are known collectively as its *philosophy*. Throughout our

Law M, Baum C, Dunn W, eds. *Measuring Occupational Performance: Supporting Best Practice in Occupational Therapy, Third Edition* (pp 1-16).

history, occupational therapy has valued occupation and performance of occupations. There have been ongoing discussions of measurement, but until the early 1990s, there was a lack of measures of occupational performance to support the profession's values and beliefs.

Adolph Meyer, a notable psychiatrist and neurobiologist who taught at Johns Hopkins University and was a proponent of occupational therapy during its early years, is widely credited with making an important contribution to the development of philosophy in the field. He also has had a major impact on measurement because he stated the first hypothesis of our discipline. In an address given at the 5th annual meeting of the National Society for the Promotion of Occupational Therapy in Baltimore, MD, in 1921, Meyer suggested that occupational therapy represents an important manifestation of human philosophy; namely, "the valuation of time and work"[1(p 6)] and the role of performance and completion in bringing meaning to life.

Meyer stated that "man learns to organize time and he does it in terms of doing things,"[1(p 6)] thus emphasizing his view of the importance of doing to achieving self-fulfillment. Meyer suggested that the view of mental illness as a problem of living rather than a structural, toxic, or constitutional disorder was an important characteristic of the field, and that occupational therapists could provide opportunities for the individual to work, plan, create, and learn to use tools and materials. These opportunities, Meyer thought, would assist patients in gaining pleasure and pride in achievement. If we were to apply these concepts in today's practice, we would provide people with an opportunity to use their minds in planning, organizing, sequencing, and carrying out a task (executive skills).

In summarizing Meyer's address, we can observe that he viewed the individual and health in a holistic rather than structural sense and believed that engagement in occupations, or doing, provided a sense of reality, achievement, and temporal organization. Meyer perceived occupational therapy as providing opportunities for engagement that would contribute to learning and improving one's sense of fulfillment and self-esteem. In doing so, he was proclaiming occupational therapy's concern for quality of life and suggesting a clear relationship between the ability to perform daily occupations and one's life satisfaction.

Meyer's themes have been repeated in more recent contributions by scholars reflecting on the unique characteristics of the field. For example, Yerxa,[7] in her Eleanor Clarke Slagle address, emphasized the role of occupational therapy in providing opportunities for fulfillment in doing when she wrote:

> In occupational therapy, the patient experiences the reality of his physical environment and his capacity to function within it. Our clinics may be chambers of horror for some individuals as they confront their physical disability for the first time by trying to do something, perhaps as simple as [eating]. Yet, if the individual is to function with self-actualization, he must discover both his limitations and his possibilities. We meet our responsibilities to the client when we provide opportunities to readjust his or her value system through the development of both new capacities and the ability to substitute for some lost capacities. We are like mirrors which can reflect, without the distortion of wish-fulfillment or self-deprecation, a true image of the client's potential.[7(p 5)]

Similarly, Fidler and Fidler[8] emphasized the role of occupation, or doing, in gaining self-actualization, when they wrote:

> The ability to adapt, to cope with the problems of everyday living, and to fulfill age-specific life roles requires a rich reservoir of experiences gathered from direct engagement with both human and non-human objects in one's environment. Doing is a process of investigating, trying out, and gaining evidence of one's capacities for experiencing, responding, managing, creating, and controlling. It is through such action with feedback from both non-human and human objects that an individual comes to know the potential and limitations of self and the environment and achieves a sense of competence and intrinsic worth.[8(p 306)]

Both Elizabeth Yerxa and the Fidlers reaffirmed Adolph Meyer's beliefs and values in the opportunities occupational therapy affords for self-actualization. They also emphasized the role of the therapist in assisting the individual to cope with problems of everyday living and to adapt to limitations that interfere with competent role performance.

Rogers[3] declared that functional independence is not only the core concept of occupational therapy theory, but also the goal of the occupational therapy process. Noting that the requirements for independence are competence and autonomy, she suggested that autonomy is reflected in the ability to make choices and have control over the environment. The opportunities afforded within occupational therapy practice for developing competence and teaching strategies for exerting autonomy make it unique among the rehabilitation disciplines. To say we influence autonomy and independence, it is necessary to use a measurement strategy that demonstrates these effects.

Occupation has always been central to the practice of occupational therapy. Writers over the decades have given direction to that practice. A sampling of these writers is presented as follows to lay the context for the measurement of occupational performance.

- "[A human] is an organism that maintains and balances itself in the world of reality and actuality by being in active life and active use... It is the use that we make of ourselves that gives the ultimate stamp to our every organ."[1(p 1)]

- Reilly[9] suggests that human beings need to produce, create, master, and improve their environment in order to achieve health and well-being.
- Fidler and Fidler[10] conceptualized activity as a valuable vehicle to acquire, maintain, or redevelop skills necessary to fulfill occupational roles and provide satisfaction.
- Individuals who perceive that they have control over their environments and can address obstacles derive satisfaction from their occupational roles.[11,12]
- Function results from a series of complex relationships among cognitive, psychological, sensory, neuromotor, and physiological capabilities as the individual interacts with his or her environment.[13]
- Occupational dysfunction can be viewed as a "breakdown in habits that leads to physiological deterioration with the concomitant loss of ability to perform competently in daily life."[14(p 30)]
- When occupational therapists present the opportunity for individuals to engage in activity, not only does the individual's functional status improve,[15] but occupational therapy makes explicit its unique contribution to the enhancement of human function.
- "...Purposeful and fulfilling occupations can provide individuals with sufficient exercise to maintain homeostasis, to keep body parts and neuronal physiology and mental capacities functioning at peak efficiency, and enable maintenance and development of satisfying and stimulating social relationships... If they are able, or encouraged to pursue this need, they will, apart from supplying sustenance for survival and safety, enhance their health."[16(p 23)]
- "Occupational therapy, at its best, is client-centered. The person receiving occupational therapy services leads the way in making decisions about the focus and nature of therapy intervention. The relationship between that person, his or her family, and the occupational therapist is a collaborative partnership whose goal is to enhance occupational performance, health, and well-being."[17(p xv)]

Bing[18] proposed the following 6 enduring values. These values can serve as hypotheses for guiding intervention and measurement and challenge students and faculty into action to empirically test these core principles.

1. Engagement in occupation is of value because it provides opportunities for individuals to influence their well-being by gaining fulfillment in living.

   Question: Does participation in occupation provide opportunities for individuals to influence their well-being?
2. Through the experience of occupation (or doing), the individual is able to achieve mastery and competence by learning skills and strategies necessary for coping with problems and adapting to limitations.

   Question: Can occupation construct opportunities for learning that yield mastery and adaptation?
3. As competency is gained and autonomy can be expressed, independence is achieved.

   Question: What is the relationship between competency, autonomy, and independence?
4. Autonomy implies choice and control over environmental circumstances. Thus, opportunities for exerting self-determination should be reflected in intervention strategies.

   Question: Is there a difference in the outcome of persons who exhibit self-determination by exercising choice and control in the design and implementation of occupational therapy services? Does changing the environment influence a person's ability to participate effectively in occupations?
5. Choice and control extend to decisions about intervention, thus identifying occupational therapy as a collaborative process between the therapist and recipient of care. In this collaboration, the patient's values are respected.

   Question: Does a collaborative, client-centered approach promote health and well-being and fewer secondary conditions?
6. Because of its focus on life performance, occupational therapy is neither somatic nor psychological, but concerned with the unity of body and mind in doing.

   Question: What is the relationship of an integrated body-mind approach to care vs a psychological approach vs a physical impairment orientation on the person's perception of his or her capacity for life and satisfaction? How does a person's spirituality affect his or her occupations?

It is useful for practitioners in occupational therapy to be familiar with these core principles[18] and to use them in assessing and planning occupational therapy services. They also guide us to important questions that are being asked as our health care systems broaden to include habilitation to support people's health.

Impact of Sociocultural Factors on Our Focus on Occupation

Despite a strong early grounding in occupation, medicine has influenced the history of occupational therapy practice. As early as the 1930s, occupational therapy practice was progressively moving away from a view of function that was holistic and occupation-centered, in favor of practice techniques that emphasized components of function such as muscle strength, range of motion, or disturbed processes of thought. By the 1960s, the focus of occupational therapy practice became inextricably linked to the medical model of health care.[19] In fact, from the mid 1960s to the mid 1980s, in the United States, occupational therapy's reimbursement was directly related to documentation of these performance components. At that time, little consideration was given to how these components affected performance in day-to-day living. In fact, findings from research indicate that there is little direct relationship between impairments (or components) and abilities.[20,21] That is, there is little transfer of skills from doing a specific action to being able to apply the action in a sequenced complex task required for participation in everyday activities. Fortunately, in the late 1970s, several prominent writers in the field expressed concern for this state of affairs and encouraged a return to the occupation-centered philosophy upon which the profession was first established.

Prominent among these was an article entitled "The Derailment of Occupational Therapy," by Philip Shannon.[22] Shannon wrote that:

> ...a new hypothesis has emerged that views man not as a creative being, capable of making choices and directing his own future, but as a mechanistic creature susceptible to manipulation and control via the application of techniques. The technique hypothesis, inspired by the principles of reductionism, subverts the occupational therapy hypothesis of man using his hands to influence the state of his own health.[(p 233)]

In the same year, Kielhofner and Burke[23] provided a detailed account of various bases for practice during the first 60 years of occupational therapy. They traced the evolution of guiding principles in the field from its humanistic roots to the competing ideas of the 1980s, noting that the paradigm of reductionism was reflected in 3 dominant intervention models that continued to influence practice. These were the kinesiological, the psychoanalytic or interpersonal, and the sensory integrative or neurological models. The authors concluded that advancement of the field would require a theoretical approach that went "beyond reductionism" and allowed an understanding of human adaptation, or "social man within a holistic theoretical framework." Today, we see the importance of this shift as all of medicine is being challenged to focus on function to foster well-being and participation, a trend that makes it all the more important for occupational therapists to return to and embrace our roots in occupation.[19]

Central Concepts for Contemporary Occupational Therapy Practice: Occupation

Just as good health is often taken for granted, so too are everyday life experiences. The satisfaction of dining with friends and family, enjoying a walk in the park, or gaining a sense of accomplishment from seeing a garden blossom can be diminished by impairments resulting from injury or disease, inability to do an activity, or lack of environmental supports, but they need not be. The remarkable adaptability of the human body, our spirituality, and the power of meaning and self-will provide many ways for people to derive satisfaction from participation in life's occupations despite temporary or permanent functional limitations. When these resources are coupled with the skillful intervention of the occupational therapist, persons can achieve health-related occupational performance.

Occupation is everything that we do in life, including actions, tasks, activities, thinking, and being. Engagement in occupation describes the interaction of the individual with their self-directed life activities. Adolph Meyer professed that individuals should attain and retain a healthful "rhythm in sleep and waking hours, of hunger and its gratification, and finally the big four—work and play and rest and sleep."[1(p 3)] Wilcock[16] challenges us to view "occupation [as] a central aspect of the human experience and unique to each individual." The definition of occupation should be basic to every occupational therapist's vocabulary. Occupation meets an individual's intrinsic needs for taking care of and expressing one's self, and finding fulfillment within the context of one's roles and environment.[24] Thus, it is through the process of engagement in occupation that people develop and maintain health and well-being.[25-30] While occupations can support one's health and well-being, recent literature highlights that occupational therapists' broad definition of occupation includes occupations that may not support one's health.[31,32] Ficher et al[31] indicate that this highlights the importance of considering the context for the occupation.

Occupational Performance

Occupational performance is doing occupations that satisfy life needs. Occupational therapy uses the word "function" interchangeably with "performance" and "occupational performance." The unique contribution of occupational therapy is that the practitioner creates the opportunity for individuals to gain the skill and confidence to accomplish activities that are meaningful and productive, and in doing so increases their occupational performance.[33]

- Occupational performance is the point when the person, the environment, and the person's occupation intersect to support the tasks, activities, and roles that define that person as an individual.[2,24]
- The concept of occupational performance has become a mainstay in the development of models of occupational therapy. It operates as a means of connecting the individual to roles and to the sociocultural environment[34]
- Occupational performance refers to the ability to choose, organize, and satisfactorily perform meaningful occupations that are culturally defined and age appropriate for looking after one's self, enjoying life, and contributing to the social and economic fabric of a community[35]
- Occupational performance results from the dynamic interaction between people, their occupations and roles, and the environments in which they live, work, and play[24]

- Occupational performance consists of meaningful sequences of action in which a person completes an occupational form[36]
- Occupational performance is the ability to perceive, desire, recall, plan, and carry out roles, routines, tasks, and sub-tasks for the purpose of self-maintenance, productivity, leisure, and rest in response to demands of the internal and/or external environment[37]
- Performance includes both the process and the result of the person interacting with context to engage in tasks[38]

The ideas underlying occupational therapy models of practice that address the inter-relationships between the person, environment, and occupation are not new. In many ways, these ideas are similar to a model (called the *ecological systems model*) proposed by occupational therapists Howe and Briggs[39] and share characteristics in common with self-determination theory, formulated by Deci and Ryan.[40] In these models, performance is viewed as the result of complex relationships between the individual as an open system and the specific environments in which activities, tasks, and roles occur. It is important to consider that a complete view of occupational performance must account for the actions, tasks, occupations, and roles of an individual as he or she goes about his or her daily life.[30,41]

David Nelson[42,43] has contributed to our thinking about occupation. Recognizing that people use the term *occupation* to mean "active doing" as well as "that which is done," Nelson proposed including both interpretations in our understanding of occupation. In his schema, *occupation* is defined as the relationship between an occupational form and occupational performance. Occupational performance consists of the "doing" of occupation, whereas occupational form concerns the context of the doing, or the other elements of a "doing situation," which provide it with purpose and meaning.

While occupational performance is a key consideration when discussing an individual's occupation, there are other elements that need to be considered. One element that has received particular attention is occupational engagement. Polatajko et al[44] define *occupational engagement* as everything that individuals do to occupy themselves. They indicate that *occupational engagement* is a broader term than *occupation performance* because humans can engage in occupations without actually doing them.

Overall, there is consensus for the term *occupational performance*. The next step in our development is for measurement models to evolve that support the occupational therapist in determining the effectiveness of occupational therapy services through the evaluation of occupational performance. The measurement of occupational performance requires the practitioner to employ 3 strategies: 1) what people do in their daily lives, 2) what motivates them, and 3) how their personal characteristics combine with the environment in which occupations are undertaken to influence successful occupational performance. Such an approach provides a framework for viewing human behavior that combines knowledge about the impairments (components) that impede performance, the environments that support or hinder performance, and the individual needs, preferences, styles, and goals.[24,30]

Occupational therapy practice must place its focus on occupational performance, assisting our clients to become actively engaged in their life activities. Basic to an occupational performance approach are the skills of the therapist to analyze tasks, activities, and occupations and propose and use learning or adaptive strategies to support the individual to perform meaningful occupations.

The Environment

The environment in which persons live, work, and play make doing and being possible. People conduct their daily lives within many different environments. Some are using the terms *environment* and *context* interchangeably. Every task and activity has a context—what is present at the time the activity occurs. The environment exists whether an activity occurs or not. For example, a community may offer curb cuts, large font (signage) for its street signs, or verbal cues at crosswalks. That city has created a universal environment, which may or may not give context to the performance of a task for an individual with a particular set of skills or limitations.

Occupational performance is always influenced by the characteristics of the environment in which it occurs. In noting this, Rogers described the qualities of the environment as important "enablers of human performance."[45] In Chapter 2, we discuss the issues of contextual measurement for contemporary occupational therapy practice.

A Client-Centered Approach to Measurement

Adolph Meyer[1] spoke of client-centered concepts in the *Philosophy of Occupation*, yet Carl Rogers was the first person to use the actual term *client-centered* to describe a health care practice that was nondirective and centered on the person's articulated needs.[46] Rogers recognized that a client-centered approach would often be at odds with a medical model approach. Indeed, the client-centered approach has often been criticized for its lack of specific techniques and inherent optimism.[47,48]

In the early 1980s, occupational therapists described the need for a practice based on a client-centered approach. The national association and occupational therapists in Canada developed client-centered guidelines for occupational therapy,[35,49] and now therapists around the world contribute to this perspective.

Client-centered occupational therapy has been defined as "an approach to service which embraces a philosophy of respect for, and partnership with, people receiving services."[49(p 253)] "The goal of the [client-] centered philosophy is to create a caring, dignified, and empowering environment in which [clients] truly direct the course of their care and call upon their inner resources to speed the healing process."[50(p 128)] Such an approach to therapy acknowledges our responsibilities to work in partnership with clients to enable them to find meaning in life through daily occupations. It also enables them to identify their needs and individualize the services they perceive they will need in order to accomplish their goals. Clients are encouraged to recognize and build on their strengths using natural community supports as much as possible. We celebrate everyone's ability to find sources of meaning and bring their resources to the occupational therapy intervention process when using a client-centered approach.

Law[17] has summarized the concepts of client-centered practice inherent in all theoretical discussion of this approach. These concepts include the following:

- Respect for clients and their families, and the choices they make
- Clients and families have the ultimate responsibility for decisions about daily occupations and occupational therapy services
- Provision of information, physical comfort, and emotional support. Emphasis on person-centered communication
- Facilitation of client participation in all aspects of occupational therapy service
- Flexible, individualized occupational therapy service delivery
- Enabling clients to solve occupational performance issues
- Focus on the person-environment-occupation relationship[17]

Using these assumptions, clients and therapists can jointly focus on their unique contribution and responsibilities and jointly select measures that will contribute to the decision-making process.[49]

What does a client-centered, occupational therapy practice mean for the way in which we measure occupational performance?

1. Occupational performance issues/problems will be identified by the client and his or her family, not by the therapist or team. If there are issues that do not surface related to safety, prevention, or health maintenance, the therapist will communicate these concerns directly to the client and family.
2. Evaluation of the success of therapy intervention will focus on change in occupational performance.
3. Measurement techniques will enable clients to have a say in evaluating the outcomes of their therapy intervention.
4. Measurement will reflect the individualized nature of people's participation in occupations.
5. Measurement will focus on both the subjective experience and the observable qualities of occupational performance.
6. Measurement of the environment is critical in helping therapists and clients understand the influence of the environment on occupational performance, as well as measuring the effects of changing environmental conditions in the home, work site, school, or community that would foster participation.

Client-centered measurement is based on the principle that effective therapy begins with a careful understanding of the individual. Each of the occupational therapy models discussed later in this chapter provides a framework for clinicians to organize information gained from interviews and formal assessments. These frameworks can form the basis for intervention that is collaborative and client-directed.

In a client-centered approach, clients and therapists work together to define the nature of the occupational performance problems, the focus and need for intervention, and the preferred outcomes of therapy. Clients will participate at different levels, depending on their capabilities, but all are capable of making choices about how they approach their rehabilitation to improve their capacity for daily life. The occupational therapist must have a fundamental respect for clients' values and visions and for their style of coping without being judgmental, as well as knowledge of the factors that influence occupational performance. During the first phase of intervention, it is important for the occupational therapist to seek information from the client about his or her perception of needs and goals. Information that is shared builds the occupational performance history, which includes information about the person, the environment, and the occupational factors that require occupational therapy intervention.

In order to be considered client-centered, occupational therapy models must consider the activities, tasks, and roles of the person[51]; the organization of services to support the individual as an active participant in his or her care[52]; and create a partnership that enables individuals to assume responsibility for their own care.[49] Each of these considerations challenges the practitioner to employ measurement strategies that go far beyond, but may include, measurement at the performance component level to fully understand the individual's capacities for occupational pursuits. The measurement process must be clinically useful and integrated into the intervention process.

A measurement model must allow the client and practitioner to jointly plan intervention. The client's knowledge of his or her condition and experience with the problem must become clear for the relationship to progress.[2] Occasionally, intervention planning must occur with a person who has a cognitive deficit, or, because of age or intelligence, does not have the capacity for independent decision making. In this case, a family-centered approach is critical. A family-centered approach is based on the same principles as a client-centered approach, with members of the family providing important information about the client's occupation and their roles and occupations as caregivers.

Why is it important for occupational therapists to use a client-centered approach to therapy measurement and intervention? As well as recognizing the fundamental respect for others inherent in this approach, there is also increasing evidence from research that client-centered practice improves not only the process, but also the outcomes of care.[17] An occupational therapy practice based on the concepts of client-centeredness is more likely to engage clients in the occupational therapy process[17] and is better able to enlist the personal and spiritual resources necessary to facilitate the healing process.[50] Researchers have also shown that a client- or family-centered approach to health services improves adherence to therapy recommendations,[53] increases client satisfaction,[54-57] and leads to enhanced functional outcomes.[58-61]

Best Practice

Best practices are a professional's decisions and actions based on knowledge and evidence that reflect the most current and innovative ideas available.[62] Many therapists, teams, and agencies engage in "standard practice," which is employing more traditional, routine, and established ways of providing services. This is a perfectly acceptable paradigm for conducting professional practice (ie, the routines or protocols are known and work). The location of practice does not determine whether one engages in best or standard practice; therapists can work in traditional or nontraditional settings and use either approach. Best practice involves thinking about problems in imaginative ways, applying knowledge creatively to solve performance problems, while also taking responsibility for evaluating the effectiveness of the innovations to inform future practices.

Remember: what is best practice today evolves into standard practice in the future. This is how knowledge advances in our profession. The standard practices of today were best practices of the past that have influenced practice. When someone continues his or her standard practices too long, it is likely that his or her practice is out of date and would not stand up to current standard practice scrutiny. As your career unfolds, watch for these transitions and recognize their contributions to the evolution of occupational therapy practice.

Interdisciplinary Systems for Participation and Quality of Life

It is important for occupational therapists to understand several key concepts to appreciate fully how occupational therapy fits into the larger context of health care and rehabilitation. Concepts from the World Health Organization (WHO) are useful here. We also acknowledge the pioneering work of Nagi,[63] who was among the first to examine the various causes and consequences of disability.

International Classification of Functioning, Disability, and Health

The International Classification of Functioning, Disability, and Health (ICF)[64] is a comprehensive rehabilitation model from WHO that offers definitions and structures for facilitating communication among health professionals and policy makers. Most health care systems models have focused on the impairment and disability aspects of the human condition; however, the introduction of the ICF has broadened this view to include personal and environmental characteristics[65] by putting forward a conceptual framework of body function and structure, activity, participation, and personal and environmental factors.[64] Through the worldwide effort to develop this classification, it was recognized that an individual's participation in society is dependent upon the interactive relationships between these elements. Over the past decade, this model has influenced collection of data that are used by policy makers to build systems of care that facilitate participation of persons with disabilities. It has also had an impact on the types of outcome measures that occupational therapists are using within their practice.[66]

We introduce the ICF here to familiarize the reader with key terms, concepts, and the factors that must be considered at each level. Table 1-1 highlights the key terminology and concepts of the new classification and contrasts the revision with the original 1980 version.[67]

In using a framework such as the ICF to organize measurement, interventions, and services, one issue is critical: occupational therapists must place their primary focus at the level of the person-environment interaction so that occupational performance issues can be assessed and addressed in the occupational therapy plan (see Vargus-Adams and Majnemer[65] for a discussion of using the ICF in childhood rehabilitation). Person-environment issues are addressed in the ICF model at the activity, environmental factors, and participation levels. Table 1-2 illustrates how this framework can be used to organize the focus of measurement in occupational therapy. When we do not focus on occupational performance, the contributions of occupational therapy are not made explicit. Because no one else has this expertise and emphasis, the result may be that the client must fend for him- or herself with occupational dysfunction that will compromise his or her function, participation, and health.

It is important for all practitioners in occupational therapy to be familiar with these principles and use them in planning services. It is also essential for educators to teach students how to measure the constructs inherent in these principles and for therapists to use occupational performance measurements in daily practice.

Occupational Therapy Models for Considering Occupational Performance Within Community Environments

The health system focuses on outcomes because of the need to be accountable—not only to the clients in need of services, but also to the government and/or the third party who provides funding for these services. With a shift in focus toward primary and secondary prevention, it is also important to know if interventions are successful in reducing the impact of secondary problems. A review of the research examining the relationship between occupation, health, and well-being indicates that occupation is a significant factor in positively influencing a person's subjective and objective health and well-being.[25]

It is within the context of performance transactions that individuals encounter the objects, people, conditions, and events that stimulate development or maturation. As Kielhofner[68] has suggested, although change is not always grossly apparent, experiences accumulate that reinforce or modify individual characteristics. Over time, changes become more evident, although the overall trend may be characterized by periods of varying organization or advancement. As the life cycle progresses, the desired course is one of greater satisfaction within one's environmental circumstances and an increasing sense of fulfillment through life's activities.

People spend most of their waking hours engaged in occupations, which include self-maintenance, and productive and leisure pursuits. Thus, to speak of performance in occupational therapy is to refer to occupational performance. Viewing occupational performance as a transaction between the individual, the occupations he or she does, and the environment provides a useful framework for viewing occupational therapy practice and measuring the occupational performance of our clients. This approach toward organizing information useful to measurement emphasizes the relationships between the person, environment, and occupation.

The following occupational therapy models can be used in a client-centered approach if the therapist places the focus on the client's goals and the client's occupational needs. Each of these models has the potential to evolve into a partnership between the occupational therapist and the client to address the client's goals. These models go far beyond the issues of performance components but do not prohibit the therapist working with the client on strategies to address component issues and environmental conditions that can influence the person's occupational performance. Each model can benefit from continued testing, and some require the development of more assessment tools; however, they all offer occupational therapy practitioners guidance in developing innovative and effective client-centered, occupation-based models of practice. We provide an overview of the key measurement issues for these models in comparison to each other; you will see both consistency and uniqueness among the models.

The Ecology of Human Performance Model

The Ecology of Human Performance Model[38,69] focuses on context and how contextual factors such as physical, temporal, social, cultural, and/or phenomenology can impact the performance of the client. The framework includes person, context, and performance variables and the interaction among them. They describe a 3-dimensional model in which you can only see the person by observing him or her in the context. A client-centered approach is central to the identification of the tasks and activities that the person does. This model helps the practitioner explore specific strategies to overcome the contextual barriers that would limit the client's performance.

Key Measurement Issues

- Tasks and activities that the person does within his or her living context
- Understanding of the social, cultural, and physical environment and its impact on the performance of the client

The Model of Human Occupation

The Model of Human Occupation (MOHO)[14,70,71] evolved from Reilly's Model of Occupational Behavior.[72] The MOHO focuses on occupational functioning and serves to guide practice in the organization or reorganization of occupational behavior. Because it focuses on the client's routines and habits, the client's perspective and motivation for activities must be determined. The person is viewed as a dynamic system influenced by the physical and social environment. MOHO has made significant contributions to occupational therapists' knowledge of clients' roles and how occupation is central to an individual's health. A number of interview measures have been developed to support the model.

Key Measurement Issues

- The routine and habits of the person
- The person's motivation for activities and tasks
- The meaning of the activity and choice of occupations

The Person-Environment-Occupation Model

This transactive Person-Environment-Occupation Model[24,73] considers the person, the occupation, and the environment in an interwoven relationship that views people in their everyday lives. The originators acknowledge that occupational performance cannot be separated from contextual influences, temporal factors, and the physical and psychological characteristics of the person. They place their model in a developmental context recognizing that environments, task demands, activities, and roles are constantly shifting. A Person-Environment-Occupation intervention seeks to enable optimal occupational performance in occupations that are defined as important by the client. The authors of this model have explicitly stated the importance of focusing on the client's goals and sharing the process of the interaction to form a partnership that will assist the client in taking responsibility for his or her own rehabilitation. This model considers the Canadian Occupational Performance Measure[74] essential to its implementation; thus, the client's goals become the focus of the intervention.

Key Measurement Issues

- The occupations that a person chooses and the goals for the therapeutic experience
- The physical and psychological characteristics of the person
- Factors in the social, cultural, physical, and institutional environment that support or hinder performance
- Temporal orientation and phase of life

The Person-Environment-Occupation-Performance Model

The Person-Environment-Occupational-Performance Model[29,30,51,75] recognizes that the person's occupational performance cannot be separated from person-centered and contextual influences. It has operationalized the intrinsic factors (psychological, cognitive, physiological, and neurobehavioral) and extrinsic or environmental factors (physical, cultural, social, and societal policies and attitudes) to understand the capacities of the individual to perform the activities, tasks, and roles that are important to the person. Additionally, the person's self-image, determined from competency, self-concept, and motivation, are considered in the overall plan for care that is driven by the client in a dynamic partnership with the clinician (and perhaps the family and others who are instrumental in the client's life). This approach requires that the practitioner determine the activities, tasks, and roles of the client to use as the central element in planning interventions and requires that the intervention engage the person in meaningful occupations as the process to support recovery or health maintenance. This model also supports an occupational performance-based approach for organization and population-based approach.

Key Measurement Issues

- The activities, tasks, and roles that are important to the person, organization, or population. The person's view of him- or herself as an occupational being
- Intrinsic factors that support performance. These include the psychological, cognitive, physiological, motor, and sensory capacities, as well as spirituality
- Extrinsic or environmental factors that serve as supports or create barriers to occupational performance, including physical, cultural, and social support and social capital as well as societal policies and attitudes

The Canadian Model of Occupational Performance and Engagement

The Canadian Model of Occupational Performance and Engagement (CMOP-E)[76] is a revised version of the CMOP, which was published by the Canadian Association of Occupational Therapists in 1997. The model describes the relationship between persons, their environments and occupations, and the process by which occupational therapists can enable clients to achieve optimal occupational performance. Spirituality, the innate essence of self, is a central construct in the model. CMOP-E also incorporates "occupational engagement," a concept that brings a broader perspective to occupation than just one's performance. As explained by the authors, "humans frequently engage in occupations without performing them."[44] This model is designed around processes to guide therapists in helping clients (individuals, groups, and organizations) achieve satisfying levels of occupational performance.

Key Measurement Issues

- Occupations that are meaningful to the client
- The internal resources of the client (physical, affective, cognitive)
- The environment of the client
- Spirituality

Kawa Model

The Kawa Model provides a perspective on occupational performance that incorporates Eastern principles of the interconnectedness of humanity and nature, and the importance of inter-relations of people.[77] The Kawa Model uses a metaphor from nature—a river or *kawa* in Japanese—to represent one's life course. Within this metaphor, the water (or one's life energy) begins at a high elevation (birth) and flows through the river, eventually ending at a larger body of water. While flowing, the water is impacted by and has an impact on elements within the river such as rocks, debris, and the walls and floor. These elements represent things within the person's life, such as personal abilities, life circumstances, and environmental factors. The ability of the water to flow effectively is determined by the interaction of the water and these river elements. Using the Kawa framework, an occupational therapist engages the client in a discussion and the client's narrative is used to depict his or her river. Specific areas for measurement are identified based on the elements that are thought to be impeding the flow of the river.

Key Measurement Issues

- Client's story of his or her day-to-day experiences
- Physical and social environmental factors (ie, the river walls and floor)
- Client's personal attributes (ie, the driftwood and debris)
- Life circumstances the client perceives to be challenging (ie, the rocks)

A review of these 6 occupational therapy models indicates their commonality in the measurement of occupational performance. All, either explicitly or implicitly, require a client-centered approach to the identification of the activities, tasks, and roles of the person (occupation). In addition, they consider the personal factors (psychological, cognitive, neurobehavioral, and physiological) and the environment (culture, social, and physical) in which the occupation is performed and the meaning that is attributed to the occupation. All of these constructs are essential to understanding the process to maximize the occupational performance of the individual. If the occupational therapy profession can consistently address the occupational performance needs of the people they serve, the public understanding of occupational therapy's contribution to health care and society will improve. As we become explicit in our use of occupational performance language, we will also facilitate the advancement of our knowledge to better serve the people who need occupational therapy services.

The Occupational Therapy Measurement Process

Measurement in occupational therapy serves multiple purposes. From an overall practice perspective, measurement is used to improve our decisions regarding specific clients or programs. As professionals, occupational therapists have an obligation to measure the need for service and evaluate the results of interventions. Information gathered through the use of measures with individual clients or groups helps occupational therapists plan therapy and evaluate the outcome of an intervention.

Measures can also be used with groups of individuals. Management and policy makers use aggregated measurement information to understand more about groups of individuals who use their services. This information can help managers and policy makers make decisions about the continuance of funding for programs or the need to establish and/or evaluate new programs or policy directions. Managers and policy makers may also be interested in using measures to evaluate whether there is change over time within a specific program in areas such as client participation in community activities. Similarly, researchers use measurement information for purposes such as investigating the effectiveness of an occupational therapy intervention or identifying patterns of participation for groups or subgroups of individuals (eg, those with and without disabilities).

In addition to being used for a variety of purposes, measurement in occupational therapy is also context specific. Occupational therapists are involved in measurement across many different systems, including health, education, and home- or community-based care, with each system presenting different challenges to implementing outcome measurement.

What Is Measurement?

Measurement is a process that involves an assessment, calculation, or judgment of the magnitude, quantity, or quality of a characteristic or attribute. Measurement is defined as the "process of obtaining a numerical description of the extent to which persons, organizations, or things possess specified characteristics."[78] In everyday living, we deal with measurements ranging from calculation of time, length, or weight to judgments of quality of life and satisfaction.

Occupational Therapy's Measurement Focus

In this book, we will consider evaluation in occupational therapy from the broad perspective of measurement of the person, occupation, and environment. Measurement of occupational performance involves evaluation of self-care, work, other productive pursuits, play, and leisure. Because of the importance of the environment for occupational performance, we also discuss the evaluation of the environmental factors that influence such performance. Because the focus of this book is on measurement of occupational performance, we do not discuss in detail or review evaluation tools that assess performance components such as range of motion, mood, endurance, or memory. Performance component testing is important as a means to gather information about why an occupational performance problem is occurring, but in an occupation-based practice, this information is used to establish capacity and not as the outcome of care.

Measurement of occupational performance includes the use of both quantitative and qualitative approaches, from the perspective of the client, his or her family or caregiver, and the occupational therapist. As occupational therapists develop an evidence-based practice, a valid measurement process is essential in providing evidence of the effectiveness and efficiency of our services. Our measurement practices need to fit within a client-centered approach where persons, their families, and therapists work in partnership to enhance occupational performance. Our clients expect, and have a right to know and receive, evidence of the outcomes of occupational therapy service provision.

What aspects of occupational performance do occupational therapists evaluate? It depends on the needs of those whom we serve. Tables 1-3 and 1-4 provide examples of the needs of potential clients and suggests the issues that occupational therapists may address from a measurement standpoint.

Implementing a measurement process within an occupational therapy practice can be challenging. There are a number of issues therapists must consider when instituting measurement within their practice—availability of time, deciding what to measure, finding an appropriate assessment tool for the measurement process, aggregating measurement information, and using the results from the measurement process to make decisions about services, all considered within a client-centered framework.[79] Using standardized measures to make decisions about individual patients has the potential to improve decision making. For example, routine administration of the Canadian Occupational Performance Measure has been associated with improvements in practice parameters such as knowledge of the patient's perspective on outcome and clinical decision making.[80] These are the issues that we will address in this book.

Planning Measurement Strategies

Occupational therapists must draw upon their knowledge of the individual, organizations, occupation, and the environment as they identify assets and limitations that affect the quality of occupational performance of the people and organizations they serve. A careful consideration of this information and the possible intervention alternatives permit the selection of various strategies for meeting client-centered goals. In each case, the particular application of an intervention process will be unique because individuals and their circumstances are unique.

Rogers[3] cautions that a therapeutic program that is right for one person is not necessarily right for another. For example, some individuals may wish to develop skills to enable occupational performance, while others may choose to modify the task or the environment, or they may choose to have someone do it for them. She suggests that clinical inquiry be individualized and focus on 3 questions: 1) What is the client's current status in occupational performance? 2) What could be done to enhance the client's performance? and 3) What ought to be done to enhance the individual's occupational performance? Such a focus demands new perspectives for outcome measurement.[81]

It is, in fact, the critical analysis of the intrinsic, extrinsic, and occupational factors and planning of intervention for the unique constellation of circumstances represented in each client's story that makes occupational therapy an immensely complex undertaking. Because of this complexity, intervention planning is one of the most challenging and critical skills for therapists to master. As Mattingly and Fleming[82] point out, what occupational therapists do appears so very simple, but the process of determining what to do is so very complex. Despite its complexities, effective intervention planning can be accomplished if careful attention is devoted to understanding the individual, what it is that he or she wants or needs to do, and the environmental context of the performance.

Identification of Occupational Performance Issues

The measurement process in occupational therapy begins and ends with occupational performance. In this process, the first step is for the client, his or her family or caregiver, or the organization to identify his or her occupational performance issues. The identification of areas of occupational performance in which the client is experiencing difficulty helps therapists to organize the rest of the measurement process. A detailed decision-making process for this purpose is discussed in Chapter 4.

Another critical aspect of quality evaluation is the person's interests and needs. In client-centered care, professionals demonstrate respect for what the individual and family wish to accomplish. Professionals then consider strengths and barriers to the performance of those tasks that the individual and family have identified. In order to provide client-centered care, professionals must depart from traditional expert models in which the professional directs the course of evaluation and planning.

Most formal testing that occupational therapists use measures the person's skills and abilities or specific task performance. However, a person's performance can vary considerably in different contexts. For example, a worker may not be able to concentrate with other workers talking, but may be able to manage the phone ringing and computer printer sounds quite well. A seamstress will need to use more primitive mending strategies for a clothing repair in a hotel room than in her sewing station. A young child may remember to wipe himself after toileting within the hygiene rituals at home, but may be distracted with peers in the early childhood center. Performance is context dependent; we must consider the impact of particular contexts as part of the data gathering process. This, along with using a client-centered approach in which a client's choices are respected, moves occupational therapy measurement away from merely a capacity approach (ie, measuring a person's best level of function in an ideal environment) toward a capability approach in which the individual's occupational performance is influenced by his or her capacity, choices, and environmental context.[83]

Summarizing Measurement Data

Following the identification of occupational performance issues, further evaluation is often completed in order to review the strengths and challenges from the perspective of the person, the environment, and occupational factors. Specific areas for measurement may include performance areas, the demands of the activities the client has selected (eg, physical, cognitive, social demands) and the environment in which the client would like to participate (eg, home, work place, community).

Table 1-1

World Health Organization's International Classification of Functioning, Disability, and Health

Body	Body Function and Structure: "physiological functions of body systems or anatomical parts of the body and their component"
Person	Activity: "the execution of a task or action by an individual"
Community/Society	Participation: "involvement in a life situation"
Environment,	Environmental Factors: "the physical, social, and attitudinal environment in which people live and conduct their lives"
Personal factors	Personal Factors: "particular background of an individual's life and living (eg, gender, race, age, fitness)"

Adapted from World Health Organization. *International Classification of Functioning, Disability, and Health (ICF)*. Geneva: WHO; 2001:212-213.

Based upon the identified occupational performance issues and a summary of strengths and challenges, a list of goals is developed with the client. These should directly relate to each identified occupational performance problem or need.

Developing Priorities

Once each occupational performance problem has an accompanying goal, the vital task of determining priorities must take place. The occupational therapist will engage the client in a discussion to determine the order in which goals will be addressed. While the most critical factor is the client's choice, other factors will influence this decision, such as availability of programs and the time or money to support the goal. Once priorities are set, further evaluation may take precedence over intervention because effective treatment is contingent on complete information.

Designing and Implementing Intervention Plans

Here, specific methods and techniques for achieving goals are determined. Strategies for addressing occupational performance problems tend to fall into 6 major categories. Two major categories relate to the environment and include making changes in a person's physical, social, and institutional environment and using technology in the form of various devices and aids. A third category focuses on modifying the activity that the client wants to do so that the activity demands better fit the client's abilities. A fourth category focuses on the person and includes various approaches to facilitating development, recovery, or adaptation of neurological, sensory, and motor deficits. The remaining 2 categories have principles that warrant specific focus in the text. These include the means of delivering services and strategies that challenge the occupational therapist to take an active role in changing attitudes, policies, and laws that shape the political and social environment.

For most goals, there will be more than one appropriate intervention strategy. The occupational therapist will work with the client to develop options and determine which strategy or strategies to try first. Throughout the intervention stage, the occupational therapist and client will engage in ongoing measurement/evaluation to determine how well the strategies are working. By implementing a variety of strategies, individualized to the client's needs, occupational therapists make it possible for the tasks and roles necessary for optimal participation in the occupations of everyday life.

Planning Ongoing Measurement Strategies

Changes within all health systems are demanding an increased focus on quality and evidence for programs gained from systematic outcome measurement.[84] By including assessment intentions within the overall intervention plan, the therapist ensures that this important aspect of intervention will be addressed. Collecting data during the intervention process is called *progress monitoring.* When therapists monitor progress systematically, they generate evidence for practice decisions.

Overall, occupational therapy intervention includes a logical flow from identified problems to goals to intervention strategies. In essence, the intervention planning process, when performed by the client and therapist together, can be likened to weaving. There is a clear design and guiding principles. The challenge is to combine the warp and weft in a way that captures opportunities for

Table 1-2

USING THE INTERNATIONAL CLASSIFICATION OF FUNCTIONING, DISABILITY AND HEALTH FRAMEWORK FOR OCCUPATIONAL THERAPY MEASUREMENT

ICF Dimension	*Body Function or Structure*	*Activities*	*Participation*	*Environmental Factors*
Occupational Therapy Classification	Performance components	Occupational performance	Occupational performance; role competence	Environmental factors
Examples of Attributes	Attention Cognition Endurance Memory Movement patterns Mood Pain Range of motion Reflexes Strengths Tone	Dressing Eating Learning Making meals Manipulation tasks Money management Socialization Shopping Walking Washing	Community mobility Education Housing Personal care Play Recreation Social relationships Volunteer work	Architecture Attitudes Cultural norms Economic Geography Light Resources Health services Institutions Social rules

Table 1-3

OCCUPATIONAL NEEDS AND AREAS FOR MEASUREMENT—INDIVIDUAL CLIENTS

Population	*Occupational Need*	*Potential Areas for Measurement*
Persons with chronic disease	Participate in community activities	Community environment (eg, availability of programs, attitudes of others, physical structures and sensory aspects), demands of the activities the person wants to do, personal abilities
Children with chronic or neurological conditions	Participate in classroom activities at school	School environment (eg, physical structures, social relationships with peers, sound and other sensory issues), demands of the school activities, personal abilities
Individuals with acute injuries	Return to paid employment	Demands of the job, aspects of the environment (eg, physical structures, attitudes of coworkers, organizational policies), personal abilities

creativity, yet yields a satisfactory outcome. The experienced weaver, like the occupational therapist in providing intervention, executes the design with a shuttle that glides smoothly, wasting neither time nor energy in pursuit of the selvage that ends this effort and marks the beginning of yet another challenge. The outcome, or the fabric of the plan, is optimal occupational performance outcomes for the client.

We have written this book to give practitioners the tools to employ an occupational performance model in evaluating their clients and to form the basis of planning care. We recognize that this best practice approach is a paradigm shift from a traditional medical or social model, but we also recognize that such an approach supports current practice guidelines and will make occupational therapists' unique contributions to care visible and contemporary with the changes in health care.

Table 1-4

Occupational Needs and Areas for Measurement—Society-Level Clients

Population	*Occupational Need*	*Potential Areas for Measurement*
Industry	Productive workers	Capacity for work, person/environment fit
Social Security Administration	Eligible recipients	Functional capacities evaluation
Hospital/community health system	Healthy communities	Community participation, absence of secondary conditions
Schools	Children with the capacity to learn	School participation, features of the environment (eg, school policies, physical, sensory, and social)
City and county government	Housing and resources for older adults	Capacity for community living, design of community environment
Architecture or engineering firm	Consumers, universal design	Person/environment fit
Retirement communities	Satisfied resident, least support	Availability of programs, design of the community environment, abilities of the residents
Day care facilities (child or adult)	Enhance performance	Demands of the activities, abilities of the children/adults, features of the environment (eg, physical, sensory, and social)
University/college	Support learning	ADA—disability—access officers, features of the environment (eg, physical, sensory, and social)

References

1. Meyer A. The philosophy of occupation therapy. *Arch Occup Ther.* 1922;1(1):1-10.
2. Baum CM, Law M. Occupational therapy practice: Focusing on occupational performance. *Am J Occup Ther.* 1997;51(4):277-288.
3. Rogers JC. Order and disorder in medicine and occupational therapy. *Am J Occup Ther.* 1982;36:29-35.
4. Brandt EN Jr, Pope AM, eds. *Enabling America: Assessing the Role of Rehabilitation Science and Engineering.* Washington, DC: National Academy Press; 1997.
5. Statistics Canada. *Participation and Activity Limitation Survey: A profile of Disability in Canada.* Ottawa, Ontario: Author; 2002.
6. Pope AM, Tarloff AR. *Disability in America: Toward a National Agenda for Prevention.* Washington, DC: National Academy Press; 1991.
7. Yerxa E. Authentic occupational therapy. *Am J Occup Ther.* 1967;21:1-9.
8. Fidler GS, Fidler JW. Doing and becoming: purposeful action and self-actualization. *Am J Occup Ther.* 1978;32:305-310.
9. Reilly M. Occupational therapy can be one of the great ideas of 20th century medicine. *Am J Occup Ther.* 1962;16:87-105.
10. Fidler G, Fidler J. *Occupational Therapy: A Communication Process in Psychiatry.* New York: Macmillan; 1963.
11. Burke JP. A clinical perspective on motivation: Pawn versus origin. *Am J Occup Ther.* 1977;31:254-258.
12. Sharrott GW, Cooper-Fraps C. Theories of motivation in occupational therapy. *Am J Occup Ther.* 1986;40(4):249-257.
13. Christiansen C. Occupational therapy: intervention for life performance. In: Christiansen C, Baum C, eds. *Occupational Therapy: Overcoming Human Performance Deficits.* Thorofare, NJ: SLACK Incorporated; 1991:4-43.
14. Kielhofner G. *Conceptual Foundations of Occupational Therapy.* Philadelphia: F.A. Davis; 1992.
15. Baum CM. The contribution of occupation to function in persons with Alzheimer's disease. *J Occup Sci: Austr.* 1995;2(2):59-67.
16. Wilcock A. A theory of the human need for occupation. *Occupational Science: Australia.* 1993;1(1):17-24.
17. Law M. *Client-Centered Occupational Therapy.* Thorofare, NJ: SLACK Incorporated; 1998.
18. Bing RK. Occupational therapy revisited: a paraphrasic journey. *Am J Occup Ther.* 1991;35(8):499-518.
19. Gillen G. A fork in the road: an occupational hazard? 2013 Eleanor Clarke Slagle Lecture. *Am J Occup Ther.* 2013;67(6):641-652.
20. Badley EM. The genesis of handicap: definition, models of disablement, and role of external factors. *Disabil Rehabil.* 1995;17:53-62.
21. Wright FV, Rosenbaum PL, Goldsmith CH, Law M, Fehlings DL. How do changes in body functions and structures, activity, and participation relate in children with cerebral palsy? *Dev Med Child Neurol.* 2008;50:283-289.

22. Shannon PD. The derailment of occupational therapy. *Am J Occup Ther.* 1977;31(4):229-234.
23. Kielhofner G, Burke JP. Occupational therapy after 60 years: an account of changing identity and knowledge. *Am J Occup Ther.* 1977;31:675-689.
24. Law M, Cooper BA, Strong S, Stewart D, Rigby P, Letts L. The person-environment-occupation model: a transactive approach to occupational performance. *Can J Occup Ther.* 1996;63:9-23.
25. Law M, Steinwender S, LeClair L. Occupation, health and well-being. *Can J Occup Ther.* 1998;65(2):81-91.
26. Stav WB, Hallenen T, Lane J, Arbesman, M. Systematic review of occupational engagement and health outcomes among community-dwelling older adults. *Am J Occup Ther.* 2012;66:301-310.
27. Wilcock A. *An Occupational Perspective of Health.* Thorofare, NJ: SLACK Incorporated; 1998.
28. Baum CM, Christiansen CH. Person-environment-occupation-performance: an occupation-based framework for practice. In Christiansen CH, Baum C, Bass-Haugen J, eds. *Occupational Therapy: Performance, Participation, and Well-Being.* 3rd ed. Thorofare, NJ: SLACK Incorporated; 2005:242-267.
29. Christiansen C, Baum C. *Occupational Therapy: Overcoming Human Performance Deficits.* Thorofare, NJ: SLACK Incorporated; 1991.
30. Christiansen C, Baum C. *Occupational Therapy: Enhancing Function and Well-Being.* 2nd ed. Thorofare, NJ: SLACK Incorporated; 1997.
31. Fischer TM, Stewart KE, Davis JA. Occupation and health, reconsidered. *Can J Occup Ther.* 2014;81(3):140-143.
32. Twinley R. The dark side of occupation: a concept for consideration. *Aust Occup Ther J.* 2013;60:301-303.
33. Baum CM, Edwards D. Occupational performance: Occupational therapy's definition of function. *Am J Occup Ther.* 1995;49:1019-1020.
34. Reed K, Sanderson S. *Concepts of Occupational Therapy.* Philadelphia: Lippincott Williams & Wilkins; 1999.
35. Canadian Association of Occupational Therapists. *Enabling Occupation: An Occupational Therapy Perspective.* Ottawa, Ontario: CAOT Publications ACE; 1997.
36. Kielhofner G. *A Model of Human Occupation: Theory and Application.* Philadelphia, PA: Williams & Wilkins; 1995.
37. Chapparo C, Ranka J. *Occupational Performance Model (Australia): Monograph 1.* Sydney: Occupational Performance Network; 1997.
38. Dunn W, Brown C, McGuigan A. Ecology of human performance: a framework for considering the effect of context. *Am J Occup Ther.* 1994;48(7):595-607.
39. Howe MC, Briggs AK. Ecological systems model for occupational therapy. *Am J Occup Ther.* 1982;36:322-327.
40. Deci R, Ryan EM. A motivational approach to self-integration in personality. *Nebraska Symposium on Motivation.* 1991;38:237-288.
41. Christiansen C, Baum CM, Bass J. *Occupational Therapy: Performance, Participation and Well-Being.* Thorofare, NJ: SLACK Incorporated; 2015.
42. Nelson D. Occupation: form and performance. *Am J Occup Ther.* 1988;42:633-641.
43. Nelson D. Therapeutic occupation: a definition. *Am J Occup Ther.* 1996;50(10):775-782.
44. Polatajko H, Davis J, Stewart D, et al. Specifying the domain of concern: occupation as core. In: Townsend EA, Polatajko HJ, eds. *Enabling Occupation II: Advancing an Occupational Therapy Vision for Health, Well-Being, & Justice Through Occupation.* Ottawa, ON: CAOT Publications ACE; 2007:13-36.
45. Rogers JC. Clinical reasoning: the ethics, science and art. *Am J Occup Ther.* 1983;37:601-616.
46. Rogers CR. *The Clinical Treatment of the Problem Child.* Boston: Houghton-Mifflin; 1939.
47. Cain DJ. Further thoughts on non-directiveness and client-centered therapy. *Person-Centred Rev.* 1990;5:89-99.
48. May R. The problem of evil: an open letter to Carl Rogers. *J Humanist Psychol.* 1983;122:10-21.
49. Canadian Association of Occupational Therapists, Department of National Health & Welfare. *Guidelines for the Client-Centered Practice of Occupational Therapy.* Ottawa, Ontario: Minister of Supply and Services; 1983.
50. Matheis-Kraft C, George S, Olinger MJ, York L. Patient-driven health care works! *Nurs Manage.* 1990;21:124-128.
51. Christiansen CH, Baum C, Bass-Haugen J, eds. *Occupational Therapy: Performance, Participation, and Well-Being.* 3rd ed. Thorofare, NJ: SLACK Incorporated; 2005.
52. Blank AE, Horowitz S, Matza D. Quality with a human face? The Samuel Planetree model hospital unit. *Jt Comm J Qual Improv.* 1995;21:289-299.
53. King G, King S, Rosenbaum P. Interpersonal aspects of care-giving and client outcomes: a review of the literature. *Ambulatory Child Health.* 1996;2:151-160.
54. Calnan M, Katsouyiannopoulos V, Ovcharov VK, Prokhorskas R, Ramic H, Williams S. Major determinants of consumer satisfaction with primary care in different health systems. *Family Practice.* 1994;11(4):468-478.
55. Caro P, Derevensky JL. Family-focused intervention model: Implementation and research findings. *Topics Early Child Spec Educ.* 1991;11(3):66-80.
56. Doyle BJ, Ware JE. Physician conduct and other factors that affect consumer satisfaction with medical care. *J Med Educ.* 1977;52(10):793-801.
57. Dunst CJ, Trivette CM, Boyd K, Brookfield J. Help-giving practices and the self-efficacy appraisals of parents. In: Dunst CJ, Trivette CM, Deal AG, eds. *Supporting and Strengthening Families (Vol. 1): Methods, Strategies and Practices.* Cambridge, MA: Brookline Books; 1994.
58. Dunst CJ, Trivette CM, Deal A. *Enabling and Empowering Families: Principles and Guidelines for Practice.* Cambridge, MA: Brookline Books; 1988.
59. Greenfield S, Kaplan S, Ware JE. Expanding patient involvement in care: effects on patient outcomes. *Ann Intern Med.* 1985;102:520-528.
60. Moxley-Haegert L, Serbin LA. Developmental education for parents of delayed infants: effects on parental motivation and children's development. *Child Dev.* 1983;54:1324-1331.
61. Rosenbaum P, King S, Law M, King G, Evans J. Family-centred service: a conceptual framework and research review. *Phys Occup Ther Pediatr.* 1998;18(1):1-20.
62. Dunn W. *Best Practice Occupational Therapy.* Thorofare, NJ: SLACK Incorporated; 2000.
63. Nagi SZ. An epidemiology of disability in the United States. *Milbank Mem Fund Q Health Soc.* 1976;54(4):439-467.

64. World Health Organization. *International Classification of Functioning, Disability, and Health (ICF).* Geneva, Switzerland: WHO; 2001.
65. Vargus-Adams JN, Majnemer A. International Classification of Functioning, Disability and Health (ICF) as a framework for change: revolutionalizing rehabilitation. *J Child Neurol.* 2014;29(8):1030-1035.
66. Wright FV, Majnemer A. The concept of a toolbox of outcome measures for children with cerebral palsy: why, what, and how to use? *J Child Neurol.* 2014;29(8):1055-1065.
67. World Health Organization. *International Classification of Impairment, Disability and Handicap.* Geneva, Switzerland: Author; 1980.
68. Kielhofner G. *A Model of Human Occupation: Theory and Application.* Baltimore: Williams & Wilkins; 1985.
69. Dunn W, Brown C, Youngstrom MJ. Ecological Model of Occupation. In: Kramer, Hinojosa J, Royeen CB, eds. *Perspectives on Human Occupation: Participation in Life.* Philadelphia: Lippincott Williams & Wilkins; 2003:222-262.
70. Kielhofner G. *A Model of Human Occupation: Theory and Application.* 4th ed. Baltimore: Lippincott Williams & Wilkins; 2008.
71. Kielhofner G, Burke JP. A model of human occupation, part one: conceptual framework and content. *Am J Occup Ther.* 1980;34:572-581.
72. Reilly, M. A psychiatric occupational therapy program as a teaching model. *Am J Occup Ther.* 1966;20:61-67.
73. Strong S, Rigby P, Stewart D, Law M, Letts L, Cooper B. Application of person-environment-occupation model: a practical tool. *Can J Occup Ther.* 1999;66(3):122-133.
74. Law M, Baptiste S, Carswell A, McColl M, Polatajko H, Pollock, N. *Canadian Occupational Performance Measure.* 5th ed. Toronto, Canada: CAOT Publication; 2014.
75. Baum CM, Bass JD, Christiansen CH. The Person-Environment-Occupation-P PEOP) Model. In: Christiansen CH, Baum CM, Bass-Haugen J, eds. *Occupational Therapy: Performance, Participation, and Well-Being.* Thorofare, NJ: SLACK Incorporated; 2015:49-56.
76. Townsend EA, Polatajko HJ. *Enabling Occupation II: Advancing an Occupational Therapy Vision for Health, Well-Being, & Justice Through Occupation.* Ottawa, ON: CAOT Publications ACE; 2007.
77. Iwama M, Rhomson N, Macdonald R. The Kawa model: the power of culturally responsive occupational therapy. *Disabil Rehabil.* 2009;31(14):1125-1135.
78. ERIC. Measurement. http://eric.ed.gov/?qt=measurement&ti=Measurement. Accessed November 6, 2014
79. Law M, King G, Russell D, MacKinnon E, Hurley P, Murphy C. Measuring outcomes in children's rehabilitation: a decision protocol. *Arch Phys Med Rehab.* 1999;80:629-636.
80. Colquhoun HL, Letts LJ, Law MC, MacDermid JC, Missiuna CA. Administration of the Canadian Occupational Performance Measure: effect on practice. *Can J Occup Ther.* 2012;79(2):120-128.
81. Zur B, Johnson A, Roy E, Laliberte Rudman D, Wells J. Beyond traditional notions of validity: selecting appropriate measures for occupational therapy practice. *Austr Occup Ther J.* 2012;59(3):243-246.
82. Mattingly C, Fleming M. *Clinical Reasoning: Forms of Inquiry in a Therapeutic Practice.* Philadelphia: F.A. Davis; 1994.
83. Morris C. Measuring participation in childhood disability: how does the capability approach improve our understanding? *Dev Med Child Neurol.* 2009;51(2):92-94.
84. Leland NE, Crum K, Phipps S, Roberts P, Gage B. Advancing the value and quality of occupational therapy in health service delivery. *Am J Occup Ther.* 2015;69(1):6901090010p1-6901090010p7.

CHAPTER 2

Measurement Concepts and Practices

Winnie Dunn, PhD, OTR, FAOTA

Chapter 2 provides detailed information about measurement concepts and principles necessary for occupational therapists to understand before conducting assessments. We will discuss ecological validity in testing the various testing perspectives and the advantages of each. We will also examine strategies for making assessment choices and maintaining the integrity of assessment processes.

Setting the Framework for Measurement

Understanding the importance of measurement as a core professional skill requires recognition about why professionals need measurement knowledge for their practice and what the central considerations are when using measurement as a tool to inform evidence-based practices.

Why Professionals Need Measurement Knowledge in Practice

There are 2 primary reasons why professionals need measurement knowledge in practice. First, measurement processes provide convincing evidence about a person's status, competencies, and challenges for both planning and documenting the effectiveness of interventions. Second, using sound measurement strategies enables professionals to include individuals and their families in the process of selecting the most compatible and effective interventions for them.

Measurement Provides Convincing Evidence

When clients need services from professionals, they have a right to expect the service providers to employ current practices and to report their activities in a systematic and consistent manner. Professionals in any discipline have a base of knowledge that enables them to view performance from a particular perspective; this base of knowledge is necessary, but not sufficient when providing evidence-based services. In addition to having mastered knowledge, professionals must find ways to document their decision-making processes for the service recipient and others as appropriate.

Measurement strategies provide the tools to ensure that the decision-making process can be recorded in a systematic manner. When professionals document their own decision-making processes and the recipient's outcomes, they take responsibility for their work because systematic measurement provides a means for others to scrutinize the professional's work. Solid measurement practices create a mechanism for analysis of the effectiveness and efficiency of the services and, when taken collectively, can inform a profession about ways to advance knowledge and practices in the profession.

Professionals Need to Engage in Evidence-Based Practice

Professionals have another responsibility related to measurement. In addition to recording our decision-making in a systematic manner, we must engage in a practice that is currently being called *evidence-based practice*. Evidence-based practice means that the professional informs the potential service recipient of what the profession knows (or does not know) about the effectiveness of the evaluations and interventions being proposed so that the recipient can make informed decisions about what services are acceptable and what the service recipient is willing to accept.

Employing evidence-based practices during planning offers professionals an additional way to establish rapport.

Law M, Baum C, Dunn W, eds. *Measuring Occupational Performance: Supporting Best Practice in Occupational Therapy, Third Edition* (pp 17-28).

Occupational therapy professionals have traditionally emphasized rapport-building as an important part of the therapeutic process. When therapists take the additional step to involve service recipients in the process of thinking through the meaning of measurement findings and the options for intervention, professionals initiate a partnership with the service recipient. This partnership establishes new roles in the therapist-client relationship and invites the service recipient to have an active voice in the therapeutic process. As a partner, the person has a bigger investment in a positive outcome, but also feels permission to speak up about plans that would be incompatible with lifestyle or be too burdensome to carry out each day. Partners also offer different perspectives on the meaning of data; the perspective of the person who has had the lived experience has unfortunately been discounted in more traditional therapeutic processes.

Central Considerations in the Measurement Process: What Parameters Matter?

A critical and often overlooked consideration when setting out to measure performance is identifying the testing strategy that will yield proper information. Sometimes, it is most important to know how often a behavior occurs (ie, frequency); other times, how long a behavior lasts is critical to measurement and planning (ie, duration); still other times, the flexibility of the behavior across time or settings is important (ie, generalizability).

Measurement parameters help professionals characterize behaviors properly. When conducting skilled observations, if a student is yelling out answers during class discussions, the teacher is probably more interested in the number of times (frequency) the student interrupts others rather than how long each interruption takes (duration). However, that same teacher needs to know the length of a student's attention for seatwork (duration) rather than the number of times the student looks at the paper or workbook (frequency).

Another key measurement parameter is applicability across situations or locations. In order to measure applicability properly, one must measure across opportunities; one type of opportunity to perform cannot inform professionals about the person's ability to use skills in various ways. For example, if a person can find things in the bedroom at home, we might hypothesize that the person can find things everywhere. However, the bedroom may be so familiar that this situation does not challenge perceptual skills (the person may be relying on memory), and when faced with "finding" tasks in other settings, performance deteriorates. Flexibility in using one's skills and the contextual resources to complete tasks is an important performance issue when managing life and, therefore, must be a central consideration in measurement. We discuss more details about context later in the chapter.

Measurement: The Process and the Outcome

In the practice of a profession, it is important to measure both the process and the outcomes of the practices. *Process measurement* (sometimes called *formative assessment*) is directed at evaluating the way that the practices are being carried out and the client's response to an intervention; *outcome measurement* evaluates the product or impact of the practices.[1] Therapists use process measurement when they wish to know how things are going. Process measures can be very focused, as in feeling tone changes as a person shifts posture, or can be programmatic, as in identifying the effectiveness and efficiency of one's scheduling system. Process measurement enables professionals to "evaluate in action" so they can adjust what they are doing to improve the experience.

Therapists use outcome measurement when they wish to know the end result or how things went. Measuring a person's successful transition to community living is a measure of the outcomes of the service system and interdisciplinary providers. Capturing accurate information as outcome data is sometimes a difficult process; it is not uncommon for professionals to "know" that a person made progress, but to have measures they selected indicate "no progress." If professionals select weak or inappropriate outcome measures, they can make the inaccurate conclusion that the services were not effective. They can also incorrectly conclude that services were effective by using very narrow measures of outcome that are not actually representative of the person's skills or satisfaction with daily life.

When we begin to apply knowledge about measurement choices within practice, we have to consider whether the measurement device is reliable, valid, and responsive to changes in the behaviors of interest. See Chapter 3 for a full discussion of reliability and validity. What we wish to emphasize here is that not all measures are appropriate for measuring changes; for instance, some measures are designed for documenting traits that remain relatively the same across time (eg, global intelligence). It is not appropriate to use trait or status measures for charting progress or planning specific features of an intervention program. For example, the Bruininks-Oseretsky Test of Motor Proficiency Second Edition (BOTMP)[2] is a norm-referenced and standardized test. *Norm-referenced* means that the BOTMP has data from a comparison sample of typical children, so we know what is inside and outside of normal expectations. *Standardized* means that there are specific methods for completing the test procedures. After administering and scoring the BOTMP, the examiner looks up the child's raw score to derive a standard score. The standard score provides a comparison of this child's performance to other children the same age, although the professional would then know generally about balance or dexterity (eg, the BOTMP does not enable the professional to know how these skills [or lack of skills] are affecting performance or how the child functions with this pattern of skills [ie, the designation "status"] without additional information from parents, the child, or the teacher).

We consider a measure responsive to change when that measure will be able to detect changes that are proportional to and accurately reflect the person's actual behavioral changes. Responsiveness can be evaluated by looking at the change in scores across time in treated and untreated groups, by calculating effect size, or by plotting change compared to chance.[3] Portney and Watkins[3] caution that practitioners must understand the behaviors they are measuring so they can determine when changes in behavior are large enough to matter for the person's life. Sometimes, a statistically significant difference in a research study can be due to large samples, and the actual amount of change in the behavior would not matter in daily life performance. Other times, a study can report no differences statistically, and yet the behavior difference would be important in the person's life. Statistical tests of significance tell us whether the numbers we report are different from a mathematical perspective. In practice, this may not be adequate information for determining whether the difference matters in the lives of the persons we are serving.

The Activities Scale for Kids (ASK) (see Table 13-1) is an example of a measure that reports on the measure's sensitivity to change. They measured across a 6-month period and found that the performance section of the ASK was more sensitive to change than the capability section.[4] We will discuss selection of outcome measures and provide additional examples of measurements that are sensitive to change throughout the book.

Performance and Criterion Measures

Measures can often be categorized as performance or criterion measures, as opposed to the norm-based measures discussed previously. These measures provide information about the person's actual performance and skill development and therefore enable the professional to plan appropriate interventions and evaluate their impact on performance. Standardized tests require the professional and person to engage in a predesigned task so that everyone has the same chance to perform. Criterion measures are designed to elicit that person's pattern of performance. Comparisons in a criterion measurement might be with that person's performance previously or with another person in the immediate setting who is more successful (ie, the gold standard for that task). The School Function Assessment (SFA) (see Table 12-10) is an example of a standardized and criterion-referenced measure of children's participation in school.

Criterion measurement is especially critical for occupational therapists for 3 reasons. First, some persons who have particular conditions cannot complete the rigors of standardized test protocols and therefore cannot be compared to a national norm. Second, the course of development and performance for persons who have particular conditions is different than for persons who are developing according to expected standards; criterion measures enable professionals to characterize these unique features of performance. For example, a person who has spasticity subsequent to nervous system trauma will move using very different postural support patterns. This person will never move the way a person who has normal tone can move, so comparing to typical patterns of movement is not useful. In fact, there are some situations in which the spasticity provides extra support for postural control that is not available to persons who have normal tone. Criterion measures provide the means to characterize the functional utility of whatever skills a person has and how these skills are used in day-to-day occupations.

Finally, there are some constructs that are so variable and so dependent on each person and environment that norms are not meaningful. Participation and quality of life are examples that fit with this aspect of measurement; each person gets to decide about what makes life meaningful, so standards would be irrelevant.

Viewpoints Offered in Various Assessment Choices

There are many perspectives about a person's participation. Scholars and professionals in practice sometimes debate about the best choices for a thorough assessment. People can report about themselves or about significant others (eg, teachers about students, parents about children, caregiver about a person cared for). In contrast, professionals can observe actual performance on standardized test items or in life activities. Finally, assessment can be with an individual or focused on a population. Let's review the options and consider the positive contributions and challenges with each choice.

Perspective Taking: Self, Proxy, and Direct Observation Measurement

Measurement can occur from many perspectives. *Self-report measures* involve a person documenting about her or his own life experiences, skills, or knowledge. Self-report data are important for documenting a person's narrative; it informs professionals how the person sees things. *Proxy measures* involve another person completing an assessment on someone's behalf; we call it a "proxy" or "other informant" report. The most common proxy reports are parents for their children, teachers for their students, and family members for each other (eg, spouse). Proxy assessments allow professionals to gather needed information when the person being served is unable to complete a self-reporting process. Critics of proxy reporting also cite the lack of objectivity in the findings. As with self-reporting, proxy information gives the care provider's point of view about the situation. We prefer "other informant" because it is easier to understand and does not presume that one person can substitute for another's perspective.

Performance Based Assessment (PBA) involves observing and documenting what a person can actually do. We employ PBA during both direct observation of the person's behavior/performance and when we administer standardized tests that have performance items that we rate for accuracy and sometimes speed.

Some argue that self- and proxy-report data do not provide objective measurement of the phenomena of interest. For example, a therapist could interview a person to find out the person's self-care abilities and strategies. This self-report method would tell us the person's view of how things go during self-care routines. Critics would say that the therapist must observe the person completing the self-care routines to document what actually happens to obtain more "objective" data. For occupational therapists, self-report is an important aspect of comprehensive measurement. Because we are concerned about the quality of life from that person's perspective, self-report provides a way to understand how life looks and feels from the person's point of view and also may be a cue that the person could be having a cognitive problem if he or she is not aware of the limitation. Taking this perspective, we accept whatever the person says as valid; we do not question the person's way of experiencing life. Even if the person is not technically "correct" about skills, it is important to know how the person sees the situation because this point of view is the person's starting point. For example, if a person says, "I can complete my personal hygiene just fine in the morning," that person may not be interested or motivated to address personal hygiene even if the therapist identifies potential difficulties in direct observation (performance assessment). Sometimes, the gap between what people perceive and can do becomes central in the intervention—particularly if the person has had a brain injury.

There are circumstances that call for performance assessment and objective information. When serving a worker who makes machine parts, precision is critical. It would not matter to the company what the person says about skills after an accident; the supervisor would want to know what the actual machine operation precision is before clearing the worker to return to the floor. In this case, the differences between the worker's perception and the precision of the work would be an important part of the worker's rehabilitation, in addition to the muscle strengthening and coordination efforts.

One more aspect of this debate is worthy of attention. Just because a professional carries out the measurements doesn't necessarily mean the resulting data are objective. In fact, many measures actually reflect the professional's perceptions of such things as dials or movements. Professionals are specially trained, yet they can make recording or interpretation errors as well. One way to reduce this potential error is to collect measurement data from multiple sources to look for consistency before making a hypothesis. Let's briefly review some recent evidence about perspective taking in assessment because there is a lot of deliberation about multiple-informant data.

Achenbach et al[5] conducted a meta-analysis of multiple-informant data used to evaluate and diagnose psychopathology. Related to children's conditions, they found a mean Pearson correlation of .22 between children and caregivers, .28 between adult informants such as a teacher and parent, .60 correlation between pairs of caregivers (eg, 2 parents, 2 teachers), .57 between 2 trained observers, and .42 between observers and teachers. They concluded that various informant ratings are not interchangeable, and suggest that each informant sees the child in different contexts and interacts related to different activities and expectations to account for the differences. In another study with children and parents, Yeh et al[6] reported that parents rate quality of life (QOL) higher than their children rated themselves during cancer treatments.

Related to adult conditions, they report a .26 overall correlation between self-report and other informant reports.[5] They found no differences between interviews and questionnaires. Klein[7] followed up with predictive testing and found that each rating (self and informant) independently predicted aspects of psychopathology, such as depression. Informant ratings uniquely predicted social adjustment in a group treated for depression. Interestingly, when evaluating a substance abuse population, correlations between self and informant ratings were much higher (.681).[5] Perhaps substance abuse involves more overt patterns of behavior, making the behaviors of interest more transparent to everyone.

Another aspect of the Achenbach et al[5] meta-analysis involved biological measures; correlations of self and collateral (ie, another person in treatment program) ratings with biological measures were lower than self and collateral (ie, another person in treatment program) report correlations with each other. Across 29 studies of pain, there was a mean correlation of .29 between self-reports and observer reports of pain behavior.[8]

Brackett et al[9] studied emotional intelligence (EI) using self-ratings and performance assessment. They found that there was a .27 correlation between a standardized test of EI and self-report on the same items. Further, they rated participant performance in an interaction based on EI parameters, and found a low relationship between self-ratings and performance in the interaction task (based on observation). They concluded "...people are particularly poor at both providing self-reports and estimating their performance on ability measures of EI, indicating that self-rated EI may not be a good proxy assessment...."[(p 785)] This conclusion reflects the authors' beliefs that their standardized assessment and the performance condition are more accurate reflections of EI than the person's self-assessment. Although this may be true, one must also consider why the differences exist and what the differences mean about our understanding of EI. Are we asking the right questions? Are we observing the behaviors that actually reflect EI? What is the person's self-rating telling us about the lived experience of EI? When dealing with human behavior, it may be more prudent to consider possibilities than presume that professionals are correct.

Another aspect of informant reporting involves clinicians as informants. McPhail et al[10] created an interesting method of examining the reports. They asked physical therapists to rate the patient from their point of view as a clinician (view 1) and from the point of view of the patient (view 2). They then compared both these perspectives to the patients' self-ratings. There was high agreement between patient self-ratings and view 2 (kappa coefficient .76-.95), and variable moderate agreement between patient self-ratings and view 1 (kappa coefficient .23-.81). Ratings were lower when the patients had lower cognitive ability. In these cases, the therapists gave lower ratings. They discuss the close daily relationship that therapists have with patients across time, suggesting that familiarity contributes to the higher ratings when compared to other studies.

Achenbach et al[5] hypothesize about the reasons for the differences found across multiple informants. They point out that each informant has a unique experience with the person being rated, and these inherent differences account for at least some of the unique data. They also suggest that individual differences of the people doing the ratings themselves are likely to contribute to differences. They caution readers about indicating that one or another rater is "wrong" or inaccurate; rather, they suggest that each rater provides an accurate assessment of different aspects of the person's functional capacity. Finally, they advocate that cross-informant data can be used to examine which information is universal (ie, everyone reports it) compared to which information seems more situation specific.

For example, people have criticized the children's versions of the Sensory Profiles for being proxy measures, stating that they are not an objective measure of sensory responsiveness. Particularly when children are sensitive to certain inputs (eg, touch or sound), exposing them to stimuli that are possibly noxious to their perceptions could seem unnecessary when family and teachers can describe the characteristics of unpleasant stimuli in some detail. Additionally, as with self-reporting, knowing the care provider's experience with the child's responses to sensory inputs is valuable for planning. In the case of sensory processing, sensory responses are contextually relevant (ie, each environment has inherent features that could be helpful or interfering to children's participation), so gathering context-specific information is useful (eg, at school, at home).

Individual Assessment

Much of the focus of professional preparation is on individual characteristics. There are many assessments that evaluate a person's individual skills and performance; documenting the individual's progress is a central tenet of many service systems. Even within the same condition, each person's response is different based on background, interests, settings, and beliefs. Individual assessment provides a clear means for documenting the course of an experience, recording impact of an intervention, and establishing a current status.

Population-Based Assessment

In recent years, the importance of population-based assessment has become clear. While tracking an individual's status and progress matters, we have also come to understand that knowing the trends of groups of people matters to health and education decisions as well. When we know the expected trajectory of a human behavior, it becomes easier to detect the onset of risk. When we understand how a particular event affects groups of people, we can establish standards or prevention strategies. Population-based assessment also provides data for identifying secondary or tertiary factors that might affect someone's outcomes.

Recognizing the growing importance of population-based assessment, the National Institutes of Health (NIH) have launched several projects to provide researchers and providers nationally with population-based data and assessment methods that can be used to further our understanding of human behavior and provide a mechanism for comparing across groups to look for similarities and differences. Two examples are the Patient-Reported Outcomes Measurement Information System (PROMIS) (www.nihpromis.org) measures and the NIH Toolbox for Assessment of Neurological and Behavioral Function (NIH Toolbox) (www.nihtoolbox.org).

The PROMIS measures provide professionals with precise ways to document physical, mental, and social well-being status from the patient's perspective. PROMIS covers several domains, including Physical Health (function, pain, fatigue, sleep), Mental Health (Depression and Anxiety), and Social Well-Being (participation in social roles and activities). The tests are available online, using item response theory so that each respondent completes a minimum number of items to get the best possible response pattern. You can request these assessments through the website: www.nihpromis.org. An example of a physical health question is, "Are you able to walk a block on flat ground?" There is a 5-point Likert scale for responding "without any difficulty" to "unable to do." There is a national database that makes it possible to know which items to select for a particular respondent. PROMIS illustrates both population-based and self-assessment working in concert for monitoring health outcomes.

The NIH Toolbox is a set of brief assessments that address cognitive, emotional, sensory, and motor functions applicable for people 3 to 85 years old. The battery is meant to document these aspects of behavior across time and facilitate understanding across domains and conditions. With a common set of brief tests that non-experts can use, the NIH Toolbox invites interprofessional team members to document many areas of interest, rather than just their expertise (eg, motor for physical therapists, cognition for psychologists). Data from the standardization study and test instruments themselves are available at the website: www.nihtoolbox.org.

Importance of Environmental Context and Ecological Validity in Measurement

Persons conduct their daily lives within the larger environment and in particular environmental contexts. Even when conducting an evaluation in a medical center clinic, the environmental context in that situation will have an influence on the person's performance. Sometimes the unfamiliar furniture and equipment will distract the person; the fact that the therapist is setting expectations for performance might cause the person anxiety. Without knowing the person's life, the therapist might construct a confusing context for the person. On the other hand, the therapist's engaging behavior could facilitate performance in areas in which the person typically performs poorly due to lack of interest.[11] We cannot derive meaning about the person's performance without considering the environmental context in which we asked the person to perform. In Chapter 1, we reviewed the frameworks in occupational therapy that include environment in their conceptualization of occupational performance.

In fact, therapists face a "validity" dilemma when they conduct assessments of component skills in isolation from the tasks of daily life. If a therapist measures range of motion and strength, is it "valid" to conclude that the person cannot eat a meal? Perhaps we know that lifting utensils requires certain component skills (under typical circumstances); we might then conclude that anyone who has less than these skills will not be able to eat with utensils. Although there is a sensible relationship here, this logic does not account for less common but successful ways of using utensils and eating. It may be invalid to conclude that a person cannot eat with utensils by only testing component skills; persons who have weakness may have constructed a different way to eat that does not require the same level of strength. Relationships among task performance, the person's interest in the task, and the skills to perform the tasks must be carefully considered to ensure that professionals construct valid hypotheses and conclusions.

A Framework to Measure Performance Within a Person's Environment

There are 4 key assumptions essential to understanding performance in context:

1. Persons and the environments in which they live are unique and dynamic
2. Contrived environmental contexts are different from natural environmental contexts
3. Occupational therapy practice involves promoting self-determination and inclusion of persons with disabilities in all aspects of society
4. Independence means meeting your wants and needs.[12]

Persons and Their Contexts Are Unique

Persons and the environmental contexts in which they perform occupations are unique and dynamic. When conducting an evaluation, we cannot understand a person without understanding the person's environment. For each occupation, the environmental context includes physical, social, cultural, and temporal features.[13-15] Even within the same family (a social and cultural environment), siblings experience life differently and develop unique interests and skills. We must consider each person's unique skills and abilities and how environmental factors influence that person's experiences. The interaction between the person and the environment forms the basis of the meaning that persons derive from their life experiences.

The person-environment interaction is dynamic. The environmental context changes when persons do occupations, and changes in the environment affect how persons react as well. For example, we set up our closets to facilitate our own dressing rituals. Our performance changes when our clothing and accessories are arranged differently (eg, when staying at a friend's house). We must also remember that persons have a range of performance abilities depending on the cues and supports or barriers they experience under different environmental circumstances.

During the evaluation process, we determine the person's performance range, not just his or her skills and difficulties. The performance range is evaluated based on what the person wants or needs to do. Although we must know the person's skills and difficulties, this knowledge is inadequate without knowing what the person is interested in and where the person is likely to be conducting various aspects of daily life.

Contrived and Natural Environments Are Different

Occupational therapists work in a variety of service systems designed for specialized services (eg, clinical settings, acute-care settings). When we conduct evaluations in these specialized settings, we must factor in the potential differences in performance that would occur in more natural settings (ie, the workplace or home). Sometimes the person will perform better in contrived settings because contrived settings control some features of the environment that might be disruptive to the person. This control might enable us to see optimal performance, but therapeutic interventions must be based on typical performance needs, not optimal ones. Conversely, we might incorrectly decide that the person cannot perform when we evaluate in contrived environments because that person needed familiarity to provide cues and supports for better performance. Ultimately, what matters to the person is the ability to perform during daily life; therefore, we must be vigilant at discovering as much as we can about the person's desired and actual performance in natural settings.

Occupational Therapy Promotes Self-Determination and Inclusion

In occupational therapy services, we want to support persons to live satisfying lives. Therefore, we must find out what persons and their families want and need to do as the first step in the comprehensive evaluation processes. In its position paper on inclusion, the American Occupational Therapy Association (AOTA)[16] states that occupational therapy personnel must advocate for all persons to have access to all of the community environments that will enable them to live satisfying lives. Therefore, a comprehensive evaluation might include visiting the workplace to identify possible adaptations or speaking to peers and supervisors about routines of the day that support or create barriers to performance.[12]

Independence Means Meeting Your Wants and Needs

Independence occurs when persons are able to manage their lives to get what they want and need. Traditionally, independence meant that persons had to actually perform the tasks of interest, yet some have taken a stand that all persons make decisions about how they want to use their resources, and this might include employing someone else to complete a necessary task (eg, getting clothing pressed), adapting the environment to make the task easier (eg, using a jar opener), or asking for help from others. The salient feature is the person's ability to know what needs to be done and finding a way to get it done; the person does not need to actually do the task to be considered independent.[16]

When conducting a comprehensive evaluation with persons who have performance needs, occupational therapists must explore adaptations in the task or environment that might support performance. We all use adaptations to support daily life (eg, pencil grips, step stools). When persons have disabilities, there is a temptation to consider typical adaptations such as these as indications that the person has the problem. A more progressive view is that the environment might need to be adjusted to make task performance easier for those who perform in that context. When we make activity or environmental adaptations, we acknowledge that the person's skills and abilities can remain the same, and the person can still improve performance.

Supporting Interaction Among Persons and Their Environmental Contexts

Some persons have limited skills (eg, coordination), abilities (eg, preparing a meal), experience (eg, using an appliance), or condition that narrows the performance possibilities (eg, arthritis). When a person has limited personal skills, this is also likely to limit possibilities when the person interacts within different environments.[12] The person may not be able to take advantage of cues and supports of each environment. A child who has developmental delays has the same environmental context as other children in the preschool but may not notice cues to guide appropriate behavior. For example, the other children might quickly notice the cues that it is snack time, but the child with developmental delays may not understand these cues and be slower to join the other children, creating a limited performance range.

The environmental context can also be limited. Each time a person tries to do something without adequate equipment or supplies, that person has a limited environmental context.[12] When support within an environment is limited, the performance range is also smaller even with good skills and abilities. A conductor will not be able to demonstrate her excellent conducting skills without an environment that contains an orchestra.

Sometimes, person skills and experience as well as environmental supports are diminished (ie, a person who has a disability and who lives in an impoverished setting). The performance range can be very restricted in this situation. Occupational therapists must attend to both person and environmental variables in comprehensive evaluation to ensure that all factors related to the performance range are considered.[12,13,15]

Comprehensive Measurement Using a Performance in Environmental Context Perspective

Occupational therapists are concerned with participation in daily life; therefore, the most important aspect of any occupational therapy evaluation is participation.[12] When using participation within the environmental context perspective in comprehensive evaluation, performance has 2 features: 1) what the person wants and needs to do and 2) assessment of actual performance. To determine what the person wants and needs to do, we talk to the person and significant others (eg, the family, friends, other care providers, a coworker, boss, minister, neighbors). Our goal is to find out what matters in the person's life. When evaluating actual performance, occupational therapists have several strategies available, including conducting interviews about how performance looks in the natural settings and how satisfying that performance is for the person. We can also observe the person's task performance, either informally or with formal assessments.

Evaluation of Person Variables

Comprehensive evaluation also requires consideration of the person's skills, abilities, and experiences. Occupational therapists examine sensorimotor, cognitive, physiological, and psychosocial features of the person's performance. We evaluate these features to determine which person variables seem to contribute to or create barriers to desired performance. There are many formal and informal methods of evaluating performance components; other references address the details of performance component assessments.

The performance within context perspective enables us to determine possible barriers and supports to participation. The interaction between these environmental variables and the person's performance is what determines the meaning persons derive from their own experiences.

Evaluation of the Environmental Context

Occupational therapists employ skilled observations and interviews to identify the physical, social, cultural, and temporal features of relevant environments.[14,17] The physical features of the environmental context include the objects, terrain, layout, and structures of the environment. Social features include the persons, interaction styles, and relationships, while culture includes the expectations of stakeholders (eg, family, community, ethnic groups, office). Temporal features of an environmental context include expectations related to age, calendar time, and stage of disability.[18]

Although the occupational therapy literature has consistently included environments as a key feature of performance, we have evaluated specific environmental contexts far less than person and performance variables. When evaluating environments, we must consider physical, social, cultural, and temporal features of the environments of interest. Then, we must identify the possible supports and barriers to participation. Finally, we must collaborate with the service recipient to identify the meaning of performance within each particular environmental context. Other sections of this text contain an analysis of environmental assessments available to professionals (see Chapter 18).

Many professionals use ecological assessments to evaluate the features of the environment. In an ecological assessment, professionals record the typical way activities occur in a particular environmental context, then the professional records what the person of interest does to complete the tasks. Finally, the evaluation team designs possible ways to bridge the gap between typical performance and the person's current performance strategies to support more effective and satisfying participation.

Supports and Barriers to Participation

Evaluation of environmental context includes consideration of how environmental features support or create barriers to participation. Each person reacts to environmental variables differently; what might provide supports to one person can be a barrier to performance for another person. For example, the noise in the street may only provide background noise for one person but may be so distracting for another person that it would be hard to concentrate on homework. Peers may successfully compel one adolescent to work harder on a group project and may have no impact on another young person. Gathering objective data about the environmental context is necessary but not sufficient to make decisions about performance; we must identify the impact of those features on the person's performance.

Identifying Meaningfulness

Experienced professionals can collect information and hypothesize about the meaning of occupations, tasks, and activities for persons. However, we cannot know meaning for others without interacting with them about their lived experiences. When inquiring about what a person wants and needs to do, we can also ask why those occupations are important or satisfying, or why doing them in a certain way or in a certain place is significant.[12] We can listen for the presence or absence of daily routines, ask about how unexpected events affect the person's performance, and identify how the person establishes priorities. This information informs us about what is meaningful to the persons we are serving and their families. Performance has different meaning when it occurs in relevant environments. When a person has poor performance in an irrelevant environmental context, this may only indicate lack of meaningfulness of the task in that context, not lack of skill for performance.[12]

The Challenge of Integrating Person, Performance, and Environmental Contextual Data

Living a satisfying life is the only thing that matters for the person and family in person-centered service provision. For some persons, living a satisfying life would include developing one's own skills, but for other persons, it might mean finding or designing environmental contexts that can support desired task performance or selecting alternative life goals. During the evaluation process, professionals must organize information and insights around the actual life the person wants to live, even if services will be provided in a center or agency (eg, hospital, clinic, senior citizen center, or shelter).

For example, it doesn't matter what the child's visual perceptual scores are on a standardized test if visual perception is not interfering with daily life activities of interest to the child and family. We only pursue visual perception testing when the teacher, child, and/or family express concern about life situations that require strong visual perceptual skills. For example, if a child wishes to participate in the family's winter leisure activity of puzzle construction and has been displaying frustration (eg, outbursts, shoving pieces off the table), it is appropriate to suspect visual perception may be a barrier to this desired socialization experience. In this example, we also recognize that participating with family members has some inherent qualities that must be considered as well. The child may feel that this is a desirable way to get parental attention; the child might also feel pressure to compete with siblings. The type of picture on the puzzle and the family's puzzle strategies (eg, sorting pieces by colors, by edges) will change the situation and supports for the child. Best practice occupational therapy would require that the therapist know as much of this information as possible to design the most successful intervention. Evaluation of visual perception is irrelevant without first considering the person's desired performance and then considering contextual features that may impact performance.

Selecting Measurement Criteria

When selecting the criterion for particular measurements, there are 5 factors to consider:

1. Relevance to the person's life
2. Comparisons to external standards
3. Application of formal evidence criteria
4. Which measures are sensitive to relevant changes
5. What levels of change are important.

Relevance to the Person's Life

The most important criterion when designing a measurement strategy is relevance. There are many measurement strategies available to us that are technically correct but would yield results that are irrelevant to the person's performance needs or desires in his or her daily life. For example, although it might be interesting to know a person's level and type of perceptual and memory skills, this information might initially be peripheral to the person's desire to cook. When someone tells us he or she wants to cook and we then measure his or her performance by asking him or her to match pictures, draw shapes, or repeat numbers, the service recipient is likely to be confused about the relationship between the 2 sets of tasks. This does not mean that perceptual and memory skills are unimportant for cooking, but the connection between them is elusive to the consumer when component skills are tested in isolation from the desired performance. Meeting the criterion of relevance would occur if the therapist listened to the person describe cooking methods and frustrations, or if the therapist watched a cooking task. Then, as perceptual and memory issues arose out of the interaction, their relationship to the desired outcome would be clear for everyone.

Comparisons of Performance to External Standards

Sometimes it is important to describe a person's performance in relation to other performance. Professionals can make comparisons between the person's earlier and current performance, between the service recipient and successful performers in the environmental context of interest, and between the service recipient and a standard performance of a like group.

Comparing to Self

It is most common and appropriate to compare a person's performance currently to that same person's performance at an earlier time or in another place. If a person can handle money and change for a purchase within the community center, we might want to know whether that person can handle money as effectively at convenience or grocery stores. If we have been working together with a man so he can dress himself, we will want to compare his current abilities with his performance at an earlier time. The "compare-to-self" paradigm is most often used to measure a person's progress in achieving performance goals and to determine the effectiveness of intervention strategies.

Comparing to Typical Models

Another measurement standard that can be used in some settings is the comparison to typical models. This means that the professional collects information about a typical performer and compares that to the performance of the service recipient in that same environmental context. School programs lend themselves readily to this type of measurement criteria. When conducting a skilled observation of the student who has been referred for assessment, the therapist can also record data on another student in the classroom who is successful at the tasks of interest. It is important to avoid the best performer; it is better to select a student who is successful in the midrange of the classroom. The advantage of this measurement criterion is that it enables professionals to frame the person's performance in the very environment that performance is expected. There is also an opportunity to be reminded of the range of behaviors that peers use while getting things done.

For example, a worker may be having difficulty getting work completed, and the supervisor thinks it is because he is up roaming around the office "all the time." However, by collecting data on another worker, the therapist can determine whether roaming around is typical behavior of many workers in this work environment. If many workers roam around and still get their work finished, then the therapist has the opportunity to provide insight about other behaviors that might be interfering with productivity. Perhaps for other workers, roaming around occurs when they have work to delegate to others, and for the target worker, roaming does not advance the work product. Knowing this can help the supervisor frame the work expectations to ensure higher work product.

Comparing to Typical Models in a Standard Sample

A more traditional external standard is a normative sample of individuals whose performance is considered collectively. Professionals are using a standard sample when they look up a person's raw score on a table to determine a standard score for that level of performance. The standard scores are derived from calculations of the scores of all persons in a particular category (eg, all 20- to 25-year-old males); the standard score that the person receives represents that person's performance in relation to all other persons in the category.

Professionals need to understand which standard score scale is used in a particular assessment. If a standard scale has a mean of 100 and a standard deviation of 10, then we can interpret the person's standard score by comparing to this scale. A score of 80 would be 2 standard deviations below the average and is likely a cause for some concern, while a 95 would be considered within average limits. However, if a standard score scale is based on a mean of 50 and a standard deviation of 10, a score of 80 would be 3 standard deviations above the mean, while a 95 would be even higher, representing the top 1% of the population.

There are advantages and disadvantages of standard sample comparisons. Standard score comparisons are most appropriate as measures of status or to establish eligibility for particular services. They are typically not appropriate for charting performance progress or for planning particular intervention strategies. Because the comparison is to an established behavioral pattern, it is sometimes easier to hypothesize about the person's performance in relation to a cohort group in that person's life settings. However, standard measures also require a more prescribed performance from the person being assessed, and this is not always possible. If a person cannot complete tasks on a standard measure in the prescribed way, it is inappropriate to compare the performance to the standard scores.

As with each measurement issue, the professional has the responsibility to select strategies and tasks based on the purpose of the measurement activities. Each of these parameters is important for certain aspects of measurement and will enhance the data available when used correctly.

Using Measurement Information for Evidence-Based Practice

The ultimate application of measurement skills and principles to practice is to partner with service recipients to consider information from measurement to select the best course of action. When service recipients and professionals can collaborate about the meaning of information and the ways to work toward a desired outcome, everyone is successful. Measurement data provide the tools for this collaboration.

Professionals engage in evidence-based practice when they actively inform the persons they are serving about the known (and unknown) benefits and risks of the intervention options. Engaging in evidence-based practice creates a vulnerability for the professional, but the process of exposing costs, benefits, and unknown factors opens the communication process as well. Service recipients are more likely to question a decision to proceed in a certain way when they understand the parameters of that plan of action. Evidence-based practice also offers the opportunity for persons to be more committed to the process of their own therapy because they will feel like a part of the process, rather than a passive beneficiary.[19,20] In addition, it provides a mechanism for professionals to think systematically and take responsibility for the relationships between plans and the person's desired outcomes.

For example, Simone, an occupational therapist, interviewed Alan, a man who wanted to improve his personal hygiene. She observed the personal hygiene ritual and noticed that Alan did not use toothpaste or a hairbrush. Although it was possible that Alan did not know about these aspects of personal hygiene, these 2 items were put away in the drawer, so the therapist suspected that Alan might need some way to remember to use these items. In a follow-up, Alan demonstrated the ability to use the toothpaste and hairbrush, so the therapist focused her planning on placement of supplies and the issue of Alan remembering the parts of the personal hygiene ritual.

When she met with Alan, Simone presented several options. She discussed a skills training approach, which would involve Alan learning a pattern of performance during hygiene. She told him that skills training had been shown to be successful with young adults with mental illness, but that professionals had not shown that skills training generalized to other patterns of task performance. Because Alan wanted to have paid work, he wanted to learn strategies for remembering the parts of the activity. The therapist also discussed cognitive retraining with Alan. She explained this approach had also been successful for improving the cognitive skill (in this case, memory), but application within daily life environments had not been tested.

The therapist also discussed adaptive strategies for supporting his task performance, such as making a list of the parts of the hygiene ritual that Alan could post or making a mat of the necessary tools on the counter to remind Alan what he needs to do in the morning. The therapist explained that adaptive strategies have been shown to support performance of desired tasks because they are designed with that task in mind. In order for this adaptive strategy to be helpful with new tasks, Alan and others would have to consider adaptations to those tasks; Alan might discover adaptive strategies that are always (or never) helpful, and he might narrow down the field of adaptations over time.

Alan decided he wanted to work on his memory skills separate from the hygiene tasks. He wanted to use adaptations for getting "regular stuff" done and work on memory to "make himself better." The therapist, caseworker, Alan, and his brother all met to hear about the plans, and the interventions proceeded.

Employing best practices in measurement is the first step to employing evidence-based practices in the course of providing services. The data from forward-thinking measurement strategies (as presented throughout this book) provide the information for current planning with individuals and the evidence for emerging best practices in the future.

The Challenges of Providing Evidence-Based Practice

There are 3 challenges in providing evidence-based practice. The professional must keep apprised of current literature, develop effective communication strategies, and understand how to evaluate the evidence available in the literature.

Keeping Current

Professionals must be apprised of current and innovative practices and the supports and challenges to those practices in the literature if they wish to engage in evidence-based practice. With the huge amount of professional literature published each month, this can seem overwhelming. It is sometimes very helpful to participate in a journal club, in which the participants take turns bringing articles to read and discuss. Professionals can also periodically conduct a search within a library system or on the Internet for current references of interest. Another strategy is to share abstracts of articles as a method of scanning for those that might inform you about your practice considerations. The team of professionals has the collective responsibility to stay current on knowledge that impacts their practice.

An example of keeping current is to review the Cochrane Collaboration databases. These reviews of studies inform professionals about the current knowledge and practices related to particular diagnoses and conditions. A limitation of the Cochrane Collaboration data is that the types of studies they accept into their databases are restricted to clinical trials. Currently, there are not many clinical trial studies in occupational therapy, so inferences must be made from the more general information provided.

There are several ways to obtain information. Universities have databases that enable you to search professional literature. You can search medical and health literature (eg, PubMed, CINAHL) resources, or educational resources (eg, ERIC). There are also other websites that provide information (eg, Bottomlines, CanChild) in a summarized way. For occupational therapists, OTSeeker (www.otseeker.com) provides a comprehensive searchable database of systematic reviews and randomized controlled trials applicable to occupational therapy. Google Scholar provides information from professional searches, and is available when other sources are harder to access.

Communicating as Partners

When engaging in evidence-based practice, professionals must find ways to clearly articulate their decision-making processes and options. This includes describing the pros and cons of certain choices and presenting a range of alternatives for a positive outcome because the decision to proceed rests collectively in the hands of the professional and other interested parties (ie, the person, family, other team members). Evidence-based practice changes the role of the "expert" in the assessment and intervention process; professionals are experts in their fields, and the service recipients are experts in living their lives. Communication must therefore be jargon free, and the professionals must distinguish factual information (ie, data) from interpretive information that the professionals derive from their experience and knowledge. In this form of conducting practice, professionals acknowledge and welcome the possibility that the intervention decisions will evolve from the communication and typically are not designed prior to the collaboration (although possibilities are presented from various perspectives as part of the interpretive process in measurement).

Evaluating Evidence

The process of evaluating the evidence available about a particular topic to decide the best course of action is complex and beyond the scope of this book. There are some general strategies that professionals can use to guide their thinking processes. First, professionals must decide how similar their service recipients are to the participants in a particular study (eg, similar ages, performance difficulties, diagnosis). This does not mean that the study participants have to be exactly like your service group, but that they are similar on issues that matter to the problem. For example, there are many diagnoses that involve hand weakness. Regardless of diagnosis, if the study addresses the interference of hand weakness, it may be applicable to your service group.

Second, you must decide how much is convincing. If everyone in the study made huge gains, this is easy to incorporate into your thinking, but this rarely happens in research. One way to evaluate "how much is convincing" is to see whether the statistical tests were significant; researchers will tell you this in the results. However, sometimes measurement data needs to be "clinically significant" (ie, important for practice decisions) separate from statistical significance. For example, Kientz and Dunn[21] reported on the Sensory Profile results with children who had autism. Although many items reached statistical significance, the researchers determined that, for practice, therapists needed to only consider items that were different by more than 1 raw score point on the Sensory Profile scale (ie, 1 to 5) because parents could only report whole points on the scale. Ottenbacher[22] discusses the opposite issue (ie, when the statistical test reveals no significance, but the change in the study is of utmost importance to practice). For example, small changes in postural control can make a very big difference in performance, but the number that is used to characterize the change is so small that the calculations do not reveal this importance. Sometimes, researchers select the wrong parameters for measurement and therefore mask a result that may be important to practice. For these situations, therapists must ask, "Would the changes reported make a difference to the persons I serve?" Professional practice requires ongoing reflection about the meaning of information for the process and outcomes of serving persons who have performance needs.

Summary

The process of measurement is a complex one. Therapists must consider the process through which they design an assessment strategy and select measurement tools. With the guidance provided in this chapter and the tools presented in this book, therapists can create a best practice method for making solid practice decisions.

References

1. Newcomer K, Hatry H, Wholey J. Planning and designing useful evaluations. In: Wholey J, Hatry H, Newcomer K, eds. *Handbook of Practical Program Evaluation.* 3rd ed. San Francisco: Josey-Bass; 2010.
2. Bruininks RH, Bruininks B. *Bruininks-Oseretsky Test of Motor Proficiency.* 2nd ed. San Antonio, TX: Pearson Global; 2005.
3. Portney LG, Watkins MP. *Foundations of Clinical Research: Applications to Practice.* 3rd ed. Upper Saddle River, NJ: Pearson Publishing; 2009.
4. Young NL, Yoshida KK, Williams JI, Bombardier C, Wright JG. The role of children in reporting their physical disability. *Arch Phys Med Rehab.* 1995;76:913-918.
5. Achenbach T, Krukowski R, Dumenci L, Ivanova M. Assessment of adult psychopathology: meta-analyses and implications of cross informant correlations. *Psychol Bull.* 2005;131(3):361-382.
6. Yeh C, Chang C, Chang P. Evaluating quality of life in children with cancer using children's self-reports and parent-proxy reports. *Nurs Res.* 2005;54:5:354-362.
7. Klein D. Patients' versus informants' reports of personality disorders in predicting 7½ year outcome in outpatients with depressive disorders. *Psychol Assess.* 2003;15:216-222.
8. Labus J, Keefe F, Jensen M. Self-reports of pain intensity and direct observations of pain behavior: when are they correlated? *Pain.* 2003;102:109-124.
9. Brackett M, Rivers S, Shiffman S, Lerner N, Salovey P. Relating emotional abilities to social functioning: a comparison of self-report and performance measures of emotional intelligence. *J Pers Soc Psychol.* 2006;91(4):780-795.
10. McPhail S, Beller E, Haines T. Two perspectives of proxy reporting of health related quality of life using the Euroqol-5D, an investigation of agreement. *Medical Care.* 2008;46:11:1140-1148.
11. Dunn W. Ecology of Human Performance Model. In: Dunbar S, ed. *Occupational Therapy Models for Intervention with Children and Families.* Thorofare, NJ: SLACK Incorporated; 2007:127-156.
12. Dunn W, McClain L, Brown C, Youngstrom MJ. The ecology of human performance: contextual influences on occupational performance. In: M. Neidstadt M, Crepeau E, eds. *Willard & Spackman's Occupational Therapy.* Philadelphia: Lippincott; 1997.
13. Christiansen C, Baum C, Bass J. *Occupational Therapy: Performance, Participation and Well-Being.* 3rd ed. Thorofare, NJ: SLACK Incorporated; 2015.
14. Dunn W, Brown C, McGuigan A. The ecology of human performance: a framework for thought and action. *Am J Occup Ther.* 1994;48(7):595-607.
15. Law M, Cooper B, Strong S, Stewart D, Rigby P, Letts L. The person-environment-occupational model: a transactive approach to occupational performance. *Can J Occup Ther.* 1996;63(1):9-23.
16. American Occupational Therapy Association. Position paper on Occupational Therapy's Commitment to Nondiscrimination and inclusion. *Am J Occup Ther.* 2014;68:S23-S24.
17. Letts L, Rigby P, Stewart D, et al. *Using Environments to Enable Occupational Performance.* Thorofare, NJ: SLACK Incorporated; 2003.
18. American Occupational Therapy Association. The Occupational Therapy Practice Framework, 3rd ed. *Am J Occup Ther.* 2014;68(suppl 1).
19. Dunn W, Cox J, Foster L, Mische-Lawson L, Tanquary J. Impact of a contextual intervention on child participation and parent competence among children with autism spectrum disorders: a pretest-posttest repeated-measures design. *Am J Occup Ther.* 2012;66(5):520-528.
20. Knight J. Coaching: the key to translating research into practices lies in continuous, job-embedded learning with ongoing support. *National Staff Development Council.* 2009;30(1):18-22.
21. Kientz M, Dunn W. A comparison of children with autism and typical children on the sensory profile. *Am J Occup Ther.* 1997;51:530-537.
22. Ottenbacher K. Use of applied behavioral techniques and an adaptive device to teach lip closure to severely handicapped children. *Am J Occup Ther.* 1986;90(5):535-539.

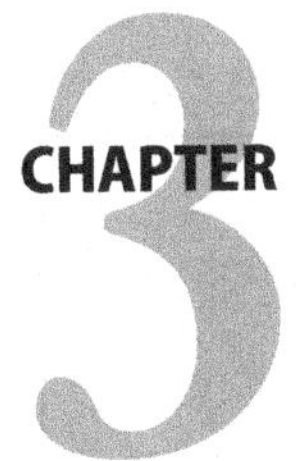

CHAPTER

Understanding Measurement Properties

Susan Magasi, PhD; Apeksha Gohil, BOT; Mark Burghart, MOT; and Anna Wallisch, MOT

Occupational therapists frequently face the need to select high-quality measurement instruments that are applicable to the client's needs and within the parameters of one's clinical environment. Selecting appropriate measurement instruments provides therapists with the ability to accurately identify problems in occupational performance, monitor change over time, and make appropriate recommendations based on predictions of future outcomes. In order to select the best measurement instrument, one must first understand the clinical applicability of the measurement instruments, as well as its properties. Knowledge regarding measurement properties allows a practitioner to understand how reproducible and consistent the measure is (reliability), as well as if the measure is providing results based on the content one wants to measure (validity).

Interpreting and reporting results from appropriate and well-designed measurement instruments can facilitate communication within treatment teams (both inside and outside of the profession), with care coordinators and funders, and with clients themselves. For example, the ability to demonstrate improvement in occupational performance can be used to communicate shared goals and challenges within the interdisciplinary team, to support the need for additional therapy time, and to motivate clients.

A proliferation of measurement instruments exists for every clinical population and setting, giving the practicing clinician a wide range of measurement options. However, not all instruments are created equal. The task of choosing the best measurement instrument for your setting and the people you serve as well as interpreting the results to support clinical decision making can be daunting. A solid understanding of measurement properties is central to occupational therapy practitioners' abilities to perform these essential tasks.

The purpose of this chapter is to provide occupational therapy practitioners with the following:

- A framework for understanding measurement properties (including reliability, validity, and responsiveness).
- A framework for interpreting scores from measurement instruments.
- A process for comparing and selecting appropriate measurement instruments for their clients and setting.

A Framework for Understanding Measurement Properties

The challenge of understanding and interpreting measurement properties is not unique to occupational therapy or rehabilitation. Indeed, different disciplines use different language and evidence to document measurement properties, making it difficult for meaningful comparisons between measures.[1] In an effort to address this conceptual confusion, an international consensus group, COSMIN (Consensus Standards for the Selection of Measurement Instruments) created uniform terminology and interpretation criteria for evaluating measurement properties in health status measures.[2] The uniform terminology and application of the COSMIN framework structures our discussion of the measurement properties throughout this chapter. Figure 3-1 provides a graphic representation of the COSMIN taxonomy.

The COSMIN taxonomy identifies 3 measurement property domains: reliability, validity, and responsiveness. Interpretability is not a measurement property but is important when selecting a measurement instrument for clinical practice and is thus included in the taxonomy.

Law M, Baum C, Dunn W, eds. *Measuring Occupational Performance: Supporting Best Practice in Occupational Therapy, Third Edition (pp 29-41).*

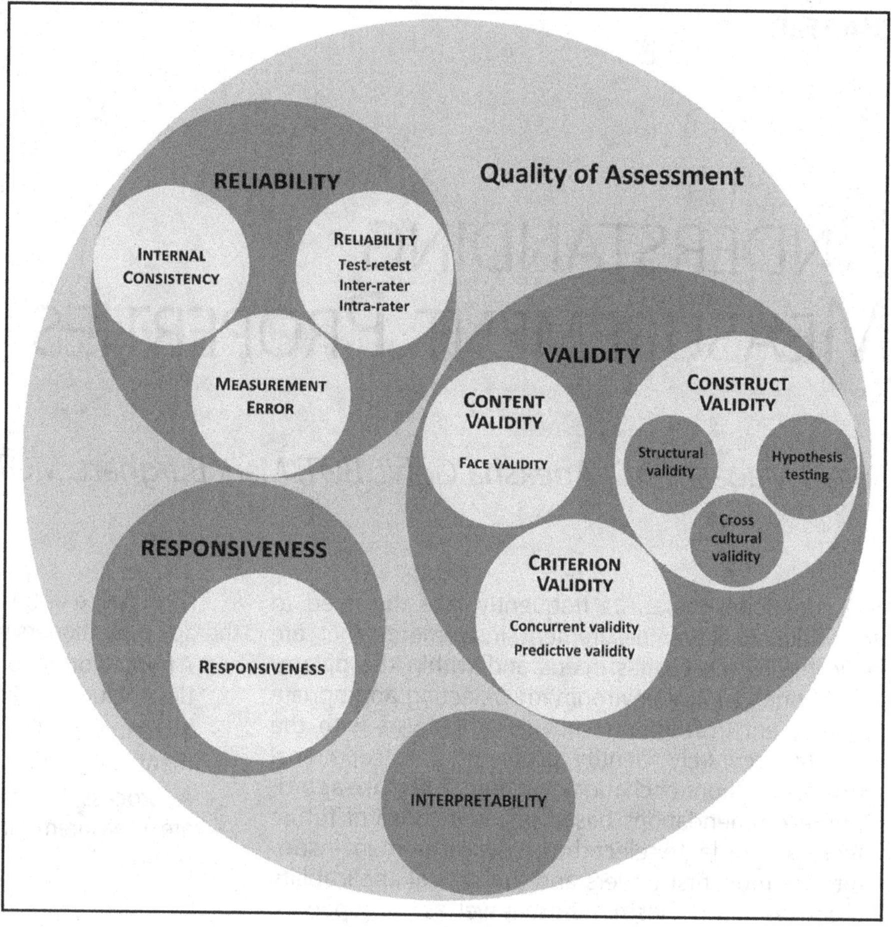

Figure 3-1. COSMIN Taxonomy.[24] (Reprinted from *J Clin Epidemiol*, 63(7), Mokkink LB, Terwee CB, Patrick DL, et al, The COSMIN study reached international consensus on taxonomy, terminology, and definitions of measurement properties for health-related patient-reported outcomes, pp 737-745, Copyright 2010, with permission from Elsevier.)

Measurement decisions should also be based on theoretical concepts. We must recognize why we are selecting a measurement approach based on occupational therapy principles. For example, checking a person's pulse is a common and conceptually driven measurement for nursing as they evaluate the person's physical status each day. Similarly, occupational therapy practitioners base the selection of measurement instruments on the relationship of the underlying constructs to occupational performance and participation. The purpose for which the measurement is used also guides the instrument selection process. Measurement instruments serve 3 main purposes in clinical practice: 1) to discriminate or differentiate between characteristics of an individual, 2) to evaluate change over time, and 3) to predict future events and needs. It is important to clarify both what constructs are being measured and why (from both a theoretical and practical perspective).

Measurement experts also have conceptual models for helping us decide about the strength and usefulness of tests. Their conceptual models describe the statistical relationships among test items, the person's competence, and item difficulty. These statistical methods help test designers select strong items and put items in a proper order when difficulty matters. The Classical Test Theory (CTT) is the basis of many widely-used occupational therapy assessments. Item Response Theory (IRT) is gaining prominence in occupational therapy and rehabilitation research and practice.[3] Many well-known and frequently used measurement instruments in occupational therapy practice, including the Functional Independence Measure (FIM), the Assessment of Motor and Process Skills (AMPS), and the Pediatric Evaluation of Disability Inventory (PEDI), are IRT-based. CTT and IRT use different statistical tests to document reliability and validity. Criteria for evaluating both CCT- and IRT-based measures will be discussed later in this chapter.

Levels of Measurement

Measurement instruments have different ways of categorizing and quantifying the construct of interest. Levels of measurement refer to properties of numbers assigned to an observation.[4] The levels of measurement provide rules for understanding, manipulating, and interpreting different types of numerical data. There are 4 levels of measurement: nominal, ordinal, interval, and ratio.

Nominal

Nominal data are constructed as named categories, and objects or people are assigned to specific named categories based on criteria and descriptors. Gender, handedness, and diagnosis are examples of nominal scales. A rule of nominal scales states that categories are mutually exclusive so that no object or person can be assigned to both groups. An additional assumption states that, when categorizing people or objects, there are exhaustive rules one follows, so every object or person can be accurately assigned to only one category. From a statistical perspective, nominal scales are for counting frequencies.

Ordinal

The next level of measurement is the ordinal scale. Ordinal scales are used to rank the phenomena. Just like running a track race, the objects or people are ranked on a first, second, or third basis, and so on, and the relationship is based on having more or less of an attribute (eg, a faster runner compared to a slower runner in track). The intervals between ranked categories in ordinal scales may be consistent or not known. For instance, the time between the first place runner and the second place runner may be different than between the second and third place runner. Because ordinal scales portray ranked categories, which are essentially labels, there are fewer statistical interpretations and manipulations one may use when working with ordinal scales. Manual muscle testing ratings are a clinical example of an ordinal scale.

Interval

Interval scales resemble ordinal scales because they depict order, but the distance between scores is known and equal. For instance, the distance between years is an equally spaced, fixed amount (ie, 365 days). Interval scales lack an absolute 0 point, thus a score of 0 does not indicate a complete lack of an attribute. For example, a temperature of 0° Fahrenheit does not mean there is a lack of temperature, it means it is cold outside. Interval scales provide researchers with a greater amount of statistics that may be applied to data on an interval scale because relative difference and equivalence may be determined.

Ratio

Ratio scales are the highest level of measurement. A ratio scale is the same as an interval scale, but it has an absolute 0 point, where a score of 0 means an individual has a complete lack of the construct being measured. For instance, when measuring the height of an individual, it is impossible to get a score of 0 and to completely lack height. Because there is an absolute 0 point, one may discuss scores as a ratio; for instance, one could discuss a child's height as half of his or her parent's height, or a parent is double the height of his or her child. Ratio scales are the highest level because one may run all statistical operations at this level.[5]

Measurement Properties

Measurement properties help end users determine whether measurement instruments are consistent, well-targeted, and sensitive enough to evaluate the constructs of interest in the population they serve. Occupational therapists must consider reliability, validity, and responsiveness when selecting a measurement instrument.

Reliability

Reliability helps occupational therapists decide whether they can trust the measurement instrument to give consistent, error-free scores. The term also denotes the reproducibility or dependability of a measurement. When an instrument is administered repeatedly under similar conditions to a person whose ability has not changed, the derived scores should be the same (or at least very similar). Reliability is thus an indication of both the consistency of the measurement and the ability to differentiate between clients.[6] From a clinical perspective, reliability is an indication of how confident you can be that the scores derived from a measurement instrument are truly accurate, and thus how confident you can be using those scores as the basis for clinical decisions. There are 2 important features clinicians should notice when interpreting the reliability of a measurement.

1. First, reliability is derived from the sample and is not an attribute of the measurement instrument itself. This is very important from both a clinical and research perspective because it means that the reliability is dependent on sample context and evaluates factors such as methods, characteristics of tested individuals, and the condition of interest. Therefore, therapists must be diligent when interpreting an instrument's reliability in the process of selecting a measurement instrument or reading a research study. As a critical consumer of the research literature, you should ask the questions, "reliable for whom?" and, "reliable for what purposes?" When selecting a measurement instrument or reporting on its reliability, you should select data from studies that most closely approximate your setting and clients.
2. Second, reliability research is conducted under strict conditions with a small number of highly trained and monitored test administrators. Clinical practice is much more variable and likely to be less precise. Therefore, the reliability reported in the literature should be considered the highest reliability possible.

According to the COSMIN taxonomy, reliability is a measurement domain that includes test-retest reliability, inter-rater reliability, intra-rater reliability, measurement error, and for a multi-item assessment, internal consistency.

Test-Retest Reliability

Test-retest reliability is the consistency of repeated measures over time in an individual who has not changed.

To further understand test-retest reliability, we will examine the 9-hole pegboard assessment, a simple performance-based measure of hand dexterity scored by the number of seconds required to place and remove pegs. If an occupational therapist tests an individual with stable hand function, his or her time (score) should be the same now, in 1 hour, and in 1 week. High test-retest reliability indicates that a measurement instrument is capable of measuring a variable with consistency. Test-retest reliability also provides confidence to practitioners that changes in test scores are due to actual changes in clients, which is useful when measuring progress.

Inter-Rater Reliability

Inter-rater reliability determines how well a measurement instrument provides the consistent results between 2 or more practitioners measuring the same construct or individual. For instance, if 2 different occupational therapy practitioners timed the client's performance on the 9-hole pegboard test, they should both get a similar time.

Perfect agreement between test administrators is difficult to achieve even with pre-determined rules and definitions for the raters to follow. In the pegboard test, each practitioner may have different reaction times when starting and stopping the timer, resulting in different scores. Additionally, when practitioners need to observe to rate a client's behavior, their individual backgrounds may result in different ratings. Thus, when high inter-rater reliability is reported by an assessment, it means the measurement the therapist has chosen yields consistent results across raters.

Intra-Rater Reliability

Intra-rater reliability determines how well an assessment provides the same scores on multiple tests within one individual rater's report. For example, if a therapist timed a 9-hole pegboard administration multiple times, he or she should get the same time on each test.

Intra-rater reliability appears easy to achieve in the 9-hole pegboard example, but often is more difficult to attain than expected. One feature that challenges intra-rater reliability is rater bias. Rater bias occurs when a therapist may be influenced by his or her memory of the first score rated, which results in good intra-rater reliability, but is not a true depiction of a measure's reliability.[5] If an assessment reports good intra-rater reliability, the test yields consistent results within a single rater.

Statistics Used to Evaluate Test-Retest, Inter-Rater, and Intra-Rater Reliability

The preferred reliability statistic for test-retest, inter-rater, and intra-rater reliability depends on the measurement instrument's response options. Intraclass Correlation Coefficients (ICC) are preferred for continuous scores because they reflect both correlation and agreement.[7-9] Cohen's kappa is the preferred statistical method for nominal scales, whereas weighted kappa is preferred for ordinal scales to show percent agreement.[7,9,10]

ICC scores typically range between 0 and 1, with larger values representing greater reliability. Kappa coefficients for nominal and ordinal scales (both weighted and unweighted) can range from -1 to 1 but typically fall between 0 and 1 in clinical assessments, with larger values representing greater reliability.[11] When evaluating the reliability of a measurement instrument, Terwee et al[12] recommend an ICC or weighted kappa of ≥0.70.

Internal Consistency

Internal consistency is the degree of inter-relatedness among items in a multi-item measurement instrument[2] and indicates the extent to which items measure aspects of the same characteristic and nothing else.[5] For instance, if an individual created a survey for parents to determine their knowledge of developmental milestones, the survey items should depict developmental milestones and not questions about child safety in the home. Unidimensionality (measuring only one construct), of the measurement instrument (or subscales within it) is a requirement for internal consistency.

Internal consistency typically measures the degree of correlation between the items with a measure. Cronbach's coefficient alpha is the preferred method for evaluating internal consistency for measures developed using CTT. Cronbach's coefficient alpha scores above 0.80 are considered to be high quality,[12] although Cronbach alpha greater than 0.90 may indicate redundancy in item content.[13] An important consideration when analyzing Cronbach's coefficient alpha is the number of items being tested. When more items are being tested, there is a greater chance they are measuring the same construct, resulting in a better Cronbach's coefficient alpha score simply because there are more items.[5]

Measurement Error

We strive for reliable measurements, but in reality, no measurement instrument is completely reliable or free from measurement error. Clients, test administrators, the environment, or the instrument itself can introduce error. For example, a client's motivation to perform the test may differ from one administration to the next. Test administrators can introduce error if they do not adhere rigidly to the test protocol. A clinician's expectations based on the client's previous performance may also introduce error. Environmental factors such as lighting, noise, and temperature can introduce variability and thus error into the assessment process. Instrumentation errors can be caused by calibration or scale issues (eg, if the battery was wearing down in the stopwatch used for a timed test, the scores may not be accurate) or by defective instruments (eg, the pegboard was poorly manufactured and the pegs did not fit smoothly in the holes). Adherence to test administration protocols, frequent retraining of clinicians, creation of a supportive environment that limits distractions, and consistent documentation in alteration or accommodations to testing protocols are strategies that can help reduce measurement error. While adherence to administration protocols is recommended, many of the clients seen in occupational therapy have physical, cognitive, and sensory issues that may impact their ability to follow administration guidelines. Clinicians should be flexible and use clinical judgment when working with clients.[14,15]

Measurement error is composed of 2 components: random error and systematic error.[2] Specifically, systematic errors are predictable errors of measurement as they usually occur by overestimating or underestimating a true score.[5] When a systematic error is detected, one may simply be able to fix the under- or overestimation. For example, if the batteries in a grip strength dynamometer are wearing down or the device needs to be recalibrated, it may consistently underreport test scores. Similarly, culturally insensitive measures that selectively disadvantage test takers from certain racial or ethnic groups are examples of systematic error. A systematic error generally affects validity (ie, the values are not true representations of the construct) more than reliability because the error is consistent.[14]

Random errors are due to chance and may affect a subject's score in an unforeseeable way from one trial to another. The random errors come from differences in client motivation, fatigue, inconsistent test administration, and inconsistent scores due to clinicians' expectations of a client. As random error diminishes, reliability increases. Because we may not always know how much a value sways from the intended value, we must estimate the measurement error through the use of reliability.[5]

The preferred statistic for measurement error in studies based on CTT is the standard error of measurement (SEM). SEM allows us to estimate the amount of error by measuring the variability of multiple scores on a single subject. Reliability and measurement error are related but distinctly separate and, when interpreting SEM, the more reliable the measurement, the smaller the error or SEM. SEM statistics also typically provide a confidence level for the derived score. For example, most SEM statistics report a 95% Confidence Interval (CI), meaning that the SEM estimates that 95% of the time, the errors from the measurement fall within the reported SEM range.

Minimal detectable change (MDC) is related to SEM. MDC is the smallest amount of change in a score that can be interpreted as real change (and not just a function of measurement error). When interpreting a measurement instrument's derived scores, it is important to consider both the score change and the standard error of measurement in order to determine the MDC. MDC provides an estimate of the error between 2 scores from 2 different assessments of the same person. For example, The Barthel Index is a commonly used performance-based measure of independence in ADL. Clients receive a score between 0 and 100, with 0 being total dependence and 100 being complete independence. The Barthel Index's measurement properties have been evaluated in people with chronic stroke.[16]

- SEM = 1.45
- MDC = 4.02

Consider a client with a chronic stroke with the following:

- Admission Barthel Index Score = 57 + 1.45 or 55.55 – 58.45
- Re-evaluation Barthel Index Score = 60 + 1.45 or 58.55 – 63.45

Did the client improve? Based on the raw scores alone, we might conclude that the client is improving. However, the difference in scores is less than the MDC, so we cannot conclude that the client has improved.

Reliability of Item Response Theory–Based Measurement Instruments

For IRT-based measurement instruments, reliability is determined by the discriminative ability of the items.[1,17] Person separation statistics indicate how well items within an IRT-based measurement instrument differentiate people. Separation statistics range from 0.0 to 1.0, with higher values being indicative of better separation. Person separation reliability values of > 0.8 are acceptable.[18] Standard error (SE) is comparable to SEM and is the recommended statistic for measurement error in IRT-based measurement instruments.[1] Smaller SE are associated with more discriminating items.

Validity

After determining a measurement instrument's reliability and that it is relatively free from error, we must determine that the assessment is valid. Validity is the degree to which an instrument measures the construct(s) it intends to assess.[2] Validity places emphasis on the ability to make inferences based on derived test scores or measurements. For example, clinicians typically use assessment scores to evaluate and predict functional performance in daily life. Assessments must have the ability to evaluate the person's current performance and accurately predict future functioning. Therefore, validity addresses what practitioners are able to do with the instrument results.

As with reliability, validity must be understood as a property of the instrument's derived scores, rather than of the instrument itself.[19] Context of use, including client characteristics, clinical settings, and conditions of measurement, all influence the validity of the scores.[6] As with reliability claims, the critical consumer must be wary of blanket statements of an instrument's validity and ask the questions, "valid for whom?" and, "valid for what purpose?"

Reliability is a necessary prerequisite for validity because validity implies that an instrument is relatively free from error. A score derived from an unreliable measure cannot be considered valid. Reliability thus defines the upper limit of validity.[6] Validity is a unitary construct,[14] but it can also be reported along a continuum.

Occupational therapy practitioners must evaluate the accumulated validity data to make informed choices when selecting and interpreting an instrument and scores.

Validity can be understood as consisting of 3 main types: content validity, construct validity, and criterion validity. Additionally, 3 measurement properties—fairness in testing, responsiveness to change, and floor/ceiling effects—help us to further understand the application of validity to clinical practice.

Content Validity

Content validity is the extent to which the domain of interest is comprehensively sampled by the items in the instrument.[12] Content validity is evaluated by making judgments about the relevance and comprehensiveness of items within a given measurement. Content validity should be evaluated in a sample similar to the target population for which the measurement will be clinically used. The context in which the instrument will be used is important to consider as not all groups may experience the measured construct in the exact same manner. Relevant experiences and manifestations of the construct must be represented; otherwise inaccurate inferences may be made based on the derived scores.

In 2009, the United States Food and Drug Administration issued the Guidance for Industry on Patient-Reported Outcome Measures, stressing the importance of direct input from people in the measured population when evaluating content validity.[20] Therefore, when evaluating content validity claims, it is important to determine that members of the target population, not just clinical or content experts, were included in the validation sample. Content validity is typically evaluated using rigorous qualitative methods.[21] Mixed methods approaches that integrate qualitative and advanced quantitative methods, such as factor analysis, structural equation modeling, and differential item functioning, are also used.[22]

Face Validity

Face validity is a component of content validity but is less rigorous. Face validity is the extent to which an instrument "appears" to test what it is intended to test. Face validity lends itself to some subjectivity and should not be considered as a significant source for instrument validity as there is no standard for judging the amount of validity an instrument possesses.

Criterion Validity

Criterion validity is the degree to which scores of an instrument are an adequate reflection of a "gold standard" measure (also referred to as the *criterion standard*).[2] By definition, criterion validity is only applicable in situations when there is an agreed upon gold standard assessment for the construct being measured. The gold standard instrument used for comparison must have previously established validity prior to comparisons because without a valid instrument serving as the comparative criterion, the instrument would not be accurate for testing.

When evaluating criterion validity, there must be convincing evidence that the comparative assessment is truly the agreed upon gold standard method for assessing the construct.[12] To assess criterion validity, the target instrument and the gold standard tool should be administered and scored independently of one another. Scores from the target instrument and the gold standard should be compared and meet a predefined level of agreement between the target instrument and the gold standard. Criterion validity is further divided into concurrent and predictive validity.[1]

- Concurrent validity establishes validity when 2 measures are taken at relatively the same time, with 1 measure being the gold standard clinical tool. If the measures are similar, we may conclude that the target assessment is as accurate or more efficient as the gold standard measure and, thus, can be used interchangeably. For example, when determining the concurrent validity of an observational balance assessment, researchers may have participants balancing on a force platform, which has been previously validated, while observing the person's posture. Concurrent validity is appropriate for instruments used for diagnostic/identification purposes (eg, to identify limitations in occupational performance) or for evaluative purposes (eg, to track change over time).
- Predictive validity establishes that derived scores from the target assessment can be used to predict future scores or clinical outcomes in the same individuals. Predictive validity is evaluated for instruments that seek to determine whether scores can predict the gold standard outcomes in the future. For example, do fall risk assessment scores predict future falls in older adults? Assessments with predictive validity are useful in identifying at-risk populations, allowing clinicians to intervene. Assessments with adequate predictive validity also help practitioners set long-term goals for the people they serve.

Construct Validity

Many constructs of interest in occupational therapy have no commonly agreed upon gold standards. In these situations, construct validation should be used to support validity claims. Construct validity is the degree to which the scores of an instrument are consistent with hypotheses with regard to internal relationships, relationships to scores of other instruments, or differences between relevant groups.[2] There are 3 aspects to construct validity: structural validity, hypothesis testing, and cross-cultural validity.

Structural validity is a relevant concept only for multi-item measurement instruments and determines the extent to which all items represent the same underlying construct.[2] If a measurement instrument is determined to measure more than one construct, then subscales scores should be reported. For example, the Bruinick-Oseretsky Test of Motor Proficiency is a comprehensive assessment of pediatric motor performance, but it includes separate subscores for strength and dexterity. For measurement instruments developed using CTT, confirmatory factor analysis (CFA) is the preferred statistical approach.[1] The factor structure and model fit are evaluated using the comparative fit index (CFI), the root mean square error of approximation (RMSEA), and the standardized root mean square residual (SRMR). Models with CFI ≥0.95, RMSEA ≤0.06, and SRMR ≤0.08 are considered to be good-fitting models.[23]

Hypothesis testing is the extent to which scores on a particular measurement instrument relate to other measures in a manner that is consistent with the theoretically derived hypothesis.[12] The construct validation of measurement instruments is based on the development and empirical testing of conceptually driven relationships between the scores of one measurement instrument with the scores from other measures. Hypotheses are evaluated by the correlation and should include both the direction and magnitude of the correlations or mean differences.[24]

There are 3 main types of construct validity described in the literature. Convergent validity claims are supported when scores from measurement instruments that purport to measure the same construct are highly correlated. Divergent validity claims are supported when scores from measurement instruments that purport to measure different constructs are weakly correlated. Known groups or discriminant validity claims are supported when samples with known differences in the constructs of interest obtain significantly different or weakly correlated scores. Construct validation is an ongoing process aimed at building a body of evidence to support construct validity claims.[25,26] Terwee and colleagues[12] suggest that the formulation of specific hypotheses and at least 75% of the results are in accordance with these hypotheses as quality criteria to substantiate construct validity claims.

Cross-cultural validity is the "degree to which the performance of the items on a translated or culturally adapted [measurement] instrument are an adequate reflection of the performance of items in the original version of the instrument."[2(p 743)] Issues of cross-cultural validity are particularly important in questionnaires and self-report instruments. Some items or constructs that are highly relevant in one culture may be quite meaningless in another. As a starting point, rigorous translation and cultural adaptation practices should be implemented in accordance with state of the science guidelines,[27] followed by cognitive and hypothesis testing in the target population.[24] A cross-culturally valid instrument should function the same way in different populations. From a clinical perspective, it is important to recognize that validity scores derived from measurement instruments cannot be assumed across cultures; rather, translations and cultural adaptations must be rigorously conducted and systematically evaluated.

Statistics Used to Evaluate Validity

Similar to reliability, the preferred validity statistic depends on the instrument's response options. When evaluating concurrent validity and both measures report continuous variables, Pearson Correlation coefficients are often reported.[7-9] When the target instrument scores are continuous and the gold standard is dichotomous (only has 2 categories), the Area Under the Receiver Operating Characteristic (ROC) Curve is commonly reported. Finally, when both measures are dichotomous, sensitivity and specificity are reported.[25] Sensitivity deals with the proportion of true positives that are correctly identified by the test, whereas specificity identifies the proportion of true negatives that are correctly identified.[28] Sensitivity and specificity are particularly important for diagnostic tests where false positives and false negatives have critical consequences. Refer to Table 3-5 for acceptable statistical ranges for validity measures.

Validity of IRT-Based Measurement Instruments

Validity in the IRT context is related to measurement accuracy, and fit statistics provide evidence of validity of the items and coherence to the construct.[18] Items that deviate from the IRT measurement model are considered to be misfitting items and are typically deleted in the instrument development process. Fit statistics are evaluated for each item via a Mean Square Statistic ratio of observed variance to expected variance from the model. Variance of 1.0 indicates perfect agreement. Fit statistics of < 2.0 are considered acceptable.

Fairness in Testing

Fairness in testing dictates that all test takers should have an unobstructed opportunity to demonstrate their standing on the construct(s) being measured.[14] Fairness in testing is a fundamental validity issue and requires attention through all stages of test development and use.[14] Issues of fairness in testing may be particularly important given that occupational therapy practitioners serve increasingly diverse populations, not only in terms of disability status, but also age, race/ethnicity, gender identity, functional literacy, and culture.

Principles of fairness in testing stress flexibility in assessment administration to provide equal opportunities for some test takers.[14] It may be appropriate to provide reasonable accommodations—alterations to the testing environment or task demands—for some people with disabilities. An in-depth understanding of the constructs being measured and the theoretical relationship between the test items (performance-based or self-report) can help ensure that accommodations do not fundamentally alter the core task demands and thereby invalidate the derived scores. Information about reasonable accommodations and modification can help end users evaluate the impact that nonstandard administrations can have on derived scores.

Responsiveness to Change

The ultimate goal of occupational therapy is to optimize occupational performance, participation, and quality of life for the people we serve. It is therefore necessary that practitioners be able to document change in performance over time. Change can be either an improvement or decrease in the person's ability to complete the measured skill. The ability of an instrument to detect change over time in the measured construct is called *responsiveness*.[2]

Responsiveness may be understood as an aspect of validity related to change in scores over time and is sometimes called *longitudinal validity*. Longitudinal studies are required to evaluate responsiveness, but the absolute time frame for the study is less important than the observation that changes in scores has occurred.[1] As with validity claims, assessing responsiveness consists of hypothesis testing by comparing change scores in known groups or by evaluating changes in measures.[12] Change scores should be obtained independently for both the comparative measure (a criterion measure, if available, or another instrument whose responsiveness has been established). The appropriate statistics for evaluating responsiveness are the correlations between change scores for the Area Under the ROC Curve for continuous variables, and sensitivity and specificity for dichotomous scales.[24]

Terwee and colleagues[12] suggest that responsive measures should also be able to distinguish important change from measurement error. Minimally clinically important difference (MCID) has become a valuable statistic when assessing changes in performance over time. The MCID is the smallest difference in the measured construct that indicates a clinically meaningful change has occurred.[29] The determination of the MCID is necessary to judge the effectiveness of treatments and interventions as clinicians rely on tracking meaningful changes in performance when comparing the effectiveness of clinical approaches.

Floor and Ceiling Effects

Floor and ceiling effects indicate that a measurement instrument may lack the ability to adequately discriminate individuals with the highest and lowest scores, thereby limiting the reliability of the results. A measurement instrument with significant floor and ceiling effects does not allow for measurement of changes at the lowest or highest ratings, limiting responsiveness and tracking functional change over time. Clinicians need to be cautious of instruments with documented floor and ceiling effects when working with individuals testing at the extremes of the assessment scale.

Practical Considerations

Interpretability

One challenge for occupational therapy practitioners using measurement instruments in clinical practice is interpreting the changes in derived scores and using them to inform treatment decisions. Statistically significant change does not necessarily translate to meaningful changes in daily life experiences and outcomes. While not strictly a measurement property, interpretability is an important consideration for use of measurement instruments in clinical practice. A variety of forms of evidence can be used to support interpretability of derived scores, including comparing means and standard deviations of subgroups that are known to be different. According to Terwee et al,[12] positive ratings for interpretability are given if mean scores and standard deviations are provided for at least 4 subgroups, regardless of the measurement approach. MCID also provides evidence of interpretability and is increasingly reported in assessment literature.[30]

Clinical Utility

Clinicians must have a thorough understanding of measurement properties in order to make informed decisions about the selection of measurement instruments and the interpretation of scores. It is also important to acknowledge the practical considerations that influence assessment use in routine clinical care. Clinical utility, or the usefulness of a clinical instrument or intervention, is related to the feasibility of administering the measurement instrument in clinical environments. Riddle and Stratford[6] have identified important considerations related to clinical utility at the clinician, client, and organizational level, including the following:

- Clinician-related factors
    - Opportunity to research and identify the best possible measurement instruments for each individual client
    - Training and certification requirements needed to properly administer the measurement instrument
    - Burden of measurement in clinicians, including the time needed to administer and score measures
    - Clinical reasoning to interpret derived scores and apply them to practice
- Client-related factors
    - Availability of appropriately targeted measurement instruments to address the construct of interest
    - Accessibility considerations when there is a mismatch between the client's functional capacity and the task demands
    - Client preferences for active treatment vs assessment. Some clients may perceive assessment processes to be less valuable than treatment.
- Organization-related factors
    - Cost of measurement instruments can limit the choices practitioners have when evaluating instruments
    - Resource requirements, such as space, equipment, and other instrument-specific requirements, can be a limiting factor in some clinical environments.

Organizational factors including policies, practices, and procedures can help or hinder measurement. Riddle and Stratford[6] suggest that a systematic and thoughtful approach to measurement can reduce the burden and increase application of appropriate instruments following a 6-step process:

1. Step 1: Clarify what you hope to assess and why
2. Step 2: State important patient-related constraints
3. Step 3: State important constraints relevant to your clinical setting
4. Step 4: Search effectively and efficiently for relevant measurement instruments
5. Step 5: Seek out measures that provide information on interpretation of score values
6. Step 6: Scrutinize measurement properties relevant to your clinical context

The following case study applies the Riddle and Stratford strategy to illustrate the identification and selection of instruments based on clinical utility and measurement property considerations.

Case Study

Felipe is a 53-year-old restaurant owner and chef who experienced a left ischemic stroke, which primarily affected his right side. After intensive inpatient rehabilitation, he was able to return to independent living. He is independent in self-care and community mobility, but he reports that he has had trouble returning to work in his restaurant. Felipe received a referral to your outpatient occupational therapy clinic for a comprehensive evaluation with a goal of returning to work at his restaurant. The assessment should also serve as a baseline measurement to track changes over time resulting from therapeutic interventions.

During the clinical interview, Felipe reports that his job involves lifting heavy supplies, reaching for pans, cutting, stirring, and dicing foods. Since his stroke, he reports feeling weak, slow, and clumsy in the kitchen. Cooking is his passion and his livelihood. His family and staff have been pitching in at the restaurant, but as a small business owner, he feels strongly that he needs to be the one in the kitchen.

Step 1: Clarify what you hope to assess and why. Based on the clinical interview, it is apparent that gross and fine motor functioning is a limiting factor in Felipe's ability to go back to work. A comprehensive performance-based instrument that addresses both fine and gross motor functioning is most appropriate for Felipe.

Step 2: State important patient-related constraints. Felipe is an action-oriented, no-nonsense kind of person who will likely respond more favorably to functional assessment with daily life tasks. His motivation and compliance with activities he considers "baby tasks" is likely to be low. Time is also a major constraint and, therefore, an assessment that can be administered within 50 minutes is needed.

Step 3: State important constraints relevant to your clinical setting. As a high-volume outpatient setting, the clinic has a quiet room for assessments. The organization is supportive of integrating new measurements into practice, but cannot allocate time or funding for training or for purchasing new assessments.

Step 4: Search effectively and efficiently for relevant measurement instruments. Based on Steps 1 through 3, a functional performance-based assessment of upper extremity function for use in adults after stroke is the most appropriate measure to find. The assessment must be free or low cost with minimal training requirements. By clearly defining these criteria in advance, the clinician can rule out instruments that are not feasible for the practice setting and the client.

The most rigorous approach to instrument identification and selection is to conduct a systematic literature search. There are a number of searchable instrument databases that provide synthesized, peer-reviewed instrument summaries. One such database is the RehabMeasures Database (RMD) (www.rehabmeasures.org). The RMD is searchable by area of assessment, diagnosis, cost, and length of time to administer the test.

Entering the search criteria in the RMD yielded a total of 5 candidate measures:

1. Nine-hole peg test (9-HPT)
2. Wolf Motor Function Test (WMFT)
3. Stroke Specific Quality of Life Scale (SSQOLS)
4. Stroke Impact Scale (SIS)
5. Action Research Arm Test (ARAT)

Brief summaries for each measurement instrument were entered into a comparison table and compared.

Based on the clinical utility information, the 2 self-report measures were eliminated from consideration as they are not performance-based. The 9-HPT is not functional and only measures finger dexterity, so it was dropped from consideration. The WMFT and ARAT were the remaining assessments under consideration.

Step 5: Seek out measures that provide information on the interpretation of score values. Based on the accumulated responsiveness and interpretability data, both the WMFT and ARAT provide guidance to the occupational therapy practitioner to direct interpretation of derived scores and to track changes in upper extremity function over time.

Both WMFT and FM have excellent reliability and validity. Therefore, our clinical reasoning to select between these 2 clinical instruments would depend on Felipe's occupational goals and job demands. The occupational therapist chose the WMFT assessment because it uses daily functional tasks, which was motivating for Felipe.

Summary

Practitioners face difficult decisions regarding the assessment and measurement of occupational performance. Reliable and valid measurement instruments must be used when assessing a person's occupational performance. By using accurate and repeatable measures, therapists can determine and assess interventional strategies to improve performance in the people they serve.

Table 3-1

STEP 4

Summary	*9-HPT*	*WMFT*	*SSQOLS*	*SIS*	*ARAT*
Constructs	Finger dexterity	Upper extremity motor ability, 2 subscales	Health-related quality of life post-stroke	Health status post-stroke, including 5-hand function items	Upper extremity function
Instrument Type	Performance-based	Performance-based	Self-report	Self-report	Performance-based
Length of Test	1 item	21 items	49 items	59 items	19 items
Time Required	<5 minutes	About 35 minutes	10 to 15 minutes	6 to 30 minutes	About 10 minutes
Functional	No	Yes	No	Yes	No

Table 3-2

STEP 5

Responsiveness and Interpretability	*WMFT*	*ARAT*
Minimal detectable change	0.1 points 0.7 seconds	Not established
Normative data	Yes	Yes
Responsiveness data	Yes	Yes
Floor/ceiling effects	Not established	Ceiling effect in people > 180 post-stroke.
MCID	Established for dominant and nondominant affected side	Established for dominant and nondominant affected side

Table 3-3

STEP 6—RELIABILITY

Reliability	*WMFT*	*ARAT*
Test-retest reliability (ICC)	.95 to .90 (stroke, n = 22)	.97 (stroke, multiple sclerosis, traumatic brain injury, n = 23)
Inter-rater reliability (ICC)	.93 to .99 (stroke, n = 10-24)	0.995 (stroke, n = 20)
Intrarater reliability (ICC)	Not reported	0.989 (stroke, multiple sclerosis, traumatic brain injury, n = 44)
SEM	0.2 seconds .1 points on the WMFT functional scale	Not established
Internal consistency (Cronbach's alpha)	.92 (stroke, n = 24)	.94 to .98 (stroke, n = 40)

Table 3-4

Step 6—Validity

Reliability	*WMFT*	*Fugl-Meyer Assessment*
Criterion validity	Fugl-Meyer, upper extremity r = -0.86-0.88	Fugl-Meyer, Upper extremity r = 0.94, p < 0.01
Construct validity	Known groups validity Able to distinguish between people with and without upper extremity impairments post-stroke	Convergent Validity (Spearman's rho) Fugl-Meyer motor 0.925 Box and Block Test 0.985 Motricity Index 0.811 Divergent Validity Fugl-Meyer sensation 0.298 Fugl-Meyer joint motion/pain 0.421 Ashworth Scale -.296 Modified Barthel Index 0.049

Table 3-5

Brief Overview of Psychometric Properties and Indices of Change

	Definition	*Clinical Bottom Line/Standards for Use*
Standard Error of Measurement (SEM)	A reliability measure that assesses response stability. The SEM estimates the standard error in a set of repeated scores.	The SEM is the amount of error that represents measurement error
Minimal Detectable Change (MDC)	A statistical estimate of the smallest amount of change that can be detected by a measure that corresponds to a noticeable change in ability	The MDC is the minimum amount of change in a client's score that ensures the change is not the result of measurement error.
Minimal Clinically Important Difference (MCID)	The smallest amount of change in an outcome that might be considered important by the client or clinician	The MCID is a published value of change in an instrument that indicates the minimum amount of change required for a client to feel a difference in the measured variable.
Test-retest	Establishes that an instrument is capable of measuring a variable with consistency	For individual decision making: ICC > 0.9 For group decisions: ICC > .7
Inter-rater reliability	Determines variation between 2 or more raters who measure the same group of subjects	Excellent reliability: ICC ≥ .75 Adequate reliability: ICC .4 to < .74 Poor reliability: ICC ≤ .4
Intrarater reliability	Determines stability of data recorded by one individual across 2 or more trials	
Internal consistency	The extent to which items in the same instrument all measure the same trait; typically measured using Cronbach's alpha	Excellent: Cronbach's alpha > .8 Adequate: Cronbach's alpha < .8 and > .7 Poor: Cronbach's alpha < .7 *Scores higher than .9 may indicate redundancy

(continued)

Table 3-5 (continued)

Brief Overview of Psychometric Properties and Indices of Change

	Definition	*Clinical Bottom Line/Standards for Use*
Criterion-related validity	Indicates that the outcomes of one instrument can be used as a substitute measure for an established test. Included concurrent and predictive validity	Excellent: correlation ≥.6 Adequate: correlation .31 to .59 Poor: correlation coefficient ≤.30
Concurrent validity	Establishes validity when 2 measures are taken at relatively the same time, often indicates that the test could be used instead of a gold-standard	
Predictive validity	The outcome of the target test can be used to predict a future outcome.	
Construct validity	Establishes the ability of an instrument to measure an abstract concept and the degree to which the instrument reflects the theoretical components of it. Includes convergent and discriminant validity	
Convergent validity	Two measures that are believed to reflect the same underlying phenomenon will correlate highly.	
Discriminant validity	Two measures that are believed to assess different characteristics will yield low correlations.	
Content validity	Items that make up an instrument adequately sample the content that defines the variable being measured.	
Face validity	An instrument appears to tests what it is supposed to test	

Reprinted with permission from Moore J, Baum C. Measuring Progress: Using the rehabilitation measures database to increase knowledge about outcome measurement. *OT Practice.* 2014;19(7):11-15.

References

1. De Vet HC, Terwee CB, Mokkink LB, Knol DL. *Measurement in Medicine: A Practical Guide.* Cambridge University Press; 2011.
2. Mokkink LB, Terwee CB, Patrick DL, et al. The COSMIN study reached international consensus on taxonomy, terminology, and definitions of measurement properties for health-related patient-reported outcomes. *J Clin Epidemiol.* 2010;63(7):737-745.
3. Velozo CA, Seel RT, Magasi S, Heinemann AW, Romero S. Improving measurement methods in rehabilitation: core concepts and recommendations for scale development. *Arch Phys Med Rehabil.* 2012;93(8 Suppl):S154-163.
4. Depoy E, Gitlin LN. *Introduction to Research: Understanding and Applying Multiple Strategies.* 5th ed. St. Louis, MO: Elsevier Health Sciences; 2015.
5. Portney LG, Watkins MP. *Foundations of Clinical Research: Applications to Practice.* Upper Saddle River, NJ: Pearson; 2009.
6. Riddle DL, Stratford PW. *Is this Change Real? Interpreting Patient Outcomes in Physical Therapy.* Philadelphia, PA: F.A. Davis Co; 2013.
7. Mokkink LB, Terwee CB, Patrick DL, et al. *COSMIN Checklist Manual.* Amsterdam: EMGO Institute for Health and Care Research; 2012.
8. Shrout PE, Fleiss JL. Intraclass correlations: uses in assessing rater reliability. *Psych Bull.* 1979;86(2):420.
9. Streiner DL, Norman GR, Cairney J. *Health Measurement Scales: A Practical Guide to Their Development and Use.* 5th ed. New York, NY: Oxford University Press; 2014.
10. Cohen J. Weighted kappa: nominal scale agreement provision for scaled disagreement or partial credit. *Psych Bull.* 1968;70(4):213.

11. Sim J, Wright CC. The kappa statistic in reliability studies: use, interpretation, and sample size requirements. *Phys Ther.* 2005;85(3):257-268.
12. Terwee C, Bot SD, de Boer MR, et al. Quality criteria were proposed for measurement properties of health status questionnaires. *J Clin Epidemiol.* 2007;60(1):34-42.
13. Tavakol M, Dennick R. Making sense of Cronbach's alpha. *Int J Med Educ.* 2011;2:53.
14. AERA, APA, & NCME. *STANDARDS for Educational and Psychological Testing.* Washington, DC: American Educational Research Association; 2014.
15. American Psychological Association. Guidelines for assessment of and intervention with persons with disabilities. *Am Psychol.* 2012;67(1):43-62.
16. Hsieh YW, Wang CH, Wu SC, Chen PC, Sheu CF, Hsieh CL. Establishing the minimal clinically important difference of the Barthel Index in stroke patients. *Neurorehabil Neural Repair.* 2007;21(3):233-238.
17. Massof RW. Understanding Rasch and Item Response Theory Models: applications to the estimation and validation of interval latent trait measures from responses to rating scale questionnaires. *Ophthalmic Epidemiology.* 2011;18(1):1-19.
18. Wright BD, Stone MH. *Measurement Essentials.* Wilmington, DE: Wide Range Inc; 1999:221.
19. Nunnally JC. *Psychometric Theory.* 2nd ed. New York: McGraw-Hill; 1978.
20. US Department of Health and Human Services Food and Drug Administration. Guidance for industry. Patient-reported outcome measures: use in medical product development to support labeling claims. 2009. www.fda.gov/downloads/Drugs/Guidances/UCM193282.pdf. Accessed June 17, 2016.
21. Patrick DL, Burke LB, Gwaltney CJ, et al. Content validity—establishing and reporting the evidence in newly developed patient-reported outcomes (PRO) instruments for medical product evaluation: ISPOR PRO Good Research Practices Task Force report: part 2—assessing respondent understanding. *Value Health.* 2011;14(8):978-988.
22. Magasi S, Ryan G, Revicki D, et al. Content validity of patient-reported outcome measures: perspectives from a PROMIS meeting. *Qual Life Res.* 2012;21(5):739-746.
23. Hu L, Bentler PM. Cutoff criteria for fit indexes in covariance structure analysis: conventional criteria versus new alternatives. *Struct Equ Modeling.* 1999;6(1):1-55.
24. Mokkink LB, Terwee CB, Patrick DL, et al. The COSMIN checklist for assessing the methodological quality of studies on measurement properties of health status measurement instruments: an international Delphi study. *Qual Life Res.* 2010;19(4):539-549.
25. Mokkink LB, Terwee CB, Knol DL, et al. The COSMIN checklist for evaluating the methodological quality of studies on measurement properties: a clarification of its content. *BMC Med Res Methodol.* 2010;10(1):22.
26. Strauss ME, Smith GT. Construct validity: advances in theory and methodology. *Annu Rev Clin Psychol.* 2009;5:1.
27. Wild D, Grove A, Martin M, et al. Principles of good practice for the translation and cultural adaptation process for patient-reported outcomes (PRO) measures: report of the ISPOR Task Force for Translation and Cultural Adaptation. *Value in Health.* 2005;8(2):94-104.
28. Altman DG, Bland JM. Diagnostic tests. 1: sensitivity and specificity. *BMJ.* 1994;308(6943):1552.
29. Redelmeier DA, Guyatt GH, Goldstein RS. Assessing the minimal important difference in symptoms: a comparison of two techniques. *J Clin Epidemiol.* 1996;49(11):1215-1219.
30. Jaeschke R, Singer J, Guyatt GH. Measurement of health status: ascertaining the minimal clinically important difference. *Controlled Clinical Trials.* 1989;10(4):407-415.

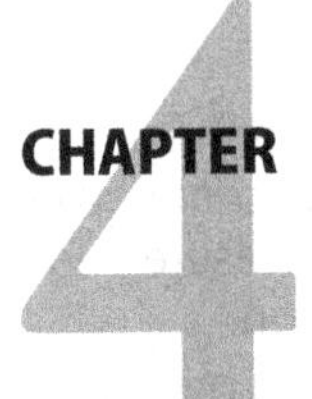

CHAPTER

Guiding Therapist Decisions for Measuring Outcomes in Occupational Therapy

Mary Law, PhD, FCAOT and Joy MacDermid, BScPT, PhD

The process of deciding how to measure occupational performance is challenging to occupational therapists for several reasons. First, while it is common for therapists in their educational programs to learn to administer many different assessments, it is less common for assessment to be learned as part of an overall measurement approach. Placing the use of assessments within a person, occupation, and environment measurement framework helps to organize our thinking about how we use measurement in practice. Second, therapists often have difficulty deciding what specific attribute(s) to measure. For example, a client has identified that he or she wants to be able to go shopping. What are the occupational performance attributes that are important to the occupation of shopping but are causing him or her difficulty—is it moving around a store, managing money, or selecting the groceries? Is the problem in performance related to where he or she will shop? The area of performance difficulty leads to a decision about the attribute to focus on for measurement. Finally, once a decision has been made about the attribute(s) to measure, what specific assessment tool is the best to use? Considerations of ease of use, time, psychometric characteristics, and cost are central to this decision.

This chapter presents a decision-making process that occupational therapists can use to guide the process of the measurement of occupational performance. We outline the decision-making process, list key questions to ask at each stage of the measurement process, and discuss important issues to consider as part of this process. Reflective questions for therapists to consider are listed for each stage of the measurement process. Although this decision-making process may seem long initially, we have purposefully described it in detail to enable student occupational therapists to learn the measurement process in a step-by-step fashion. As therapists become more skilled in measurement, they will find that the process flows smoothly from the identification of occupational performance issues to further assessment to intervention and outcome measurement.

Outcome measures selected for client evaluation and decisions should be valid and reliable and able to measure the impacts of the rehabilitation interventions provided to patients. Desirable qualities of these measures include the following:

- Easy for the practitioner to access/apply, and provide minimal inconvenience or discomfort for the clients
- Relevant and applicable across different contexts (clinical conditions/severity, language/literacy, cultures, environments)
- Have clearly defined standardized procedures to allow consistent application and interpretation
- Have the ability to assist with diagnosis/classification, goal-setting, prognosis, treatment planning, discharge planning, and/or measurement of treatment effectiveness for individual clients
- Reflect domains of client's health that may be affected by rehabilitation
- Provide a consistent numeric metric that can accurately quantify treatment effects associated with different interventions
- Have sufficient comparative data to others with similar conditions
- Have strong consistent measurement properties across different client populations and contexts.

Any single outcome measure is unlikely to fulfill all measurement purposes because the measurement

Law M, Baum C, Dunn W, eds. *Measuring Occupational Performance: Supporting Best Practice in Occupational Therapy, Third Edition (pp 43-56).*

properties that optimize different measurement purposes may compete against each other. Fortunately, a spectrum of outcome measures are available that evaluate relevant aspects of occupational therapy practice. While the evidence is incomplete on most measures with respect to all of the criteria listed previously, we have a strong tradition of evaluating clinical measurement as one of its foundational scientific principles. Thus, there is a substantial but imperfect body of evidence to form how we evaluate the outcomes of our interventions. Clinicians should be able to understand the properties of different outcome measures and apply an evidence-based approach to selecting and interpreting the scores obtained from an outcome evaluation process. When evaluating the impact of a clinical decision, it is important to match the evaluation indicator to the type of decision that was made and to the focus of intervention.

Basic Purposes of Clinical Measurement

Clinical measurement can serve 4 different purposes:

1. Identify strengths, limitations, barriers, or facilitators that can inform the intervention (decision making)
2. Evaluate change over time (treatment effectiveness, maturation, and decline in status)
3. Discriminate between or amongst different groups (diagnosis or classification)
4. Predict future status (diagnosis or outcome)

A measure is labeled an *outcome measure* if it is used to evaluate change following interventions (treatment effectiveness). This type of use for a measure is the most common clinical purpose of measurement. Outcome measures can help us determine whether a change occurs in an aspect of functioning and/or health following rehabilitative intervention. Evaluation over time also may be used to measure maturation effects, as is sometimes required in pediatrics, or decline, which can be measured as an indication of the functional implications of aging or disease. The form of validity that is most relevant to this function is responsiveness—the ability of a measure to detect change over time.

The second most common purpose for using a measure of client status is to discriminate between subgroups. Discrimination can result in classification into clinically meaningful diagnostic or classification subgroups. Classification can also separate different clinical subgroups to establish their treatment needs or functional capability. For example, it has been shown that a classification system is useful to divide patients with low back pain into different clinical subgroups that require different treatment approaches.[1] Others have developed a staging system for functional independence across the activities of daily living (ADL), mobility, and executive-function domains (ASME) using the Functional Independence Measure (FIM) in a manner consistent with the ICF model as a method for "assessment and goal setting in terms that are meaningful to patients and their care givers."[2(p 29)] Discriminative (known groups) validity is the most related measurement property for this type of clinical tool application.

Lastly, measures are sometimes used to predict a patient's future status. For example, the Movement Assessment of Infants (MAI), a neuromotor assessment tool, has been used to predict which infants will be diagnosed with cerebral palsy at a future follow-up.[3] The FIM has been used to predict discharge status for stroke patients, correctly predicting outcome in 70% of cases.[4] Predictive validity is the most related measurement property for this type of clinical tool application.

Aren't Outcome Measures Just for Research?

Evaluation of outcomes is distinct from clinical research. In fact, it is important that clinicians not think that measuring outcomes is performed for research purposes, but rather to choose standardized measures that are primarily used for decision making on individual patients. However, "practice-based evidence" can be an important driver of evidence-based practice. Evidence derived from practice can identify priority areas for research where outcomes are suboptimal, or identify practice variations that suggest that optimization of care might be improved. Further, with the increasing acknowledgment of the importance of effectiveness research, the importance of observational research documenting the clinical outcomes achieved in practice increasingly is being valued.[5]

Measuring Occupational Performance Outcomes for a Person and/or His or Her Family

I. Identification of Occupational Performance Issues by the Person

The first stage in the measurement process requires an occupational therapist to identify the client's perspectives about the reasons for referral to occupational therapy and the issues to be addressed during occupational therapy intervention. The goal is for the therapist to learn about the client, his or her occupations, and any difficulties he or she is having in performing the occupations that he or she needs to, wants to, or is expected to do.[6]

How is this identification of occupational performance issues accomplished? Because it is the person's perspective and experiences that are most important, this information is best gained through an interview, narrative, or other self-report method with the person receiving occupational therapy services. Several methods used to enable a person to identify occupational performance issues are discussed in detail in Chapter 7. If the person is unable to participate in the identification of occupational performance issues, it is necessary to find an alternative source of information. This could be a family member, friend, or caregiver (see Stage II of this measurement process).

Therapists need to ensure that there is time and a suitable place for such assessment. For example, it is very difficult for a person to identify occupational performance issues quickly in a rushed outpatient clinic. In such a situation, finding a quieter room and more time will facilitate a more positive experience and lead to a more valid identification of issues.

The primary purpose of this stage of the measurement process is to identify occupational performance issues that will be the focus of intervention. This stage serves as a screening process. If the person is competent to respond and does not identify any occupations that he or she needs to do and is having difficulty in performing, then occupational therapy services are not required. It may be that occupational therapy services will be required at a later time, or they are not necessary at all. If there are occupational performance issues identified, then this stage of the process serves to describe the status of the person's performance from his or her perspective. Using this information, the therapist can begin to make hypotheses about the reasons for performance difficulties. Decisions about further assessment of specific performance areas, components, and environmental conditions flow directly from these hypotheses.

Some of the reflective questions at this stage of the process center on the clinical usefulness, reliability and validity, and applicability of the assessment to specific populations. These topics have already been discussed in some detail in Chapter 2, and specific methods to critically review measurement tools regarding these properties are described later in this chapter. However, it is important for therapists to consider the clinical utility and psychometric properties of a quantitative measure at every stage of the measurement process. If a measure has not been shown to provide consistent (reliable) and accurate (valid) information, its use in identification of occupational performance issues is not warranted. It is often tempting for a therapist to use a home-grown checklist or make a few changes to a published measure before using it. Checklists and adapted measures are not reliable or valid unless extensively tested, so a therapist using them will never be certain if the information that he or she obtains is accurate. Likewise, there are specific methods to ensure that qualitative assessments are consistent and dependable (see Chapter 6).

II. Identification of Occupational Performance Issues for This Person by Another Individual or Group

Because family and friends are so often central to the occupational therapy service plan, they will be included in this stage of the process. In fact, in instances such as young children or persons with significant cognitive impairments, family or friends are the primary source of information about a person's occupational performance. In other situations, another service provider may be the source of issue identification. For example, a service provider in a skilled nursing facility may indicate a need for assistance with feeding a resident or transferring him or her from a wheelchair to a toilet. In Chapter 7, methods to assess occupational performance from the perspective of others are described in detail.

III. Further Assessment of Specific Occupational Performance Areas

Once the person, family, or others have identified the occupational performance issues that will be the focus of occupational therapy intervention, further assessment of these specific performance attributes is often required. For example, a 26-year-old woman recovering from a brain injury resulting from a motor vehicle accident wants to be able to look after her apartment, cook meals, do laundry, shop for groceries and household items, and get around her community. Using an assessment of instrumental ADL (IADL), the therapist assesses actual performance in these activities. This assessment provides specific information about the woman's initial level of performance so that intervention can focus on appropriate tasks and provide a comparison for future assessments of progress during therapy. The information from such an assessment also contributes to the clinical reasoning process about why performance difficulties are occurring.

IV. Assessment of Environmental Conditions and Performance Components

Using information from the referral for occupational therapy services, the person's (or other's) identification of occupational performance issues, and further assessment of occupational performance attributes, the therapist forms a hypothesis about the reasons for the difficulties in occupational performance. To confirm this hypothesis, assessment of specific performance components and/or environmental conditions that are barriers to performance is often required. For example, information about strength and range of motion of a worker with a hand injury is important in planning intervention. If the parents of a 3-year-old girl with spina bifida want their daughter to be able to play on an outdoor playground in her neighborhood, information about the physical accessibility of the playground is necessary before planning intervention.

The purpose of assessment of performance components and environmental conditions is to provide information about the reasons for performance difficulty and help to identify the focus of intervention. The most important consideration is how further information will contribute to knowledge about the person and help determine the focus of therapy intervention. Is the time taken for these assessments worth the benefit gained from increased knowledge? Let's consider the young girl and the outdoor playground. If a physical accessibility assessment indicates that the playground is fully accessible, then the focus of intervention would be on ensuring that the girl had sufficient outdoor mobility to use the playground. However, if the playground is not accessible, then the most beneficial focus of intervention will be on changing the playground environment to increase accessibility for all children with disabilities.

V. Selection of Outcome Measures

One of the most challenging decisions in measurement is deciding what specific assessment tool(s) to use for the evaluation of occupational performance. Issues of theoretical compatibility, specific purpose for measurement, clinical utility, reliability, and validity are important to consider.

First, let's consider where you might look to find an appropriate outcome measure for use in a specific clinical situation. Potential sources of information include textbooks (including this text), published test critiques, journals, and published reviews of measures in the occupational therapy field (see References for more information about these sources).

Occupational therapists use theory and models of practice to guide their clinical practice. In Chapter 1, we described several theoretical approaches to occupational therapy practice that use a person-environment-occupation perspective as the way of understanding occupational performance and planning occupational therapy services. Using one of these approaches leads to the use of assessments that measure a person's occupational performance in the context of his or her everyday life. In selecting assessment tools to use, a therapist will want to ensure that the assessment measures occupational performance from this broad perspective so that the assessment fits with his or her approach to practice.

In current health care practice, therapists have a limited amount of time for measurement. It is important to use assessments that provide useful information in the shortest time frame possible. One also must consider whether doing an assessment initially will save or increase time later on in the occupational therapy intervention process. For example, the identification of specific occupational performance issues by the client may take longer initially but can lead to more focused further assessment and intervention, thus saving time in the long run. Other issues of clinical utility to consider include the availability and cost of an assessment manual; training required to learn the assessment, and ease of administration, scoring, and interpretation. Clinical utility is often overlooked by developers of measures, but it is one of the most significant influences on actual use of an outcome measure in a clinical situation.

Finally, it is important to review the reliability and validity of a measure. It is here that the purpose for using a particular outcome measure will guide decisions about which measure is best. Do you want the assessment to describe the current status of a person, to predict his or her performance in the future, or to assess change in performance over time? If you wish to describe a person's current status, you will want evidence that the measure is reliable between observers and can discriminate between persons who do or do not have performance difficulties. For prediction of performance in the future, a measure should have reliability between observers and over time, and evidence that it can accurately predict future performance. In the increasingly important area of evaluation of change over time, a measure needs to have reliability between observers and over time, as well as evidence that it is sensitive to and will pick up actual changes in performance over time.[7] Use of the measurement review form in Appendix B will aid therapists in evaluating the clinical utility, reliability, and validity of an outcome measure.

VI. Carry Out the Assessment

The next stage in the measurement process is the actual use of the assessment. Whether that assessment is used for initial identification of occupational performance issues or further assessment of components or environmental conditions, there are several important factors to consider.

Research on assessment practices indicates that the environmental location or context of the assessment has a significant influence on the validity of the findings.[8] Performance of specific activities is dependent on the context, so an assessment is best if carried out where the activity will be done most often by that person. With an increased emphasis on community-based interventions and concerns about the lack of generalization of acquired skills, it is most appropriate to measure outcomes in home and community environments. When this is not possible, the therapist must remember that the observed performance accurately reflects function only in the testing environment.

As we have learned earlier, it is important for outcome measures to have evidence of consistency or reliability. However, information that a measure has excellent reliability does not mean that you, as the therapist using the measure, will be able to administer it in a reliable manner. To ensure consistency in your measurement practices, take the time to learn and practice each new assessment tool that you begin using. Work with your colleagues to train each other. Test consistency (reliability) between therapists by both administering an assessment with the same client(s) and comparing the agreement between your scores. To test consistency with yourself for assessments involving scoring of performance, one suggested method is to videotape clients performing the assessment, score these tapes a few weeks apart, and compare the agreement between scores. The limitation of this method is that scoring an assessment on a videotape is not the same context as scoring with a person right there with you. However, if you score the assessment at the same pace, the use of videotapes can tell you about your consistency while minimizing the measurement burden for the client.

VII. Interpret Measurement Results

Interpreting and communicating the results of a measurement to your client and others is the last step in the measurement process. Each time an assessment is completed, a therapist spends time making sense of the information and how it informs the therapy process. Do the results of the assessment indicate that the person is having difficulty performing certain tasks? Are there specific performance components (eg, organizing, planning) that are barriers to performance? This information is discussed with the client, the family, and others such as the rehabilitation team. Decisions are made about what therapy should be provided, or if it has already been provided, whether it was successful.

Using the Decision-Making Process for a Person

Let's use an example to consider how this decision-making process is implemented in occupational therapy practice. Mrs. Talbot recently had a stroke, affecting the left side of her body. She was in the hospital for 10 days and is now returning home. Although she is able to move around her house using a cane and can dress and feed herself, she and her family are concerned about her ability to look after herself on a day-to-day basis.

I. Identification of Occupational Performance Issues by the Person

The occupational therapist uses the Canadian Occupational Performance Measure (COPM)[6] to enable Mrs. Talbot to identify the occupational performance issues most important to her as she returned home. Through this assessment, she identifies making meals, housework, taking the bus to the grocery store, grocery shopping, and working in her garden as the 5 most important issues to her. Doing the COPM with Mrs. Talbot took about 45 minutes. By the end of that time, both the therapist and Mrs. Talbot knew the focus of occupational therapy intervention.

II. Identification of Occupational Performance Issues for This Person by Another Individual or Group

The occupational therapist, with Mrs. Talbot's permission, contacts her son and daughter-in-law after the first visit in order to ask them about their concerns for their mother. In this instance, the concerns of the son are very similar to those of Mrs. Talbot.

III. Further Assessment of Specific Occupational Performance Areas

Initially, Mrs. Talbot wants to focus on household activities. The therapist uses the Performance Assessment of Self-Care Skills (PASS)[9] to assess her performance in the activities of meal preparation, finances, use of the telephone, shopping, and housekeeping. The results of this assessment indicate that performance is decreased in the areas of meal preparation and shopping.

IV. Assessment of Environmental Conditions and Performance Components

Mrs. Talbot indicates that making meals is the first task on which she wants to focus in occupational therapy intervention. Using the Kitchen Task Assessment (KTA),[10] the occupational therapist assesses Mrs. Talbot's cognitive abilities to plan and carry out a cooking task. Through observation during this assessment, the therapist is also able to identify any limitations in performance caused by movement difficulties. The results of this assessment indicate that Mrs. Talbot can plan and organize a cooking task without difficulty. She does, however, have problems in carrying out tasks requiring the use of both hands together. It is also difficult for her to move around the kitchen to obtain cooking utensils. Using this information, the therapist and Mrs. Talbot develop an intervention plan that includes making changes to the organization of her kitchen and the use of some adaptive strategies for 2-handed activities.

V. Selection of Outcome Measures

As we have seen in Stages II, III, and IV of this example, the occupational therapist chooses specific assessment tools to use with Mrs. Talbot. The decision to use the specific assessments is based on the therapist's theoretical model of practice and her knowledge of the psychometric properties of different assessments. This occupational therapist uses a client-centered approach to occupational therapy assessment and intervention. The use of the COPM fits with this perspective because it enables a client to identify the occupational performance issues that are most important to him or her at a particular time. The therapist, through reading the COPM manual, knows that the COPM has good to excellent test-retest reliability and excellent validity in detecting change over time.

This therapist uses a person-environment-occupation approach to practice that focuses on the assessment of client-identified tasks within his or her own environment. Both PASS and KTA assessments enabled the therapist and Mrs. Talbot to determine the reasons for difficulties in performance. For example, in meal preparation, the primary difficulties relate to the environmental layout of her kitchen and performance of 2-handed activities.

VI. Carry Out the Assessment

In this example, performing the assessments in a contextually appropriate location is easy because Mrs. Talbot is seen in her home. Prior to using the assessments cited in this example, the occupational therapist has ensured that she received appropriate training in assessment administration. In the case of the COPM, she worked with a colleague and used the COPM training video to learn how to do the measure. For the other assessments, she and her colleagues practiced together before using them with a client.

VII. Interpret Measurement Results

After each assessment is completed, the therapist shows Mrs. Talbot the results, carefully pointing out areas of performance that are accomplished without difficulty and areas in which performance is decreased. A short report on the results of each assessment is given to Mrs. Talbot, along with a copy for her son and the home-therapy program. When the therapist and Mrs. Talbot feel that intervention directed toward improving meal preparation is completed, the COPM is used for Mrs. Talbot to rate change in performance. Again, these results are shared with Mrs. Talbot, her son, and other members of the home-therapy team.

The fundamental questions posed are as follows:

1. What does the score on this outcome measure tell me about the client's status?
2. What is the error associated with the measured value?
3. How much will the score need to change on subsequent assessments so I can be confident that a real change has occurred?
4. How much will the score need to change on a subsequent assessment so I can be confident that an important amount of change has occurred?
5. What is my long-term treatment goal and how does it relate to a score on its outcome measure?

To be confident that a measured value is useful in clinical decision making, we must have some idea of the consistency of the score. In other words, we need to know the amount of error associated with the score that we achieve when we assess our patients. The standard error of mean (SEM) can be used to describe the error associated with a reported value expressed in the original units of the measure. The SEM is related to the variability of the underlying population and the reliability of the scores on that particular outcome measure in a similar group. Although there are several methods for calculating the SEM, the most popular method is as follows:

$$\text{SEM} = (\text{sample standard deviation}) \sqrt{1 - \text{reliability coefficient}}$$

Although a measure has been shown to have high reliability coefficients across a broad number of conditions, the standard deviation can be expected to vary between different conditions and even within conditions over time as the level of disability changes. Thus, SEM is an estimate. When faced with a lack of data indicating the SEM is appropriate to our client's condition and level of disability, we can extrapolate from data that most closely approximates our patient. When one is interested in estimating the error associated with a score at a single point in time, internal consistency coefficients are used to indicate stability.

Once you determine the SEM, you must decide on the level of precision or your estimate. One SEM is associated with a 68% confidence interval (for a description of the sampling distribution and z-values, see any standard statistical text). To obtain higher confidence levels, the SEM can be multiplied by z-values associated with different confidence levels. For example, 1.65 is the z-value associated with the 90% confidence level and 1.96 is the z-value associated with the 95% confidence level. By multiplying the SEM for the measures taken by this level of confidence (z-value), you can establish a range within which a patient's true score is likely to lie, at the specified confidence level. Traditionally, research studies often use a 95% confidence. However, in clinical practice, we are often happy with a 90% level for estimation because this is "high confidence" but not so rigorous that we would establish very wide confidence intervals that would be practical to achieve in clinical practice.

For example, a SEM (for one point in time) of 4.4 points has been reported for an outcome measure. Multiplying the SEM of 4.4 points by the z-value of 1.65 provides a 90% confidence level, yields a value of 7.3 points. The interpretation is that at the time of assessment, there is a 90% chance that a client's true score is within 7.3 points of the measured score.

Measurement of the Decision-Making Process: Evaluation of Outcomes for a Program

When developing a measurement approach to evaluate the outcomes of an occupational therapy intervention program, there are additional issues to consider. Programs usually include groups of clinical activities that are delivered in a package to a specific group of clients. For example, a day program for seniors with dementia often includes a variety of activities designed to engage group members in occupation and thus maintain everyday functioning. In evaluating outcomes for the program, the primary interest is in information about the average amount of change in clients who participate in the program. The outcomes that are measured relate to the specific goals of the program, rather than to the specific goals of each client.

I. Identification of Occupational Performance Goals for the Program

The first stage in the measurement process for evaluation of a program requires those who are running the program to identify the long-term occupational performance goals of the program. Designing an evaluation strategy for a program takes time and is best started by a review of the mission of the organization and the goals of the program.[11] Reviewing the mission of the organization that is delivering the program provides a direction for the types of outcomes that will be measured. For example, if the mission of the program is to facilitate community integration, the outcomes that will be measured for program evaluation will focus on attributes that reflect integration into the community. It is important at this stage to describe who delivers the program and which clients receive the program. It is also important to ensure that people in the program are delivering services in a consistent manner. All of this information will help you to decide the feasibility of evaluating the program. The resources (both time and people) that are required to evaluate a program are often overlooked in the enthusiasm to get started. It is important to include all stakeholders, both service providers and clients, in the process of developing an evaluation of a program. Without this inclusion, implementation of changes based on the evaluation results will be more difficult.

Following a review of the mission and the structure of the program, the long-term occupational performance goals and attributes to be measured are specified. For example, a program to provide therapy services to children with disabilities in schools has a long-term goal of improving the children's function within the school environment. The specific attributes to be measured in this situation include functional mobility, handwriting, and socialization. Once the specific attributes have been selected, the most appropriate respondents for the assessment are identified. For example, in a school therapy program, do you want to measure outcomes from the perspective of teachers, therapists, parents, or the children themselves (if old enough)? Outcomes assessments from the perspective of teachers or therapists is often completed, while the perspective of parents or children receiving those services is not gathered as often.

II. Selection of Assessment Tool(s) to Use

In selecting appropriate assessment tools for the evaluation of programs, many of the issues to consider are the same as a measurement process for individuals. Issues of theoretical compatibility, the specific purpose of the assessment, clinical utility, reliability, and validity all influence the selection of the assessment to use. Please refer back to Stage V of the individual decision-making process for a discussion of these issues. The use of standardized assessment tools that have previously been used in the evaluation of programs is recommended. Using individualized tools such as goal attainment scaling is more difficult in evaluating programs because aggregation of individualized data is difficult to interpret.

III. Carry Out the Assessment

The goal for measurement in the evaluation of a program is to do outcome assessment in the context (place) that will most accurately reflect a person's performance. In evaluating the outcomes of a school therapy program, the most appropriate context in which to do the evaluation is in the school itself. On the other hand, for a program focused on community reintegration, evaluation is best done out in the community rather than in the location of the program.

If more than one person is administering assessments in evaluating a program, it is important to ensure a satisfactory level of agreement between evaluators. At a minimum, agreement between evaluators on at least 5 assessments should be over 75%. For large evaluations, reliability statistics for evaluators should be calculated.

Before beginning the evaluation, a data collection process is developed. A data collection form can be developed to capture the relevant information for the evaluation of the program. This process works best if it is simple, accessible, and short.

IV. Interpret Measurement Results

Once the assessment information for a program evaluation is collected, the next step is analysis and interpretation of the data. Decisions to be made at this stage include how the data will be aggregated and analyzed. Often, program evaluations simply calculate average change for each client and for the group. These results can be displayed in charts or graphs so that they are easily interpreted. If further statistical analysis is desired, one may need to seek out other resources, such as a statistician to help with that analysis.

It is essential to communicate the results of your outcome measurement to the program clients and other stakeholders (eg, managers, funders). They will want to know if, overall, there are positive changes in the attributes that are measured. Are the results of the evaluation consistent with the goals of the program? Finally, you and others involved in the evaluation can address how the program should be changed based on the evaluation results. It is at this point that you need to be creative and look at options for change supported by the data that are gathered. Any decisions about change are communicated to the clients, families, service providers, and others involved with the program. For the results of a program evaluation to have impact, it is important to use the information that is collected to improve the effectiveness of the program.

Using the Decision-Making Process for a Program

How would the decision-making process for outcome measurement with programs be implemented in a sample occupational therapy program? Consider the school-based therapy program discussed earlier. You work in a program providing occupational therapy services to children ages 5 to 12 years in the school system. The overall mission of this program is to maintain and enhance functioning of the children within the school. The program is delivered by 3 therapists within a school district.

I. Identification of Occupational Performance Goals for the Program

The goals for the program are improved functioning in the school setting, as indicated by changes in ability to move around the school, do classroom activities, and socialize with other children and school staff.

II. Selection of Assessment Tool(s) to Use

Based on a review of the measurement literature, you determine that the School Function Assessment (SFA)[12] is the most appropriate measure to use to evaluate your program. The SFA is a relatively new measure that focuses on children's abilities in a school setting and has been well supported in terms of reliability and validity.

III. Carry Out the Assessment

All of the therapists in the program attend a course focused on using the SFA. You then train with each other and together administer the assessment to a few children. This enables you to compare results and ensure that all of you are administering and scoring the assessment in a consistent manner. During the course of 1 year of the program, the SFA is administered to each child in the program before he or she begins occupational therapy and after therapy is finished. By the end of 1 year, you have results from 85 children.

IV. Interpret Measurement Results

The data from the SFA, as well as demographic information such as age, referral problem, and diagnosis, is recorded on a data collection form. Using a computer spreadsheet, you calculate the average scores of the group of children before and after therapy, enabling you to determine the average change in scores on the SFA. These change scores are graphed according to age and referral problem to determine whether there are differences in outcomes according to these factors. If you wish to do further analysis, you will contact someone who is more knowledgeable about statistics. The written results from this evaluation are shared with the families, the schools, and the school administrators.

How to Use Outcomes Measures to Help Make Clinical Decisions on Programs

Many clinicians can see the benefit of using outcome measures on individual clients, but are unsure of how to use them to evaluate their clinic outcomes. Outcomes research, program evaluation, and bench-marking share some commonality in that large pools of observational data on outcomes are used to make decisions about services or programs. Some areas such as inpatient rehabilitation have moved toward use of standard measures that are collected in many centers to facilitate these comparisons (eg, the FIM). There is increasing pressure from payers to demonstrate outcomes, making it essential that clinicians be prepared to show that meaningful outcomes were achieved for patients and those outcomes compare favorably to those reported when alternative health care providers or interventions are selected. For those without access to established databases or software, clinic databases can be established using routine office software.

With the move toward outcomes databases, it will be important to keep in mind the limitations of observational data. Outcome studies, or effectiveness research, often depend on observational data (not randomized studies). Observational data, no matter how meticulously gathered, is at risk of bias. That means it is always possible that considerations other than the treatment are responsible for the observations in outcomes. Differences between groups may exist because of treatment. However, alternative sources of difference might be driving the observed differences. The reasons or pathway taken for individuals to end up in a certain subgroup may be the real factor(s) that determines the outcomes achieved. These factors are usually called *biases* because they contaminate the ability to ascribe differences between groups to the (treatment) factor. Differences between and amongst groups drawn from an outcome database may be due to variation in the distribution of these "risk factors." Common factors that might vary between subgroups include age (and associated differences in comorbidity and physical demands), sex/gender, severity of the disorder, variations in comorbidity/physical health, occupational demands, access to timely services, and socioeconomic, geographical, or environmental factors. When comparisons are made across different health care systems, this can create another source of potential covariation, thus limiting the ability to define a causal relationship between outcomes achieved and interventions provided.

Searching for Outcome Measures

One of the first steps in using outcome measures is selecting the appropriate measure. Many of the strategies that have been devised for refining search strategies do not apply very well to outcome measures. Finding studies of outcome measures does not necessarily lead to finding the measure itself. Many outcome measures may be mentioned in treatment studies or psychometric studies, but it is less common for the instruments themselves to be readily accessible.

The overall process of selecting an outcome measure for practice is to do the following:

1. Identify the conceptual framework and/or concepts that are important to measure (achieve alignment between your conceptual framework, your client's issues, and your measurement purpose).
2. Search scientific articles on outcome measures, articles addressing treatment effectiveness in a similar patient population, and textbook and online outcome measure resources to identify a potential list of outcome measures/instruments.
3. Remove any outcome measures that are not standardized, clearly not suited to your purpose or situation, or that have been shown to be unreliable or invalid for your purpose.
4. Critically appraise your potential outcome scale(s) using a standardized process or instrument, or evaluate fundamental measurement principles.
5. Determine whether the instrument can evaluate change, discriminate, or predict in the manner required for your population and purpose.
6. Obtain the measures of interest, and determine the scoring mechanism and any specific instructions on administration (including whether valid translations are available).
7. Identify copyright or reimbursement issues, and ensure compliance.
8. Devise and document a strategy regarding what procedures will be followed in implementing outcome measures into practice (when they will be applied, who will provide them, how/when they will be scored, where the data will be retained, how the data will be used). Ensure that all parties involved participate in devising the implementation strategy and understand their roles.
9. Pilot test 1 or 2 instruments for a specified period and re-evaluate the instrument's performance, feasibility, and implementation process.
10. Finalize your choice and a set time frame to review outcomes data.

A number of practical issues must be considered when attempting to incorporate new measures into practice. Expect and prepare for a learning curve. Lack of adequate preparation will inevitably lead to frustration and an inability to use outcome measure scores in clinical decision making. Strategies for success include making the instruments readily available for use when needed, engaging clinicians throughout the process of adopting and implementing the measure, identifying the benefits to the clinic/clinician and client for measurement, providing the measures to clients in a standardized way that fits with clinic flow, and having a strategy to ensure that forms are completely and accurately completed by all respondents. Certain payers or regulatory bodies may have predetermined outcomes measures to be used within the context of care to their enrollees. If you choose to veer from that, document what is needed so the person who will approve rehabilitation has a clear understanding of your choice and rationale for a selected client.

Developers of outcome measures have intellectual property rights with respect to their instruments, so it is important that these be respected. Many developers do not charge for the use of their instruments. In this case, it is advisable to contact the developer to request permission to use their instrument and inquire whether there is any documentation regarding proper administration or interpretation. In some cases, outcome measures and/or their supporting documentation must be purchased. Usually, this is a one-time cost, but in some cases, there can be ongoing charges for a license, for the measure forms, and/or for scoring. These practical issues may determine which measures are feasible in your practice. Some companies have developed platforms for administering, scoring, and providing interpretation of outcome measures in a computer-based format. Ongoing license fees for software and for reports are common in this case.

The Critical Review of Measures

Occupational therapists, in selecting measures to use in their practice, want to use the best available measures in their practice. To ensure this, it is important to determine the clinical utility, standardization, reliability, and validity of potential measures. How can therapists find out information about measures? The most obvious choice is to find a critical review of a measure. Sources of these types of reviews include textbooks[13,14] or measurement review books.[15,16] The Internet is also a source of information about measures. An example is the Educational Resource Information Clearinghouse (ERIC), which has published reviews on the Internet. Finally, there is educational software (available on CD-ROM) that provides critical reviews of outcome measures used in rehabilitation.[17]

There is always a chance that a critical review of a measure is not available. It is important, therefore, that students and therapists develop an understanding of the process of reviewing a measurement tool. To aid in this process, we have provided rating forms for this purpose that have been developed and tested over the past 15 years. The rating forms and accompanying guidelines were used in the review of all measures described in this book and can be used by students and therapists to review measures for their practice. See Appendix E for Outcome Measures Rating Forms and Guidelines.

Table 4-1

Measuring Occupational Performance Outcomes: Stage I

Stage in the Measurement Process	*Key Questions*
Identification of occupational performance issues by the person	• How will I enable the person to identify the occupational performance issues that are the reasons for seeking occupational therapy services? • Is the client able to complete this assessment? If not, who has the best information about these issues? (see Table 3-2) • What assessment method will I use? • Where will I do the assessment? • Why am I evaluating occupational performance—to screen; to identify that there are occupational performance issues; to describe the person's status in performing occupations that they need to, want to, or are expected to do? • Is the assessment method reliable and valid? • Is the assessment method clinically useful? • Is the assessment method valid for client(s) with this type of problem? • How will the results of this assessment of occupational performance issues guide decisions about further assessment and occupational therapy intervention?

Table 4-2

Measuring Occupational Performance Outcomes: Stage II

Stage in the Measurement Process	*Key Questions*
Identification of occupational performance issues for this person by another individual or group	• Why has another person or group identified potential occupational performance issues? • Have I discussed this issue with the person and their family? • What assessment method will I use? • Why am I evaluating occupational performance to screen for issues or to describe occupational performance status? • Is the assessment method reliable and valid? • Is the assessment method clinically useful? • Is the assessment method valid for use with client(s) with this type of problem? • How will the results of this assessment of occupational performance issues guide decisions about occupational therapy assessment and intervention?

Table 4-3

Measuring Occupational Performance Outcomes: Stage III

Stage in the Measurement Process	*Key Questions*
Further assessment of specific occupational performance areas	• What specific occupational performance attribute(s) will I assess? • What assessment method will I use—individualized or standardized; quantitative or qualitative? • Who will complete the assessment? • Where will the assessment occur? • What is the age of the person? • Is the assessment method reliable and valid? • Is the assessment method clinically useful? • How will I use the results of this assessment?

Table 4-4

Measuring Occupational Performance Outcomes: Stage IV

Stage in the Measurement Process	*Key Questions*
Assessment of environmental conditions and performance concepts	• What specific aspects of the environment and performance components are potential barriers to performance and need further assessment? • Who will complete the assessment? • Where will the assessment occur? • Is the assessment method reliable and valid? • Is the assessment clinically useful? • How will I use the results of this assessment to focus occupational therapy intervention?

Table 4-5

Measuring Occupational Performance Outcomes: Stage V

Stage in the Measurement Process	*Key Questions*
Selection of assessments to use	• Where do I look to find measures to use? • Does this assessment fit with my theoretical approach to occupational therapy? • What is the purpose of this assessment—to describe a person's status, to predict future performance, to evaluate change in performance over time?

(continued)

Table 4-5 (continued)

Measuring Occupational Performance Outcomes: Stage V

Stage in the Measurement Process	*Key Questions*
Selection of assessments to use	• What is the cost of the assessment? • How long does it take to administer? • How much training do I require before I can administer the assessment in a reliable manner? • Is there a manual available to guide the assessment? • How easy is it to administer the assessment, score it, and interpret the results? • Does the assessment have evidence of reliability—over time, between raters? • Does the assessment have evidence of validity—content, criterion, and construct? • If I am using the assessment to evaluate change over time, does it have evidence of responsiveness?

Table 4-6

Measuring Occupational Performance Outcomes: Stage VI

Stage in the Measurement Process	*Key Questions*
Carry out the assessment	• How do I ensure a contextually accurate assessment? • How do I ensure a reliable assessment?

Table 4-7

Measuring Occupational Performance Outcomes: Stage VII

Stage in the Measurement Process	*Key Questions*
Interpret measurement results	• How do I involve my client in assessment interpretation? • Am I trained to interpret the assessment results? • Do I need assistance in analyzing trends in assessment data? • Who will receive the assessment results? • What will occur based on the assessment results?

Table 4-8

Evaluation of Outcomes for a Program: Stage I

Stage in the Measurement Process	*Key Questions*
Identification of occupational performance goals for the program	• What are the overall goals/mission of your organization? • What are the long-term goals for the program (in occupational performance terms)? • Who is involved in delivering the program? • Who are the clients who receive the program? • What specific occupational performance attribute(s) do you want to assess? • Who will be the respondent(s) for the assessment? • Who has the best information about these issues? • How will the results of this assessment of occupational performance issues guide decisions about occupational therapy intervention?

Table 4-9

Evaluation of Outcomes for a Program: Stage II

Stage in the Measurement Process	*Key Questions*
Selection of assessments tool(s) to use	• Where do I look to find assessment tool(s) to use? • Does this assessment fit with the program's theoretical approach to occupational therapy? • Will this assessment fit with my purpose—to describe a person's status prior to entry into a program, or to evaluate change in performance over time? • What is the cost of the assessment? • How long does it take to administer? • How much training do I require before I can administer the assessment in a reliable manner? • Is there a manual available to guide the assessment? • How easy is it to administer the assessment, score it, and interpret the results? • Does the assessment have evidence of reliability—over time, between raters? • Does the assessment have evidence of validity—content, criterion, and construct? • If I am using the assessment to evaluate change over time, does it have evidence of responsiveness?

Table 4-10

Evaluation of Outcomes for a Program: Stage III

Stage in the Measurement Process	*Key Questions*
Carry out the assessment	• How do I ensure a contextually accurate assessment? • Have I shown that the evaluators can administer the assessment tool(s) in a consistent (reliable) manner? • Have I developed a process/forms for data collection?

Table 4-11

Evaluation of Outcomes for a Program: Stage IV

Stage in the Measurement Process	*Key Questions*
Interpret assessment results	• How will you be aggregating assessment results across clients? • Am I trained to interpret the assessment results? • Do you need assistance in analyzing trends in assessment data? • How do I involve my clients in assessment interpretation? • Who will receive the assessment results? • What will occur based on the assessment results?

References

1. Fritz JM, Delitto A, Erhard RE. Comparison of classification-based physical therapy with therapy based on clinical practice guidelines for patients with acute low back pain: a randomized clinical trial. *Spine.* 2003;28:1363-1371.
2. Stineman MG, Ross RN, Fiedler R, Granger CV, Maislin G. Functional independence staging: conceptual foundation, face validity, and empirical derivation. *Arch Phys Med Rehabil.* 2003;84:29-37.
3. Harris SR, Swanson MW, Andrews MS, et al. Predictive validity of the "Movement Assessment of Infants." *J Dev Behav Pediatr.* 1984;5:336-342.
4. Mauthe RW, Haaf DC, Hayn P, Krall JM. Predicting discharge destination of stroke patients using a mathematical model based on six items from the Functional Independence Measure. *Arch Phys Med Rehabil.* 1996;77:10-13.
5. Jette AM, Keysor JJ. Uses of evidence in disability outcomes and effectiveness research. *Milbank Q.* 2002;80:325-345.
6. Law M, Baptiste S, Carswell A, McColl M, Polatajko H, Pollock N. *Canadian Occupational Performance Measure.* 5th ed. Ottawa, Ontario: CAOT Publications; 2014.
7. Law M. Criteria for the evaluation of measurement instruments. *Can J Occup Ther.* 1987;54:121-127.
8. Park S, Fisher AG, Velozo CA. Using the Assessment of Motor and Process Skills to compare performance between home and clinical settings. *Am J Occup Ther.* 1993;48:519-525.
9. Rogers IC, Holm MB, Goldstein G, McCue M, Nussbaum PD. Stability and change in functional assessment of patients with geropsychiatric disorders. *Am J Occup Ther.* 1994;48:914-918.
10. Baum CM, Edwards D. Cognitive performance in senile dementia of the Alzheimer's type: the Kitchen Task Assessment. *Am J Occup Ther.* 1993;47(5):431-436.
11. Letts L, Law M, Pollock N, et al. *A Programme Evaluation Workbook for Occupational Therapists: An Evidence-based Practice Tool.* Ottawa, Ontario: CAOT Publications; 1999.
12. Coster W, Deeney T, Haltwanger I, Haley S. *The School Function Assessment.* San Antonio, TX: The Psychological Corporation; 1998.
13. Law M, Baum C, Dunn W. *Measuring Occupational Performance: Supporting Best Practice in Occupational Therapy.* Thorofare, NJ: SLACK Incorporated; 2000.
14. Van Deusen I, Brunt D. *Assessment in Occupational Therapy and Physical Therapy.* Orlando, FL: W.B. Saunders; 1998.
15. Impara JC, Plake BS. *The Thirteenth Mental Measurements Yearbook.* Lincoln, NE: University of Nebraska Press; 1998.
16. Murphy LL, Impara JC, Plake BS. *Tests in Print V. Buros Institute of Mental Measurements.* Lincoln, NE: University of Nebraska Press; 1999.
17. Law M, King G, MacKinnon E, Russell D, Murphy C, Hurley P. *All About Outcomes* (CD-ROM). Thorofare, NJ: SLACK Incorporated; 1999.

Mine the Gold

Occupational therapists must be aware of contributions from the physiology, psychology, neuroscience, child development, and aging literature as well as assessments from these disciplines. Information about the cognitive, motor, sensory, psychological, and language capacities of our clients can give the practitioner more confidence in occupational performance assessment findings and adds an important dimension to the development of a client- and family-centered plan.

Become Systematic

Systematic assessment of key person factors that may influence assessment results and occupational performance has the potential to yield valuable information to guide the evaluation and intervention planning process. If a person has an unrecognized visual, auditory, motor, psychological, cognitive, or language deficit, the validity of the occupational performance assessment will be threatened and the absence of such information may produce data that implies excess disabilities.

Use Evidence in Practice

As we strive to implement evidence-based practice in the context of client-centered care, use of standard tools and clinical observations to assess person factors plays an important role in clinical and research protocols. Insights into limitations impacting assessment results and occupational performance can be considered when planning and modifying interventions and shared during the client and family education process.

Make Occupational Therapy Contributions Explicit

Occupational therapists offer the unique perspective of assessing the impact of person and environment factors on occupational performance. Results of person factor assessments are utilized to design interventions that enable performance of valued activities and to guide remediation of limitations.

Engage in Occupation-Based, Client-Centered Practice

Assessment of vision, hearing, cognition, motor factors, language, and literacy can yield valuable information that will guide the evaluation and intervention planning process and help the client perform meaningful activities and enhance quality of life.

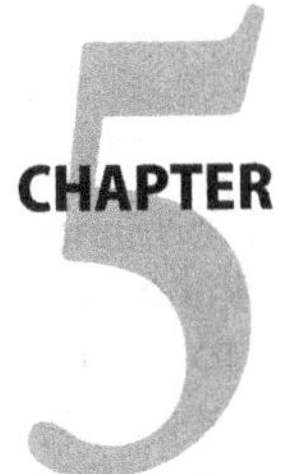

CHAPTER 5

Identifying Person Factors That Impact Occupational Performance Assessment

Monica S. Perlmutter, OTD, OTR/L, SCLV, FAOTA and Meredith P. Gronski, OTD, OTR/L

Throughout this text, the importance of the person's performance in daily life is emphasized as the central feature of occupational therapy evaluation. Occupational therapists are trained to identify factors that may limit the person's capacity to engage in his or her occupations by observing the person, the environment, and the task to determine what contributes to and what limits successful performance.

Occupational therapists must recognize the impact impairments may have on an individual's ability to fully participate in valued activities, as well as his or her performance during the evaluation process. For example, if a person has difficulty participating in an assessment, possible causes may include decreased visual acuity, hearing loss, motor performance, depression, memory loss, or low literacy. The validity of our occupational therapy evaluation may be threatened by such impairments that potentially interfere with the individual's ability to demonstrate his or her capacity.

Occupational therapists' knowledge of anatomy, neuroscience, and physiology prepares practitioners to assess and identify impairments that could create an excess disability (ie, an unnecessary disability) for clients and their families. This body of knowledge enables us to modify the evaluation approach to accommodate particular impairments; we just need to recognize what the potentially limiting factors might be. The occupational therapy evaluation process must include assessment and documentation of key person factors that may affect the individual's ability to participate in the occupational therapy evaluation and in daily occupations. Information about the cognitive, motor, sensory, psychological, and language capacities of our clients can give the practitioner more confidence in occupational performance assessment findings and adds an important dimension to the development of a client- and family-centered plan.

Key Concepts

- The overarching purpose of the occupational therapy evaluation process is to determine the client's level of occupational performance, goals, and priorities; and develop client centered intervention. To accomplish this, occupational therapists must consider person factors that may influence assessment performance.
- Clinical observations play a key role in providing clues about possible influence of person factors on assessment performance and, ultimately, occupational performance.
- The occupational therapy evaluation process is very fluid; occupational therapists utilize clinical reasoning skills continually to observe client behaviors that are indicative of intrinsic limitations. These observations may prompt need for follow up with a more thorough and targeted assessment.
- Targeted assessment of person factors that are suspect for influencing assessment and occupational performance can yield valuable information to guide the evaluation and intervention planning process.

Importance of Identifying Person Factors That May Influence Assessment Performance and Validity of Results

- Allows for more accurate interpretation of assessment results

Law M, Baum C, Dunn W, eds. *Measuring Occupational Performance: Supporting Best Practice in Occupational Therapy, Third Edition (pp 59-68).*

- Promotes intervention planning that better meets the needs of clients because assessment approach can be modified to accommodate for intrinsic/personal impairments
- Insights into impairments impacting assessment and occupational performance can be shared during the client and family education process
- Physicians and other health care team members can be apprised of findings and plan medical care accordingly
- Clients and families can be referred to other health care professionals and community resources to address concerns

Person Factors That May Limit Assessment Performance

As we strive to implement evidence-based practice in the context of client-centered care, standardized assessment tools play an important role in our clinical and research protocols, along with careful clinical observations. We must ask the questions: Can the client see the task, hear the directions, and read and retain the instructions? Is it possible that the client's performance could be influenced by depression or anxiety? Could the person's depression confound the planning process? Do strength, ROM, and endurance limitations limit the client's ability to participate in non-motor assessments? Does the client have aphasia, use a different language, or have low literacy and, if so, could this influence assessment performance? The occupational therapist must have access to this information prior to the evaluation process and implementation of client-centered intervention strategies. If a person has an unrecognized visual, auditory, motor, psychological cognitive or language deficit, or cannot read, the validity of the assessment will be threatened and the absence of such information may produce data that implies excess disabilities. In the following section, each of these potentially influential impairments will be considered in detail.

Determining the Impact of Cognition on Occupational Performance Assessment

The degree of cognitive capacity is central to the occupational nature of humans who go beyond survival needs in their pursuit of occupation.[1] Cognition encompasses many inter-related processes, both static and dynamic. Self-awareness, attention, planning, initiation, and inhibition of behaviors support an individual's ability to execute a plan, evaluate his or her task performance, and problem solve. Higher level executive function (EF) skills begin to develop in the preschool years, with functional gains optimizing during the ages of 15 and 19 years and again at 20 to 29 years of age. Declines in performance on EF tasks occur for 50- to 64-year-olds, providing support for the vulnerability of executive skills due to normal aging.[2] By the time people reach older adulthood, they have had significant neuronal loss in many areas of the brain.[3] Cognition in adulthood may also be limited by sensory deficits,[4] medication, trauma, chronic conditions, and neurologic episodes.[5,6] The ability to pursue activities that are meaningful to individuals across the lifespan, perform academically, participate in complex IADLs, and engage socially is supported, and sometimes limited, by cognitive capacity.

Meaningful, goal-directed activities rely on high-level cognitive processes.[7] For example, very young infants and toddlers use developing cognition to interact with their environment, develop social bonds with caregivers, and establish cause-and-effect-based routines. School-age children utilize developing EF skills to transition between activities or thoughts throughout the day. In addition, the ability to manage time, schedules, and assignments is driven by EF. Throughout adulthood and older adulthood, a high level of cognitive capacity is required in order to safely and independently perform IADLs, accurately perform essential job functions of paid work, and participate in leisure activities.

Implications of Decreased Cognitive Function on Occupational Therapy Assessment

Deficits in high-level cognitive functions may be suspected, but are not always apparent in everyday interactions with a client of any age, nor are they typically detected with global cognitive screening instruments. Thus, it is important for the occupational practitioner to be aware of this possibility and investigate through formal evaluation or by reviewing existing interdisciplinary reports, such as IQ and achievement reports in an educational setting. Therapists should recognize the potential influence of cognitive impairment on the evaluation process and take steps to ensure that assessment results are not confounded by cognitive deficits.

Often, therapists are directly testing specific aspects of cognition; however, at other times, the focus of the assessment is on task performance or movement. During these times, it is essential to be aware of the impact that cognition may be having on these other functions. For example, a child in school may have difficulty with producing written work on a line due to poor attention rather than motor control or visual processing. Further, an older adult with poor working memory may not complete a cooking task due to her inability to remember the steps. The practitioner can utilize strategies during the assessment process, such as testing in a quiet environment, taking frequent breaks, and modifying cueing strategies. Use of these strategies should be documented in the interpretation of the overall occupational performance assessment results.

Determining the Impact of Motor Performance on Occupational Performance Assessment

Movement arises from interactions among many body structures and systems, and the vast majority of occupational performance requires a motor response.[8] The development and performance of fundamental motor skills are considered the building blocks of more complex movements and occupational performance. The ability to perform basic and complex movement activities is supported by factors such as muscle tone, motor planning and control, and coordination. Changes and abnormalities in muscle tone may be related to an inefficiency of the neuromuscular system[9] and have the potential to limit an individual's ability to make accurate and controlled movements. Age-related neuromuscular impairments such as decreased muscle strength, reduced number of motor units, decreased speed of movement,[10] as well as stroke, arthritis affecting the knees, gait disturbances, and body sway are associated with postural changes and falls.[11]

Children must engage with their environment, interact with toys, and navigate a variety of terrains in order to learn and produce skilled motor responses for play, academic assignments, and social interaction during games and sports. Movement development progresses from primitive reflex patterns to voluntary, controlled movement.[12] Infants and young children rely on reflex patterns as their first method of environmental interaction, and these are essential to life. Children with delayed motor milestones will have subsequent delays in strength and coordination that may lead to difficulty utilizing school tools successfully later in childhood.[13] A lack of motor coordination often leads to the student fatiguing more easily, turning in messy work, and limiting his or her effort due to frustration.[14] Adults with motor impairments due to chronic conditions, such as multiple sclerosis, may have difficulty with endurance and balance during leisure and work activities.[15] In older adults, poor balance, fatigue, and limited flexibility may lead to restricted participation due to fear of falling.[16]

Implications of Decreased Motor Function on Occupational Therapy Assessment

Many assessments require motor responses regardless of the fact that the purpose of the assessment is unrelated to motor performance. Some tests have motor requirements, such as writing or pointing; these actions may be challenging for people with motoric challenges. Additionally, eye movements, head turning, and mouth movements might be embedded into an assessment and can be challenging for some people. When measuring occupational performance, it is critical for therapists to consider whether the individual can physically perform the required motor response and whether the client has the postural control and endurance to complete the task in the standard position and allotted time frame. If a child cannot maintain an upright posture in a chair, it will be difficult for him or her to performed skilled fine motor tasks. Similarly, if an older adult with arthritis cannot grasp the spoon handle with sufficient strength, he or she will likely have difficulty completing a complex cooking task.

Muscle and grip strength tests can be used to establish a baseline, but occupational therapists should also determine whether the person has enough power to perform daily activities such as transferring to the tub or carrying groceries.[17] The therapist can also consider an alternative position, frequent rest breaks, or use of adaptive equipment. Additionally, the occupational therapy evaluation can be scheduled at a time when the client has optimal endurance.

Determining the Impact of Sensory Function on Occupational Performance Assessment

Sensations contribute to occupational performance and quality of life by providing information about the surrounding environment and possible hazards, allowing for enjoyment of the positive sensations, offering protection against painful stimuli, and promoting well-coordinated motor performance. Sensory receptors begin development and functioning in utero.[18,19] Children and youth may experience sensory impairment with regard to stimuli reception and interpretation, as well as sensory modulation.[20,21] Adults reach peak sensory capacity during the second decade and then gradually decline, with a rapid descent after 45 to 55 years of age.[3] Sensory modality loss can result from body structure and nervous system changes, environmental factors,[22] medication, and various health conditions.

Children must be able to receive sensory stimuli, process it accurately, and modulate appropriate responses as they engage in play, academic pursuits, and social interaction. Infants with vision impairment may have difficulty with maternal bonding and future social interactions.[23] A school-age child who is over-reactive to physical touch may be unable to tolerate the hardness of his chair or feel classmates brushing against him in the hallway. Additionally, children with vision or hearing loss are at risk of participating in fewer activities than their peers. Children with hearing loss may be specifically limited in social opportunities with peers due to associated language delays.[24]

Adults experience sensory loss for a variety of reasons. Adults with sensory loss due to carpal tunnel syndrome may have difficulty with IADL and work performance.[25] In older adults, age-related vision loss due to macular degeneration and glaucoma are associated with difficulty with performance of near vision tasks, community mobility, and leisure activities as well as psychosocial and emotional implications.[26-28] Moderate to severe hearing loss is associated with decreased ability to interact with others, difficulty paying attention, loss of feeling close to others, and greater likelihood of depression than non–hearing impaired individuals.[29]

Implications of Decreased Sensory Function on Occupational Therapy Assessment

When measuring occupational performance, it is critical for therapists to consider whether the individual can hear directions, see objects that need to be manipulated, and feel the shape and texture of testing materials so that testing procedures can be modified accordingly. For example, if a child is consistently overstimulated by his therapist's voice, the feel of his socks on his feet, and the proximity of his classmates, he is likely to have difficulty focusing on the assessment activities. If an adult has an undetected hearing loss, incorrect following of test instructions may be misinterpreted. Quiet testing environments, use of task lighting and magnifiers, and pairing tactile input with auditory or visual cues can facilitate optimal assessment performance and accurate interpretation of results.

Determining the Impact of Psychological Issues on Occupational Performance Assessment

Development of basic emotions, such as happiness, anger, and fear, begins in the first year of life[30]; emotional self-regulation does not begin to develop until well into the preschool years.[31] Twenty percent of children and adolescents have a behavior or emotional disorder; the most common disorders include anxiety, depression, attention-deficit hyperactivity disorder, and conduct disorder.[32] In addition, children with physical health concerns are at greater risk for emotional and behavioral conditions.[33]

Throughout adulthood and older adulthood, individuals encounter a variety of potential stressors including decline in physical health and cognitive capacity, role changes, and loss of social support.[22] In addition, presence of comorbid mental health conditions has the potential to influence occupational therapy assessment outcomes.[34] Depressive and anxiety-related symptoms can be expressed in a variety of ways that may influence performance on occupational performance assessments, including fatigue, reduced concentration, sleep disturbances, and sense of feeling "slowed down."[35,36] Additionally, engaging in cognitively challenging activities while under psychological stress creates a multitasking situation, and the amount of attention that can be directed toward information processing required by the assessment may be reduced.[37]

Psychological disorders and personality components have a significant effect on participation in meaningful occupations for individuals across the lifespan. Personality characteristics, such as introversion, confidence, and agreeableness, as well as psychosocial skills, range and stability of emotion, and self-efficacy can either facilitate or prohibit a child's participation during play and school experiences.[38] Additionally, a child's play patterns and ability to perform at school can be influenced by the parent-child relationship and psychological state of the primary caregiver.[39,40]

The relationship between well-being and activity participation for adults and older adults is well documented. Menec[41] found that social and productive activities were related to happiness, function, and mortality, while solitary activities were only related to happiness. Engagement in productive activities has been linked to a sense of self-competence, and leisure activity participation is related to a greater sense of social self, both of which positively affected well-being.[42] In addition, volunteering is associated with higher levels of well-being[43] as well as physical activity.[44]

Implications of Psychological Issues on Occupational Performance Assessment

Children with emotional and behavioral problems may have difficulty cooperating during the occupational therapy evaluation process. Children and youth with decreased impulse control, inattention, and/or hyperactivity may have greater need for structure, redirection, behavior ground rules, and breaks in order to optimally perform.[45] Conducting assessments in naturalistic settings may be the ideal approach to evaluate behavior, family dynamics, and child-parent interactions.[46] Practitioners can build a positive rapport, promote a safe atmosphere, and use reinforcement strategies to optimize evaluation performance.

In adults and older adults, performance on occupation-based assessments may be affected by competing thoughts related to depression and anxiety. Establishing a strong rapport with the person being evaluated can provide an anchor point for determining the person's psychosocial condition. Asking the person how he or she felt about the performance will also inform the interpretation process. When therapists sense that a person's psychosocial status is interfering, changing the evaluation time, offering breaks, and providing options for the client may reduce the impact of psychosocial factors on the occupation-based assessment performance.

Determining the Impact of Language and Literacy on Occupational Performance Assessment

Language includes reading, writing, talking, and listening. Although assessment and intervention of language and literacy skills are often delegated to other disciplines, communication and literacy is inextricably linked to daily occupational performance and quality of life. Individuals with language deficits are at risk for social isolation, challenges with relationships, barriers in the community and at work, and decreased independence.[47,48]

Infants first use noises to begin babbling and express themselves. By listening to phonemes and sounds from the environment, infants learn about patterns of speech and caregivers' reactions through social interactions.[49] As children have more experiences with listening to and producing sounds, they enhance their ability to articulate syllables and form words. Early auditory experiences provide a type of "auditory scaffolding" that allows a child to gain information from the environment and practice creating noise while receiving information from caretakers.[50]

Literacy levels of clients and family members of all ages must also be considered as practitioners embark on the occupational therapy evaluation process. According to the 2011 American Community Survey of 291.5 million people regarding language use in the United States, 60.6 million (21%) speak a language other than English at home.[51] Approximately 80 million US adults are considered to have lower health literacy, which is associated with reduced understanding of health-related knowledge.[52] In addition, a variety of health conditions encountered throughout the lifespan may impact expression and comprehension of language, including cerebral palsy,[53] stroke,[54] dementia, and other progressive neurologic diseases.[55]

The ability to process and utilize language is essential for participation in many of the occupations of childhood such as bonding with caregivers, following directions, interacting with peers, and responding to requests for information as a mark of academic learning. Adults with low literacy or language deficits will have difficulty with medication management, following recipes, and maintaining a shopping list or budget. Modest changes in language, particularly with naming objects, have been identified in the normal aging population.[56] Even slight changes as the result of aging or a neurological injury may interfere with the individual's ability to effectively communicate with family, friends, and physicians.

Implications of Limitations in Language and Literacy on Occupational Performance Assessment

Occupational therapists must identify the potentially significant impact that language impairments and low literacy may have on assessment and occupational performance. Language is required for most assessment procedures, even when it is not the focus of the assessment. Following simple instructions requires listening skills, and responding to assessment questions requires comprehension and expression to form an answer.

Self- and proxy-report measures are particularly at risk for misinterpretation from clients and family members who have low literacy levels, language barriers, or language comprehension deficits. Some pediatric and older adult evaluations rely heavily on parent or caregiver report measures. Thus, occupational therapy practitioners must be aware of the caregiver's reading level and language preferences. Adults with aphasia or hearing loss may need instructions or interview questions in written format. Reading acuity and comprehension can be facilitated by changing font size and style as well as spacing parameters.[57] Interpreters may be used to facilitate the evaluation process. Practitioners working with clients with low literacy can utilize plain language during verbal communication, revise written materials, ask clients to repeat assessment directions to ensure understanding, and keep in mind that head nodding does not always imply understanding.[58] Therapists may also want to observe spontaneous, demonstrated task performance and compare with performance based on standardized verbal instructions.

Identifying Person Factors That May Limit Assessment Performance

Targeted assessment of person factors that may influence assessment of occupational performance may be an important first step in the occupational therapy evaluation process. Assessment of vision, hearing, cognition, motor factors, language, and literacy can yield valuable information that will guide the evaluation and intervention planning process and help the client seek help to resolve identified impairments. Practitioners should first investigate whether the information may already be available in their setting because there is no need to duplicate testing. For example, speech pathologists and neuropsychologists may evaluate some of these constructs. However, if vision, audition, memory, depression, and literacy are not assessed in a formalized way, then the occupational therapist can collect data. Table 5-1 includes example assessments for use across the lifespan for the range of person factors. All identified measures are intended to be used as screening tools to help quantify the client's capacity for participation in the occupational therapy evaluation and activity performance. For example, an occupational therapist in a school setting may choose to utilize the BOT-2 Short Form to gain a general sense of the client's gross and fine motor skill capacity before evaluating performance of functional educational tasks. Following the occupational performance assessment, the occupational therapist may choose to continue with more extensive motor skills assessment, if it is warranted. References and links to public domain sources are also provided. Refer to Tables 5-2 and 5-3 for case-based illustrations of how use of selected person factor assessments can inform the occupational therapy evaluation and intervention planning process.

Case 1: Identifying Person Factors That Impact Occupational Performance Assessment to Support Analysis of Capacity and Limitations in a Child

Peter is a 6-year-old boy who is diagnosed with Autism Spectrum Disorder and Attention Deficit Hyperactivity Disorder (ADHD). He enjoys talking about elevators and likes to draw buildings with elevators. Peter lives at home with his mom, dad, and 2-year-old brother. Both of his parents work full time and have high expectations for their children. Peter attends his local public school and receives 60 minutes per day of special education services for positive behavioral supports, written expression, and pragmatic communication goals. Peter's first grade teacher recently requested an occupational therapy evaluation due to Peter's poor attention during structured lessons, difficulty understanding and following directions, struggle with using school tools, and challenges at recess and in the cafeteria.

The occupational therapist wants to understand Peter's educational history and functional capacity prior to making a recommendation for services, so she chooses to review his school records and administer several assessments to gain a sense of the factors that may influence his performance during classroom observations. These results will assist the occupational therapist to interpret the results of occupational profile measures such as the School Function Assessment (teacher) and COPM (parent).

Equipped with this information, the occupational therapist proceeds to administer the School Function Assessment with Peter's teacher and the COPM with his parents, and conducts skilled observations of his educational performance in the classroom, lunchroom, hallways, and playground. The following adjustments were made during the occupational performance assessments:

- Peter will need simple, repeated verbal instructions from his teacher and parents to facilitate cognitive processing
- Peter should be asked to repeat directions and information shared to ensure understanding
- Peter's family could consider a referral to a developmental optometrist to support his reading, writing, and coordination
- Peter should be positioned in the front of the classroom or in close proximity to written materials during the occupational therapy assessment to support his visual skills
- Peter may need the support of adaptive supplies during assessment of writing and other educational tasks that require a motor-based response
- Peter will need frequent movement breaks or other strategies to facilitate his self-regulation skills during the occupational therapy evaluation process

Information from these person factor assessments allowed the occupational therapist to gain more accurate evaluation results as well as a clearer understanding of Peter's capacity and limitations. This information was also useful as the occupational therapy and educational team collaborated regarding the development of his client-centered Individualized Education Plan. The occupational therapy practitioner also shared the assessment results with Peter's family, with a particular focus on how the impairments impact their son's occupational performance at home and how they can be addressed to foster his participation and success at home through use of strategies used at school.

Case 2: Identifying Person Factors That Impact Occupational Performance Assessment to Support Analysis of Capacity and Limitations in an Older Adult

Mrs. Wheeler is a 68-year-old woman who had a stroke 6 months ago. After 2 weeks of inpatient rehabilitation, she went home. She recently visited her physician and indicated that she was having difficulties doing what she needed to do at home and indicated she was no longer going out into the community. She was referred to an occupational therapist for an in-home visit.

Mrs. Wheeler lives in a single-story home that is accessed by 5 steps to the front door and 4 to the back. Her daughter visits 2 to 3 times per month; she has little social support other than those visits. The occupational therapist wants to understand Mrs. Wheeler's goals and her occupational history prior to helping her develop a plan, so she decides to administer several assessments to gain a sense of the factors that may influence her performance on assessments such as the Activity Card Sort (ACS) and the COPM.

Equipped with this information, the occupational therapist proceeds to administer the ACS, COPM, and other relevant measures. The following adjustments were made while administering the assessments:

- Speaking in a loud tone of voice and positioning self across from Mrs. Wheeler so she can benefit from lip reading and gestures
- Positioning ACS cards in the right visual field to enable Mrs. Wheeler to attend to testing materials
- Use of the enlarged version of the COPM rating cards and placement in right visual field
- Repeating and clarifying directions as needed to facilitate cognitive processing
- Asking Mrs. Wheeler to repeat directions and information shared to ensure understanding
- Use of clear, simple terminology in view of literacy level

Table 5-1

Person Factor Assessments

Person Factor	*Children, Youth, and Families*	*Adult*	*Older Adult*
Cognition	BRIEF Connors-3	MOCA	SB MOCA
Motor	Bayley-3 BOT-2 PDMS-2 Beery VMI	UE ROM MMT screen	UE ROM MMT screen
Sensory	Hearing screen from health record Sensory Processing Measure Sensory Profile Vision screen (locate, fixate, track, convergence)	Lighthouse NA Whisper Test	Lighthouse NA Whisper Test
Psychological	CBCL CDI	Beck Depression Scale DASS	GDS DASS
Language/literacy	Vineland Adaptive Behavior Communication Sub-Test Bayley-3 Language Sub-Test	FAST REALM	FAST REALM

Information from these person factor assessments allowed the occupational therapist to gain more accurate evaluation results as well as a clearer understanding of Mrs. Wheeler's capacity and limitations. This information was also useful as they collaborated regarding the development of her client-centered intervention plan. The occupational therapy practitioner also shared the assessment results with Mrs. Wheeler's daughter, with a particular focus on how the impairments impact her mother's occupational performance, how they will be addressed to foster her mother's participation, and implications for the daughter in terms of how she assumes and manages the caregiving process. In addition, concerns regarding Mrs. Wheeler's low mood and hearing loss were reported to the referring physician for further management.

Future Directions in Practice and Research

As the landscape of health care evolves, more and more individuals with disabling conditions and injuries will seek occupational therapy services. Practice is evolving from inpatient and outpatient medical models of care to community- and home-based models of care that address everyday performance. Additionally, these policy changes are heavily focused on the promotion of preventative care and self-management. Individuals will be required to take control of their own health and occupational therapists can empower clients to be proactive in their health care and develop partnerships with their health care providers. Occupational therapists can provide further support by sharing information about specific impairments with clients, their families, and their health care team so that specific deficits can be addressed. For example, reading glasses can be prescribed or medical treatment can be pursued to address depressive symptoms. The occupational therapy evaluation process must include documentation of person factors that limit or support overall performance so that the intervention planning process and discharge to community resources remains targeted and client-centered across the continuum of care.

Table 5-2

Case 1

Assessments	*Results*	*Interpretation*
Developmental Vision Screening	Acuity (per school health record): 20/25 Visual tracking: fair to poor Saccades: moderate Unilateral cover test: normal R / L	Normal visual acuity. Difficulty focusing and tracking. Overall attention to task, reading skills, and art and writing may be impacted by this.
Annual School Hearing Screening	WNL	Normal hearing acuity
Sensory Profile-School Companion	Auditory: probable difference Visual: definite difference Movement: definite difference Touch: typical performance Behavior: definite difference Registration: probable difference Seeking: definite difference Sensitivity: typical performance Avoiding: definite difference	Probable difficulty with self-regulation due to differences in sensory processing. May also have difficulty retaining directions or be distracted by visual or auditory input and have a high need for movement.
Educational Record Review of Psychometric Evaluation: • Weschler Abbreviated Scale of Intelligence-WASI • Woodcock-Johnson Tests of Achievement-WJ-III	Verbal IQ SS=99 Nonverbal IQ SS=112 Broad reading SS=86 Broad math SS=90 Broad written exp SS=72 Total achievement SS=80	Average Intelligence Below average academic achievement. This gap indicates the presence of a learning disability, specifically in written expression.
Behavior Rating Inventory of Executive Function	Behavior regulation (T)=72 Metacognitive (T)=78 Global executive (T)=76	Clinically significant difficulty with global executive function skills in the classroom may be impacting behavior and academic performance.
Record Review of Expressive and Receptive Language Evaluation Report from SLP • Clinical Evaluation of Language Fundamentals (CELF-4)	Receptive language SS=85 Expressive language SS=95	Average expressive language and slightly below average receptive language.
Bruininks-Oseretsky Test of Motor Proficiency-2 Short Form	Short form SS=37	Below average motor skills may be impacting performance of daily school tasks and recess participation.

Table 5-3

CASE 2

Assessments	*Results*	*Interpretation*
Lighthouse Near Acuity Card	20/80 OU with glasses on	Low vision; the physician needs to know she needs a referral for visual services
Rivermead Behavior Inattention Test	43/54	Probable left neglect
Montreal Cognitive Test	23/30	Mild cognitive loss; may not retain new information easily, have reduced concentration and be a possible safety risk
Boston Naming Test	10/14	Some limitations in naming; may indicate mild cognitive loss
Rapid Assessment of Adult Literacy in Medicine (REALM)	155	7.7 grade reading level; may need to modify verbal instructions and written materials

REFERENCES

1. Wilcock A. A theory of the human need for occupation. *J Occupational Science.* 1993;1(1):17-24.
2. DeLuca CR, Wood SJ, Anderson V, et al. Normative data from the CANTAB. I: development of executive function over the lifespan. *J Clin Exp Neuropsychol.* 2003;25(2):242-254.
3. Hooyman NR, Kiyak HA. *Social Gerontology: A Multidisciplinary Perspective.* 7th ed. Boston: Allyn and Bacon; 2005.
4. Heyl V, Wahl HW. Managing daily life with age-related sensory loss: cognitive resources gain in importance. *Psychol Aging.* 2012;27(2):510-21.
5. Tran D, Baxter J, Hamman R, Grigsby J. Impairment of executive cognitive control in type 2 diabetes, and its effects on health related behavior and use of health services. *J Behav Med.* 2014;37(3):414-422.
6. Sinha S, Gunawat P, Nehra A, Sharma BS. Cognitive, functional, and psychosocial outcomes after severe traumatic brain injury: a cross-sectional study at tertiary care trauma center. *Neurol Indial.* 2013;61(5):501-506.
7. Baum C, Katz N. Occupational therapy approach to assessing the relationship between cognition and function. In: Marcotte TD, Grant I, eds. *Neuropsychology of Everyday Functioning (Science and Practice of Neuropsychology).* New York: Guilford Press; 2009:62-91.
8. Chapparo C, Ranka J. The occupational performance model (Australia): a description of constructs and structure. In: Chapparo C, Ranka J, eds. *Occupational Performance Model (Australia): Monograph 1.* Sidney: Occupational Performance Network; 1997:1-22.
9. Woodward RL, Surburg PR. The performance of fundamental movement skills by elementary school children with learning disabilities. *The Physical Educator.* 2001;58(4):198-205.
10. Bonder B, Bello-Hass V. *Functional Performance in Older Adults.* Philadelphia: F.A. Davis Co; 2009.
11. Campbell AJ, Borrie MJ, Spears GJ. Risk factors for falls in a community-based prospective study of people 70 years and older. *J Gerontol.* 1989;44(5):M112-M117.
12. Case-Smith J, O'Brien JC. *Occupational Therapy for Children.* Maryland Heights, MO: Mosby/Elsevier; 2010.
13. Sullivan MC, McGrath MM. Perinatal morbidity, mild motor delay, and later school outcomes. *Dev Med Child Neurol.* 2003;45:104-112.
14. Case-Smith J. Effectiveness of school-based occupational therapy intervention on handwriting. *Am J Occup Ther.* 2002;56(1):17-25.
15. Nilsagård Y, Denison E, Gunnarsson LG, Boström, K. Factors perceived as being related to accidental falls by persons with multiple sclerosis. *Disabil Rehabil.* 2009;31(16):1301-1310.
16. Arfken CL, Lach HW, Birge SJ, Miller JP. The prevalence and correlates of fear of falling in elderly persons living in the community. *Am J Public Health.* 1994;84(4):565-570.
17. Dean E, DeAndrade AD. Cardiovascular and pulmonary function. In: Bonder BR, Bello-Hass VD, eds. *Functional Performance in Older Adults.* 2nd ed. Philadelphia: FA Davis; 2009:65-100.
18. Bradley RM, Mistretta CM. Fetal sensory receptors. *Physiol Rev.* 1975;55(3):352-382.
19. Lecanuet JP, Schaal B. Fetal sensory competencies. *Eur J Obstet Gynecol Reprod Biol.* 1996;68:1-23.
20. Tomchek SD, Dunn W. Sensory processing in children with and without autism: a comparative study using the Short Sensory Profile. *Am J Occup Ther.* 2007;61(2):190-200.
21. Cosbey J, Johnston SS, Dunn ML. Sensory processing disorders and social participation. *Am J Occup Ther.* 2010;64(3):462-473.
22. Foster E, Perlmutter M, Baum CM. Evaluating occupational performance of older adults. In: Coppola S, Elliott S, Toto P, eds. *Strategies to Advance Gerontology Excellence: Promoting Best Practice in Occupational Therapy.* Bethesda: AOTA Press; 2008:349-382.

23. Robson KS. The role of eye-to-eye contact in maternal-infant attachment. *J Child Psychol Psychiatry.* 1967;8(1):13-25.
24. Engel-Yeger B, Hamed-Daher S. Comparing participation in out of school activities between children with visual impairments, children with hearing impairments and typical peers. *Res Dev Disabil.* 2013;34(10):3124-3132.
25. Katz JN, Gelberman RH, Wright EA, Lew RA, Liang MH. Responsiveness of self-reported and objective measures of disease severity in carpal tunnel syndrome. *Med Care.* 1994;32(11):1127-1133.
26. Lamoureux EL, Hassell JB, Keefe JE. The impact of diabetic retinopathy on participation in daily living. *Arch Ophthalmol.* 2004;22:84-88.
27. Noe G, Ferraro J, Lamoureux E, Rait J, Keeffe JE. Associations between glaucomatous visual field loss and participation in activities of daily living. *Clin Experiment Ophthalmol.* 2003;31:482-486.
28. Scilley K, Jackson GR, Cideciyan AV, Maguire MG, Jacobson SG, Owsley C. Early age-related maculopathy and self-reported visual difficulty in daily life. *Ophthalmology.* 2002;109(7):1235-1242.
29. Strawbridge WJ, Wallhagen JI, Seema SJ, Kaplan GA. Negative consequences of hearing impairment in old age: a longitudinal analysis. *Gerontologist.* 2000;49:320-326.
30. Berk LE. *Child Development.* 6th ed. Boston: Allyn and Bacon; 2003.
31. Rothbart MK, Sheese BE, Rueda MR, Posner MI. Developing mechanisms of self-regulation in early life. *Emot Rev.* 2011;3(2):207-213.
32. Koppelman J. Children with mental disorders: making sense of their needs and the systems that help them. *NHPF Issue Brief.* 2004;4:1-24.
33. Fleischfresser S. Wisconsin Medical Home Learning Collaborative: a model for implementing practice change. *WMJ.* 2004;103(5):25-27.
34. Crawford MJ, Robotham D, Thana L, et al. Selecting outcome measures in mental health: the views of service users. *J Ment Health.* 2011;20(4):336-346.
35. Bierman EJ, Comijs HC, Jonker C, Beekman AT. Effects of anxiety versus depression on cognition in later life. *Am J Geriatr Psychiatry.* 2005;13(8):686-693.
36. O'Donnell C. The greatest generation meets it greatest challenge: vision loss and depression in older adults. *J Vision Impairment Blindness.* 2005;99:197-208.
37. Stawski RS, Sliwinski MJ, Smyth JM. Stress-related cognitive interference predicts cognitive function in old age. *Psychol Aging.* 2006;21(3):535.
38. Tucker-Drob EM, Briley DA, Harden KP. Genetic and environmental influences on cognition across development and context. *Curr Dir Psychol Sci.* 2013;22(5):349-355.
39. Champagne FA. Early adversity and developmental outcomes interaction between genetics, epigenetics, and social experiences across the life span. *Perspectives on Psychological Science.* 2010;5(5):564-574.
40. Shonkoff JP. Leveraging the biology of adversity to address the roots of disparities in health and development. *Proc Natl Acad Sci U S A.* 2012;109(suppl 2):17302-17307.
41. Menec VH. The relation between everyday activities and successful aging: a 6-year longitudinal study. *J Gerontol B Psychol Sci Soc Sci.* 2003;58(2):S74-S82.
42. Herzog AR, Franks MM, Markus HR, Holmberg HR, Holmberg D. Activities and well-being in older age: effects of self-concept and educational attainment. *Psychol Aging.* 1998;13:179-185.
43. Morrow-Howell N, Hinterlong J, Rozario PA, Tangl F. Effects of volunteering on the well-being of older adults. *J Gerontol Soc Sci.* 2003;58B:S137-S145.
44. Fukukawa Y, Nakashima C, Tsuboi S, et al. Age differences in the effect of physical activity on depressive symptoms. *Psychol Aging.* 2004;19(2):346-351.
45. Lambert WL. Mental health of children. In: Cara E, McRae A, eds. *Psychosocial Occupational Therapy: A Clinical Practice.* Clifton Park, NY: Delmar; 2005:384.
46. Stewart KB. Purposes, processes, and methods of evaluation. In Case-Smith J, O'Brien JC, eds. *Occupational Therapy for Children.* 6th ed. Maryland Heights, MO: Mosby; 2010:193-211.
47. Cruice M, Worrall L, Hickson L, Murison, R. Finding a focus for quality of life with aphasia: social and emotional health, and psychological well-being. *Aphasiology.* 2003;17(4):333-353.
48. Ross K, Wertz R. Quality of life with and without aphasia. *Aphasiology.* 2003;17(4):355-364.
49. Tronick E. *The Neurobehavioral and Social-Emotional Development of Infants and Children.* New York: W. W. Norton & Company; 2007.
50. Pisoni DB, Conway CM, Kronenberger WG, et al. Efficacy and effectiveness of cochlear implants in deaf children. *Deaf Cognition: Foundations and Outcomes.* 2008;52-101.
51. Ryan C. (2013). Language Use in the United States: 2011; American Community Survey Reports. United States Census Bureau. http://www.census.gov/prod/2013pubs/acs-22.pdf. Accessed June 18, 2016.
52. Kutner M, Greenberg E, Jin Y, Paulsen, C. *Health Literacy of America's Adults: Results from the 2003 National Assessment of Adult Literacy (NCES 2006-483).* Washington, DC: US Department of Education, National Center for Education Statistics; 2006.
53. Pirila S, van der Meere J, Pentikainen T, et al. Language and motor speech skills in children with cerebral palsy. *J Commun Disord.* 2007;40(2):116-128.
54. Pedersen PM, Vinter K, Olsen TS. Aphasia after stroke: type, severity and prognosis. The Copenhagen aphasia study. *Cerebrovasc Dis.* 2004;(17):35-43.
55. Illes J. Neurolinguistic features of spontaneous language production dissociate three forms of neurodegenerative disease: Alzheimer's, Huntington's, and Parkinson's. *Brain Lang.* 1989;137(4):628-642.
56. Kirshner HS, Bakar M. Syndromes of language dissolution in aging and dementia. *Compr Ther.* 1995;21(9):519-523.
57. Garrett KL, Huth C. The impact of graphic contextual information and instruction on the conversational behaviours of a person with severe aphasia. *Aphasiology.* 2002;16(4-6):523-536.
58. Smith DL, Gutman, SA. Health literacy in occupational therapy practice and research. *Am J Occup Ther.* 2011;65:367-369.

CHAPTER 6

Using Naturalistic Measurement Methods to Understand Occupational Performance

Mary A. Corcoran, PhD, OTR/L, FAOTA; Carolyn Baum, PhD, OTR/L, FAOTA; and Winnie Dunn, PhD, OTR, FAOTA

Occupational therapists continue to feel the effects of increasingly greater demands from organizations, payers, and decision makers for clinical outcomes to justify occupational therapy intervention. The costs of health care in the United States and many other countries are spiraling upward at the same time that the health care marketplace is being extended through the Affordable Care Act to millions of previously uninsured patients. At the same time, access to information and demographic changes has resulted in better informed clients who expect individualized outcomes that return them to meaningful roles. This has proven to be a source of tension for the occupational therapy profession. On one hand, reimbursable parameters for clinical outcomes often remain narrowly focused on performance that can be measured with standardized tools; on the other hand, the profession and many consumers are beginning to understand the power of occupation-based practice, the importance of understanding the client's narrative experience, and critical role of establishing a client-centered therapeutic relationship.

Occupation-based therapy depends on an accurate understanding of the client's occupational profile and performance. Although many therapists strive to obtain this information for every client, 2 nagging questions persist. How do we know that the right questions are being asked, and how do we ensure that we have conducted and interpreted our observations and interviews accurately? This measurement dilemma is compounded by the fact that often there are few rating scales or tests that quickly and accurately assess many of our concepts of interest, including important aspects of the therapeutic process (such as collaboration). When measurement tools do exist, they may be lengthy to administer, making them impractical in a busy practice setting. In addition, many concepts that are central to occupation, such as habits, role balance, and meaning, are difficult to measure without a precise definition that clearly distinguishes each concept from similar concepts.

Naturalistic research designs and data analysis methods are a likely choice when clinical questions include concepts that are not well defined and are difficult to measure. These methods also fit well into any practice setting. In fact, occupational therapists are already widely using 2 data collection methods that are central to naturalistic research: observation and interviews. The problem with use of naturalistic methods to assess occupation is that techniques to assure rigorous use are not well understood by many health care providers. Without understanding how to conduct interviews and observations to assure trustworthiness in the results, the therapist runs the risk of missing important information or being criticized for using an unscientific approach to assessment. Therefore, the purpose of this chapter is to help therapists refine and expand their use of naturalistic methods to systematically assess occupational performance, validate practice, and build new knowledge. To this end, material will be presented to do the following:

- Define naturalistic methods
- Discuss the application of naturalistic methods to practice
- Describe the process for analyzing narrative data
- Introduce the use of mixed methods (integrating qualitative and quantitative data) in occupational therapy

This chapter is not meant to be a substitute for texts on therapist-client interaction, in-depth interviewing, or naturalistic research methods. Rather, the chapter provides

Law M, Baum C, Dunn W, eds. *Measuring Occupational Performance: Supporting Best Practice in Occupational Therapy, Third Edition (pp 69-81).*

selected introductory material about the nature of naturalistic research and adding rigor to the use of observation and interview techniques during the occupational therapy process. This information is offered as a way of reliably gaining insight about a client's occupational profile and supporting occupation-based practice.

Why Use a Naturalistic Approach to Understand Occupation?

We have been fortunate in our profession to count among our members a number of highly skilled naturalistic researchers. These researchers, such as Elizabeth Yerxa and Betty Hasselkus, not only add to the body of literature, but also issue a call to action for the use of naturalistic methods as "a relevant, ethical, and realistic way of knowing..."[1(p 199)] Many in the occupational therapy and occupational science literature have turned to naturalistic methods as the natural choice for understanding occupation.

What are the characteristics of occupation that lend themselves to study from a naturalistic perspective?

- Occupation is complex and nuanced
- Occupations are processes in that they are the means to an end (activity) and involve active doing
- Occupations are meaningful and therefore can only be understood from the participant's perspective. Similarly, occupations are an individual experience at a particular time. Although the individual may be engaging in an occupation within a group of individuals who are all doing exactly the same thing, the experiences of each are unique
- Occupations are dynamic, changing, and developing over time, and even in subtle ways, from day to day
- Occupations are formed by cultural backgrounds; they are shaped by personal interests, desires, and values
- Occupations are highly influenced by environment, including physical, social, spiritual, cultural, personal, temporal, and virtual environmental contexts[2]

Thus, we have an ethical and scientific responsibility to study occupation using methods that preserve the specific environmental context, clarify meaning and complexity, and reflect a basis in cultural beliefs and values. Occupational therapy researchers have responded to that responsibility using a wide range of naturalistic designs, including use of life history,[3] life review,[4] grounded theory,[5] single-case research,[6] autoethnography,[7] and video microanalysis.[8] Occupational therapy is a profession with a rich heritage of naturalistic study. A prominent example is Florence Clark's Eleanor Clarke Slagle lecture[9] in which she offered a narrative analysis of Penny Richardson, an active, intelligent woman who struggled to regain occupational health after a stroke. Clark's purpose in her lecture was to offer a unique design for scientific inquiry in occupational science, a design based in the ethnographic tradition. In doing so, she drew on a substantial history of research within and outside the field of occupational therapy that seeks the meaning of occupation in the "...deep richness of mundane affairs."[10(p 162)]

In order to gain this insight into the meanings associated with occupation, the tradition of naturalistic (or qualitative) research must be understood. In particular, what is a naturalistic tradition, how is it different from an experimental tradition, and what strategies are used to increase our ability to trust the results (trustworthiness)?

Naturalistic Research Tradition

A naturalistic research tradition seeks to gain an in-depth and complex understanding of some poorly understood phenomena within a particular group. This understanding cannot be generalized beyond the individuals who participated in the study but does offer rich insight that may have compelling implications for a larger group. Although it is beyond the scope of this chapter to discuss all these differences, several of particular relevance are examined here.

Purpose: Complexity and Meaning Versus Predicting and Explaining

The client's choices about activities, competence, environment, and every other aspect of occupation set the parameters for occupational therapy; therefore, it is reasonable that an approach must be adopted that will clarify those expectations and desires. In her book entitled *Qualitative Research in Occupational Therapy*,[2] Dr. Joanne Cook provides a compelling connection between the values, beliefs, and language of occupational therapy and qualitative research. Cook asserts that understanding the complexities and nuances of occupation requires the in-depth and context-based approach of naturalistic inquiry. Occupational therapy and naturalistic research are also congruent in terms of their very purpose, which is to understand feelings, attitudes, experiences, and behaviors, as opposed to predicting behaviors. Cook[2] quotes Maxwell[11] regarding the purposes of research for which a naturalistic approach is appropriate. The purposes of a naturalistic approach are to do the following:

- Understand the meaning for participants in the study of the events, situations, and actions they are involved with and of the accounts that they give of their lives and expectations
- Understand the particular environmental context within which the participants act and the influence that this environment has on their actions
- Identify unanticipated phenomena and influences and generate new grounded theories about the latter
- Understand the process by which events and actions take place

Thus, naturalistic research methods are an appropriate choice for learning about the meanings of life events, from the participant's perspective, in such a way as to preserve the complexities and environmental context.

The Setting: Natural Versus Controlled

Investigators use naturalistic designs to study things in their everyday settings, as opposed to an experimental tradition where everyday settings are not necessarily desirable. For example, if you were administering a highly standardized test to a group of children, you would want a controlled classroom setting with minimal distractions. If you test the child in his home, any unusual occurrence, such as a pet entering the room or a sibling playing with an attractive toy, can introduce confounding variables and change the outcome of the test.

In a naturalistic study, the everyday setting is necessary because investigators want to describe social occurrences in order to make sense of them and the meanings people associate with them.[12] For example, to describe the experience of caring for a spouse with dementia at home, Corcoran interviewed caregiving husbands and wives in their homes to understand caregiving style (ways of thinking about and conducting care tasks).[5] The environment (both physical and social) was a vital part of understanding what and why caregivers enacted care as they did on a daily basis. For example, a woman who was caring for her husband talked about his inability to help her in the kitchen as he used to do. She was very upset about this change in her husband and talked about how fixing a meal together was meaningful to their relationship. Now that meaningful activity was gone and the woman was sure that this was a sign that her husband was one step closer to death. As she showed the interviewer around the kitchen, she pointed out her new mini-blinds, which replaced the "ugly roll-up type of blind." The interviewer noticed the glare from this new window covering and made a notation about it. When the last research visit was completed just 2 weeks later, the interviewer suggested to the woman that she close the mini-blinds whenever she worked in the kitchen with her husband. This suggestion was based on the possibility that her husband was susceptible to the glare created by the mini blinds and unable to see well in the kitchen. Although the outcome of this suggestion is not known, it is certain that without visiting the woman in her home, the suggestion may not have occurred to the interviewer. Interviewing in the home provided an opportunity to observe what was happening and rely less on being told what was happening.

Types of Data: Words Versus Numbers

The potential sources of data are quite extensive, but how the data are managed once collected is different in a naturalistic vs an experimental study. The purpose of data management is to convert "raw" data into a form that lends itself to analysis. If the purpose of analysis is to predict behavior (or other phenomena), the type of study is probably experimental and data are reduced to numbers. However, if the purpose of the study is to understand more about the meanings associated with events (or other phenomena), the type of study is probably naturalistic and non-numeric (narrative, auditory, or visual) data are reduced to codes, and then codes are assembled into themes. The 2 examples that follow help to illustrate that difference.

An occupational therapist wants to know what differences exist in types of leisure activities of individuals with stroke compared with individuals with brain injury. He interviews a large number of clients and asks each to "Tell me about your leisure activities during the past month."

Example 1

In order to predict the type of leisure activities based on diagnosis, the occupational therapist would use an experimental design and analyze his or her data with statistical tests. Statistical tests require numbers, so the occupational therapist would need to assign numerical codes to the different types of leisure activities that emerged from the interviews. Let's say the occupational therapist assigns the following codes to the information he collected through interviews:

- 0 = No leisure activities are reported
- 1 = More than 50% of reported activities primarily involve playing sports
- 2 = More than 50% of reported activities primarily involve games or puzzles
- 3 = More than 50% of reported activities are primarily passive
- 4 = More than 50% of reported activities are primarily social

If the occupational therapist sorts the data in terms of diagnosis, the result of analysis would be a comparison of types of activities reported by individuals with stroke to leisure activities reported by individuals with brain injury.

Example 2

In order to understand the meanings associated with these leisure activities, the occupational therapist would sort the phrases (retained as words) into several categories. Let's say the occupational therapist hears the following types of information:

- Activities that stretch my abilities (such as sports and puzzles)
- Activities that help me relax (such as visiting friends/family, listening to music, reading)
- Activities that are done for fun (building model cars, playing games)
- Activities that pass the time (watching television, surfing the internet)

Again, keeping track and sorting by diagnosis, the result of analysis would indicate the meaning associated with leisure activities of individuals with stroke and individuals with brain injury. They are the same activities, but different questions yielded different outcomes.

See the difference? In example 1, the data were reduced to numbers and the results answered the question of *what* was done for leisure. In example 2, data were reduced to phrases and the results answered the question of *why* participants engaged in leisure activities. One approach is not better than the other; they are simply different questions.

Sources of Accuracy: Trustworthiness Versus Validity and Reliability

The mix of in-home observation and interview discussed previously in the caregiving style study[5] actually increases the validity of the results because it provides a way to check on conclusions from 2 sources—what was seen and what was heard. This technique for increasing the validity of naturalistic inferences is one type of triangulation. *Triangulation* is a method used by naturalistic researchers to "...get a better fix on the subject matter at hand."[12(p 2)] An interesting example of triangulation is found in historical analysis in which data are collected from archival materials, including letters, photographs, diaries, books, films, and manuscripts. Triangulation consists of a range of interconnected approaches, including many forms of observation and interview, which enable the researcher to view the phenomena from several angles. Interviews can involve anything from one-on-one conversations to group discussions, and formats range from completely open-ended to highly structured. Likewise, observations take many forms, ranging from photographs or field notes of naturally occurring social scenes to simulated interactions in role plays. If a therapist cannot travel to a client's home, there are any number of creative methods for understanding the physical attributes of the home, including floor plans, photographs, and videos.

What other principles of naturalistic research, such as triangulation, exist and can potentially be applied to practice? Traditionally these include credibility, transferability, dependability, and confirmability. Each is defined next.

Credibility involves establishing that the results of the naturalistic inquiry are credible or believable from the perspective of the participant in the research. Because the purpose of naturalistic research is to describe or understand the phenomena of interest from the participant's viewpoint, the participants are the only ones who can legitimately judge the "correctness" of the results. One popular way to assure credibility is *member checking*. With member checking, the results of the analysis are communicated to the participants so they can clarify, correct, revise, or verify.

Transferability refers to the degree to which the results of naturalistic research can be transferred to other contexts or settings. From a naturalistic perspective, transferability is primarily the responsibility of the one doing the transferring. The naturalistic researcher can and should enhance transferability by doing a thorough job of describing the participants, research context, and assumptions that guided the research. The person who wishes to "transfer" the results to a different context is then responsible for judging the sensibility of the transfer.

Dependability emphasizes the need for the researcher to account for the ever-changing context within which research occurs. The researcher is responsible for describing the changes that occur in the setting and how these changes affected the way the researcher approached the study.

Confirmability refers to the degree to which the results could be confirmed or corroborated by others. There are a number of strategies for enhancing confirmability. The researcher can document the procedures for checking and rechecking the data throughout the study. Another researcher can take a "devil's advocate" role with respect to the results, and this process can be documented. The researcher can actively search for and describe negative instances that contradict study conclusions, also known as looking for "disconfirming cases." After the study, the researcher can conduct a data audit that examines the data collection and analysis procedures and makes judgments about the potential for bias or distortion.

Naturalistic questions require the researcher to make many notes and reflect on similarities and differences in the context. These notes are not always used by others to "check" on the veracity of the findings, so one additional strategy for assuring trustworthiness includes use of multiple interviewers who are also involved in analysis. Teams of interview-researchers spend many hours talking about what they are hearing and seeing, then coming to a consensus about what it all means. Many readers would consider these team approaches to be among the most rigorous of naturalistic designs.

Role of the Investigator: Involved and Subjective Versus Uninvolved and Objective

Many new researchers and others using naturalistic methods worry about injecting too much of their own viewpoint and assumptions into the data analysis. This concern is rooted in the fact that experimental studies require the investigator to remain totally objective in order to avoid introducing bias to the study. In fact, the most highly controlled and valid design is considered the randomized 2-group double blind study, in which everyone, including the investigator, has no idea of group assignment until the end of the study. Although controlling for bias is important and addressed through mechanisms such as those in the preceding paragraph, the naturalistic investigator must take a very involved and subjective role in the research process. The naturalistic investigator chooses those topics with which he or she has familiarity, if not substantial expertise. This expertise allows the investigator to draw on a bank of knowledge to direct questions and interpret data. Further, and perhaps more importantly, the investigator becomes a research tool in that his or her expertise and experiences lead to insightful, creative, and informed hunches. In naturalistic research, the investigator maintains a careful balance between inserting him- or herself into the data and forcing the data to his or her will.

Stake[13,14] discusses 6 common researcher roles seen in naturalistic work. The investigator's primary purpose, according to Stake, is reflected in the following roles:

1. Teacher: Learn what the target audience needs to know, then inform, sophisticate, increase competence, socialize, or liberate the group.
2. Evaluator: Give careful attention to data's merits and shortcomings based on a specific set of criteria.
3. Theorist: Use the uniqueness of the data to illustrate a solution, or new understanding for the data.
4. Advocate: Discover the best arguments against assertions and provide data to counter them.
5. Biographer: Chronicle a life history explored against a thematic network (ie, a set of issues).
6. Interpreter: Recognize and substantiate new meaning; find new connections and make them comprehensible to others.[13]

Notice how well these researcher roles overlap with the roles occupational therapists often assume in a therapeutic relationship. Perhaps this overlap further reflects one of the points in this chapter—there is a natural and consistent purpose between naturalistic research and occupational therapy.

Practice-Based Uses for Naturalistic Approaches

Up to this point, the content of this chapter has reasoned that much of occupational therapy involves minimally defined and understood concepts, and that measuring these concepts calls for applying naturalistic approaches to occupational therapy practice. An overview of selected principles of naturalistic research has been presented (purpose, setting, data type, sources of accuracy, and researcher roles) as the basis for applying these principles in practice.

Despite the long tradition of "special harmony" between occupational therapy and naturalistic study,[10] the range of possible ways that naturalistic designs can be applied to everyday practice has not been fully explored. However, naturalistic methods are already an important clinical tool in occupational therapy. In this section, use of naturalistic methods to support 4 practice-related efforts will be described. They are evaluation and treatment planning, case studies, clinical reasoning, and program evaluation.

Evaluation and Treatment Planning

Therapists are probably most familiar with the use of naturalistic methods to gather information for purposes of evaluation and treatment planning, such as interviewing to understand a client's goals. For example, how often have you asked a new client the open-ended question, "What is a typical day like for you?" Occupational therapists gather vital insight into routines, activity choices, performance, social systems, and resources with just this simple interview question. This is one example of many informal ways that occupational therapists use the basics of naturalistic methods in everyday practice. Another example is careful observation. Occupational therapists watch clients engaged in daily activities in order to understand issues such as safety, fatigue, problem solving, and performance. Thus, much of the information used to evaluate performance and plan treatment are naturalistic methods. Later, we'll talk about principles for improving the trustworthiness of these methods.

Case Studies

In another familiar clinical application, naturalistic methods are used in case studies to gather relevant occupational performance and profile data, which are derived at least partially from interviews and observations. Case reports are a regular feature in the major occupational therapy journals around the world and are valued for their ability to illustrate complex and dynamic relationships. Think about how occupational therapists choose the best illustration of occupation or a change in occupation. Often, the case is chosen because it is classic—the person in the case demonstrates characteristics or is residing in contexts that are typical of the situation encountered. Other cases are chosen because they are so unusual, either in terms of the presenting circumstances or the outcomes. Both of these decisions are similar to the goals of a naturalistic study, which might involve quoting a typical informant or looking for a disconfirming case.

Clinical Reasoning

Naturalistic methods have also been used on an informal basis to guide clinical reasoning. For example, ethnographic principles can be used as a framework by which an occupational therapist can identify and describe occupation from the client's perspective, including its meaning.[15,16] "Ethnography is the work of describing a culture. The central aim of ethnography is to understand another way of life..."[17(p 3)] Culture as the basis of occupation was a relationship recognized by the founders of the profession,[18] although the ability to understand and apply cultural concepts to therapeutic interventions remains a contemporary focus for inquiry.[8,18] Occupational therapy is one of only a few health professions to actively shape clinical decisions based on the client's beliefs and meanings. For this reason, many occupational therapists function as informal ethnographers without really being aware of the connection. Occupational therapists conduct these ethnographies in several settings. Therapists engage in narrative analysis with each other over lunch and between treatment sessions, sharing clinical successes and puzzles in an effort to better understand their clients' occupational performance. Clark named these lunchroom discussions "occupational storytelling," which she describes as important to understanding the "spirit of the survivors with whom they [occupational therapists] work."[9(p 1074)]

Mattingly and Fleming[19] also speak of storymaking between occupational therapist and client during which a future story is created for the client. This type of storytelling is crucial for building a therapeutic partnership between client and therapist and for guiding the clinical reasoning of the occupational therapist. In the beginning, the therapist's contribution to the story may be sketchy and largely based on past experiences and technical knowledge. Over time, details that individualize the story are added so that the client's unique experiences and meaning shape the intervention.

Evaluating Programs

Although most therapists are familiar with naturalistic data for describing single cases and puzzling through practice issues, fewer are aware of the clinical application of naturalistic methods to evaluate clinical programs. A primary goal of program evaluation is typically to determine whether the program is effective. While effectiveness is often measured by calculating a numerical change score, naturalistic methods are a useful approach when tests and surveys are not appropriate. Sometimes, the effectiveness of a program can only appropriately be understood from the viewpoint of the individuals who experienced it. In these cases, data would be gathered through focus groups, open-ended questions, or individual interviews. The evaluator would sort the responses in terms of "codes" or types of experience or opinions expressed. In doing so, the evaluator performs a thematic analysis by organizing, reducing, and describing the data.[20] In program evaluation, naturalistic methods can be used alone or in a mixed methods approach combining quantitative (numerical) data. Besides testing a program's effect, it is also important to understanding how a program was implemented, the participants' opinions, unexpected effects, and the program's strengths and weaknesses from a number of perspectives.[21-24] This information, which is critical to replication, is sometimes only available in narrative form through interviews or observations.

Patton identified 5 types of program evaluations that have particular relevance to the clinic and can be conducted at least partially through naturalistic methods:

1. *Process* evaluations measure the internal operations of the program, including how the clients accessed and moved through the program, client-therapist interactions, and program strengths and weaknesses. Because the evaluator is interested in how the program operated, detailed information is required from clients, therapists, and program administrators. The evaluator is looking for information about formal and informal activities that give the program its character.
2. A second type of program evaluation involves outcomes that are highly individualized. *Evaluating individualized outcomes* is necessary when a range of effects and experiences can be appropriately expected. Usually, this type of evaluation involves interview and observation of the client before, during, and after the program. The evaluator is seeking evidence of the effect of the program for that particular client.
3. A third type of program evaluation includes detailed *case studies* of unusual circumstances. Although there are many reasons for presenting cases as an example of usual treatment, new knowledge about the program can be gained from an in-depth study of situations that were not typical (outstanding successes, unusual failures, or dropouts). A naturalistic approach helps the evaluator to understand the unique set of circumstances at play in unusual cases as the basis for making programmatic changes.
4. *Program implementation* information is the fourth type of potential evaluation data; this is also known as *treatment fidelity*.[25] If a program is not implemented as it was designed, predicted outcomes may not be achieved. Therefore, it is important to gather data about what the therapist actually did in treatment and compare this information to the intended treatment. Qualitative data are especially appropriate to program implementation evaluation because few program designers can accurately anticipate the effect of client characteristics and contextual attributes on treatment implementation.
5. *Quality improvement* is the fifth type of program evaluation that can be conducted partially through naturalistic methods. Although it is important to know how much adaptive equipment was issued and how long clients were treated, the evaluator will also want to know more about how clients experienced or were affected by treatment. For instance, it would be a useful indicator of quality to know if and how clients used strategies introduced as part of their occupational therapy experience.[24]

Use of naturalistic methods to evaluate occupational performance and clinical programs can result in rich information that falls between and beyond the points on a standardized scale. The next section outlines broad decisions and methods for applying a naturalistic approach to measurement in occupational therapy practice.

Principles for Applying Naturalistic Methods to Occupational Therapy Practice

For discussion purposes, this section is organized according to 6 broad principles related to the use of naturalistic methods to evaluate occupational performance and clinical programs. They are as follows:

1. Choose the most knowledgeable informants
2. Ask the right questions, watch the right behaviors
3. Keep the setting natural

4. Document your observations or interview information
5. Analyze your data for themes
6. Confirm your findings

Each of these topics is represented by a wealth of conceptual and technical information in the literature. In fact, books are available that address each one of these questions in detail. The purpose of the following discussion is to provide a broad overview of how to approach these questions and to pique interest in learning more. Therapists who are committed to applying naturalistic methods to practice are encouraged to read any of a number of excellent publications on the topic, especially Miles and Huberman,[26] Denzin and Lincoln,[12] or Charmaz.[27] The occupational therapy literature also contains many excellent examples of a naturalistic approach to exploring occupation, clinical reasoning, and professional behaviors.

It is highly recommended that therapists seek out and partner with a researcher who is familiar with naturalistic methods. It is not necessary that this person is an occupational therapist, but his or her knowledge of technique will be beneficial to develop the therapist's approach and answer questions.

Choose the Most Knowledgeable Informants

Informants are knowledgeable sources of information that can provide an insider's perspective.[28] In the clinic, this would obviously include the client as the recipient of occupational therapy services. However, the richness and detail of naturalistic methods is partially due to the fact that information is gathered from many sources; plus, this serves as a triangulation strategy. Therefore, it is important to think about others, such as family, who may be good informants by virtue of having a unique perspective on the questions at hand.

To develop a list of potential informants, keep clearly in mind what you want to know. For instance, if you are questioning the benefits of occupational therapy for a particular individual, you may wish to interview only a caregiver or family member in addition to the individual receiving treatment. However, if you want to know the strengths and weaknesses of an occupational therapy program, then the list grows longer. First, think about the types of individuals who are in a position to comment knowledgeably. Your list may include clients, family members, interventionists, clerical staff, and administrators. Second, because you cannot interview everyone on the list, think about which individuals within each type will provide information that is unique. You may want to speak with the most satisfied and least satisfied clients. In naturalistic designs, the investigator looks for informants who will represent a wide range of experiences. Don't forget to ask each of your informants to recommend someone for an interview who feels differently about the topic than he or she does. This strategy, called *snowballing*, provides entry into those valuable disconfirming cases.

Ask the Right Questions; Watch the Right Behaviors

As with all aspects of research, deciding how to gather information must be driven by the clinical question and the amount of time the therapist has available. To decide among the range of possible data collection techniques, the occupational therapist must keep his or her questions clearly in mind. To do otherwise usually adds time and effort to the project without adding substantial gain. After a short list of appropriate data collection techniques has been developed, the occupational therapist must carefully examine each for its costs in terms of time and materials. For instance, data collection and analysis from interviews with 5 clients for 30 minutes each over a 2-month time frame may be more cost-effective than videotaping 10 hours of treatment. While videotaping sounds easier, it represents a high initial cost in materials, and analysis is time-consuming. It is important to remember when choosing a method that in-depth information can be effectively collected with just a few well-chosen interview questions or observations, as opposed to a large number (as would be needed in a experimental-type study).

As has been indicated, naturalistic methods yield non-numeric data. These data may be in the form of observations, interviews, or other visual information.

Observation is a vital part of the therapeutic process. Occupational therapists constantly observe their clients for many reasons, including assessment of progress, response to therapy, adverse effects, and level of challenge. Deciding what, when, and how to observe must be driven by the clinical questions asked. In addition, the therapist may either participate in the activity being observed while making notes about observations, or stand back and observe without participating. The determinant for participation or non-participation depends on the extent to which the observed phenomena can occur or will be changed by the occupational therapist's presence. For example, think about observations of self-feeding with or without the occupational therapist's presence. If the therapist wants to observe for the effect of a particular piece of adaptive equipment on performance, he or she will want to participate. However, if the therapist wants to see how well the client uses the equipment independently at lunch, the occupational therapist should not be involved.

Interviews can proceed in a number of ways depending on many factors, including setting, allotted time, complexity of information being sought, and characteristics of the informant and interviewer. Interviews raise a host of critical decisions to consider thoughtfully, especially decisions about the setting, interview questions, and interviewer's actions. As always, it is important to remind yourself of the question because it establishes the purpose, goals, and direction of the interview. Next, it may help to consider the informant's characteristics. Children require short, simple questions or the opportunity to look at objects (pictures, toys) that are relevant to the discussion. Based on your knowledge of the informant, plan other aspects of the interview, including order of the questions, their level of complexity, and needed attributes of the setting.

An important but often overlooked consideration is the interviewer's approach, including how friendly, talkative, and casual the interviewer appears. Interviewers must avoid asking questions in such a way as to promote or suggest a particular response, which is labeled a *leading question.* An example of a leading question is "Did that make you upset?" instead of "How did that make you feel?" As an interviewer, the therapist also has a special challenge to avoid: offering treatment advice during the interview. If information comes up that could potentially lead to a therapeutic suggestion, make a note and return to it during a treatment session. A final consideration involves the interviewer's actions during the interview. Although we will discuss documenting information in more detail later, it is important to consider what the interviewer will be doing during the interview, such as taking extensive field notes or recording the interview.

Decisions about interviews also include interview format and content. Format refers to the plan for organizing data collection, ranging from group interviews to individual interviews. With a limited amount of time, interviews may be done in groups. A focus group format is especially popular but requires special knowledge because this format combines expertise in interviewing with expertise in group dynamics. Anyone wishing to use a focus group approach should refer to a number of excellent texts, especially Krueger and Casey[29] and Kamberelis and Dimitriadis.[30] Interviews may also be conducted in other formats, such as one-on-one, small group, telephone, or Internet interviews. However, each of these formats introduces other decisions. For example, use of telephone or Internet interviewing may lack depth because the atmosphere does not involve direct human contact. Analyzing existing blogs and diaries offers a ready source of data, but it can be difficult to engage in the spiral process of data collection, analysis, and research question refinement that is the hallmark of the naturalistic inquiry process.

Interview content refers to the composition of the questions, or what is being asked, and their order. In an open-ended interview, a few carefully chosen *stem questions* or statements are posed to the participants to establish the topic, such as "Describe your morning routine." The interviewer then uses *probes* to get more in-depth and detailed information about the participant's response to the stem question. Probes are questions that ask for clarification ("Tell me more about how that goes"), similarities ("What other situations make that happen?"), dissimilarities ("How is that different from other mornings?"), and elaboration ("Can you give me some examples of when that happens?"). Some naturalistic researchers regard the probes as more important than the initial stem question, so practitioners should be very familiar and comfortable with their use. An alternative to the use of stem questions is an invitation to the informant to tell a story that illustrates a significant experience. The practitioner can use probes to delve more deeply for meaning. For example, interviewing parents of a child with a disability may include a request to relate a story about an event when the child's disability influenced decisions about how to spend the family vacation.

Visual data can be gathered from sources other than interview and observation. Potential sources of narrative data may be found in archival material (photographs, recordings, film, diaries) or more contemporary materials, such as informant blogs. A good source of visual data for therapists to consider is medical records, in particular, evaluations or discharge summaries from key team members.

Keep the Setting Natural

While it is not always possible to interview someone in the environment where an activity primarily occurs, this is the ideal. In Corcoran's caregiving style study,[5] some spouses were concerned about the reactions of other family members, so the interview was conducted in a local coffee shop or a library. The interviewer attempted to get as close to the natural setting as possible, both because information could be provided by seeing the immediate area of an informant's home, and also out of courtesy to the caregiver. On these occasions, caregivers were asked to bring photo albums of recent events so that the interview could involve clarifying and understanding aspects of the environmental context.

For those occupational therapists who do not work in the community, the following strategies may be helpful:

- Make generous use of visuals such as photographs, videotapes, or floor plans. Ask the client to look at the visuals with you and tell you what you're seeing. Remember that environments are dynamic, so ask about times when the picture might look different, such as on a busy day.
- When interviewing, try to talk in an area that is private and comfortable. The point is to make the client comfortable enough to trust you with his or her innermost feelings and concerns. Sometimes the best place is the client's room when no staff or other patients are around.
- Remove any symbols that will remind the client of the institution or your position as a health care provider, such as a white lab coat or a medical records file.

In an institutional setting, sometimes just one member of the team conducting a home visit can have a large effect on treatment planning and problem solving. Consider a proposal to the administration of the institution for a home visit for each client that meets certain criteria, such as lacking a full-time caregiver.

Document Your Observations or Interview Information

There are a number of choices about how to record qualitative data. As with all choices in naturalistic research, data collection methods should be guided by what the occupational therapist wants to know (the clinical question). It is usually not important for the purposes of clinical evaluation to have information recorded verbatim, so the expense of recorded data collection may not be justified. The occupational therapist may choose to use field notes if the information sought is very focused, such as a review of a typical daily routine to understand use of pacing. Field notes are familiar to most therapists as a method for documenting the contents of an interview or observations and the therapist's impressions. A safe method is to take field notes and audiotape so that information can be verified from a number of sources. Be aware, however, that your plans for audiotaping need to be approved by the compliance officer at your institution or the institutional review board. No matter which recording method is chosen, be sure to accurately record the date and client initials in notes and on tape labels. Preserve the informant's confidentiality by using his or her initials only and by locking materials in a secure place. Destroy these tapes as soon as their information has been analyzed.

Analyze Your Data for Themes

By far, the best way to become familiar with drawing conclusions from qualitative data is by working with someone who has experience in the area of qualitative data analysis. There are many computer software programs that make qualitative analysis manageable. These programs are useful, flexible, and powerful tools that save time and expand the interviewer's ability to explore the data. However, for everyday clinical practice, these programs may not be necessary or even feasible. Regardless of the methods used, qualitative analysis is conducted by sorting information based on similarities (coding), which eventually forms themes. Practitioners may find that it is sufficient to keep a running log or journal that summarizes the emerging themes.

If you take nothing else away from this chapter regarding analysis, the most important point to understand is that collecting and analyzing data are simultaneous tasks. Never make the mistake of collecting information without attempting to understand what you are seeing and hearing. Naturalistic designs are spiral, so that analysis of data leads to refinement of understanding, and that refinement leads to more focused and relevant data collection.

According to Wolcott,[31] the purpose of qualitative analysis is to transform data from their original form (transcripts of interviews, videotapes) to new knowledge. This transformation occurs as a result of 3 overlapping processes: description, analysis, and interpretation.[31] These processes do not particularly proceed in a linear fashion because the process of analysis may reveal the need for further description, and so on. In description, data are described generally through a summarizing narrative; a short memo that attempts to capture the gist of what is being said. To get started, think about answering the basic questions of who, what, when, where, and how. Morse and Richards[32] also talk about describing data in terms of gathering material that relates to selected topics of interest to the researcher (or occupational therapist), such as daily routines or social outings.

Description provides the groundwork for analysis, during which data are examined for concepts or themes among key elements and relationships. Analytic coding is used to identify and define "common threads that run through the data."[32(p 113)] By identifying themes, a researcher begins to understand what is important or meaningful about the topic. The third process involved in transforming data is interpreting themes for meanings and implications. In this process, the themes are compared and contrasted to develop an overarching theory about what is happening in this study. For example, in Corcoran's caregiving study,[5] the themes that appeared initially seemed to be related to the concept of caregiver self-care. However, on further analysis, this theme emerged as a subtheme to the overarching narrative of control.[5]

An important contribution to transforming data comes from the insights and hunches of anyone who reviews or collects the data. These insights and hunches are captured in memos to oneself that are documented immediately as they occur. Often, memos from another person who is in contact with the client provides a vital idea that can jump-start an analysis in new and interesting directions.

Confirm Your Findings

Earlier in this chapter, information was presented regarding strategies that can help a researcher dig below the surface to reveal interesting and important information, as well as to assure trustworthiness. Many of those strategies can and should be used by occupational therapists who are interviewing or observing for clinical reasons. *Triangulate* the data by finding several perspectives on the same phenomena. For example, you could ask a family member about the same events or behaviors on which the client commented, not as a way of confirming or refuting, but just simply to get a more nuanced picture of that event. Alternately, you could interview and observe the same actions, thereby getting an idea of how the client talks about performance and then carries out the activity. If necessary, use simulation or role play. A third way of triangulating data is by asking another staff member to interview the client. This may not be as feasible in a busy setting, but if you keep the questions brief and focused, it may be possible in a short amount of time. Finally, triangulate by testing the same skills or performance areas that the client has told you about. For example, Leibold and colleagues[33] used the Activity Care Sort[34] to structure the task of recalling daily activities and as a resource for triangulation.

We finish this chapter with 2 contemporary strategies that are tools for the occupational therapist.

Coaching Practices With Children and Families: A Method for Collecting Qualitative Information

When we examine the intimacy that grows from the interactions during coaching, we see that coaching methods are a specific way to collect qualitative information about families and individuals. By emphasizing reflective questions and comments, therapists frame the person's goals to invite deep thinking. Therefore, coaching becomes an in situ way to collect qualitative information about the person or family's situation and how they experience everyday routines. Let's examine the characteristics of coaching to see how it contributes to qualitative assessment practices.

Originally, professionals used coaching practices to address organizational performance at work.[35] In recent years, people from many disciplines have applied the principles of coaching to address health and well-being.[35,36] Coaching practices take advantage of learning theory by creating opportunities for individuals to recognize their values, assumptions, and expectations about a situation as a basis for developing meaningful solutions. Coaching emphasizes equality in the relationship between the coach and the person being coached (sometimes called the *coachee*) by employing reflective comments and questions to uncover the best personal solutions for the challenges that the coachee faces. Summarizing the interdisciplinary literature on coaching, Dunn et al identified 5 key components of coaching[37]:

1. The relationship is based on reciprocal communication.
2. The coachee identifies the issues.
3. Communication is focused on solving a problem, facing a challenge.
4. Solutions grow out of the coachee's insights.
5. Solutions are situated within authentic environments and activities.

For example, educators have studied coaching and found effectiveness. Knight and Cornett[38] found that teachers employ new evidence-based methods in their classrooms at a significantly higher rate (86%) when they have had coaching, compared to traditional professional development. In another study, Tay[39] demonstrated that teachers were very satisfied and reported self-efficacy after coaching to support children with self-regulatory problems.

Based on the ideas from interdisciplinary literature, Graham[40] developed Occupational Performance Coaching (OPC) to emphasize the integration of the coaching literature with occupational therapy approaches and expertise. As is also true with person-centered practices, OPC invites the parents, teachers, and/or children to identify their priorities and goals. Two key points of OPC include: 1) striving for satisfying occupational performance in the areas identified by parents, teachers, and/or children; and 2) building capacity to manage occupational challenges independently in the future.

In a case report, Graham et al[41] showed efficacy of OPC using a pre-/post-test design and postintervention interviews. The results showed that coaching could be a useful method. Following up with a one-group time-series design in 2013, Graham et al[42] investigated the effect of coaching on children's performance and parent self-efficacy. Both children and parents improved significantly, with many of the performance goals sustained across time after the OPC intervention. Following this line of thought, Missiuna et al[43] designed a model called "Partnering for Change," which is a school and family partnership based on coaching practices at school.

Dunn et al[37] used a baseline, pre-/post-test, follow-up design to investigate the effectiveness of OPC on children's participation and parents' efficacy with 20 families who have a child with Autistic Spectrum Disorder (ASD). They found that children had significant improvements in family identified goals, and parents reported significant improvements in their sense of competence as parents. Kientz and Dunn[44] followed a similar research design with adolescents who had ASD and also found that they increased participation in chosen activities significantly after 8 coaching sessions. Foster et al[45] used a qualitative design to investigate the effect of coaching on mothers of children with ASD. The themes that emerged from their discussion about their experience with OPC were relations, analysis, reflection, awareness, and self-efficacy.

Kessler et al[46] used a randomized trial design to test OPC for individuals who had a stroke. They compared ordinary care to 10 sessions of OPC and found that those receiving OPC showed a significant improvement in engagement in occupations.

The evidence is growing that reflective discussions are an effective method for gaining insights and achieving significant changes in participation. Simultaneously, coaching practices provide a structure for qualitative data gathering that deepens our understanding about the people we serve while documenting changes that matter to the people's lives. Learning how to skillfully engage in this type of dialogue is a useful tool for assessment that supports effective interventions.

In other fields of study, professionals discuss motivational interviewing; you will see that many of the same basic principles are the same as coaching practices. It is important to know all the ways that evidence-based ideas are discussed in the literature; this makes more resources available to you in your practice.

Introduction to Motivational Interviewing and Its Relationship to Occupational Therapy

The occupational therapy process begins with the clinician having a conversation with the client to conduct an occupational interview. This interview leads to the goals the client wants to achieve in the occupational therapy intervention. This interview serves as the narrative and provides a means to understand the client's problems and

Table 6-1

Comparisons of Naturalistic and Experimental Traditions

Characteristics	*Naturalistic*	*Experimental*
Type of reasoning	Inductive	Deductive
Epistemology	Holistic perspectives	Logical positivism
Purpose	Reveal complexity and meanings; generate theory	Predict, explain, test theory
Research process	Spiral	Linear
Setting	Naturalistic	Controlled
Role of the investigator	Involved; subjective	Uninvolved; objective
Type of data	Pictures; text; observation	Numbers
Sources of accuracy	Strategies to assure trustworthiness	Validity and reliability
Use of writing	Analysis	Dissemination

what these challenges mean within the broader context of their lives. Motivational interviewing and occupational therapy's focus on client-centered care share an important beginning.[47] Rogers challenged clinicians to take a client-centered approach where the approach is centered on the client's perspective, as well as his or her interests, values, and concerns. Occupational therapists use qualitative interviewing techniques to collect this important client-centered information.

Information must be collected, relationships must be established. Motivational interviewing is a means of communication that facilitates the client's intrinsic motivation and encourages the clinician to look for and choose the client's experiences and goals to guide treatment and promote change[48] (in our case, we would look for the client to guide their own treatment to achieve a change in occupational performance). In a motivational interview, the clinician engages the client in a reflective dialogue. Table 6-2 contrasts a traditional approach with a motivational interviewing approach.[49,50]

The motivational approach might seem familiar to the occupational therapist as the approach that was first published in occupational therapy in the early 1990s[51] and reflects how occupational therpaists relate to their clients.

Sumsion and Law[52] identify 5 core elements of client-centered practice in occupational therapy:

1. A shift in the balance of power in favor of clients
2. Joint partnership between therapist and client in decision making
3. Active listening as a validation of the importance of the client's voice
4. Client choice in the goals and process of therapy
5. Hope, an emotional investment in the future

See Chapter 7 for a comprehensive review of client-centered care and its measurement.

Conducting a Motivational Interview

Miller and Rollnick[53] established some guidelines for motivational interviewing because they believed that its value rested in persons discovering the advantages and disadvantages for themselves. Early work in motivational interviewing emphasized conditions that require changes in behavior (addiction, medication management, obesity). It has recently become central to work that is focused on enhanced rehabilitation.[54]

There are a few motivational interviewing techniques that can be of great value to the occupational therapist. The literature on motivational interviewing is growing and readily available. This brief introduction illustrates this systematic method for gathering qualitative data in partnership with those we serve; motivational interviewing also provides a way to change behavior. As we learn more about participation (see Chapter 9), we will see that motivational interviewing is a way of helping clients recognize and do something about their current or potential problems. Because it taps the client's intrinsic motivation, it arises from within rather than being imposed from others.[53]

Where Do We Go From Here?

Clinical questions come in many forms and may be asked about an individual client or a whole group. Hopefully, the reader understands from this chapter that the clinical question determines the type of measurement approach taken and details about data collection and analysis. When clinical research questions involve underdeveloped concepts, therapists should consider the merits and feasibility of applying a qualitative approach. A qualitative approach is useful for examining questions ranging from an individual's occupational preferences to program evaluation. With their skilled use of observation

Table 6-2

Comparison Between Traditional Approaches and Motivational/Coaching Approaches

Traditional Approach	*Motivational Approach*
Clinician as expert	Clinician develops partnership with client and exchanges information to facilitate informed decision making
Clinician tells client what to do	Clinicians match the client's capabilities with the environment to highlight the client's success with tasks. Client has the right to decide his or her own care
Clinician expects respect from client	Practitioner earns respect from the client

Table 6-3

Motivational/Coaching Process

Asking permission communicates respect for the client	Do you mind if we talk about your [accident, stroke] ...?
Eliciting change, the person gives voice to the need or reason for change	What would you like to see different about your current situation?
Exploring importance of the activity	How important is it for you to do this activity again?
Open-ended questions build empathy	What brought you here today? What has happened since we last met? Can you say more about that?
Emotion-seeking skills reveal the person's point of view	How did that make you feel? Is your condition having an impact on others?

and interview, occupational therapists are in a unique position to use qualitative inquiry in everyday practice. A substantial literature on naturalistic research methods is available to further inform practitioners, and contact with an experienced researcher is highly recommended. With practice, therapists may find themselves publishing case studies that illustrate clinical phenomena, and designing more opportunities to examine occupation through the use of naturalistic approaches.

References

1. Yerxa E. Seeking a relevant, ethical, and realistic way of knowing for occupational therapy. *Am J Occup Ther.* 1991;45(3):199-204.
2. Cook JV. *Qualitative Research in Occupational Therapy: Strategies and Experiences.* Albany NY: Delmar; 2001.
3. Frank G. Life history model of adaptation to disability: the case of a "congenital amputee." *Soc Sci Med.* 1984;19(6):639-645.
4. Chippendale T, Bear-Lehman J. Effect of life review writing on depressive symptoms in older adults: a randomized controlled trial. *Am J Occup Ther.* 2012;66:438-446.
5. Corcoran MA. Caregiving styles: a cognitive and behavioral typology associated with dementia family caregiving. *Gerontologist.* 2011;51(4):463-472.
6. Price-Lackey P, Cashman J. Jenny's story: reinventing oneself through occupation and narrative con-figuration. *Am J Occup Ther.* 1996;50(4):306-314.
7. Neville-Jan A. Encounters in a world of pain. An autoethnography. *Am J Occup Ther.* 2003;57(1):88-98.
8. Burke JP. What's going on here? Deconstructing the interactive encounter (Eleanor Clarke Slagle Lecture). *Am J Occup Ther.* 2010;64:855-868.
9. Clark F. Occupation embedded in a real life: interweaving occupational science and occupational therapy. Eleanor Clarke Slagle Lecture. *Am J Occup Ther.* 1993;47(12):1067-1078.
10. Kielhofner G. Qualitative research: part two—methodological approaches and relevance to occupational therapy. *Occup Ther J Research.* 1982;2:150-164.
11. Maxwell J. *Qualitative Research Design: An Interactive Approach.* Thousand Oaks, CA: Sage; 1996:17-19.
12. Denzin NK, Lincoln YS. *Handbook of Qualitative Research.* Newbury Park, CA: Sage Publications; 1994.
13. Stake RE. *The Art of Case Study Research.* Thousand Oaks, CA: Sage Publications; 1995.
14. Stake RE. *Qualitative Research: Studying How Things Work.* New York, NY: Guilford Press; 2010.

15. Lawlor MC, Mattingly CF. Beyond the unobtrusive observer: reflections on researcher–informant relationships in urban ethnography. *Am J Occup Ther.* 2001;55:147-154.
16. Magasi S, Hammel J. Women with disabilities' experiences in long-term care: a case for social justice. *Am J Occup Ther.* 2009;63:35-45
17. Spradley JP. *Participant Observation.* New York: Holt, Rinehart, and Winston; 1980.
18. Bonder BR, Martin L, Miracle AW. Culture emergent in occupation. *Am J Occup Ther.* 2004;58:159-168.
19. Mattingly C, Fleming M. *Clinical Reasoning: Forms of Inquiry in a Therapeutic Practice.* Philadelphia: F.A. Davis; 1994.
20. Schwandt TA. *Dictionary of Qualitative Inquiry.* 2nd ed. Thousand Oaks, CA: Sage Publications; 2001.
21. Creswell J, Plano-Clark VL. *Designing and Conducting Mixed Methods Research.* Thousand Oaks CA: Sage Publications; 2011.
22. Funnell SC, Rogers PJ. *Purposeful Program Theory: Effective Use of Theories of Change and Logic Models.* San Francisco, CA: Jossey-Bass; 2011.
23. Gitlin LN, Corcoran MA, Martindale-Adams J, Malone C, Stevens A, Winter L. Identifying mechanisms of action: why and how does intervention work? In: Schultz R, ed. *Intervention Approaches to Dementia Caregiving.* Oxford Press; 2000.
24. Patton MQ. *How to Use Qualitative Methods in Evaluation.* Newbury Park, CA: Sage Publications; 1987.
25. Burgio L, Corcoran MA, Lichstein KL, et al. Judging outcomes in psychosocial interventions for dementia caregivers: the problem of treatment implementation. *Gerontologist.* 2001;41(4):481-489.
26. Miles MB, Huberman AM. *Qualitative Data Analysis.* 2nd ed. Newbury Park, CA: Sage Publications; 1994.
27. Charmaz C. *Constructing Grounded Theory: A Practical Guide Through Qualitative Analysis.* Thousand Oaks, CA: Sage Publications; 2006.
28. Crabtree BF, Miller WL. *Doing Qualitative Research.* Newbury Park, CA: Sage Publications; 1992.
29. Krueger RA, Casey MA. *Focus Groups: A Practical Guide for Applied Research.* 5th ed. Newbury Park, CA: Sage Publications; 2015.
30. Kamberelis G, Dimitriadis G. *From Structured Interviews to Collective Conversations.* New York, NY; Routledge; 2013.
31. Wolcott HF. *Transforming Qualitative Data.* Newbury Park, CA: Sage Publications; 1994.
32. Morse JM, Richards L. *Readme First for a User's Guide to Qualitative Methods.* Thousand Oaks, CA: Sage Publications; 2002.
33. Leibold ML, Holm MB, Raina KD, Reynolds CF III, Rogers JC. Activities and adaptation in late-life depression: a qualitative study. *Am J Occup Ther.* 2014;68:570-577.
34. Baum CM, Edwards DF. *Activity Card Sort.* St. Louis, MO: Washington University; 2001.
35. Pentland W. Conversations for enablement: using coaching skills in occupational therapy. *Occupational Therapy Now.* 2012;14(2):14-16. http://www.caot.ca/otnow/March12/pages%2014-16.pdf. Accessed June 18, 2016.
36. Rush DD, Shelden MLL. *The Early Childhood Coaching Handbook.* Baltimore, MD: Brookes Publishing Company; 2011.
37. Dunn W, Cox J, Foster L, Mische-Lawson L, Tanquary J. Impact of a contextual intervention on child participation and parent competence among children with autism spectrum disorders: a pretest–posttest repeated-measures design. *Am J Occup Ther.* 2012;66(5):520-528.
38. Knight J, Cornett J. *Studying the Impact of Instructional Coaching. Manuscript.* University of Kansas Center of Research on Teaching; 2009.
39. Tay HY. Setting formative assessments in real-world contexts to facilitate self-regulated learning. *Educational Research for Policy and Practice.* 2015;14(2):169-187.
40. Graham F, Rodger S, Ziviani J. Coaching parents to enable children's participation: an approach for working with parents and their children. *Austr Occup Ther J.* 2009;56(1):16-23.
41. Graham F, Rodger S, Ziviani J. Enabling occupational performance of children through coaching parents: three case reports. *Phys Occup Ther Ped.* 2010;30(1):4-15.
42. Graham F, Rodger S, Ziviani J. Effectiveness of occupational performance coaching in improving children's and mothers' performance and mothers' self-competence. *Am J Occup Ther.* 2013;67(1):10-18.
43. Missiuna CA, Pollock NA, Levac DE, et al. Partnering for change: an innovative school-based occupational therapy service delivery model for children with developmental coordination disorder. *Can J Occup Ther.* 2012;79(1):41-50.
44. Kientz M, Dunn W. Evaluating the effectiveness of contextual intervention for adolescents with autism spectrum disorders. *J Occup Ther, Schools, Early Intervention.* 2012;5(3-4):196-208.
45. Foster L, Dunn W, Lawson LM. Coaching mothers of children with autism: a qualitative study for occupational therapy practice. *Phys Occup Ther Pediatr.* 2013;33(2):253-263.
46. Kessler D, Ineza I, Patel H, Phillips M, Dubouloz CJ. Occupational Performance Coaching adapted for stroke survivors (OPC-Stroke): a feasibility evaluation. *Phys Occup Ther Geriatrics.* 2014;32(1):42-57.
47. Rogers CR. *Client-Centered Therapy: Its Current Practice, Implications and Theory.* Boston: Houghton Mifflin; 1951.
48. Lussier MT, Richard C. The motivational interview in practice. *Can Fam Physician.* 2007;53(12):2117-2118.
49. Rollnick S, Mason P, Butler C. *Health Behavior Change: A Guide for Practitioners.* London: Churchill Livingstone; 1999.
50. Miller WR, Rollnick S. *Motivational Interviewing: Preparing People for Change.* 2nd ed. New York: Guilford Press; 2002.
51. Law M, Baptiste S, Mills J. Client-centred practice: what does it mean and does it make a difference? *Can J Occup Ther.* 1995;62(5):250-257.
52. Sumsion T, Law M. A review of evidence on the conceptual elements informing client-centred practice. *Can J Occup Ther.* 2006;73(3):153-162.
53. Miller WR, Rollnick S. *Motivational Interviewing: Preparing People to Change Addictive Behavior.* New York: Guilford Press; 1991.
54. Lenze EJ, Host HH, Hildebrand MW, et al. (2012). Enhanced medical rehabilitation increases therapy intensity and engagement and improves functional outcomes in post-acute rehabilitation of older adults: a randomized-controlled trial. *J Am Med Dir Assoc.* 2012;13(8):708-712.

Mine the Gold

Client-centered assessment sets the tone for the entire therapeutic relationship with the client. It does not overstate the importance of client-centered assessment to say that it is the basis for all future interactions with the client.

Become Systematic

The 6 measures reviewed in this chapter all depend on self-report, all have similar administration times between 20 and 40 minutes, all yield results that are reported in both narrative and quantitative/scored formats, and all have desirable psychometric properties.

Use Evidence in Practice

The 6 measures reviewed in this chapter all have desirable psychometric properties.

Make Occupational Therapy Contributions Explicit

A client-centered assessment shows belief in the potential of the client and enthusiasm about his or her ability to achieve goals and overcome occupational performance problems.

Engage in Occupation-Based, Client-Centered Practice

Client-centered assessment unconditionally accepts the client's identification of problems and rating of performance and also accepts when the client says that something is not a problem.

CHAPTER 7

Measuring Occupational Performance Using a Client-Centered Perspective

Mary Ann McColl, PhD, MTS and Nancy Pollock, MSc, OT Reg. (Ont.)

This chapter focuses on assessing occupational performance using a client-centered approach. We will begin by defining and discussing client-centered practice, and then review 4 measures designed for adults and 2 for children.

Defining Client-Centered Assessment

Client-centered practice is an "orientation to practice" rather than a theory or a framework.[1] It is a way of thinking about the relationship between clients and therapists. Client-centered practice was first defined by Carl Rogers[2,3] as an approach to therapy characterized by 3 essential elements: empathic understanding, unconditional positive regard, and therapeutic genuineness. In order for therapy to be successful, Rogers claims that 6 conditions need to be present: a warm and trusting rapport, freedom to express feelings without judgement, recognition and acceptance by the client of his or her spontaneous self, responsibility for choices, developing insight, and supported growth toward maturity and independence.[4]

Since the early 1980s, client-centered practice has become the default assumption of how occupational therapists relate to their clients, and the implicit best practice in occupational therapy. Occupational therapists have calibrated the classic definition of client-centered practice to speak to the context of occupational therapy. Sumsion and Law identify 5 core elements of client-centered practice in occupational therapy:

1. A shift in the balance of power in favor of clients
2. Joint partnership between therapist and client in decision making
3. Active listening as a validation of the importance of the client's voice
4. Client choice in the goals and process of therapy
5. Hope, an emotional investment in the future[5]

Even with this focus, numerous commentators have suggested that client-centered occupational therapy amounts to little more than rhetoric.[6-8] Richard and Knis-Matthews[9] found only 35% agreement between the goals set by therapists and those set by their clients. Bright and colleagues[10] engaged in critical reflection on their practice in a rehabilitation setting, and were surprised to discover the extent to which the therapeutic relationship was governed by system and profession priorities, rather than client priorities. Kjellberg and associates[11] surveyed clients in a mental health facility, and found that only 12% to 14% identified problems and set goals for therapy autonomously. In the remaining cases, therapists made decisions, either unilaterally (20% to 22%) or in consultation with clients (66%).

Barriers to Client-Centered Assessment

Although broadly endorsed, it seems that client-centered practice is not easy to implement. Various authors have enumerated the barriers to a client-centered orientation to practice. These typically can be classified as originating in the client, the system, or the therapist.[12] While we acknowledge that some systems and some clients make it more difficult to practice from a client-centered orientation, we are most interested in the therapist-level barriers—that is, those factors that affect the day-to-day

Law M, Baum C, Dunn W, eds. *Measuring Occupational Performance: Supporting Best Practice in Occupational Therapy, Third Edition* (pp 83-94).

choices therapists make that characterize their practice as client centered or not.[9]

Perhaps the most common objection to a client-centered approach is that it takes more time.[10] It is more laborious to engage clients in a process of naming and claiming problems and identifying the desire to work on those problems than it is to simply tell them what the therapist observes to be wrong and the best way to fix it. Bright and colleagues[10] noted the extent to which they felt the pressure of time in their therapeutic relationships. They attributed the sense of urgency to organizational goals, such as early discharge, efficient use of resources, and funder restrictions. As a result, they set small "realistic" goals, rather than engaging with clients about their hopes and dreams for the future. They acknowledged that they had been co-opted by the system within which they worked, at the expense of their clients. The question is whether the time spent in client-centered assessment and practice is an investment in a better outcome or is wasted.

Another impediment often cited to client-centered practice is the perception that some types of clients simply lack the insight or ability to participate actively in their own assessment and decision making.[11] In particular, clients with mental illnesses or cognitive impairments are often questioned as to their ability to identify the most pressing problems and collaborate in figuring out the best way to address those problems. In these instances, therapists perceive that they are acting in the best interests of their clients by taking charge of the therapeutic agenda and process, but are they really just underestimating the resources that lie within clients, or are they unprepared to invest the time required to uncover those resources?[4] Colquhoun and colleagues[13] showed that 100% of their clients with cognitive impairments could identify occupational performance problems, and 94% could score those problems on importance, performance, and satisfaction.

Therapists are particularly keen to be explicitly in charge when therapy involves issues of risk or legal liability.[12] They take their responsibility for their clients very seriously and often adopt a very low tolerance for any form of risk in the therapeutic process. Although this appears benevolent on the surface, it can act to significantly undermine the autonomy and development of clients who may feel that they are being treated like children.

A fourth major objection to client-centered practice has to do with power and professionalism. As Brodley[14] puts it, the tenets of client-centered practice are in conflict with the conventional forces in professions. Professions are established to assert power and control over a domain of knowledge and practice. Client-centered practice acknowledges the power that professions and institutions have, but it asks professionals to use their power responsibly, to uphold the power that clients have to control their own destiny. Often in discussions of client-centered practice, professionals endorse the idea of "giving power" to clients. Despite the benevolent intent of this statement, it betrays an underlying assumption that power lies with the professional and that he or she may choose to bestow some of it on the client under certain circumstances.

Brodley further suggests that client-centered practice is a "disciplined expression of the therapist's character, values and attitudes."[14(p10)] In so doing, she implies that not all therapists will be up to the task. Crocker and Johnson[15] distinguish between fixing, helping, and serving. *Fixing* involves doing something for another person; *helping* involves doing something with another person. In both instances, the other is assumed to be incapable, or at least less capable. *Serving*, on the other hand, means offering what is needed to allow the other to do. Serving focuses on the served rather than the server. It assumes his or her capability, provided the necessary support. The client-centered therapist serves—a therapeutic stance that requires setting aside the ego.

A final barrier to client-centered practice is the paucity of tools that support this type of practice. Despite the broad endorsement of client-centered practice in occupational therapy, we were able to find only 4 assessments for adults and 2 for children that truly embraced a client-centered orientation. Assessment often represents a therapist's first interaction with a client. As such, it takes on considerable importance in establishing the therapeutic relationship.

Characteristics of Client-Centered Assessments

Client-centered assessments have a number of key features that render them eligible for inclusion in this chapter. First and foremost, they are self-report measures, assuming that clients know what they want. Therapists using a client-centered approach to assessment implicitly trust clients to identify the problems that will form the basis for therapeutic engagement.[16] For therapists who function from a client-centered perspective, there is no question of conflict between the problems that the therapist identifies and those that the client identifies. Only the problems that are troubling the client have status in the therapeutic process. The therapist understands his or her job in assessment as uncovering the problems for which the client is seeking help.

A second feature of the client-centered assessment is that there is no corroboration or validation by the therapist (or anyone else for that matter). The only relevant frame of reference for therapy is that of the client. Although the therapist may have knowledge and expertise about certain aspects of disability and therapy, he or she can never fully understand the values, beliefs, and experiences of the client and must therefore accept the client's reports as the most relevant source of information.

A third feature of client-centered assessments is that they are often more open-ended, affording greater opportunity to hear the client's unedited, uncensored experience of occupation. Client-centered assessment acknowledges that there is an affective component to assessment. Not all that needs to be known can be communicated as pure information. Much meaning and information is conveyed in the words chosen, the tone in which a response is delivered and the time taken to produce a response. Consider the difference between the following 2 answers to the question, "How are things going for you at work these days?"

1. "I hate that place!"
2. "Not so well, actually. I've been having trouble getting up for it each day."

Both are admittedly negative responses, but they are significantly different in the emotional tone conveyed and the amount of information exchanged. Now, compare both of these with a less open-ended format, where the same clients are asked to rate their productivity as positive, neutral, or negative. Both would say negative, but we would fail to capture the qualitative differences in their 2 experiences of occupational performance.

Two final criteria were applied when choosing the measures to be reviewed in this chapter on client-centered assessment of occupational performance. The measures chosen had to be widely used by occupational therapists in practice, education, and research. They also had to have published evidence of acceptable psychometric properties.

Client-Centered Assessment With Adults

Canadian Occupational Performance Measure

The Canadian Occupational Performance Measure (COPM)[17] is a semi-structured interview aimed at identifying problems in occupational performance. The COPM was designed to correspond to the Canadian Model of Occupational Performance (CMOP)[18] and is also compatible with the Canadian Model of Occupational Performance and Engagement (CMOP-E).[19] The COPM has 3 sections: self-care (made up of personal care, community management, and functional mobility), productivity (made up of education/training, work, and school/play), and leisure (active recreation, quiet recreation, and socialization). The COPM offers 2 scores: performance and satisfaction with performance, both of which are self-rated by the client. In addition, identified occupational performance problems are weighted in terms of the importance of those activities. This serves to establish the client's priorities and leads very naturally into goal setting and treatment planning.

The COPM has been used with clients in a wide variety of settings. It has been officially translated into 30 languages and is used in over 40 countries. The COPM has been shown to have excellent psychometric properties, with more than 45 studies providing evidence of reliability, validity, responsiveness, and utility.[17]

Two measures have been published that are very similar to the COPM and based on the identical structure. The Client-Oriented Role Evaluation[20] focuses on roles and assesses each in terms of importance, performance, and satisfaction. The Self-Identified Goals Assessment (SIGA)[21] incorporates fixed alternative questions, thus significantly compromising the client-centered aspect of the measure. A recent study found that COPM performance scores correlated very highly with SIGA scores (goals: $r=.76$; overall: $r=.62$; $p<.0001$).[22] The same study found moderate correlation between the COPM Performance Score and the OSA Competence score ($r=.54$).

Occupational Circumstances Assessment Interview and Rating Scale

The Occupational Circumstances Assessment Interview and Rating Scale (OCAIRS) (Version 4.0)[23] is based on the Model of Human Occupation (MOHO). It assesses occupational participation on the basis of a semi-structured interview and therapist ratings. The interview covers 12 major areas derived from MOHO concepts, including roles, habits, personal causation, values, interests, skills, short- and long-term goals, interpretation of past experience, physical and social environments, and readiness for change. The interview typically takes 20 to 30 minutes, with an additional 5 to 20 minutes for therapist rating. Ratings require therapist judgment to interpret statements made in the interview to assess whether they Facilitate, Allow, Inhibit, or Restrict occupational participation. The rating scales provide a template for deciding whether the individual needs minimal, moderate, or extensive occupational therapy. Three different versions of the OCAIRS are available for mental health, physical disability, and forensic settings.

Although it depends entirely on self-report data from the interview, the OCAIRS is scored by the therapist and explicitly dependent on therapist judgment of the nature and extent of problems. As such, it can be considered only partially client centered.

Results from the OCAIRS have been shown to compare very favorably with those on the Assessment of Occupational Functioning, and this is offered as proof of concurrent validity for both.[24] Studies by the authors and colleagues have shown moderate levels of inter-rater reliability and discriminant validity.[25-28] A recent study confirms the unidimensionality of the underlying construct of occupational participation and affirms the reliability and validity of the measure.[29]

Occupational Performance History Interview

The Occupational Performance History Interview (Version 2.0; OPHI-II) was included in the previous edition; however, only part of the measure qualifies as client centered. The OPHI-II is a 3-part measure based on the MOHO,[30] consisting of the following:

1. A semi-structured interview covering occupational roles, daily routine, occupational settings, occupational choices, and critical life events
2. Three rating scales completed by the therapist: Occupational Identity Scale (11 items), Occupational Competence Scale (9 items), and Occupational Settings (9 items)
3. A life history narrative co-created by the therapist and client, designed to situate occupational performance issues in historical context and to assess the trajectory of past, present, and future occupational performance.

The semi-structured format of this measure contributes to client-centered practice, and the narrative history is composed jointly by the therapist and respondent; however, the rating scales are completed by the therapist independently based on the information gleaned from the interviews. Thus, like the OCAIRS, the OPHI-II cannot be considered fully client centered.

The OPHI-II was designed to be used in conjunction with the MOHO and has been shown to be amenable to use with other theoretical perspectives.[31] Like any interview, it is dependent on the therapist's skill at establishing rapport and eliciting information. Reliability studies showed the original OPHI to be moderately stable, with high utility reported by therapists for assessing occupational performance.[31,32] International studies using the OPHI-II have shown that the 3 subscales are valid measures across cultures and languages.[33]

Occupational Self-Assessment

The Occupational Self-Assessment (Version 2.2; OSA)[34] is a 21-item self-report paper-and-pencil measure designed to conform with the MOHO[30] and with the Canadian definition of client-centered practice.[35] The OSA asks clients to rate themselves on a 4-point scale on competence and importance of issues related to volition (5 items), habituation (5 items), and performance (11 items). It further invites clients to identify those areas where they seek to make a change.

Based on a large international study using Rasch analysis, scoring keys were developed for the Competence and Value Scales, and items were aggregated into subscales: Basic Tasks of Living; Managing Life & Relationships; and Satisfaction, Enjoyment, Actualization. This analysis also confirmed the construct validity of the measure.[36] Subsequent research confirms the reliability, validity, and sensitivity of the measure.[34,37,38]

Client-Centered Assessment With Children

The ability to understand the subjective experience of children is often more difficult given their level of cognitive and language development. The ability to reflect on one's self-efficacy develops with age.[39] Efforts to develop self-report measures for children have shown that the provision of a more structured approach can support them in assessing their competence and in identifying areas important to them.[40] The addition of pictorial items or rating scales using familiar symbols such as happy faces can assist the young child in understanding the concept of self-assessment and scoring. For these reasons, client-centered assessments for children are less open-ended than adult measures.

It is important to adapt self-report tools for the child to be able to understand and complete them because the alternative has been to ask the parent to complete measures on behalf of the child. Several studies have shown that, not surprisingly, parent and child perspectives are very different.[41,42]

The COPM can be used with children, but given its open-ended interview format, it can be difficult for young children to grasp. Most of the studies in which the COPM has been used have interviewed the parents rather than the child.[43] In studies where children were the respondents, those children were typically at least 8 years of age.[44-46] Given the cognitive demands of the COPM and the requirement for self-awareness, this need for a higher level of development makes sense. Two measures developed specifically for use with children meet the criteria for inclusion in this chapter.

Child Occupational Self-Assessment

The Child Occupational Self-Assessment (COSA)[47] is an adaptation of the OSA. Designed for children from ages 8 to 13 years, this measure is also based on the MOHO frame of reference. Children respond to statements about their competence in everyday activities and the value they place on those activities. The COSA can be completed as a paper-pencil task or as a card sort. A 4-point scale for competence uses a range of sad to happy faces, and the importance value is assigned using a range of 1 to 4 stars. The results can inform the focus of therapy because the child has indicated the areas where he or she feels less competent and the value he or she places on those activities.

The COSA has been used with a variety of children experiencing occupational challenges due to physical, cognitive, and affective problems.[42,47,48] Research on the psychometric properties of the COSA using the RASCH Rating Scale Model showed that the measure has good evidence of item reliability, is sensitive enough to detect differences in respondents, and has good content and construct validity.[49-51]

Perceived Efficacy and Goal Setting System

The Perceived Efficacy and Goal Setting System (PEGS)[52] is designed for use with young children ages 5 to 10 years. Using cards with drawings of children performing typical daily activities, the child rates his or her perceived efficacy in performing those activities by sorting the cards. The cards where the child has indicated that he or she is less competent are then reviewed and are used to allow the child to decide on goals for therapy based on the importance of that activity to the child. Within the 24 test items are activities representing the areas of self-care, productivity, and leisure. Parallel teacher and parent questionnaires allow for caregiver perspectives to be included. Blank cards also permit the addition of other activities important to the child.

The PEGS has been used with populations with a wide variety of developmental disorders and disabilities.[53-57] Research focused on the psychometric properties of the PEGS indicates good internal consistency, test-retest reliability, and support for the content, construct, and discriminative validity of the measure.[58-60]

Since the publication of the PEGS, cross-cultural validation studies have been completed in Sweden and Austria,[53,59] and researchers in other countries have made suggestions for adaptation of the cards to depict more culturally relevant activities within their context.[57] A second edition of the PEGS is in development to reflect some of these findings.

Discussion

The chapter has reviewed 6 measures of occupational performance, all of which offer at least a partially client-centered approach. The measures have a number of notable similarities; for example, all depend on self-report, all have similar administration times between 20 and 40 minutes, all yield results that are reported in both narrative and quantitative/scored formats, and all have desirable psychometric properties.

The client-centered approach to assessment has a number of significant advantages. The main advantage is its tendency to enhance the sense of mastery and control among clients.[61,62] This is accomplished in a number of ways: through communication of interest in the client's perceptions of his or her problems, through the therapist's commitment to assist the client with those problems, and through the therapist's communication of confidence in the client's ability to identify and solve problems. A client-centered therapist conveys during the assessment that he or she is not going to take over the process, assume sole responsibility for the success of therapy, or impose his or her will on the client. The dominance of professionals in the process of assessment and therapy has been shown to be counter-therapeutic.[62] Professional dominance creates dependency, disempowerment, and perhaps even institutionalization. Instead, a client-centered relationship shows belief in the potential of the client, shows enthusiasm about his or her ability to achieve goals and overcome problems, and offers knowledge and experience that may be marshalled to help.

A second advantage of the client-centered approach to assessing occupational performance is the extent to which it supports an individualized approach to therapy.[63] Because clients identify occupational performance problems that are pertinent to their unique circumstances and context, occupational therapy interventions become explicitly framed in the context of that individual's life.

The third advantage of the client-centered approach is the opportunity that it presents for the therapist's own personal and professional growth and development. Unlike the traditional model, where the therapist is the only expert, client-centered therapy provides an opportunity for the therapist to learn more about occupational performance from each new client.

Given these advantages, why wouldn't every therapist subscribe to the client-centered approach? There are, of course, also challenges to assessing occupational performance from a client-centered perspective.

According to Rogers,[3] the success or failure of client-centered assessment is often a function of the therapist's personality. He acknowledges that it is not for everyone; particularly, it is not an acceptable approach for those therapists who have difficulty with a belief in the expertise of clients and their ultimate resourcefulness and adaptiveness.

It is possible that it does not work as well for all clients. Some clients appear to expect therapists to tell them what their problems are; for example, some clients from non–Western cultures are unaccustomed to being decision makers and active participants in their therapy. The client-centered approach was developed with the North American and European health care environments in mind and may not be suitable with people from other cultures. For these clients, a therapist who will not take charge may be perceived as less skilled, less effective, or less cooperative.[64-66] It is also important when assessing clients from different cultures to be aware of views of disability and illness held by the client and by other members of his or her community. Other considerations with people from non-Western cultures include cultural assumptions and expectations about therapy; roles in society; family obligations and duties; relationships with professionals; and comfort in expressing needs, setting goals, and accepting help.

It is also challenging to sustain a client-centered approach to assessment when the client has diminished cognitive capacity. There may be difficulties dealing with abstract ideas and particularly with scoring procedures, such as self-rating. The numerical rating scale has become a familiar part of Western culture; however, the idea of assigning an abstract number to occupational performance may not be suitable for all. Some clients may require the therapist to be more creative in how scores are generated. Alternative symbolic ways to illustrate the intent of the scale should be considered to facilitate clients' understanding and engagement.

Table 7-1

CANADIAN OCCUPATIONAL PERFORMANCE MEASURE (COPM)

Source	www.thecopm.ca; www.caot.ca
Key References	Law et al[17]
Purpose	• The COPM was developed to accompany the Canadian Model of Occupational Performance, and to identify problems in occupational performance.
Type of Client	• All types of clients, all ages
Test Format	• Semi-structured interview
Procedures	• Five-step process including identifying problems, weighting importance, scoring performance and satisfaction, reassessing after therapy interval.
Time Required	• Average 20 to 30 minutes
Reliability	
Inter-rater	• Seven reliability studies showing highly acceptable scores for test-retest reliability between .67 and .93. See manual for details of these studies, as well as McColl et al.[43]
Test-retest	
Internal Consistency	
Validity	
Content *Construct* *Criterion*	• Sixteen studies identified showing all types of validity of COPM in relation to common measures, such as Reintegration to Normal Living, Satisfaction with Performance Scaled Questionnaire, Functional Independence Measure
Utility	• Twenty-one utility studies showing COPM responsive to change and useful in clinical practice in a wide variety of settings and populations around the world.
Strengths	• Focuses on explicit model of occupation and occupational therapy. • Therapists report that communicates effectively with clients, families and teams about what occupational therapists do • Supports collaborative goal setting • Available in hard copy and electronic format, and in many languages.
Complexities	• Requires good interviewing skills and well-developed sense of occupation.

Client-centered assessment is also challenging when an interpreter is needed to overcome a language barrier. The ideal interpreter is someone who can communicate fluently with both therapist and client, is impartial to the outcome of the assessment, has no preconceived notions about the client, and is a good listener. Furthermore, he or she is someone in front of whom the client can tell the whole truth. Assessing the degree to which someone can act as an interpreter, knowing his or her relationship to the client, and ensuring that the interpreter is not editorializing are all important issues in obtaining the best possible information. Further, it may be useful to try to discover and take into account the interpreter's bias, if one is suspected.

A somewhat more complex situation arises when the client is noncommunicative and requires a proxy respondent rather than an interpreter. Most important in the case of proxy respondents is to be clear that they are expected to place their own wishes and impressions to one side and attempt to answer as though they were the client. From their privileged position of knowing the client, they are asked to tell us how they think the client would answer the question if he or she were able.

Client-centered assessment is also challenged when the client is too acutely ill to be able to readily identify problems. In some instances, the future may look so threatening and overwhelming that a therapeutic process may be necessary in order to help an individual get to the stage where he or she is able to identify problems. Occupational therapy may offer activities, simulations, discussions, or outings that assist the individual to begin

Table 7-2

Occupational Circumstances Assessment Interview and Rating Scale (OCAIRS—Version 4)

Source	MOHO Clearinghouse: http://www.cade.uic.edu/moho/
Key References	Haglund & Forsyth[29]; Forsyth et al[67]
Purpose	• The OCAIRS was designed to gather information on 12 concepts associated with MOHO.
Type of Client	• Three versions of the OCAIRS are available for mental health, physical disability and forensic settings.
Test Format	• Semi-structured interview and therapist-scored rating scales
Procedures	• Client is interviewed and therapist assigns ratings regarding strengths and weaknesses.
Time Required	• Interview 20 to 30 minutes and 5 to 20 minutes for therapist ratings
Reliability	
Inter-rater	• Moderate levels of inter-rater reliability[25-28]
Test-retest	• Affirms the reliability of the measure[29]
Internal Consistency	
Validity	
Content	• Concurrent validity based on Assessment of Occupational Functioning[24]
Construct	• Uni-dimensionality of the underlying construct of occupational participation and affirms the validity of the measure[29]
Criterion	• Discriminant validity—differentiates different types of psychosocial dysfunction using Global Assessment Scale[29]
Utility	• The rating scales provide a template for deciding if the individual needs minimal, moderate, or extensive occupational therapy.
Strengths	• Provides comprehensive assessment of MOHO concepts
Complexities	• Requires good interviewing skills. Ratings completed based on therapist judgment, although data come from client self-report.

to conceptualize the demands of his or her life, together with the potential pitfalls and obstacles.

Attention and memory problems make any form of assessment difficult, and with client-centered assessment, these deficits make it doubly important to find a space that is free from distractions and minimally stimulating. In order to obtain useful information, it may be necessary to complete the interview in multiple sittings if fatigue or distractibility becomes apparent.

Summary

This chapter reviews 6 measures of occupational performance that are at least partially client-centered—4 for adults and 2 for children. Client-centered assessment differs from professionally directed assessment in that it unconditionally accepts the client's identification of problems and rating of performance, and also accepts when the client says something is not a problem. Client-centered assessment is the basis for client-centered practice. In the first encounter with a client, the therapist reveals him- or herself as client-centered or not. The therapist either accepts the client's view of the situation or challenges it based on his or her own observations and evaluation. Client-centered assessment sets the tone for the entire therapeutic relationship with the client. It does not overstate the importance of client-centered assessment to say that it is the basis for all future interactions with the client.

Table 7-3

Occupational Performance History Interview (Version 2; OPHI-II)

Source	MOHO Clearinghouse http://www.cade.uic.edu/moho/
Key References	Kielhofner et al[33,68]
Purpose	• The OPHI-II is designed to assess 3 constructs of occupational adaptation: occupational identity, occupational competence, and the impact of occupation behavior settings.
Type of Client	• Occupational therapy clients who are capable of responding to an in-depth interview
Test Format	• 3 scales: occupational identity, occupational competence, occupational behavior settings
Procedures	• Life History Narrative: qualitative data from interview. Therapist interviews client and completes rating scales and Life History Narrative.
Time Required	• Approximately 1 hour
Reliability	
Inter-rater	• Not reported
Test-retest	• Rater separation statistics indicate raters have the same degree of severity and leniency.
Internal Consistency	• Not reported
Validity	
Content	• Using RASCH analysis methods, strong evidence that test items captured underlying traits. Low percentage of misfit statistics (8% to 9%) indicate validity across different subjects.
Construct	• Separation statistics indicate OPHI-II detects meaningful differences between persons and levels of competence.
Criterion	• Not reported.
Utility	• Five thematic areas: occupational roles, daily routine, environment, choices, life events
Strengths	• OPHI-II can be readily learned through the manual and used with a wide variety of clients.
Complexities	• Therapist rather than client assigns the scores.

Table 7-4

Occupational Self-Assessment (OSA)

Source	MOHO Clearinghouse http://www.cade.uic.edu/moho/
Key References	Baron et al[34]; Kielhofner et al[38]
Purpose	• The OSA was designed to measure self-rated occupational performance and environmental adaptation, according to the Model of Human Occupation.
Type of Client	• All occupational therapy clients who can self-report
Test Format	• Two-part questionnaire, with 3 response options for each question
Procedures	• Self-administered
Time Required	• 10 to 20 minutes
Reliability	
Inter-rater	• Not reported
Test-retest	• Both subscales stable over time[38]

(continued)

Table 7-4 (continued)

Occupational Self-Assessment (OSA)

Reliability	
Internal Consistency	• Not reported
Validity	
Content *Construct* *Criterion*	• Using Rasch analysis, no item misfits indicating that all 4 scales have internal Criterion validity. Scales valid for most subjects and order of item calibrations performed as Construct expected. Scores positively correlated with Falls Efficacy Scale scores[69]
Utility	• Competence and values scales, stable over time
Strengths	• Client self-report
Complexities	• Scoring very complex

Table 7-5

Perceived Efficacy and Goal Setting System (PEGS)

Source	CanChild Centre for Childhood Disability Research, www.canchild.ca
Key References	Missiuna et al[52,58]
Purpose	• The PEGS was developed as a goal-setting instrument for use with young children.
Type of Client	• Children ages 5 to 10 years.
Test Format	• Interview, card sort and questionnaires.
Procedures	• Children self-assess their perceived efficacy using pictures of daily activities and then set goals. Parallel parent and teacher questionnaires can be used.
Time Required	• Average of 15 to 20 minutes to administer, 30 minutes to score and interpret
Reliability	
Inter-rater	• Not reported
Test-retest	• Adequate Pearson coefficient .77. Swedish version reported 71% to 100% agreement.[60]
Internal Consistency	• Excellent Alpha coefficient .80.[58]
Validity	
Content	• Excellent based on the process of development and cross cultural validation studies[52,53,60]
Construct	• Excellent, hypotheses supported in validation study.[52]
Criterion	• Adequate—expected correlations with other related measures of performance and self-efficacy.[58]
Utility	• Primary use in practice to allow children to articulate what is important to them and what they want to work on in therapy.
Strengths	• Children enjoy doing the PEGS • Therapists reported value as a negotiating tool and for increasing parent and teacher understanding of the scope of occupational therapy practice. • Supports collaborative goal setting
Complexities	• Children need to be at a cognitive level of at least 5 years of age to respond.

Table 7-6

Child Occupational Self-Assessment (COSA)

Source	MOHO Clearinghouse http://www.cade.uic.edu/moho/
Key References	Keller et al[47,49,50]
Purpose	• The COSA is designed to facilitate client-directed practice through the children self-assessing their competence in performing everyday activities.
Type of Client	• Children ages 8 to 13 years
Test Format	• Checklist form or card sort form—child completed.
Procedures	• Children self-assess their competence on a list of 24 everyday activities and rate the importance of each activity to them. This is done either on a checklist form or through a card sort of items. Scoring key uses happy faces and star.
Time Required	• Estimated 10 minutes for child to complete. Not reported in manual. Time for suggested discussion of the results to aid in interpretation and development of a plan will vary.
Reliability	
Inter-rater	
Test-retest	• Item reliability through Rasch analysis for competence scores was 0.97 and 0.85 for the values scores.
Internal Consistency	• Person separation index had reliability of 0.83 for competence and 0.91 for values.
Validity	
Content	• Results for item hierarchies fit theoretical expectations. All items on competence scale meet Rasch fit requirements, while only one item on values scale does not meet requirements.
Construct	• Able to differentiate children on competence and values scales. For competence, fit on the scale for children was not significantly related to age, gender, ethnicity, diagnosis, or country.
Criterion	• Items on competence scale shown to be unidimensional, with 11.75% misfit in Rasch analysis. Values scale is not unidimensional and has an 15.3% misfit rate.
Utility	• COSA assists the therapist in understanding the child's sense of competence and facilitates collaborative goal setting with the child.
Strengths	• Children were able to understand and complete the measure. Therapists reported the COSA was valuable in helping them to get to know their clients. • The COSA includes items across occupational performance areas.
Complexities	• Children need adequate cognitive abilities for self-reflection and the desire to collaborate in goal setting.

References

1. Taylor R. *The Intentional Relationship.* Philadelphia, PA: F.A. Davis Co; 2008.
2. Rogers C. Significant aspects of client-centered therapy. *Am Psychol.* 1946;1(10):415-422.
3. Rogers C. *Client-Centered Therapy: Its Current Practice, Implications and Theory.* Boston: Houghton-Mifflin Co; 1965.
4. Rogers C. Significant Aspects of Client-Centered Therapy. Webb D. (Ed.) 2013. http://www.all-about-psychology.com/client-centered-therapy.html. Accessed June 18, 2016.
5. Sumsion T, Law M. A review of evidence on the conceptual elements informing client-centred practice. *Can J Occup Ther.* 2006;73(3):153-162.
6. Rebeiro KL. Client perspectives on occupational therapy practice: are we truly client-centred? *Can J Occup Ther.* 2000;67(1):7-14.

7. Whalley-Hammell KR. Client-centred practice in occupational therapy: critical reflections. *Scand J Occup Ther.* 2013;20:174-181.
8. Whalley-Hammell KR. Client-centred occupational therapy in Canada: refocusing on core values. *Can J Occup Ther.* 2013;80(3):141-149.
9. Richard LF, Knis-Matthews L. Are we really client-centred? Using the Canadian Occupational Performance Measure to see how the client's goals connect with the goals of the occupational therapist. *Occup Ther Mental Health.* 2010;26(1):51-66.
10. Bright F, Boland P, Rutherford SJ, Kayes NM, McPherson KM. Implementing a client-centred approach in rehabilitation: an autoethnography. *Disabil Rehabil.* 2012;34(12):997-1004.
11. Kjellberg A, Kahlin I, Haglund L, Taylor R. The myth of participation in occupational therapy: reconceptualizing a client-centred approach. *Scand J Occup Ther.* 2012;19:421-427.
12. Sumsion T, Lencucha R. Balancing challenges and facilitating factors when implementing client-centred collaboration in a mental health setting. *Br J Occup Ther.* 2007;70:513-520.
13. Colquhoun H, Letts L, Law M, MacDermid J, Edwards, M. Feasibility of the Canadian Occupational Performance Measure for routine use. *Br J Occup Ther.* 2010;73(2):48-54.
14. Brodley BT. *Practicing Client-Centred Therapy.* Ross-on-Wye, UK: PCCS Books; 2011.
15. Crocker L, Johnson B. *Privileged Presence.* Boulder, CO: Bull Publishing Co; 2006.
16. Dickerson AE. Should choice be a component in occupational therapy assessments? *Occup Ther Health Care.* 1996;10(3):23-32.
17. Law M, Baptiste S, Carswell A, McColl MA, Polatajko H, Pollock N. *The Canadian Occupational Performance Measure.* 5th ed. Toronto, Ontario: CAOT Publications; 2014.
18. Canadian Association of Occupational Therapists. *Enabling Occupation.* Ottawa: CAOT Publishing; 1997.
19. Townsend EA, Polatajko HJ. *Enabling Occupation II: Advancing an Occupational Therapy Vision of Health, Well-being, & Justice Through Occupation.* Ottawa: CAOT Publications ACE; 2007.
20. Toal-Sullivan D, Henderson PR. Client-Oriented Role Evaluation (CORE): the development of a clinical rehabilitation instrument to assess role change associated with disability. *Am J Occup Ther.* 2004;58(2):211-220.
21. Link-Melville L, Baltic TA, Bettcher TW, Nelson D. Patients' perspectives on the self-identified goals assessment. *Am J Occup Ther.* 2002;56:650-659.
22. Stuber C, Nelson DL. Convergent validity of three occupational self-assessments. *Phys Occup Ther Geriatrics.* 2010;28(1):13-21.
23. Forsyth K. *A User's Manual for the Occupational Circumstances Assessment Interview and Rating Scale: OCAIRS (Version 4.0).* Chicago, IL: Model of Occupational Performance Clearinghouse; 2005.
24. Brollier C, Watts JH, Bauer D, Schmidt W. A content validity study of the Assessment of Occupational Functioning. *Occup Ther Mental Health.* 1989;8(4):29-47.
25. Brollier C, Watts JH, Bauer D, Schmidt W. A concurrent validity study of two occupational therapy evaluation instruments: the AOF and OCAIRS. *Occup Ther Mental Health.* 1989;8(4):49-60.
26. Haglund L, Henriksson C. Testing a Swedish version of OCAIRS on two different patient groups. *Scand J Caring Sci.* 1994;8:223-230.
27. Haglund L, Thorell L-H, Walinder J. Assessment of occupational functioning for screening of patients in occupational therapy in general psychiatric care. *Occup Ther Mental Health.* 1998;18(4):193-206.
28. Deshpande S. *A User's Manual for the Occupational Circumstances Assessment Interview and Rating Scale: OCAIRS (Version 2.0).* Chicago, IL: Model of Occupational Performance Clearinghouse; 2002.
29. Haglund L, Forsyth K. The measurement properties of the Occupational Circumstances Interview and Rating Scale—Sweden (OCAIRS-S V2). *Scand J Occup Ther.* 2013;20:412-419.
30. Kielhofner G. *A Model of Human Occupation: Theory and Application.* 4th ed. Baltimore: Williams & Wilkins; 2008.
31. Kielhofner G, Henry AD, Walens D, Rogers ES. A generalizability study of the Occupational Performance History Interview. *OTJR.* 1991;11:292-306.
32. Kielhofner G, Henry AD. Development and investigation of the Occupational Performance History Interview. *Am J Occup Ther.* 1988;42:489-498.
33. Kielhofner G, Mallinson T, Forsyth K, Lai J. Psychometric properties of the second version of the Occupational Performance History Interview (OPHI-II). *Am J Occup Ther.* 2001;55:260-267.
34. Baron K, Kielhofner G, Ienger A, Goldhammer V, Wolenski J. *Occupational Self-Assessment.* Chicago: Model of Human Occupation Clearinghouse; 2002.
35. Law M, Baptiste S, Mills J. Client-centred practice: what does it mean and does it make a difference? *Can J Occup Ther.* 1995;62(5):250-257.
36. Kielhofner G, Forsyth K. Measurement properties of a client self-report for treatment planning and documenting occupational therapy outcomes. *Scand J Occup Ther.* 2001;8:131-139.
37. Taylor R, Wook Lee S, Kramer J, Shirashi Y, Kielhofner G. Psychometric study of occupational self-assessment with adolescents after infectious mononucleosis. *Am J Occup Ther.* 2011;65:e20-e28.
38. Kielhofner G, Dobria L, Forsyth K, Kramer J. The occupational self-assessment: stability and the ability to detect change over time. *OTJR.* 2010;30(1):11-19.
39. Bandura A. *Self-Efficacy: The Exercise of Control.* New York: W.H. Freeman & Co; 1997.
40. Harter S. Issues in the assessment of the self-concept of children and adolescents. In: La Greca A, ed. *Through the Eyes of the Child: Obtaining Self-reports From Children and Adolescents.* Newton, MA: Allyn and Bacon; 1990:293-325.
41. McGavin H. Planning rehabilitation: a comparison of issues for parents and adolescents. *Phys Occup Ther Pediatr.* 1998;18:69-82.
42. O'Brien JC, Bergeron A, Duprey H, Olver C, St. Onge H. Children with disabilities and their parents' views of occupational participation needs. *Occup Ther Mental Health.* 2009;25:164-180.

43. McColl MA, Law M, Baptiste S, Carswell A, Polatajko H, Pollock N. *Research on the COPM: An Annotated Resource.* Ottawa: CAOT Publications; 2006.
44. Miller LT, Polatajko HJ, Missiuna C, Mandich AD, Macnab JJ. A pilot trial of a cognitive treatment for children with developmental coordination disorder. *Hum Mov Sci.* 2001;20:183-210.
45. Palisano R. A collaborative model of service delivery for children with movement disorders: a framework for evidence-based decision making. *Phys Ther.* 2006;86(9):1295-1305.
46. Reid DT. Benefits of a virtual play rehabilitation environment for children with cerebral palsy on perceptions of self-efficacy: a pilot study. *Pediatr Rehabil.* 2002;5(3):141-148.
47. Keller J, Kafkes A, Basu S, Frederico J, Kielhofner G. *The Child Occupational Self-Assessment (Version 2.1).* Chicago, IL: MOHO Clearinghouse; 2005.
48. Kramer J. Using mixed-methods to establish the social validity of self-report assessment: an illustration using the Child Occupational Self-Assessment (COSA). *J Mix Methods Res.* 2011;5:52-76.
49. Keller J, Kafkes A, Kielhofner G. Psychometric characteristics of the Child Occupational Self-Assessment (COSA), part one: an initial examination of psychometric properties. *Scand J Occup Ther.* 2005;12:118-127.
50. Keller J, Kielhofner G. Psychometric characteristics of the Child Occupational Self-Assessment (COSA), part two: refining the psychometric properties. *Scand J Occup Ther.* 2005;12:147-158.
51. Kramer J, Kielhofner G, Smith E. Validity evidence for the Child Occupational Self-Assessment. *Am J Occup Ther.* 2010;64:621-632.
52. Missiuna C, Pollock N, Law M. *The Perceived Efficacy and Goal Setting System.* San Antonio, TX: PsychCorp; 2004.
53. Costa U. Translation and cross-cultural adaptation of the Perceived Efficacy and Goal Setting System (PEGS): results from the first Austrian-German PEGS version exploring meaningful activities for children. *OTJR.* 2014;34(3):119-130.
54. Dunford C, Missiuna C, Street E, Sibert, J. Children's perceptions of the impact of Developmental Coordination Disorder on activities of daily living. *Br J Occup Ther.* 2005;68(5):207-214.
55. Engel-Yeger B, Nagauker-Yanuv L, Rosenblum S. Handwriting performance, self-reports, and perceived self-efficacy among children with dysgraphia. *Am J Occup Ther.* 2009;63:182-192.
56. Engel-Yeger B, Weissman D. A comparison of motor abilities and perceived self-efficacy between children with hearing impairments and normal hearing children. *Disabil Rehabil.* 2009;31:352-358.
57. Missiuna C, Pollock N, Josman N, et al. *Giving Children a Voice: Cross-cultural validation of the Perceived Efficacy and Goal Setting (PEGS) System in Eight Countries.* Poster presented at the 15th International World Federation of Occupational Therapy Congress, Santiago, Chile; 2010.
58. Missiuna C, Pollock N, Law M, Walter S, Cavey N. Examination of the Perceived Efficacy and Goal Setting System (PEGS) with children with disabilities, their parents, and teachers. *Am J Occup Ther.* 2006;60:204-214.
59. Vroland-Nordstrand K, Krumlinde-Sundholm L. The Perceived Efficacy and Goal Setting System (PEGS), part I: translation and cross-cultural adaptation to a Swedish context. *Scand J Occup Ther.* 2012;19:497-505.
60. Vroland-Nordstrand K, Krumlinde-Sundholm L. The Perceived Efficacy and Goal Setting System (PEGS), part II: evaluation of test–retest reliability and differences between child and parental reports in the Swedish version. *Scand J Occup Ther.* 2012;19:506-514.
61. Emener WG. Empowerment in rehabilitation: an empowerment philosophy for rehabilitation in the 20th century. *J Rehabil.* 1991;57(4):7-12.
62. Goodall C. Preserving dignity for disabled people. *Nurs Stand.* 1992;6(35):25-27.
63. Brown SJ. Tailoring nursing care to the individual client: Empirical challenge of a theoretical concept. *Res Nurs Health.* 1992;15:39-46.
64. Jaffe Y, Kipper DA. Appeal of rational-emotive and client-centered therapies to first-year psychology and non-psychology students. *Psychol Rep.* 1982;50:781-782.
65. Schroeder DH, Bloom LJ. Attraction to therapy and therapist credibility as a function of therapy orientation. *J Clin Psychol.* 1979;35:683-686.
66. Wanigaratne S, Barker C. Clients' preferences for styles of therapy. *Br J Clin Psychol.* 1995;34:215-222.
67. Forsyth K, Deshpande S, Kielhofner G, et al. *User's Manual for the OCAIRS—Version 4.* Chicago: MOHO Clearinghouse; 2006.
68. Kielhofner G, Mallinson T, Crawford D, Nowak M, Rigby M, Henry A. *User's Manual for the OPHI-II.* Chicago, IL: Model of Occupational Performance Clearinghouse; 1998.
69. Nakamura-Thomas H, Kyougoku M. Application of occupational self assessment in community settings for older people. *Phys Occup Ther Geriatr.* 2013;31(2):103-114.

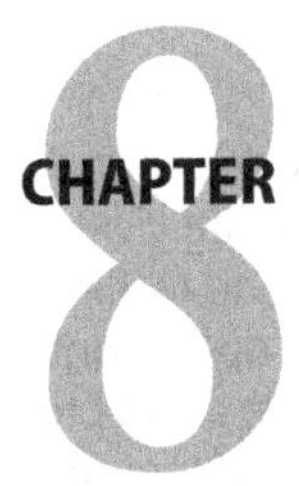

CHAPTER 8

Self-Determination and Self-Management

Joy Hammel, PhD, OTR/L, FAOTA; Danbi Lee, PhD, OTD, OTR/L; Jenna Heffron, PhD, OTR/L; and Kira Meskin, OTD, OTR/L

Two central tenets of occupational performance involve 1) being able to choose and determine the meaningful activities and roles in which you engage, and 2) being able to manage the interaction between you and environments in which you live and seek to participate.[1,2] The 2 interrelated concepts of self-determination and self-management give us a client-centered, consumer-directed, and evidence-based framework for assessing and working on these key occupational performance concepts within occupational therapy practice.

Self-determination has emerged in large part from within the grassroots disability community, especially from within the community of people with intellectual and developmental disabilities. The assessments in this area were designed to be used by people with disabilities to identify needs and issues related to choice, control, decision-making, and power. The knowledge gained from them can not only lead to increased choice and control of people with disabilities, but it also has the potential to influence emotional and physical health and quality of life outcomes for individuals and their families and social support networks, and people with disabilities as a social group in our society.

Self-management emerged as a central tenet of Bandura's self-efficacy and social cognitive learning theory that posited that people learn best from the social world around them, especially from other people going through the same issues or problems in life.[3] This social role modeling, vicarious learning, and shared problem-solving approach focuses on developing this increased self-efficacy or confidence in self that then leads to improved performance and sustained engagement. Self-management then involves socially learning several key skills such as managing symptoms of chronic conditions as they occur, communicating with health care professionals on your health needs, and managing environmental resources (social, cultural, physical, economic, information) needed to support your health and participation. Self-management builds upon self-determination by offering a systematic evidence-based approach to goal setting and action planning. Self-management assessments then focus on measuring how confident a person is in managing their everyday life and world around them so they can live life well with a chronic condition or disability.

Together, these 2 concepts and assessments related to them can inform and guide occupational therapy interventions in a socially and ecologically valid way that actively involves people with disabilities in all decision making throughout the process.

Overview of Self-Determination

Key Concepts

Self-determination is based on the belief that people with disabilities have the right to: 1) choose how they want to live; and 2) be supported in a way that facilitates their preferences.[4] In this way, self-determination is a matter of social and occupational justice.[2,4,5] Although self-determination is an important outcome for all people with disabilities, it is most commonly emphasized within education and intellectual/developmental disability (I/DD) research and practice. Supporting the development of self-determination in students with I/DD is considered best practice in secondary education and transition services and is associated with positive school, community, and adult outcomes.[6-10]

The functional model of self-determination has driven the development of assessment methods, strategies, materials, and supports for professionals to utilize in practice.[11] The functional model defines self-determined behavior as volitional actions that allow a person to be the primary causal agent in their life and to maintain or

Law M, Baum C, Dunn W, eds. *Measuring Occupational Performance: Supporting Best Practice in Occupational Therapy, Third Edition (pp 95-112).*

improve their quality of life.[12,13] *Causal agency* refers to the person exerting control over outcomes in his or her life by consciously engaging in certain actions.[7] These self-determined actions are characterized as having 4 essential characteristics: 1) the person acted autonomously; 2) the behaviors are self-regulated; 3) the person initiated and responded in a psychologically empowered manner; and 4) the person acted in a self-realizing manner.[12] In other words, if the person's actions have these 4 essential characteristics (and therefore enable them to act as a causal agent), the person can be said to have acted in a self-determined manner.[7]

Self-determination can emerge across the lifespan as children and adolescents learn to develop skills and attitudes that enable them to become causal agents.[9,10] These skills and attitudes are considered component elements of self-determination and consist of choice making; decision making; problem solving; goal setting and attainment; self-regulation/self-management; self-advocacy and leadership; positive perceptions of control, efficacy, and outcome expectation; self-awareness; and self-knowledge. Teaching these skills, creating opportunities, and providing the necessary supports are crucial to enabling people with disabilities to develop and acquire component elements, which can lead to the development of self-determined behavior.[9,10]

Self-determination is dependent both on a person's individual capacity and on opportunities available to him or her. Wehmeyer and Field[11] developed a set of quality indicators of school-wide and classroom factors that support the development of students' self-determination. Their quality indicators include the following:

- Knowledge, skills, and attitudes for self-determination are addressed in the curriculum
- Students, parents, and staff are involved participants in individualized educational decision making and planning
- Students, families, faculty, and staff are provided with opportunities for choice
- Students families, faculty, and staff are encouraged to take appropriate risks
- Supportive relationships are encouraged
- Accommodations and supports for individual needs are provided
- Students, families, and staff have the opportunities to express themselves and be understood
- Consequences for actions are predictable
- Self-determination is modeled through the school environment

Although these indicators are specific to school and classroom environments, they can be applied to other settings as well.

Several studies have shown the impact of both individual and environmental factors on a person's level of self-determination.[13-17] Further, research shows that individuals who have higher levels of self-determination achieve more positive academic, employment, and independent living outcomes and report a higher quality of life.[14,18-21] Thus, by fostering self-determination through the facilitation of individual capacity and environmental opportunities, occupational therapy practitioners can help clients to achieve desired occupational and quality of life outcomes. See Table 8-1 for a summary of key concepts related to self-determination.

Importance of Measurement in Self-Determination

Occupational therapy practitioners strive to maintain a client-centered and holistic practice and are particularly attuned to collaborating with and gathering information about clients with disabilities to gain a greater understanding of what is currently important and meaningful to them.[1] During evaluation, practitioners consider clients' desires and needs in relation to what they want to do both in the present and future. In doing so, practitioners can promote clients' sense of self-determination by providing opportunities for greater decision-making power, choice, and control related to goal identification, intervention planning, and discharge planning.[1]

However, specifically measuring clients' self-determination using standardized and informal assessments can help occupational therapy practitioners to identify their current capacities and opportunities for exerting choice and control over their lives. By understanding the facilitators and barriers to self-determination in a client's life, practitioners can be better attuned to how to utilize the facilitators and mitigate the barriers. In this way, measuring self-determination can allow practitioners to help clients obtain or maintain desired levels of control and support throughout the therapeutic process. Moreover, measuring clients' capacities and opportunities for self-determination can improve our ability to help them achieve desired levels of choice and control over their participation in life's many occupations outside of the therapeutic context, both in the present and in the future.

Overview of Self-Management

Key Concepts

Self-management has been receiving a growing interest in health care, reflecting the large health care expenditure on chronic conditions and the recognition that people with long-term conditions and disabilities need the knowledge and skills to make day-to-day decisions about their health.[22-24] Self-management also recognizes that clients are the ones who know the most about the impact of their chronic conditions and that they should have control over their health and health care.[25]

Unlike acute conditions (eg, broken leg, flu) that have known prognosis and usually a cure, chronic conditions (eg, diabetes, asthma, arthritis) and long-term disabilities (eg, stroke, cerebral palsy, multiple sclerosis) have unpredictable progress and no cure. Because of that, people with chronic conditions need to engage in daily and lifelong medical management, role management, and emotional management to monitor their conditions and fully live their life with the conditions they have.[23] Self-management refers to this "dynamic and continuous process of self-regulation" to manage the impact of the chronic conditions in everyday life.[26(p 178)]

The heart of self-management is to enable and empower people with chronic conditions to confidently manage their own health and to reduce unnecessary involvement of health care professionals. People with chronic conditions gain confidence as a self-manager by acquiring the knowledge and skills needed to manage their health and care, by trying out positive behavior changes, and by building their own strategies to maintain their behaviors despite challenges and potential setbacks. Hibbard et al[27] found that empowered and activated self-managers have the following characteristics:

- They believe that patients have important roles in self-managing care and collaborating with providers
- They have the knowledge needed to manage and maintain their condition
- They exhibit the skills and strategies to manage their condition, collaborate with their health providers, and access appropriate and quality health care

To make people with chronic conditions an activated self-manager, self-management interventions emphasize skills such as self-monitoring, problem solving, decision making, and finding and utilizing resources.[25] With these skills, individuals with chronic conditions learn how to manage symptoms and how to maintain or improve their health conditions. While traditional self-management programs have not focused beyond symptom and health management, there are programs developed by occupational therapists that focus on environment and task modification skills as means to manage the impact of long-term disabilities and chronic conditions on performance and participation.[28,29] Various measures have been used to evaluate the impact of these self-management programs or to assess individual's self-management behaviors to inform self-management interventions.[30]

Importance of Measurement in Self-Management

Self-management approaches and interventions may be used at different times in the rehabilitation process and across the continuum of health care delivery services. Occupational therapy practitioners often work with people with disabilities or people with co-morbid conditions such as diabetes, arthritis, and fatigue that require everyday and long-term management. However, occupational therapy practitioners do not work with those clients extensively or follow them across different settings (eg, from in-patient to out-patient setting). Therefore, it is important to provide self-management supports to clients while occupational therapy practitioners are part of the clients' recovery or transition.[23]

Self-management measures are important beginning points for self-management support. Using assessments, occupational therapy practitioners can evaluate and understand the clients' abilities to self-manage their health and care, which will inform the therapists how to best support their skill development.[23] For programs entailing one-to-one collaboration between a client and therapist, self-management measures such as Patient Activation Measure (PAM) can be used to tailor self-management supports to the individual needs and level of readiness. Self-efficacy scales or other health behavior scales can inform the practitioner with areas the client is more or less confident to manage. Measures such as health- or participation-related measures can be used to show whether and how self-management impacted important health and participation outcomes.

Selecting and Using Self-Determination and Self-Management Measures

See Tables 8-2 through 8-4.

Future Directions for Practice and Research in Self-Determination and Self-Management

The movement behind the development of self-determination and self-management assessment has several implications for future occupational therapy practice and research. These include the following:

- Occupational therapy practitioners now have more sophisticated and validated measurement tools to consider clients' desires, needs, and goals in relation to what they want to do now and in the future, as well as the skills they may need to confidently manage the environment and sustain their outcomes over time. Practitioners have the opportunity to promote self-determination and self-management in occupational and social role performance, and to research the impact of this development on long-term health and wellness.[1]
- Although occupational therapy practitioners know how to measure self-determination and self-management–related choice, control, and confidence in individual symptom management, less is known about how people learn how to self-manage everyday home, community, work, and social participation;

the strategies they use to do this; and the impact upon their occupational performance and health over time. These represent rich areas for further research and testing and measurement development.

- Occupational therapy practitioners need to critically examine their own power in therapeutic relationships,[31-34] and how they can shift that power back to people with disabilities and their support networks via use of self-determination and self-management approaches and instruments. Data from these instruments also can help us to evaluate our role as consultants in supporting people to make their own informed decisions.[4,5,35,36]

Overview of Measures of Self-Determination

Capacity (the individual's knowledge, skills, and perceptions) and opportunity (the individual's chances to utilize their knowledge, skills, and perceptions) are the 2 major components measured by self-determination assessments. Self-determination should be measured using a combination of informal and standardized procedures and should emphasize the input of multiple stakeholders, such as the person and his or her family, teachers, and employers. Informal procedures can include observational reports from teachers, family members, and employers; interviews with the person and his or her teachers and family; employability and independent living rating scales; and vocational skill assessments.[37] Standardized procedures can include measures such as The Arc's Self-Determination Scale (SDS),[38] Quality of Life Questionnaire (QOL.Q),[39] and Community Participation Indicators (CPI) Enfranchisement Scale.[40] Together, these informal and standardized measures can provide a holistic view of the person's capacity and opportunity for self-determination.

In addition to the measures reviewed in this chapter, several other assessments are available that measure self-determination across populations and settings. These include the American Institutes for Research (AIR) Self-Determination Scale[41] (available at http://education.ou.edu/zarrow), Field Hoffman Self-Determination Assessment Battery[42] (available at https://www.ghaea.org), Express Yourself! Assessing Self-determination in Your Life[43] (available at www.uic.edu), Wellness Recovery Action Plan[44] (WRAP; available at www.mentalhealthrecovery.com/wrap/), Personal Preference Indicators Assessment[45] (available at http://education.ou.edu/zarrow), and Money Follows the Person Quality of Life Scale.[46]

Selection Criteria for Review

The standardized measures reviewed in this chapter were selected based on the following 3 factors:

1. The measure's usefulness in evaluating the 4 essential characteristics of self-determination across different populations and in different contexts
2. The level to which the measure includes self-report indicators and involves key stakeholders in the evaluation process
3. The measure's ability to be conducted alongside other self-determination measures and procedures in order to create a holistic view of the individual's capacity and opportunities for self-determination

Each measure meets the necessary criteria for reliability and validity. Although all measures are evidence-based, some are well established while others are emerging as relevant and important tools for assessing self-determination.

List of Measures Reviewed in This Chapter

- The Arc's SDS (Table 8-5)
- QOL.Q (Table 8-6)
- CPI Enfranchisement Scale (Table 8-7)

Overview of Measures of Self-Management

Most common constructs that are measured to evaluate self-management interventions are self-efficacy, health behavior/attitude, health status, health service utilization, quality of life, and psychological indicators.[30] While self-efficacy and health behavior/attitude measure self-management behaviors, other constructs assess the outcomes or the following impact when one maintains self-management behaviors.

Measures to Assess Self-Management Behaviors

The major construct measured specific to self-management is self-efficacy. Self-efficacy theory represents the most commonly cited and studied theory guiding self-management interventions. Self-efficacy is a person's belief and confidence to perform specific behaviors.[3] A person with a strong sense of efficacy enhances personal accomplishment and well-being as he or she maintains strong commitment to master skills and challenges and quickly recover after failures or setbacks.[3] Therefore, a confident person is more likely to take an action to initiate and maintain behavioral changes. Various self-efficacy scales are available to measure confidence in areas requiring management:

Table 8-1

SUMMARY OF KEY CONCEPTS RELATED TO SELF-DETERMINATION

Key Concept	*Definition*
Self-determination	The state of acting volitionally in a way that causes a person to be the primary causal agent in his or her own life and to maintain or improve his or her quality of life. A person's current capacity for self-determination can be defined as the degree to which he or she possesses a set of skills needed to exert choice and control, but moreover, this capacity is impacted by environmental (eg, physical, social, political) characteristics that serve as barriers to and/or opportunities for the exertion of such choice and control.
Occupational justice	A person's right to full participation in everyday occupations, regardless of disability status
Causal agency	*Causal* refers to expressing or indicating a purpose, intent, or cause. *Agent* means one who acts or has the authority to act. Thus, *causal agency* implies that individuals who make or cause things to happen in their lives do so with the intended outcome of achieving a specific end or creating change, acting in a volitional and purposeful manner.
Autonomy	Having choice and control over decisions and actions in one's life does not necessarily mean acting on one's own without help from others
Empowerment	The obtainment of power by a marginalized or oppressed group (such as people with disabilities).[47] People with disabilities can become empowered as they advocate for themselves and become self-determined. Occupational therapy practitioners cannot empower clients, but they can support their clients throughout their empowerment process
Advocacy	Includes self-advocacy (expressing one's own needs, wants, and preferences) and collective advocacy (a group of people rallying around a common cause, often a political position related to disability rights). Occupational therapy practitioners can promote clients' self-determination by supporting their self-advocacy skills and by advocating alongside them.
Dignity of risk	The right of people with disabilities to take risks as they see fit rather than have their decisions and actions controlled by others
Environmental opportunities and supports	A key requirement for self-determination, the environment can be set up to either support or inhibit an individual from obtaining a desired level of self-determination.

- Symptom management: Chronic disease, arthritis, and diabetes self-efficacy scales (see www.patienteducation.stanford.edu for complete forms), Fall Self-Efficacy scale[48]
- Activity/participation management: Participation Strategies Self-Efficacy Scale,[49] Daily living Self-Efficacy scale,[50] Reasonable Accommodation Self-Efficacy Scale[51]

An emerging measure in self-management is the PAM. The PAM serves as a measure of self-management supports with a belief that activated and engaging people are more likely to have better health outcome.[52] Other more objective self-management behavior measures include frequency of engagement in physical activities, use of self-management techniques, and adherence to doctor's recommendations.[30] These are important outcomes as they indicate whether the person utilizes and performs management skills to manage conditions, assessing the actual behavioral change. Stanford Patient Education Research Center offers various assessments to document self-management behaviors such as exercise, communication with physicians, relaxation, and eating breakfast with protein (see www.patienteducation.stanford.edu for complete forms).

Measures to Assess Outcomes of Self-Management Behaviors

Positive behavior changes may influence health status, health service utilization, or quality of life of a person with chronic conditions. Other frequently used measures in the area of self-management thus include those indicators. Health status can be assessed with self-rated health, pain, fatigue, social/role activity limitations, sleep, and stress.[30]

Table 8-2

STRATEGIES FOR SELECTING MEASURES OF SELF-DETERMINATION AND SELF-MANAGEMENT

Select Measures That Do the Following:
• Include self-report indicators
• Involve key stakeholders (eg, client, family member, educator, and/or service provider)
• Are well-researched and proven to be reliable and valid
• Assess environmental conditions (eg, supports and barriers)
• Evaluate the effectiveness of the service delivery program presently being employed (eg, empowerment program evaluation)
• Assess a full range of performance abilities across different contexts and areas of the client's life
• Can be conducted alongside other self-determination measures and procedures
Consider the Following:
• The client's perspective and experiences (eg, meaningful occupations, reason for referral, issues to be addressed during therapy)
• The measure's intended setting and targeted population (ie, some measures are appropriate for specific settings or populations)
• Cognitive accessibility of the assessment tool
• The time involved to conduct the assessment
• Searching outside the field of occupational therapy (eg, special education, nursing) for applicable measures
• The purpose of using the assessment (eg, baseline information, change over time)

Health care utilization is generally measured through frequency of visits to physicians and the emergency department, hospitalization, and readmission. Other outcomes of self-management are related to changes in performance, participation, and well-being. Informed and effective self-managers can build and maintain routines and manage their roles and occupations by controlling or managing the impact of chronic conditions in their everyday lives, which results in improved performance, participation, and well-being. Those constructs can be assessed using other performance, participation-based assessments, or quality of life measures introduced in other chapters in this book.

Selection Criteria for Review

As described in the previous section, there are various measures available to be used alone or in combination according to the different goals of evaluation.[30] Out of these many constructs that can be measured, the measures reviewed in the following tables include assessments that directly measure self-management behaviors. Most of them are self-efficacy scales that are most commonly used and can be useful in occupational therapy practice. The PAM is also included as it is gaining more attention in the area of self-management and shows strong psychometric evidence and strong correlation with health outcomes.[52]

List of Measures Reviewed in This Chapter

- Falls Self-Efficacy Scale (Table 8-8)
- Chronic Disease Self-Efficacy Scale (Table 8-9)
- PAM (Table 8-10)
- Daily living Self-Efficacy Scale (Table 8-11)
- Participation Strategies Self-Efficacy Scale (Table 8-12)

ACKNOWLEDGMENT

The authors gratefully acknowledge Katherine E. McDonald, PhD for her input on the self-determination portion of this chapter.

Table 8-3

Factors to Remember When Measuring Self-Determination and Self-Management

Issues With Self-Report

- Although self-reporting measures can support clients' participation in the therapeutic process, self-reports have been critiqued for their ability to obtain objective data (eg, the person's responses may depend on how he or she was feeling at the time of completion, the person may report answers he or she deems to be socially desirable, etc).

Issues With Proxy Report

- Although a proxy report can provide valuable information about a client that may not be obtained otherwise, it may not be as accurate as if the client were reporting for him- or herself.
- Using a proxy report should be used as a final resort; that is, steps should be taken to modify/adapt an existing assessment, create an informal assessment that is accessible to the client, and/or conduct an assisted interview before using a proxy report. Proxy reports should NOT be used for convenience purposes or in an effort to save time.

Cognitive Accessibility Issues

- Even assessments that have been created with cognitive accessibility in mind may not be accessible to all clients with disabilities
    - Assessments may need to be modified, such as by simplifying language, instructions, and/or using pictures/visual supports (be sure to follow the assessment's guidelines in regard to modifying standardized assessments for accessibility)
    - If you are unable to locate an assessment that meets your client's cognitive accessibility needs, consider using an informal assessment and/or pairing a standardized (and potentially adapted) instrument with an informal one.

Self-Determination

Measurement Results Are Not Absolute Truths

- Even if measurement results indicate low levels of self-determination in a client, do not allow this information to limit the opportunities that you make available to him or her. You might be surprised by what your client can actually do when provided with a just-right challenge and given opportunities for self-determination.
- As Calculator and Black noted, it is "preferable to set expectations that may be later proven to be too high than to aim low and underestimate students' capabilities."[53(p 330)]

Self-Management

Issue With Self-Efficacy Scales

- There may be challenges in using a self-efficacy scale as a self-report outcome measure. Clients may overestimate their own confidence at baseline and later come to the realization that they were not as knowledgeable and skilled as they thought. As such, increased self-awareness can lead to decreased ratings of confidence, although it is likely that confidence will build and maintain over time. It is important to be aware of such possibility and to attempt to collect outcomes over time and flexibly through multiple means, including a combination of self-report and performance-based clinical assessments.

Table 8-4

Strategies for Reporting About Self-Determination and Self-Management

- Utilize a strengths-based approach in the written and verbal reports.
    - Emphasize the person's abilities rather than focusing on deficits.
- Structure and format the written and/or verbal report in an accessible manner.
    - Use plain language that is familiar and accessible to the client and his or her family/caregivers. Do not use jargon.
    - Use graphics or photographs to depict a topic or word, text that is at least size 14 font, short sentences with 1- and 2-syllable words when possible, and examples from your time with the client.

Self-Determination

- Use the measure as a tool to support the client's participation in the meeting, particularly during reporting and decision making.
    - Discuss with the person ahead of time how he or she wants to be involved, such as by using his or her responses and results from the measure (eg, preferences, strengths, limitations, goals) to guide goal setting and intervention planning/transition planning.
- Use the measure as a tool to help the client be more in control of his or her own therapy progress and outcomes.
    - Using the results, gain feedback from the client about therapy interventions, and initiate or continue conversations with the client about barriers and facilitators to self-determination that they are experiencing.

Self-Management

- Use the measure as a tool to motivate the client to make lifestyle changes
    - Using the results, discuss areas of lack of confidence/action and strategies to increase confidence or promote behavioral changes.
    - Use with self-management support techniques such as motivational interviewing.

Table 8-5

The Arc's Self-Determination Scale (SDS)

Source	Available for free download at http://education.ou.edu/zarrow
Key References	Wehmeyer & Kelchner[38]; Wehmeyer[54]
Purpose	• Measures overall self-determination • Provides information on each of the 4 essential characteristics of self-determination: autonomy, self-regulation, psychological empowerment, and self-realization

(continued)

Table 8-5 (continued)

The Arc's Self-Determination Scale (SDS)

Type of Client	• Adolescents with mild cognitive disabilities
Test Format	• Scale consists of 72 items • Subscale scores as well as a total self-determination score can be calculated. Higher scores indicate higher levels of self-determination.
Procedures	• The student provides responses using a 4-point Likert scale measure; other items require the student to complete a story, identify goals, and make a choice between 2 options.
Time Required	• Approximately 30 minutes to 1 hour to complete
Standardization	• The measure was field-tested with a sample of 500 adolescents with cognitive disabilities.
Reliability	
Test-Retest	• Not reported
Internal Consistency	• The measure has good internal consistency: α=.90 for the scale as a whole (α=.90 for the Autonomy domain, α=.73 for the Psychological Empowerment domain, and α=.62 for the Self-Realization domain). The lower alpha levels for the last 2 domains are not unexpected for measures that assess perceptions and beliefs.
Inter-Rater	• Not reported
Validity	
Content	• Not reported
Construct	• The measure has discriminative validity. The scale differed in most skill measurement areas by chronological age (older students did better), and differentiated between students with cognitive disabilities and students without disabilities.
Criterion	• Concurrent criterion-related validity was established by showing relationships with conceptually related measures, including measures of locus of control, academic achievement attributions, and self-efficacy. Most relationships to other measures are moderate to strong (.25 to .5), and relationships are strongest in the predictable areas.
Utility	
Research Programs	• Can be used to evaluate outcomes of self-determination programs and interventions
Practice Settings	• Can be used to generate discussion with students about things that they find interesting or problematic, or that they want to discuss further • The normed data can provide information about student strengths and weaknesses and, therefore, guide intervention.
Strengths	• Can be used with ease in various settings beyond the school system. For example, the adult version of the SDS is identical to the student version, with the exception of minor changes to reflect outcomes appropriate for adults (eg, addresses work instead of school). • Suited for both individual and group administration
Complexities	N/A

Table 8-6

Quality of Life Questionnaire (QOL.Q)

Source	IDS Publishing Corporation, P.O. Box 389, Worthington, OH 43085
Key References	Schalock et al[39,55]
Purpose	• To measure the overall quality of life of people with intellectual and developmental disabilities (I/DD)
Type of Client	• Adults with I/DD
Test Format	• 40-item scale, interview style format
Procedures	• The respondent chooses the most appropriate response to his or her life situation from 3 possible responses. Response scores range from 1 (low) to 3 (high). • Overall QOL.Q score consists of scores from 4 subscales: (1) satisfaction, (2) competence/productivity, (3) empowerment/independence, and (4) social belonging.
Time Required	• Completion time not reported
Standardization	• The measure was standardized for people with intellectual disabilities. • Lachapelle et al[19] tested the measure with an international sample of 182 adults with mild I/DD living in community settings (with family, independently, or in a supported living setting). • Caballo et al[56] also validated the measure for use with Mexican and Spanish populations.
Reliability	
Test-Retest	• Very good test-retest ($r=.87$) reliability
Internal Consistency	• Very good internal consistency ($\alpha=.90$)
Inter-Rater	• Very good inter-rater reliability ($r=.83$)
Validity	
Content	• Has been shown to have good structural validity using factor analysis
Construct	• Evidence of construct validity • Has a strong history of construct validation with other populations, including visually disabled adults
Criterion	• Has a strong history of criterion validation with other populations, including visually disabled adults • Lachapelle et al's[19] correlational analyses determined significant positive correlations between this measure's overall QOL.Q scores and the Arc's SDS's overall SD scores ($r=0.49$, $P<0.01$), as well as on all of the subscale scores except one.
Utility	
Research Programs	• Can be used to evaluate outcomes of self-determination interventions
Practice Settings	• Can be used to initiate discussions about the interconnectedness of the client's self-determination and quality of life • Can be used to evaluate outcomes of self-determination interventions
Strengths	• Useful for determining client satisfaction with his or her quality of life • Can be useful in initiating conversations between professionals and clients, and can help the team to get at the core of barriers and facilitators to self-determination
Complexities	N/A

Table 8-7

Community Participation Indicators (CPI) Enfranchisement Scale

Source	Instrument is available from authors upon request
Key References	Heinemann et al[40,57]
Purpose	• To assess the environmental context of participation; specifically, it measures enfranchisement, a complex construct that reflects people's subjective assessments of whether the communities in which they participate value their full participation.
Type of Client	• Adults (age 18 years or older) with and without disabilities
Test Format	• 48 items with 5-point Likert scale response options (all the time, frequently, sometimes, seldom, almost never)
Procedures	• The respondent completes the items on this self-report measure.
Time Required	• Completion time not reported
Standardization	• Heinemann et al[40] pilot tested the initial draft measure with 258 adults with and 68 adults without disabilities. The revised version was evaluated with 461 adults with and 451 without self-identified activity limitations. • Heinemann et al[57] tested the measure with 1163 adults with different types and degrees of disabilities.
Reliability	
Test-Retest	• Not reported
Internal Consistency	• Cronbach's alpha was $\alpha = .96$
Inter-Rater	• Not reported
Validity	
Content	• Eighteen focus groups with 63 people with disabilities were conducted to develop conceptual framework and inform item development. • Sixteen cognitive interviews were done to ensure item comprehension.
Construct	• Heinemann et al[40] reported that people without self-identified disabilities reported higher levels of enfranchisement than did people with disabilities, thus supporting the instrument's construct validity • Heinemann et al[57] found that Rasch analysis confirms the items fit. The importance and control items also correlated with disability severity.
Criterion	• Not reported
Utility	
Research Programs	• Can be used as an outcome measure for self-determination interventions focusing on improving community participation
Practice Settings	• Can be used to assess a client's perceived opportunities for self-determination in their community
Strengths	• Can help gain useful information about how the environment can either support or hinder self-determination • Unique in that it assesses the environmental context from the perspective of people with disabilities themselves, which places the onus of change on the environment rather than on the person him- or herself
Complexities	N/A

Table 8-8

FALLS SELF-EFFICACY SCALE (FES)

Source	Rehab Measure: http://www.rehabmeasures.org/PDF%20Library/Falls%20Efficacy%20Scale.pdf
Key References	Tinetti et al[48]
Purpose	• To assess self-efficacy of balance and stability during activities of daily living and fear of falling in the elderly population
Type of Client	• Older adults, individuals with brain injury, multiple sclerosis, Parkinson's disease, spinal cord injury, and stroke
Test Format	• 10-item paper questionnaire
Procedures	• The rater reads the questions and records the client's responses. The client can also self-administer the questionnaire.
Time Required	• Approximately 10 to 15 minutes to complete
Standardization	• Tinetti et al[48] and Powell and Myers[58] tested the measure with community-dwelling older adults with a sample size of 74 and 60, respectively. • Hellström and Lindmark[59] recruited 30 individuals with stroke to test the measure. • Medley et al[60] tested the measure with 26 individuals with brain injury. • Cakt et al[61] tested the FES with 45 adults with multiple sclerosis. • Wirz et al[62] tested the measure with 42 adults with spinal cord injury. • Rahman et al[63] tested the measure with 110 adults with Parkinson's disease.
Reliability	•
Test-Retest	• Tinetti et al[48] reported adequate test-retest reliability ($r=0.71$) with older adults. • Hellström and Lindmark[59] reported excellent test-retest reliability (ICC=0.97) with people with stroke.
Internal Consistency	• Tinetti et al[48] reported strong internal consistency ($\alpha=0.91$).
Inter-Rater	• Not reported
Validity	
Content	• Not reported
Construct	• Medley et al[60] reported adequate correlation coefficients with the Berg Balance Scale, Assistive Device, and Dynamic Gait Index Score ($p<0.05$) with people with brain injury. • Rahman et al[63] demonstrated that the measure discriminated fallers and non-fallers (fallers showed significantly lower confidence) among people with Parkinson's disease.
Criterion	• Powell and Myers[58] reported excellent correlation with the Activities Specific Balance Confidence Scale (ABC) ($r=0.84$) among community-dwelling older adults. • Wirz et al[62] reported excellent concurrent validity with the Berg Balance Scale and the 16-item FES-I ($r=-0.81$) among people with spinal cord injury. • Cakt et al[61] reported excellent correlation with 10-meter walk test, Dynamic Gait Index, Functional Reach, and Beck Depression Inventory among people with multiple sclerosis.
Utility	
Research Programs	• Can be used to evaluate outcomes of falls prevention self-management interventions
Practice Settings	• Can be used as a tool to assess fear or risk of falling before/during treatment sessions • Recommended to be used in inpatient rehabilitation with people with stroke to evaluate their confidence level in mobility and balance
Strengths	• Has a long history and has been tested with various populations • Is a short questionnaire to assess fear of falling or risk of falling
Complexities	N/A

Table 8-9

Chronic Disease Self-Efficacy (6-Item Short Form Is Available)

Source	Stanford Patient Education Research Center: http://patienteducation.stanford.edu/research/secd32.html
Key References	Lorig et al[64,65]
Purpose	• To assess self-efficacy to perform self-management behaviors
Type of Client	• Individuals with chronic conditions
Test Format	• 32-item paper questionnaire with 10 subscales (exercise regularly; get information on disease; obtain help from community, family, friends; communication with physician; manage disease in general; do chores; do social/recreational activities; manage symptoms; manage shortness of breath; and control/manage depression)
Procedures	• The rater reads the questions and records client's responses. The client can also self-administer the questionnaire.
Time Required	• It takes approximately 20 minutes to administer the test. Scoring may take an additional 5 to 10 minutes for calculating subscales.
Standardization	• Lorig et al[64] tested the measure with baseline information of 1130 individuals with existing chronic conditions who were enrolled in the randomized control trial of the Chronic Disease Self-Management Program (CDSMP).
Reliability	
Test-Retest	• Test-retest reliability ranged from 0.72 to 0.89 for 9 subscales.
Internal Consistency	• Internal consistency ranged from .77 to .92 for 8 subscales (2 subscales include 1 item only).
Inter-Rater	• Not reported
Validity	
Content	• Not reported
Construct	• Not reported
Criterion	• Not reported
Utility	
Research Programs	• Particularly developed to evaluate Stanford Chronic Disease Self-Management programs • Can be used to evaluate self-management behavior outcomes for other self-management–based interventions and with various populations
Practice Settings	• Can be used to evaluate confidence in self-management behaviors of clients with comorbid conditions such as diabetes, arthritis, or asthma
Strengths	• Widely used to evaluate the CDSMP • Can be used across different chronic conditions
Complexities	N/A

Table 8-10

Patient Activation Measure (PAM)

Source	Purchase through Insignia Health: http://www.insigniahealth.com
Key References	Hibbard et al[27,66]
Purpose	• To assess the extent to which clients with chronic conditions are activated (the knowledge, skills, and confidence integral to managing one's own health and health care)
Type of Client	• Adults and older adults with chronic conditions • Adults with mental health condition • Employees with and without chronic conditions
Test Format	• 22-item paper questionnaire
Procedures	• The rater reads the questions and records the client's responses. The client can also self-administer the questionnaire. • The total score can be categorized into 4 different levels of activation.
Time Required	• Approximately 15 minutes to complete
Standardization	• Hibbard et al[27] tested the measure via telephone surveys with national sample of 1515 people age 45 years and older. • Hibbard et al[66] developed a short form of PAM by reducing the number of items to 13 items. • Fowles et al[67] tested the measure with 625 employees to test whether the measure can be used with a broader population. • Green et al[68] tested the PAM with people with mental health conditions with an adapted version PAM-MH. • Skolasky et al[69] further tested the measure with 855 older adults who have multimorbidity.
Reliability	
Test-Retest	• Hibbard et al[27] reported good test-retest reliability based on 95% confidence interval (CI) estimate. • Green et al[68] reported good test-retest reliability ($r=0.74$) of the PAM-MH.
Internal Consistency	• Hibbard et al[27] and Skolasky et al[69] show high internal consistency with both adults with chronic conditions and older adults with multiple conditions ($\alpha=0.87$ and 0.91, respectively).
Inter-Rater	• Not reported
Validity	
Content	• Items were developed based on literature review, expert consensus process, and 2 patient focus groups.[27]
Construct	• Hibbard et al[27] reported strong construct validity (higher activation was significantly associated with better health, less health care utilization, better health behaviors, and lower fatalism). • Skolasky et al[69] supported construct validity by showing that PAM scores are positively associated with physical activity, structured exercise, and adaptive health behavior among older adults. • Green et al[68] reported that the PAM-MH has concurrent validity (strong relationship with Recovery Assessment Scores).
Criterion	• Hibbard et al[27] reported strong criterion validity.

(continued)

Table 8-10 (continued)

Patient Activation Measure (PAM)

Utility	
Research Programs	• Can be used as an outcome measure of self-management interventions
Practice Settings	• Can be used to assess activation level of the client to tailor self-management support matching client's level
Strengths	• Shows consistently good psychometric properties at individual patient level and across different populations • Shows strong association with health behavior outcomes • Level of activation predicts health care outcomes such as medication adherence and hospitalization
Complexities	N/A

Table 8-11

Daily Living Self-Efficacy Scale (DLSS)

Source	Maujean et al[50]
Purpose	• To assess self-efficacy in daily functioning
Type of Client	• Tested with people with stroke, but can be used with people with any type of disabilities
Test Format	• 12-item paper questionnaire with 2 subscales (psychosocial functioning and activities of daily living)
Procedures	• The rater reads the questions and records the client's responses. The client can also self-administer the questionnaire.
Time Required	• Approximately 10 minutes to complete
Standardization	• The measure was tested with 2 groups: 259 people with stroke and 165 caregivers and community members who did not have a stroke.
Reliability	
Test-Retest	• Maujean et al[50] reported good to excellent temporal stability when administered twice, with a mean interval of 8.76 days (ICC > 0.75).
Internal Consistency	• Internal consistency ranged between 0.91 and 0.95 for the overall scale and 2 subscales.
Inter-Rater	• Not reported
Validity	
Content	• Items were developed based on literature review, review of existing measures, and clinical experiences with people with stroke.
Construct	• The measure has convergent validity: high positive correlation with the Patient Competency Rating Scale and moderate positive correlation with the Generalized Self-Efficacy Scale (p < 0.001). • The measure has discriminant validity: a nonsignificant correlation with the Telephone Interview for Cognitive Status—Modified (TICS-M) and low relationship with Barthel Index. • The measure discriminated the stroke and non-stroke groups on the overall scale and subscales.
Criterion	• Not reported

(continued)

Table 8-11 (continued)

Daily Living Self-Efficacy Scale (DLSS)

Utility	
Research Programs	• Can be used to assess function level self-efficacy outcomes of self-management programs
Practice Settings	• Can be used to assess confidence in effectively functioning in the community before discharge or in community-based settings
Strengths	• Unique in that it measures self-efficacy on a functional level
Complexities	N/A

Table 8-12

Participation Strategies Self-Efficacy Scale (PS-SES)

Source	Instrument is available from authors upon request
Key References	Lee et al[49]
Purpose	• To assess self-efficacy in utilizing strategies to live and participate in the community
Type of Client	• Tested with people with stroke, but can be used with people with any type of disabilities
Test Format	• 35-item paper questionnaire with 6 subscales (managing home participation; staying organized; planning and managing community participation; managing communication; and advocating for resources)
Procedures	• The rater reads the questions and records the client's responses. The client can also self-administer the questionnaire.
Time Required	• Approximately 20 minutes to complete
Standardization	• The instrument was tested with 166 adults with mild to moderate stroke.
Reliability	
Test-Retest	• Not reported
Internal Consistency	• The measure shows high internal consistency ranging between 0.86 and 0.93 for 6 subscales.
Inter-Rater	• Not reported
Validity	
Content	• Items were developed based on literature review and expert panel reviews.
Construct	• Not reported
Criterion	• Not reported
Utility	
Research Programs	• Can be used as an outcome measure for self-management interventions focusing on improving participation in the community
Practice Settings	• Can be used to assess confidence in participation management before discharge or in a community-based setting • Provides a set of strategies that can be taught to clients to improve their management in home, community, work, and communication participation
Strengths	• Is the only measure that evaluates self-efficacy in managing participation level activities with an emphasis on environmental and activity modifications
Complexities	N/A

References

1. American Occupational Therapy Association. Occupational therapy practice framework: domain & practice, 3rd ed. *Am J Occup Ther.* 2014;68(suppl 1):S1-S51.
2. Hammel J, Charlton J, Jones R, Kramer J, Wilson T. Disability rights and advocacy: partnering with disability communities to support full participation in society. In Boyt Schell BA, Gillen G, Scaffa ME, eds. *Willard & Spackman's Occupational Therapy.* 12th ed. Baltimore, MD: Lippincott, Williams & Wilkins; 2014:1031-1050.
3. Bandura A. *Self-Efficacy: The Exercise of Control.* New York, NY: W.H. Freeman; 1997.
4. Pennell RL Self-determination and self-advocacy: shifting the power. *J Disabil Policy Stud.* 2001;11(4):223-227.
5. Kielhofner G. Rethinking disability and what to do about it: disability studies and its implications for occupational therapy. *Am J Occup Ther.* 2005;59(5):287-496.
6. Handley-More D, Wall E, Orentlicher ML, Hollenbeck J. Working in early intervention and school settings: current views of best practice. *Early Intervention School Special Interest Section Quarterly.* 2013;20(2):1-4.
7. Wehmeyer ML. Assessment and intervention in self-determination. In Scruggs TE, Mastropieri MA, eds. *Advances in Learning and Behavioral Disabilities.* Bingley, UK: Emerald Group Publishing Limited; 2011.
8. Wehmeyer ML, Abery B, Mithaug DE, Stancliffe RJ. *Theory in Self-Determination: Foundations for Educational Practice.* Springfield, IL: Charles C. Thomas Publisher Ltd; 2003.
9. Wehmeyer ML, Agran M, Hughes C, Martin J, Mithaug DE, Palmer S. *Promoting Self-Determination in Students With Intellectual and Developmental Disabilities.* New York, NY: The Guilford Press; 2007.
10. Wehmeyer ML, Palmer SB, Soukup JH, Garner NW, Lawrence M. Self-determination and student transition planning knowledge and skills: predicting involvement. *Exceptionality.* 2007;15:31-44.
11. Wehmeyer ML, Field SL. *Self-Determination: Instructional and Assessment Strategies.* Thousand Oaks, CA: Corwin Press; 2007.
12. Wehmeyer ML. Self-determination and individuals with severe disabilities: re-examining meanings and misinterpretations. *Res Pract Persons Severe Disabl.* 2005;30(3):113-120.
13. Shogren KA, Wehmeyer ML, Palmer SB, et al. Understanding the construct of self-determination: examining the relationship between the Arc's self-determination scale and the American Institutes for Research self-determination scale. *Assessment Effect Intervention.* 2008;33(2):94-107.
14. Nota L, Ferrrari L, Soresi S, Wehmeyer ML. Self-determination, social abilities, and the quality of life of people with intellectual disabilities. *J Intellect Disabil Res.* 2007;51:850-865.
15. Stancliffe RJ, Abery BH, Smith J. Personal control and the ecology of community living settings: beyond living-unit size and type. *Mental Retardation.* 2000;105:431-454.
16. Wehmeyer ML, Bolding N. Self-determination across living and working environments: a matched-samples study of adults with mental retardation. *Mental Retardation.* 1999;37:353-363.
17. Wehmeyer ML, Bolding N. Enhanced self-determination of adults with intellectual disabilities as an outcome of moving to community-based work or living environments. *J Intellect Disabil Res.* 2001;45:371-383.
18. Fowler CH, Konrad M, Walker AR, Test DW, Wood WM. Self-determination interventions' effects on the academic performance of students with developmental disabilities. *Educ Train Dev Disabil.* 2007;42(3):270-285.
19. Lachapelle Y, Wehmeyer ML, Haelewyck MC, et al. The relationship between quality of life and self- determination: an international study. *J Intellect Disabil Res.* 2005;49:740-744.
20. Martorell A, Gutierrez-Recacha P, Perda A, Ayuso-Mateos JL. Identification of personal factors that determine work outcome for adults with intellectual disability. *J Intellect Disabil Res.* 2008;52(12):1091-1101.
21. Wehmeyer ML, Palmer SB. Adult outcomes for students with cognitive disabilities three-years after high school: the impact of self-determination. *Educ Train Dev Disabil.* 2003;38(2):131-144.
22. Bodenheimer T, Lorig K, Holman H, Grumbach K. Patient self-management of chronic disease in primary care. *J Am Med Assoc.* 2002;288(19):2469-2475.
23. Hammel J, Finlayson M, Lee D. An organization-centered strategy: self-management: an evolving approach to maintain health, participation and wellbeing. In Christiansen CH, Baum CM, Bass-Haugen J, eds. *Occupational Therapy: Performance, Participation, and Well-Being.* 4th ed. Thorofare, NJ: SLACK Incorporated; 2014.
24. Holman H, Lorig K. Patient self-management: a key to effectiveness and efficiency in care of chronic disease. *Public Health Reports.* 2004;119(3):239.
25. Lorig KR, Holman HR. Self-management education: history, definition, outcomes, and mechanisms. *Ann Behav Med.* 2003;26(1):1-7.
26. Barlow J, Wright C, Sheasby J, Turner A, Hainsworth J. Self-management approaches for people with chronic conditions: a review. *Patient Educ Couns.* 2002;48(2):177-187.
27. Hibbard JH, Stockard J, Mahoney ER, Tusler M. Development of the Patient Activation Measure (PAM): conceptualizing and measuring activation in patients and consumers. *Health Serv Res.* 2004;39(4p1):1005-1026.
28. Wolf TJ, Baum CM, Lee D, & Hammel J. The development of the Improving Participation after Stroke Self-Management Program (IPASS): an exploratory randomized clinical study. *Top Stroke Rehabil.* 2016;23(4):284-292.
29. Finlayson M, Garcia JD, Preissner K. Development of an educational programme for caregivers of people aging with multiple sclerosis. *Occup Ther Int.* 2008;15:4-17.
30. Du S, Yuan C. Evaluation of patient self-management outcomes in health care: a systematic review. *Int Nurs Rev.* 2010;57(2):159-167.
31. Longmore PK. *Why I Burned My Book and Other Essays on Disability.* Philadelphia, PA: Temple University Press; 2003.
32. Couser GT. What disability studies has to offer medical education. *J Med Humanities.* 2011;21:21-30.
33. Phelan, S. Constructions of disability: a call for critical reflexivity in occupational therapy. *Can J Occup Ther.* 2011;78:164-172.
34. Linton S. *Claiming Disability: Knowledge and Identity.* New York, NY: New York University Press; 1998.

35. Hammel J, Magasi S, Heinemann A, Whiteneck G, Bogner J, Rodriguez E. What does participation mean? An insider perspective from people with disabilities. *Disabil Rehabil.* 2008;30(19):1445-1460.
36. Spassiani NA, Sawyer AR, Abou Chacra MS, Koch K, Muñoz YA, Lunsky Y. "Teaches People That I'm More Than a Disability": using nominal group technique in patient-oriented research for people with intellectual and developmental disabilities. *Intellect Dev Disabil.* 2016;54(2):112-122.
37. Clark GM. Transition planning assessment for secondary-level students with learning disabilities. In Patton JR, Blalock G, eds. *Transition and Students With Learning Disabilities: Facilitating the Movement From School to Adult Life.* Austin, TX: ProEd; 1996:131-156.
38. Wehmeyer ML, Kelchner K. *The Arc's Self-Determination Scale.* Arlington, TX: Arc National Headquarters; 1995.
39. Schalock RL, Keith KD. *Quality of Life Questionnaire.* Worthington, OH: IDS Publishers; 1993.
40. Heinemann AW, Lai JS, Magasi S, et al. Measuring participation enfranchisement. *Arch Phys Med Rehabil.* 2011;92:564-571.
41. Wolman JM, Campeau PL, DuBois PA, Mithaug DE, Stolarski VS. *AIR Self-Determination Scale and User Guide.* Washington, DC: American Institutes for Research; 1994.
42. Field S, Hoffman A. Self-determination in secondary transition assessment. *Assess Eff Interv.* 2007;32(3):181-190.
43. Cook J, Petersen C, Jonikas J. *Express Yourself! Assessing Self-Determination in Your Life.* Chicago, IL: University of Illinois at Chicago National Research & Training Center on Psychiatric Disability; 2004.
44. Copeland ME. *Facilitator Training Manual: Mental Health Recovery.* West Dummerston, VT: Peach Press; 2012.
45. Moss J. *Personal Preference Indicators.* Oklahoma City, OK: Center for Learning and Leadership/UCEDD, University of Oklahoma Health Sciences Center; 2006.
46. Sloan M, Irvin C. *Money Follows the Person Quality of Life Survey.* Prepared for Centers for Medicare and Medicaid Services (CMS). Washington, DC: Mathematica Policy Research, Inc; 2007.
47. Charlton JI. *Nothing About Us Without Us: Disability Oppression and Empowerment.* Berkeley, CA: University of California Press; 1998.
48. Tinetti ME, Richman D, Powell L. Falls efficacy as a measure of fear of falling. *J Gerontol.* 1990;45(6):P239-243.
49. Lee D, Fogg L, Baum C, Hammel J, Wolf T. Validation of the Participation Strategies Self-efficacy Scale (PS-SES). *Disabil Rehabil.* 2016:1-6. [Epub ahead of print]
50. Maujean A, Davis P, Kendall E, Casey L, Loxton N. The daily living self-efficacy scale: a new measure for assessing self-efficacy in stroke survivors. *Disabil Rehabil.* 2013;36(6):504-511.
51. Rumrill PD. *Increasing the Frequency of Accommodation Requests Among Persons With Multiple Sclerosis: A Demonstration of the Progressive Request Model.* Fayetteville, AK: University of Arkansas; 1993.
52. Hibbard JH, Mahoney ER, Stock R, Tusler M. Do increases in patient activation result in improved self-management behaviors? *Health Serv Res.* 2006;42(4):1443-1463.
53. Calculator SN, Black T. Validation of an inventory of best practices in the provision of augmentative and alternative communication services to students with severe disabilities in general education classrooms. *Am J Speech Lang Pathol.* 2009;18:329-342.
54. Wehmeyer ML. Student self-report measure of self- determination for students with cognitive disabilities. *Educ Train Mental Retardation Dev Disabil.* 1996;31:282-293.
55. Schalock RL, Keith KD, Hoffman K, Karan OC. Quality of Life: its measurement and use. *Mental Retardation.* 1989;27:25-31.
56. Caballo C, Crespo M, Jenaro C, Verdugo MA, Martinez JL. Factor structure of the Schalock and Keith Quality of Life Questionnaire (QOL-Q): validation on Mexican and Spanish samples. *J Intellect Disabil Res.* 2005;49(10):773-776.
57. Heinemann AW, Magasi S, Bode RK, et al. Measuring enfranchisement: importance of and control over participation by people with disabilities. *Arch Phys Med Rehabil.* 2013;94(11):2157-2165.
58. Powell LE, Myers AM. The Activities-Specific Balance Confidence (ABC) scale. *J Gerontol A Biol Sci Med Sci.* 1995;50A(1):M28-34.
59. Hellström K, Lindmark B. Fear of falling in patients with stroke: a reliability study. *Clin Rehabil.* 1999;13(6):509-517.
60. Medley A, Thompson M, French J. Predicting the probability of falls in community dwelling persons with brain injury: a pilot study. *Brain Injury.* 2006;20(13-14):1403–1408.
61. Cakt BD, Nacir B, Genç H, et al. Cycling progressive resistance training for people with multiple sclerosis: a randomized controlled study. *Am J Phys Med Rehabil.* 2010;89(6):446-457.
62. Wirz M, Müller R, Bastiaenen C. Falls in persons with spinal cord injury: validity and reliability of the Berg Balance Scale. *Neurorehabil Neural Repair.* 2010;24(1):70-77.
63. Rahman S, Griffin HJ, Quinn NP, Jahanshahi M. On the nature of fear of falling in Parkinson's disease. *Behav Neurol.* 2011;24(3):219-228.
64. Lorig K, Stewart A, Ritter P, Gonzalez V, Laurent D. *Outcome Measures for Health Education and Other Health Care Interventions.* Thousand Oaks: Sage Publications; 1996.
65. Lorig KR, Sobel DS, Ritter PL, Laurent D, Hobbs M. Effect of a self-management program for patients with chronic disease. *Effective Clinical Practice.* 2001;4:256-262.
66. Hibbard JH, Mahoney ER, Stockard J, Tusler M. Development and testing of a short form of the Patient Activation Measure. *Health Serv Res.* 2005;40(6p1):1918-1930.
67. Fowles JB, Terry P, Xi M, Hibbard J, Bloom CT, Harvey L. Measuring self-management of patients' and employees' health: further validation of the Patient Activation Measure (PAM) based on its relation to employee characteristics. *Patient Educ Couns.* 2009;77(1):116-122.
68. Green CA, Perrin NA, Polen MR, Leo MC, Hibbard JH, Tusler M. Development of the Patient Activation Measure for mental health. *Administration Policy Mental Health Mental Health Serv Res.* 2010;37(4):327-333.
69. Skolasky RL, Green AF, Scharfstein D, Boult C, Reider L, Wegener ST. Psychometric properties of the patient activation measure among multimorbid older adults. *Health Serv Res.* 2011;46(2):457-478.

Mine the Gold

The World Health Organization acknowledges the importance of participation as an indicator of health and well-being. There is an increasing emphasis on participation in criteria for funding health care outcomes and educational programs as well.

Become Systematic

By using participation measures consistently in practice, we inform our clients and colleagues that this is a central feature of occupational therapy practice. By linking other measurement data to participation data, we demonstrate our clinical reasoning processes and our unique perspective as occupational therapists.

Use Evidence in Practice

Evidence from occupational therapy literature on participation indicate that we can characterize aspects that support or interfere with a child's or adult's ability to participate in specific situations. Evidence from other disciplines indicate that it is important to measure both the person's methods of participating and the experiences with participation in his or her life.

Make Occupational Therapy Contributions Explicit

Occupational performance is the central construct of occupational therapy. By measuring participation directly, therapists are clearly indicating the purpose of occupational therapy practice, and other information can serve to inform the participation focus.

Engage in Occupation-Based, Client-Centered Practice

The concept of participation clearly reflects the importance of the person's experience with daily life. With a focus on participation, therapists are less likely to contrive activities that are inconsistent with that person's actual life pattern and are more likely to engage their clients in activities that are motivating and have meaning to the individual.

CHAPTER

General Measures of Participation Across the Lifespan

Mary Law, PhD, FCAOT; Winnie Dunn, PhD, OTR, FAOTA; and Carolyn Baum, PhD, OTR/L, FAOTA

Participation has been a central concept to occupational therapy since our profession began in the early 1900s. One of the founders of occupational therapy, Adolph Meyer, spoke eloquently about how persons used their time and organize themselves in order to participate in occupations across the lifespan.[1] In 1977, Tristam Engelhardt stated:

> Occupational therapy does not seem to be bound to the concept of disease, instead it focuses upon the success of individuals in finding fulfillment through human activity. [By] viewing humans as engaged in activities, realizing themselves through their occupation, occupational therapy supports a view of the whole person in function and adaptation [and participation].[2(p 666)]

Participation is derived from the Latin words *participatus* (meaning "part") and *capere* (meaning "to take").[3] As defined today, participation means taking part in something, sharing, being involved, or experiencing something.[4] From an occupational therapy perspective, participation can be defined as taking part in the occupations of everyday life. Participation is the ultimate goal of occupational therapy intervention.

Over the past 2 decades, participation has become a central and important concept in the field of health and disability worldwide. The World Health Organization (WHO), in revising their classification of disability, focused on participation as the important goal for persons with health. The areas of participation described within the International Classification of Functioning (ICF)[5] include Learning & Applying Knowledge, General Tasks and Demands, Communication, Movement, Self-Care, Domestic Life Areas, Interpersonal Interactions, Major Life Areas, and Community, Social, and Civic Life.

For occupational therapists, participation has been defined by Coster and Khetani as "sets of organized sequences of activities directed toward a personally or socially meaningful goal."[6(p 643)] A person's participation does not occur in isolation; thus, it can only be considered in relationship to that person's skills and abilities and the environment in which he or she lives. In the ICF, the complexity of participation is recognized by stressing the interrelationships between body function and structure, activity, personal factors, and environmental characteristics.[5] In occupational therapy, the complexity of participation in occupations is acknowledged in all occupational therapy theoretical models, which emphasize the transactional relationships between person, occupations, and environment.

The WHO's conceptual model for disability and health emphasizes participation, and the Person-Environment-Occupation (PEO) model we are using in this text also focuses on participation as the result of the interaction of person, occupations, and environments. Figure 9-1 illustrates the similarities in these conceptual models by superimposing them; the unique contribution of occupational therapy's perspective about occupation is notable.

Participation and Occupational Performance

This book focuses on issues and strategies to measure occupational performance. As described in Chapter 1, occupational performance is the result of a person's effort to engage in activities central to daily living, which include, but are not limited to, activities of self-care (eg, grooming, bathing, feeding), productivity (eg, vocational pursuits, maintaining a home, communicating with others), and leisure (eg, play, hobbies, recreational activities). *Occupational performance* is a term unique to the profession of occupational therapy to describe how a person functions in his or her environment.

Law M, Baum C, Dunn W, eds. *Measuring Occupational Performance: Supporting Best Practice in Occupational Therapy, Third Edition (pp 115-151).*

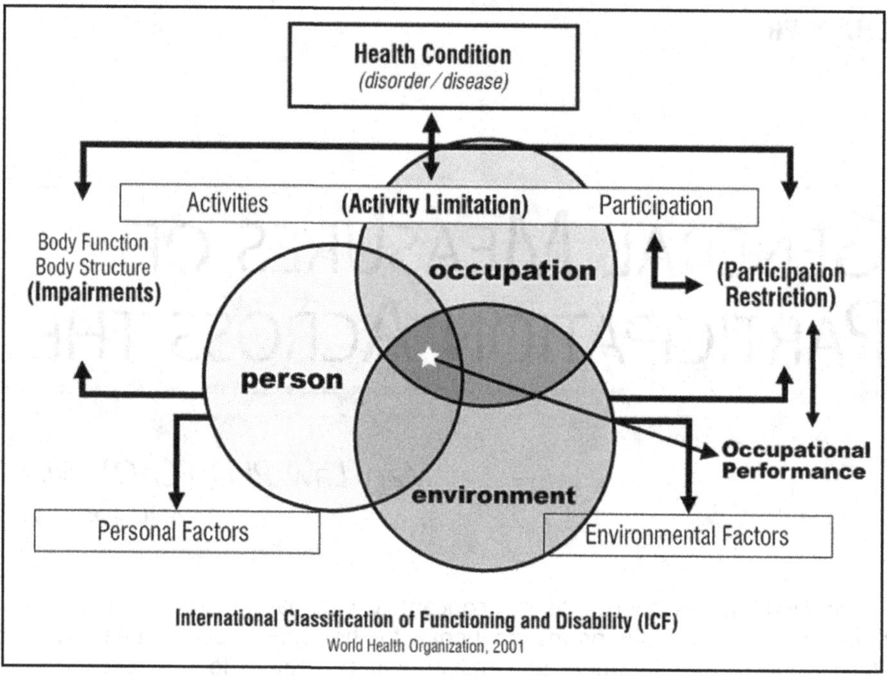

Figure 9-1. International Classification of Functioning and Disability (ICF).

Occupational therapists do not separate the physical act of doing from the meaning or purposeful intent of the act. When examining occupational performance, occupational therapists strive to understand how the dynamic relationship between person, environment, and occupation, as well as a person's developmental stage, culture, and societal roles, impact on his or her ability to perform the tasks and activities that are important to the person. Defined simply, successful occupational performance occurs when a person is able to complete an occupation in a manner that achieves the goal of the occupation, while satisfying the person. Occupational therapists understand occupational performance to be the point at which the "person, environment, and occupation intersect to support the occupations (including tasks and activities) and roles that define that person as an individual."[7] As detailed in Chapter 2, occupational performance has both objective, observable components and subjective, experiential components.

What then is the relationship between occupational performance and participation? Both of these terms are used to describe and classify important concepts. Participation has been defined as involvement in a life situation, whereas occupational performance describes the act of doing an occupation and the experience of those moments in time. We can see that these descriptions share many similarities. In fact, as occupational therapists, our goal is to support a person's participation in occupations that they want or need to do.[8,9]

From the point of view of measurement, an outcome of participation is very similar to the outcome of occupational performance. Although the ICF specifies 10 categories of participation, most occupational therapy conceptual models classify occupational performance into 3 to 8 primary categories. For example, the categories of self-care, productivity/work, and leisure are used in the Canadian Model of Occupational Performance and Engagement,[10] while the American Association of Occupational Therapists has 8 categories ranging from activities of daily living to social participation.[11] The majority of items within the WHO participation categories would fit into these categories of occupational performance (see Figure 9-1).

Participation, Quality of Life, and Health

Participation in occupations meaningful to a person has a direct and substantial impact on health and quality of life for children, adults, and older adults.[12-14] Anne Wilcock[15] details how participation in occupations has been a vital part of humankind throughout history. It is through participation in everyday occupations that people grow and develop, connect with other humans, make a living, learn, contribute to society, and enjoy life.[16-18] For children and youth, participation has a substantial influence on optimal development. Through participation in everyday occupations, children and youth develop skills, learn to socialize with others, gain improved physical and mental health, and engage in activities that are meaningful.[13] Research also indicates that participation benefits children who are at risk for developmental and/or behavioral difficulties.[19,20]

Participation is also central to theories of healthy aging because activity engagement is associated with physical, emotional, and cognitive health. By assessing the participation of older adults, occupational therapists can help them select rewarding and meaningful activities to optimize their experiences. By knowing what is important to older adults, the occupational therapist can help them compensate for losses by finding other ways to accomplish occupations that are important and necessary for them to do.

Measuring Participation

The assessment of participation is challenging. As Law states:

> Because participation in occupations is complex, weaving a pattern across time and space, capturing its essence through measurement is challenging. Think about it. Participation in occupations has several dimensions—a person's preferences and interests, what they do, where they do it, with whom they do it, and how much they enjoy and find it satisfying. In considering person, environment, and occupation, the measurement of participation occurs at the transactions among these domains.[21(p 642)]

Many assessments of participation have been developed through population-based time use surveys. Information from these surveys contributes to our knowledge about how populations in different countries spend their time.[13,22] Occupational therapists can use this information to augment their knowledge about typical patterns of occupational performance. These surveys, however, are not as useful in doing assessments for individual clients or groups because they only provide general conclusions about what is typical. Occupational therapy intervention is designed to address the specific issues that a particular client or group exhibits, and so measurement must uncover those specific characteristics.

Csikszentmihalyi[23] has used individual strategies for identifying patterns of participation. He asked participants to record their experiences at randomly selected times triggered by a pager signal. His work led him to conclude that people need a balance of task difficulty and personal skill during participation to experience what he termed *flow.* During flow, persons are absorbed in their activities and are not aware of time passing. His work provides us with insight about characteristics of successful participation, and also demonstrates a way to measure the experience of participation as it is occurring. However, this strategy for collecting information requires an expanse of time that may not be feasible in many practice settings. Additionally, occupational therapists are also concerned with personal strategies people use to engage in their occupations, and this measurement strategy does not provide a means for uncovering these data.

Whiteneck and Dijkers[24] have described the challenges in measuring participation because the concept is individual in nature, but also multidimensional and subjective. Because of the personal nature and complexity of participation, most participation measures have used self-report or proxy-report formats. Such a measurement strategy fits with a social model of disability and acknowledges the intimate relationships between participation and the environment. The majority of participation measures focus more on the observable characteristics of participation rather than a person's subjective experiences. Few measures assess the broad nature of participation, including what is done, where participation takes place, how often it occurs, and how enjoyable it is for the person.

Participation Measures Reviewed in This Chapter

The task of choosing participation measures for reviewing this chapter was easier than the previous edition because more measures are being developed. There are still few measures that have been developed specifically to focus on participation as defined by the WHO.[5] On the other hand, there are many measures that include some or all of the items and categories found within the participation dimension of the ICF. For example, dozens of quality of life measures exist within the health and social sciences literature. Because of these challenges, we develop criteria to guide the selection of measures to be reviewed within the chapter.

All measures reviewed within the chapter cover a broad range of participation categories within the ICF (starting with Table 9-1). Many assessments in other chapters contain participation aspects that are consistent with the ICF; we are not repeating them here, but would rather refer you to the specific chapters of interest to your topic. Chapter 6 focuses on client-centered measures of occupational performance; the results of these assessments often identify participation issues. For example, a client may identify participation in several occupations on the Canadian Occupational Performance Measure (COPM). For full reviews of these client-centered measures, please see Chapter 6. Chapters 9 and 14 focuses on measures that primarily assess play and leisure activities, while Chapter 10 focuses on the area of work.

The other criteria used to select measures for this chapter include the following:

- Currently available and in use in occupational therapy practice, education, and/or research
- Fit with a client-centered approach to occupational therapy practice
- Noncategorical in nature; not focused on one diagnosis
- Evidence of recent research about the measure or using it in a study
- Evidence of acceptable psychometric properties
- Observable or self-report, but focused on the nature and experience of participation

Table 9-1

Activity Card Sort (ACS)

Source	Baum and Edwards[25]
Key References	Baum and Edwards[26]; Laver-Fawcett and Mallinson[27]; Hamed and Holm[28]; Jong et al[29]; Eriksson et al[30]; Packer et al[31]; Doney and Packer[32]; Chan et al[33]; Katz et al[34]; Sachs and Josman[35]
Purpose	• The Activity Card Sort (ACS) is a comprehensive instrument for assessing participation in occupation. The original version (1995) was intended for use with older adults with cognitive deficits; however, it has since been used across diverse adult populations to assess participation, establish functional treatment goals and record changes in activity patterns.
Type of Client	• Adults with and without cognitive loss.
Test Format	• The ACS is a client-centred, interview-based activity measurement that assesses current, previous, and percent retained of activities. Photographs are categorized into 4 domains: instrumental activities, low-demand leisure activities, high-demand leisure activities, and social activities. It can be performed with a client or with a parent or caregiver. The ACS has 3 formats that utilize different sorting strategies: community living, institutional, and recovering versions.
Procedures	• The 89 photographs have been classified into 4 domains: (1) Instrumental activities of daily living (IADL); (2) Social activities (SC); (3) High-demand leisure activities; and (4) Low-demand leisure activities. The client or caregivers sort 89 photograph cards, one at a time, into groups reflective of whether the activity is or has been done by the client in their regular daily life. These groups may vary depending on the version of the tool being used. Scoring: Categorization enables the calculation of scores for current activity, activities done previously, and activity retained. The sum total of current activities is divided by the sum total of previous activities. This provides a percent of retained activity level. In all 3 formats, the client is asked to identify their 5 top activities as a guide for goal setting and intervention.
Time Required	• Average completion time is 20 minutes. More time is required if the clinician asks probing questions about activities retained, lost, or desired.
Standardization	• The photographs can be tailored to the specific population of interest. Numerous versions of the ACS have been developed that are specific to the population of interest (eg, Israeli, UK, Australian, Puerto Rican, Hong Kong, Arabic and Dutch versions are now available).
Reliability	
Test-Retest	• Baum and Edwards[26] reported a test-retest coefficient of 0.897 in a sample of 20 older adults living within the community with a one week test-retest interval. • Everand et al[36] reported high test retest reliability for the instrumental (r = 0.95), social (r = 0.83), low demand leisure (r = 0.91), and high demand leisure (r = 0.88) subscales (time interval of 74 days). • High intra-class correlation coefficient values have been reported for the Hong Kong version (ACS-HK) with ICC = 0.98 (CI 0.97 to 0.99).[33] • For the Puerto Rican version,[37] the test–retest reliability for total score current activity level was ICC = 0 .82 (n = 20 community-dwelling older adults). Test-retest reliability was high for instrumental activities of daily living (ICC = 0.82), low physical demand leisure activities (ICC = 0.84), for high physical demand leisure activities (ICC = 0.71) and for sociocultural activities (ICC = 0.81). • Hamed and Holm[28] reported that the Arabic ACS (A-ACS) demonstrates good test–retest reliability (r = 0.80, p < .00) over a period of 1 month. Internal consistency for the A-ACS was excellent (α = 0.90).

(continued)

Table 9-1 (continued)

ACTIVITY CARD SORT (ACS)

Reliability	
Internal Consistency	• Katz et al[34] reported high internal consistency for the Israeli version ACS on instrumental activities of daily living (IADL; α=0.82) and social-cultural activities (α=0.80) and moderate internal consistency for low and high physical leisure activities (α=0.66 and 0.61 respectively). • Internal consistency of the United States ACS[36] reported α=0.71 for IADL, α=0.77 for social-cultural, α=0.71 for low demand leisure and α=0.85 for high demand leisure activities.[28] • Internal consistency for the ACS-Hong Kong was excellent (r=0.89).[33]
Inter-Rater	• Jong et al[29] reported inter-rater agreement for the Dutch version (ACS-NL) total score and sub test scores were ICC=0.79 (high physical leisure) to ICC=0.87 (IADL) activities.
Validity	
Content	• Content validity for the original US version comprised 2 studies: 1) Photographs were shown to an initial sample of 120 older adults, 2) a second sample of 40 older adults provided feedback and an additional 7 activities were added to the original ACS, to bring the total of the second edition of the ACS to 89. The ACS has been adapted for use with older adults in other countries, including Arab countries (A-ACS)[28]; Australia (ACS-Australia)[31]; Hong-Kong (ACS-HK)[33]; Israel[34,35]; Korea[30]; Puerto Rico[38]; the Netherlands[29]; and most recently, the UK.[27] The total activities in each version reflect the cultural differences of each country in which the tool was validated. • For total retained activity level and individual activity areas , the ACS (Israeli version) differentiated between healthy adults and older adults, individuals with multiple sclerosis, spouses or caregivers of individuals with Alzheimer's, and stroke survivors (1 year post-stroke) ($p<0.001$).[34]
Construct	• Factor analysis of the Israeli version of the ACS found young and older adults ($n=184$) classify activities into domains different from those suggested by the author. However, a modified scoring system was used in this study.[34,35] • Orellano et al[37] reported scores for total current activity level of the PR-ACS differed between individuals with MS and healthy older adults ($t=6.86$; $p<.001$). This suggests the PR-ACS can adequately discriminate between 2 different groups on levels of current activity participation. • The Hong Kong version (ACS-HK) is reported to be able to differentiate activity levels of adults at different functional levels, post-stroke ($n=60$; $t=-14.24$; $p\leq.001$).[33] • The A-ACS was able to discriminate between individuals with MS and healthy adults on current and retained levels of participation ($F=5.09$, $p<0.03$; $F=6.01$, $p<0.02$, respectively).[28]
Criterion	• Everand et al[36] evaluated the concurrent validity of the Activity checklist with the Activity Card Sort in 20 adults with high correlations for instrumental (r=0.90), social (r=0.78), low demand leisure (r=0.82), and high-demand leisure (r=0.72) activity subscales. • Moderate correlations were reported between the Israeli version of the ACS category "doing now" and the number of hours a person reported being active on the Occupational Questionnaire (r=0.54).[34] • Moderate correlations (r=0.66, $p<.001$) were reported between average scores for total current activity level on the PR-ACS and total mean scores of the PR RAND SF-36 (health-related quality of life)[37]

(continued)

Table 9-1 (continued)

Activity Card Sort (ACS)

Criterion	• For the Arabic ACS (A-ACS)[28] reported moderate correlations with the participation index of the Mayo-Portland Adaptability Inventory ($r=0.458$, $p<0.00$) and the Arabic version of the Performance Assessment of Self-care Skills ($r=0.581$, $p<0.00$)[28] • Doney and Packer[32] reported moderate correlations between the ACS-Australia (ACS-Aus) and the Adelaide Activities Profile ($r=0.434$, $P=0.000$). Pearson product–moment correlations between the ACS-Aus and the Personal Well-Being Index were also moderate ($r=0.354$, $P=0.010$) • Pearson's correlation coefficients between the ACS-HK and the ComQoL were high ($r=0.86$; $p=.00$) demonstrating convergent validity with measures of quality of life.[33]
Utility	
Research Programs	• Useful for research directed at examining the occupational performance patterns of different age and diagnostic groups, as well as between genders. • To date, the ACS has been used to investigate the participation of (for example) older adults living in the community,[36] adults transitioning with a disability,[39] adults experiencing cognitive deficits,[40] stroke,[41] and vision problems.[42]
Practice Settings	• Cross-cultural research has demonstrated that the ACS has improved validity and utility when the activities depicted are relevant to people's culture and environment. • Is a comprehensive assessment of participation in instrumental, social cultural, low, and high physical leisure activities. • Can help the client select goals to guide interventions • Provides information on patterns of participation and changes in engagement in activities over time. • The institutional version allows the therapist to create a preadmission status for treatment planning and triggers ideas for intervention that include the person's prior experiences and interests. • The recovering version allows clinicians to record changes in activity patterns.
Strengths	• Is user friendly, particularly for people with cognitive and/or language difficulties. • Support occupation focused, client-centered practice. • Can be adapted to different cultural populations, enabling cross cultural research.
Complexities	• Should not be the sole measure used to establish treatment goals. • More research is necessary to determine whether the scores capture a change in behavior.

Table 9-2

Assessment of Preschool Children's Participation (APCP)

Source	CanChild
Key References	Bult et al[43]; Chen et al[44]; Law et al[45]
Purpose	• Document a child's participation in areas of play, skill development, active physical recreation, and social activities. This measure captures the intensity and diversity of a preschool child's participation by identifying which activities he or she has participated in over the past 4 months and how often.

(continued)

Table 9-2 (continued)

Assessment of Preschool Children's Participation (APCP)

Type of Client	• Children aged 2 to 5 years, 11 months
Test Format	• Paper and pencil, parent/caregiver completed questionnaire. 45 drawings of everyday activities organized into 4 activity domains: play (9 items), skill development (15 items), active physical recreation (10 items), and social activities (11 items).
Procedures	• Parents/caregivers complete the APCP by looking at drawings of children performing 45 different activities. Parents/caregivers then identify whether their child has participated in the activity during the past 4 months and rated how often they participated using a 7-point ordinal scale ranging from once in the past 4 months (1 point) to once or more daily (7 points). They will also record where the activity was done most often, with whom it was done most often, and how much enjoyment they perceive their child is having. • Scoring: Two scores are generated for each item: participation diversity (a count of the total number of activities in the past 4 months; or as a percentage of activities overall and by activity type) and participation intensity (average amount of time spends participating in activities across the total number of possible activities)
Time Required	• Administration time is approximately 30 to 40 minutes
Reliability	
Test-Retest	• In the Dutch version, Bult et al[43] reported insufficient test-retest reliability for play (Intraclass Correlation Coefficient=0.63 and 0.68) and the intensity in skill development (0.67) for children with physical disabilities. Test-retest reliability was found in all other areas for groups of patients but not as individuals (0.73 to 0.91)
Internal Consistency	• Law et al[45] reported varied internal consistency of the APCP with Cronbach's alpha scores ranging from good to excellent for diversity (0.73 to 0.85) and moderate for intensity (0.52 to 0.70) in a sample of 120 children with cerebral palsy. • Bult et al[43] reported varied internal consistency in the Dutch version of the APCP. Significant Cronbach's alpha coefficients were found only in the areas for the total scores for participation diversity, intensity, and in both areas of active physical recreation (0.07 to 0.86).
Inter-Rater	• Not reported
Validity	
Content	• Measure is modeled after the Children's Assessment of Participation and Enjoyment (CAPE) that has shown adequate test-retest reliability, and varied internal consistency and construct validity.[46] 23 of 45 items are identical to the CAPE and 15 similar items were modified to fit preschool children. Only 7 items were not in the CAPE • Item generation was based on review of developmental literature and existing measures of participation. Pilot testing was conducted with 57 parents of children with typical development who attended 4 local day care centers in southern Ontario. Initial tests used 48 items, 3 of which were eliminated for being endorsed less than 10% of the time and resulted in improved levels of internal consistency during the pilot test.[45] • ICF-CY analysis of content of the APCP showed that all but one meaningful concept was linked together. The 45 activities in the APCP were classified into 7 of 9 activities and participation domains of the ICF-CY. The APCP is different from other measures of participation in that it does not include the domain of self-care.[47]

(continued)

Table 9-2 (continued)

Assessment of Preschool Children's Participation (APCP)

Validity	
Construct	• Law et al[45] reported construct validity of the APCP with a relatively small group of children with cerebral palsy (n = 120). ¤ Significant differences in participation diversity and intensity based on age, with children 4 years of age and above participating in a greater variety and more frequently. Medium effect size was found for participation diversity (ω2 = 0.07) in all areas except play activities (0.02), which was small. ¤ Significant differences in participation diversity and intensity were found in children based on their GMFCS classification with those classified as GMFCS I to III participating in a greater range of activities and more frequently than children with GMFCS IV to V. Large effect size (0.21 to 0.23) in all areas except overall diversity and intensity of social activities, which was medium to large (0.08 to 0.16). ANOVA calculations found similar effect size (0.07 to 0.33) when accounting for child age, sex, and family income. ¤ Small to medium significant differences in participation diversity and intensity of play and skill development activities were found between income levels (0.03 to 0.07). No significant differences were found in participation intensity for social and active physical recreation activities. ¤ Small differences were found between boys and girls with girls participating in a broader range of activities and more frequently (0.03 to 0.05). Girls participated more intensely in social activities and more diversely in active physical recreation activities (0.03). • Tested using a Dutch version of the APCP with a small group of parents of children (n = 126) with physical disabilities (n = 59) and without (n = 67). ¤ Children with physical disabilities participated in significantly fewer activities than those without ($p < 0.001$), confirming hypothesis ¤ Partial confirmation of hypothesis in participation vs sex or age was found. Boys and girls participated at an equal level in all areas except in skill development, where girls participated more intensely ($p = 0.02$)—partial confirmation of hypothesis. Children aged 4 years and above significantly participated in more activities and at a greater intensity ($p < 0.001$). However, for specific activity types, there were only significant differences in scores in skill development and social activities ($p < 0.001$).
Criterion	• Chen et al[44] utilized the Taiwanese version of the APCP with 89 children with cerebral palsy. It was found to have fair to excellent correlations with the criterion-related measures of the GMFM-66 (r = 0.43-0.85, $p < 0.01$) and WeeFIM (r = 0.39-0.73, $p < 0.01$). Fair to excellent predictive capacities at baseline was found with the GMFM-66 (r = 0.51-0.77, $p < 0.01$) and at follow-up with the WeeFIM (r = 0.46-0.82, $p < 0.01$)
Responsiveness	• Chen et al[44] reported that changes in the Taiwanese version of the APCP from baseline to follow-up was statistically significant (t = 1.82-7.43, $p < 0.05$) and markedly responsive (standardized response mean = 0.8 – 1.3).
Standardization	• The APCP can be administered by the parent/caregiver or interviewer-assisted. • Poor manual. Manual is available but information is lacking. No evidence of reliability or validity given. No scoring or interpretation information was given.

(continued)

Table 9-2 (continued)

Assessment of Preschool Children's Participation (APCP)

Utility	
Research Programs	• Can be used to assess diversity and intensity of a child's participation • Can evaluate changes in participation over time • Has been used in studies to assess participation in children with and without disabilities[48-50]
Practice Settings	• Can capture overall level of participation, including level of diversity and intensity of a client • Similar in purpose to the Children's Assessment of Participation and Enjoyment (CAPE) except it is meant for children under 6 years of age and is completed by the caregivers.
Strengths	• User friendly for parents • Accessible and engaging tool to use with parents of children of different age ranges, disability levels, and cultures.
Complexities	• Validity of the score is dependent on the parent's ability to read the questions accurately. • Parent-completed questionnaire therefore may not capture the overall diversity and frequency of activities that a child may participate in. Activities completed in daycare, kindergarten, or playgroups may be missed. • Questions about diversity and intensity of participation are in relation to the past 4 months, which may be subject to seasonal variations in participation and activity. • There may be differences in relevance of the activities based on culture[47] • Currently no normative data to which comparisons can be made.

Table 9-3

The Child and Adolescent Scale of Participation (CASP)

Source	The CASP and also the CASP Youth Version are available for free on the webpage of its author, G. Bedell: http://sites.tufts.edu/garybedell/measurement-tools/
Key References	Bedell[51-53]; de Kloet et al[54]; Hwang et al[55]; McDougall et al[56]
Purpose	• The CASP was originally created as a part of a larger measure—the Child and Family Follow-up Survey (CFFS)—but independent administration and scoring guidelines are available so that the CASP can be used as a caregiver report of a child's participation for research and practice purposes. It is meant to measure participation across 3 settings (home, school, and the community) and identify associated barriers and supports. Possible uses of the CASP include personal intervention planning, program evaluation, and multi-site and populated-wise research. A youth version of the CASP, to be filled out by the young people themselves, also exists. • It is used both as a descriptive and an evaluative measure and will therefore be evaluated as such following the criteria established by Law[57] in this report.
Type of Client	• The CFFS, of which the CASP began as a part, was designed to measure the outcomes of children and youth with brain injuries. The guidelines suggest it is used for school-aged children age 5 years or older.[51]

(continued)

Table 9-3 (continued)

The Child and Adolescent Scale of Participation (CASP)

Type of Client

- Initial psychometric testing with the CASP was carried out by Bedell[52] on children and youth with acquired brain injuries who were discharged from a inpatient rehabilitation facility (n=60)
- Further psychometric testing was carried out by Bedell[53] on 313 children and youth, aged 3 to 22 years, with and without disabilities (n=313).
- The Youth Version of the CASP was tested on youth with a variety of chronic conditions/disabilities ages 11 to 17 years by McDougall et al[56] (n=430). The Youth Version is appropriate for all young people with the cognitive capacity to answer the questions posed in the CASP.

Test Format

- The CASP contains 4 subsections: 1) Home Participation (6 items), 2) Community Participation (4 items), 3) School Participation (5 items), and 4) Home and Community Living Activities (5 items). Each item is rated on a 4-point ordinal scale (4="Age Expected (Full participation)," 3="Somewhat restricted," 2="Very restricted," 1="Unable," 0="Not Applicable"). The CASP also contains open-ended questions designed to elicit information from caregivers about supports and barriers to their child's participation.[51]
- The Youth Version of the CASP is very similar to the adult version with minor changes in wording.[56]
- Individual item scores, subsection setting scores, and total summary scores can be used for research and practice. The higher score, the greater the age-related participation.[51]
- Scoring of the Youth Version of the CASP is identical to the original.[56]

Procedures

Administration

- No specific training is required to administer the CASP although those using the measure for a specific purpose should be familiar with the theory, psychometric properties, and rating scales of the measure.[51]
- The CASP can be administered in 2 different ways: 1) caregivers of children and young people with disabilities independently complete the CASP by answering the questions and following the instructions that accompany the measure (whether a paper or electronic copy) or 2) the CASP is administered by interviewer in person or over the phone.[51]
- The Youth Version of the CASP is meant to be completed by the young people themselves, either independently or via interviewer, although the administration and scoring manual for the measure is not yet available according to Bedell's website.

Scoring

- To calculate the CASP Total Summary Score: divide the sum of all "Applicable" items by the maximum possible score of all applicable items (80 if all 20 items are applicable), then multiply the percentage by 100 to produce a score out of 100.[51]
- To calculate the CASP Subsection Score: divide the sum of all "Applicable" items in a particular subsection or setting by the maximum possible score of all applicable items (eg, 24 for Home Participation if all 6 items in the subsection are applicable), then multiply the percentage by 100 to produce a score out of 100.[51]
- To calculate the CASP item-level scores, take the rating provided for each item (eg, 1=unable to participate, 2=very limited, 3=somewhat limited, 4=age expected/full participation).[51]
- The open-ended questions at the end of the CASP can be analyzed and summarized when the CASP is administered on a large scale to inform program planning.[51]
- The Youth Version of the CASP is scored in the same way described previously.[56]

(continued)

Table 9-3 (continued)

The Child and Adolescent Scale of Participation (CASP)

Type of Client

Time Required

Interpretation

- The CASP has not been formally tested to establish its responsiveness as an evaluative measure nor has its minimally significant clinical difference been noted. However, Agnihotri et al[58] (n = 4) used the CASP to evaluate an arts-based intervention for youth with ABI. In so doing, they established "ranges of summary scores" to describe levels of participation (75 to 100 = "Age Expected," < 75 to 50 = "Somewhat limited," < 50 to 25 = "Very limited," < 25 to 0 = "Unable," 0 = "Not Applicable").

Administration

- The CASP takes about 10 minutes to administer.[51]
- The Youth Version of the CASP, when administered via interviewer, took 30 to 60 minutes to complete in one study.[56]

Scoring

- The time it takes to score the CASP is not explicitly stated. However, given the simplicity of the calculation, the CASP could likely be scored in anywhere from 5 to 10 minutes, assuming that the open-ended questions at the end of the CASP are not being content-analyzed.

Reliability

Test-Retest

- Bedell[52] (n = 60) found that the CASP has excellent test-retest reliability (Interclass correlation coefficient = 0.94).[53] However, given that the CASP uses an ordinal scale, this writer believes that the Spearman rank coefficient may have been a more appropriate statistic given the criterion established by Law.[57]
- Test-retest reliability is not yet available for the Youth Version of the CASP.
- de Kloet et al[54] (n = 35) found that the Dutch translation of the CASP (CASP-DLV) had adequate test-retest reliability (Interclass correlation coefficient = 0.90). However, given that the CASP uses an ordinal scale, this writer believes that the Spearman rank coefficient may have been a more appropriate statistic given the criterion established by Law.[57]

Internal Consistency

- Bedell[52] (n = 60) found that the CASP has excellent internal consistency (Cronbach's alpha = 0.98).[53]
- Bedell[53] (n = 313) found that the CASP has excellent internal consistency (Cronbach's alpha = 0.96).
- McDougall et al[56] found that the Youth Version of the CASP has adequate internal consistency (Cronbach's alpha = 0.87)
- Hwang et al[55] found that the traditional Chinese version of the CASP (CASP-C) has good internal consistency overall (Cronbach's alpha = 0.96) and for all 4 subsections (home, alpha = 0.96; neighborhood and community, alpha = 0.89; school, alpha = 0.90; home and community living activities, alpha = 0.88).
- de Kloet et al[54] (n = 147) found that the Dutch translation of the CASP (CASP-DLV) had excellent internal consistency (Cronbach's alpha = 0.95)

(continued)

Table 9-3 (continued)

The Child and Adolescent Scale of Participation (CASP)

Validity	
Content	• Scale construction is excellent. The CASP was based on the ICF; a literature review; and input from families, children, clinicians, and researchers.[53] • Chien et al[59] reviewed 16 instruments measuring children's participation examining the extent to which the measure captured participation or whether the items "captured the meaning of children's participation such as involvement in certain life situations that include sets of organized sequences of activities directed toward a personally or socially meaningful goal".[59(p 143)] 91.8% of the participation items of the CASP were found to capture participation.
Construct	• Bedell[52] (n=60) reports that CASP summary scores are significantly correlated to the Paediatric Evaluation Disabilities Inventory subscale scores. Children with greater age-related participation tend to have higher mobility ($r=0.51$, $p<0.01$), social ($r=0.65$, $p<0.01$) and self-care functioning ($r=0.72$, $p<0.01$).[53] • Bedell[52] (n=60) reports that CASP summary scores are negatively correlated with the Child and Adolescent Factors Inventory scores ($r=-0.58$, $p<0.01$) indicating children with greater participation tend to have fewer functional impairments.[53] • Bedell[52] (n=60) reports that CASP summary scores are negatively correlated with the CHILD and Adolescent Scale of Environment scores ($r=-0.57$, $p<0.01$) indicating that children with greater participation have fewer physical, social and attitudinal barriers in their environments.[53] • Bedell[53] (n=313) found through analyses of variance and t tests that the CASP was able to differentiate between disability groups ($F=35.67$; $p<0.001$). • Anderson et al[60] (n=136) used the CASP to measure the social participation of children with TBI 6 months post-injury and found a significant difference in CASP scores compared to a control group. • Bedell[53] (n=313) found that CASP summary scores are significantly correlated to the Paediatric Evaluation Disabilities Inventory scores ($r=-0.66$, $p<0.001$). • Bedell[53] (n=313) reports that CASP summary scores are negatively correlated with the Child and Adolescent Factors Inventory scores ($r=-0.43$, $p<0.001$) indicating children with greater participation tend to have fewer functional impairments. • Bedell[53] (n=313) reports that Rasch analysis of CASP results support the hypothesis that children with a "greater extent of participation...should participate in more difficult or challenging life situations"[53(pp 345-347)] with only the individual items of "Shopping/Managing Money" and "Using Transportation" falling outside the model of participation trends postulated by researchers. • McDougall et al[56] (n=430) found that the Youth Version of the CASP was able to discriminate between disability groups ($F=4.33$, $p<0.0001$). Through post-hoc analysis, this same study found that CASP results indicated that youth with an amputated limb had significantly higher participation scores than those with cerebral palsy ($p<0.01$) or ASD ($p<0.0001$). Finally, this study found that CASP results suggested that youth with communication disorders/cleft lip and/or palate had significantly higher participation scores than youth with ASD ($p<0.01$). • Hwang et al[55] found that the Traditional Chinese version of the CASP (CASP-C) found significant differences for all subsections apart from home and community living activities between children with mild intellectual disability and those with severe intellectual disabilities. • de Kloet et al[54] (n=147) found that the Dutch Translation of the CASP (CASP-DLV) total score correlated significantly with the score of the Pediatric Quality of Life Inventory ($r=0.451$, $p<0.05$) and the Pediatric Stroke Outcome Measure ($r=-0.497$, $p<0.05$). All subsection measures were also significantly correlated with these 2 alternative outcomes measures.

(continued)

Table 9-3 (continued)

The Child and Adolescent Scale of Participation (CASP)

Standardization	• The CASP and the Youth Version of the CASP can be self-administered or administered via interviewer. The manual for the CASP provides instructions and scoring instructions for the original measure. No manual is yet available for the Youth Version of the CASP, although the original manual's administration and scoring instructions provide guidance as both versions are scored the same way.
Utility	• Bedell[53] reports that the CASP's psychometric properties support its use as a discriminative or evaluative tool although researchers and clinicians must keep the measure's ceiling effect in mind. • Badge et al[61] selected the CASP based on its psychometric properties and clinical utility (i.e. its relevance to clinical priorities and following feedback from clinicians) as 1 of 3 chosen measures out of an original 44 possibilities to measure outcomes of the New South Wales Brain Injury Rehabilitation program. • Ziviani et al[62] note in their systematic review of participation measures that the CASP has strong clinical utility given that it is readily available, does not require any training to administer, and is simply and quick to administer. • It is one of the few measures that has both a parent version and a youth one[56]
Strengths	• Good psychometric evidence for its use: in their systematic review of 8 participation questionnaires using a standardized taxonomy, Rainey et al[63] found that the CASP had been most extensively evaluated out of all studied measures with moderate positive results on all assessed measurement properties. • Quick to administer, which makes the measure well-suited for large research studies and busy practice environments • Can be used for children and youth of various ages • The CASP has been translated into several languages: Spanish, French, German, Hebrew, and Mandarin.
Complexities	• As Bedell[51] reports, consensus has not yet been established on how to treat "not applicable" items on the CASP, although current practice tends to be to disregard those items when scoring. • Bedell[53] ($n=313$) reports that the CASP has ceiling effects for children without disabilities (14% of sample of children without disabilities) and children with disabilities (10% of sample of children with disabilities). • To a certain extent, the CASP may measure both the "participation" and "activity" constructs of the ICF as it asks caregivers both whether their child participates and also the "amount of assistance the child needs to be able to participate" or their child's ability.[53] It does not discriminate between the 2 concepts. • Although the CASP has been used as an evaluative measure by Agnihotri et al[58] and Catroppa et al,[64] it requires further psychometric testing to fully establish the measure's responsiveness and a minimally significant clinical difference before it can be a strong evaluative measure. • The CASP measures the objective experience of participation by asking caregivers whether their child engages in a specific type of activity (eg, "structured events and activities in the neighbourhood") in comparison with other children their age.[51(p 3)] This does not take into account the subjective component of participation. After all, the desired level of participation in a particular activity by a certain child will be determined in part by personal preference rather than being a "normal" amount of expected participation. The measure also fails to capture whether caregivers regard a low score in a particular item or subsection as an area in which they would like to see change. • The point above is underlined by the results of McDougall et al,[56] who compared CASP scores generated by parents to the Youth Version CASP scores generated by the teenage children of these parents. McDougall et al[56] ($n=430$) found moderate agreement between youth and parent scores ($ICC=0.63$, 95% $CI=0.41$ to 0.75), but that youth tended to rate themselves significantly higher than their parents ($t=10.93$, $p<0.0001$).

Table 9-4

Craig Handicap Assessment and Reporting Technique (CHART)

Source	Dave Mellnick, Craig Hospital Research Department, 3425 S. Clarkson Street, Englewood, CO, 80110; 303-789-8202; www.craighospital.org.
Key References	Tozato et al[65]; Walker et al[66]; Dijkers[67]; Hall et al[68]; Rintala et al[69]; Whiteneck[70]; Whiteneck et al[71]; WHO[72,73]
Purpose	• To measure the level of handicap experienced by an individual in a community setting.
Type of Client	• Designed for clients with spinal cord injuries. The Revised CHART has also been used in research for people with traumatic brain injury, stroke, multiple sclerosis, amputations, and burns.
Test Format	• Twenty-seven questions belonging to 5 subscales: 1) physical independence, 2) mobility, 3) occupation, 4) social integration, and 5) economic self-sufficiency. There are 2 to 7 items per subscale. Subscales correspond to 5 of 6 areas of handicap identified by ICIDH.[72] • Scoring: Each subscale has a maximum score of 100 points, which corresponds to the typical performance of an average person without disability. High subscale and total scores indicate less handicap. The maximum economic self-sufficiency score corresponds to US median income
Procedures	• Self-report questionnaire that asks client to indicate time spent performing items. Can also be completed by caregiver as proxy.
Time Required	• Estimated to be 30 minutes.
Reliability	
Test-Retest	• Tozato et al[65] found test-retest reliability coefficients of CHART-J range from 0.57 to 1.00. Dijkers[67] found subscale coefficients to be in excellent range (r=0.80 to 0.95), as well as the coefficient for the total score (r=0.93).
Internal Consistency	• Not reported
Validity	
Content	• Based on ICIDH[73]—Ensured domain of handicap areas are covered in full, without overlap with impairment and disability.
Construct	• Distinguished between groups (ie, based on culture, age, education, injury level, time since injury); however, the authors recommend that group differences should be interpreted with caution.[68] • Rasch analysis supported underlying structure and linearity of CHART.
Criterion	• Concordance of CHART scores with therapist ratings of high vs low handicap.
Standardization	• Not standardized. Revised CHART was developed with additional "cognitive independence" scale to increase applicability to stroke population.
Utility	
Research	• Useful for measuring community reintegration of broad populations such as SCI clients. • Useful in rehabilitation program evaluation.
Clinical	• May be useful for measuring change in performance (before vs after intervention), although does not appear to have been specifically tested for this.
Strengths	• Focuses on objective, observable criteria to limit interpreter bias. • Normative data has been established with large sample sizes. • Views occupation in a manner similar to occupational therapy perspective.
Complexities	• The CHART has a ceiling effect, particularly for the SCI population. • Economic self-sufficiency scale is based on US income, limiting international interpretation. • Large percentage of incomplete data for the economic self-sufficiency subscale in large studies, which impacts total scores reported in research. • Reliance on total scores may mask important differences at the subscale level.

Table 9-5

COMMUNITY PARTICIPATION INDICATORS (CPI)

Source	Allen Heinemann, Rehabilitation Institute of Chicago http://www.ric.org/research/centers/cror/publications/cpi/
Key References	Heinemann et al[74,75]; Hammel et al[76]; Magasi et al[77]
Purpose	• To measure the level of engagement, satisfaction, and enfranchisement (eg, choice, opportunity, access, fulfillment, etc) experienced by an individual in a community setting.
Type of Client	• Developed for people with a variety of impairments, including mobility, communication, learning, cognitive, hearing, or vision.
Test Format	• Forty-eight questions belonging to 4 subscales: 1) importance of participation; 2) social connection, inclusion, and membership; 3) control over participation; and 4) access to transportation and communication services. Scoring: Instructions for scoring are located at www.ric.org.
Procedures	• Self-report questionnaire that asks client to estimate the frequency of time spent on items.
Time Required	• Estimated to be less than 30 minutes.
Reliability	
Test-Retest	• Not reported
Internal Consistency	• Item-total correlations ranged from .18 to .73. No Chronbach's alpha reported.
Validity	
Content	• Based on ICF and developed using a grounded theory approach to understand the perspective of people with disabilities.
Construct	• Factors were developed using Exploratory Factor Analysis, Confirmatory Factor Analysis, Item Response Theory, and Rasch analysis. The factors distinguished between groups based on severity, type, and number of disabilities; however, authors suggested more work needed to be done using samples that differed across environments, socioeconomic status, and access to community resources.[74]
Criterion	• Not reported
Standardization	• Not reported
Utility	
Research	• Useful in measuring perception of enfranchisement for a broad range of populations. • Measures perceived importance of participation; social connection, inclusion, and membership; control over participation; and access to transportation and communication services.
Clinical	• May be useful for understanding how much choice and control a person feels they have. May be useful in understanding barriers to a person's participation. May be useful in goal setting or discharge planning
Strengths	• Measures choice and control of participation for a broad range of populations. • Community-based tool that can help a therapist understand barriers to participation. • Tool is freely available from www.ric.org.
Complexities	• Needs more evidence for reliability. • Tool was developed using a population from one metropolitan area, so need to use caution when generalizing results to people living in other regions and from diverse backgrounds. • Clear scoring procedure not available on the form. • Will need to read measurement article to score factor structures.

Table 9-6

Impact on Participation and Autonomy Questionnaire (IPAQ)

Source	Paula Kersten, PhD, Senior Lecturer in Rehabilitation School of Health Professions and Rehabilitation Sciences University of Southampton Highfield; P.Kersten@soton.ac.uk
Key References	Cardol et al[78-80]
Purpose	• The IPAQ is a generic self-report questionnaire, focusing on person-perceived autonomy and participation for individuals with chronic disorders. The scale was developed for use as a profile for disease severity assessment, needs assessment, and outcomes assessment (evaluation).[79]
Type of Client	• Individuals with chronic disorders, such as neuromuscular disease, traumatic brain injury, stroke, spinal cord injury, rheumatoid arthritis, and fibromyalgia
Test Format	• Consists of 5 testing domains: social relations, autonomy in self-care, mobility and leisure, family role, and work and educational opportunities[79] • Consists of 39 self-report items, with 31 related to perceived participation (using a 5-point likert scale) and 8-items related to the perceived problem (using a 3-point likert scale)[79]
Procedures	• Providing a self-report IPAQ to an individual with a chronic disorder to complete
Time Required	• Approximately 30 minutes
Reliability	
Test-Retest	• Good test-retest reliability with weighted kappa ranged from 0.56 and .90 for the perceived participation items and .59 to .87 for the problem experience items[79] • Weighted Kappa showed moderate agreement with 2 items addressing family role (0.56 to 0.59) and 1 item addressing perceived problem in self-care (0.59)[79]
Internal Consistency	• Intraclass correlation coefficient (ICC) ranged from .83 (family role) to .91 (autonomy outdoors)[79] • Homogeneity of the domains was good with Cronbach's alpha considered at .91 (autonomy outdoors), .86 (social relations), .90 (family role), and .91 (work and educational opportunities)[79]
Validity	
Content	• Factor analysis indicated that the factors could be best interpreted according to the following domains of participation: autonomy indoors, family role, autonomy outdoors, and social relations. With this factor solution, 67% of the total variance could be explained. Most of the variance (43%) was explained by the factor addressing autonomy indoors indicating good construct validity.[79]
Construct	• Discriminant validity was best supported when comparing the IPAQ and the London Handicap scale (LHS) and 2 domains of the LHS[79] • Correlations between all domains of the IPAQ and the domains "economic self-sufficiency" and "orientation" on the LHS were low (r=-.01 to -.29) demonstrating good discriminant validity[79] • Discriminant validity between the IPAQ and the domains of the Sickness Impact Profile 68-item version (SIP68) and the Short-Form Health Survey (SF-36) was only demonstrated by a low correlation between the domain "social relations" on the IPAQ and the physical domain of the SF-36 (r=-.26) and the physical domain of the SIP (r=.16)[79]
Utility	• Provides person-perceived health status information that many other health status assessments do not assess (ie, Rankin Scale, the Craig Handicap Assessment and Reporting Technique (CHART), and the London Handicap Scale (LHS).[78]
Strengths	• Minimal time required • Easy to administer
Complexities	• Items regarding perceived problems appear less sensitive to change than other participation items.[80]

Table 9-7

ASSESSMENT OF LIFE HABITS SCALE (LIFE-H)

Source	International Network on the Disability Creation Process, A108-525 Wilfrid-Hamel Blvd E, Quebec City, Quebec G1M 2S8
Key References	Chien et al[59]; Desrosiers et al[81]; Figueiredo et al[82]; Fougeyrollas et al[83]; Gagnon et al[84]; Magasi and Post[85]; Noreau et al[86,87]; Poulin and Desrosiers[88]; Roy-Bouthot et al[89]; Sakzewski et al[90]
Purpose	• LIFE-H assesses the quality of social participation of people with disabilities. It covers the 12 domains of life habits proposed by the Disability Creation Process (DCP): 6 relating to daily activities (nutrition, fitness, personal care, communication, housing, and mobility) and 6 relating to social roles (responsibilities, interpersonal relationships, community life, education, employment, and leisure)
Type of Client	• Adults age 18 years or older with or without disabilities • Children age 5 to 13 years
Test Format	• LIFE-H is an assessment tool, though the short form has also been used as a screening tool. • Various forms of this outcome measure are available covering all 12 domains ¤ LIFE-H 2.1 (1997) contains 58 items ¤ LIFE-H 3.0 (1998) has a long form that contains 242 items, which can be used as a whole or as subsections. The short form contains 77 items and is a general measure of handicap ¤ LIFE-H 3.1 (2001) has 77 items ¤ LIFE-H for Children (2007) has 197 items in the long version and 64 items in the short form.
Procedures	Can be self or clinician administered. Has also been given to proxies of clients in stroke rehabilitation. • Each item is rated for the following: ¤ The level of perceived difficulty (using a 5-point ordinal scale: not applicable, not performed, performed by substitution, with difficulty, or no difficulty) ¤ The type of assistance required (4-point ordinal scale: no aides, technical aids, adaptation, human assistance—beyond expectation for age in children) ¤ The satisfaction for each item (5-point scale; 0 = very dissatisfied and 4 = very satisfied). Satisfaction is rated from 1 to 5 for the children's version. • When a life habit is not performed because it is not part of their daily life and the person does not wish for it to be part of their life, it is scored as "non-applicable" **Scoring** • An accomplishment score is calculated using the combined and weighted level of difficulty and types of assistance: (Sum of Scores x 10) / (number of applicable life habits x 9) • Total scores for each life habit category range from 0 to 9, where a score of 0 indicates total handicap or total disruption to participation and a score of 9 represents optimal participation.
Time Required	• LIFE-H 3.0 = 40 to 120 minutes (long form); 30 to 60 minutes (short form)

(continued)

Table 9-7 (continued)

Assessment of Life Habits Scale (LIFE-H)

Reliability	

Test-Retest	• Review of psychometric properties of LIFE-H in stroke rehabilitation found *excellent* test-retest reliability (Interclass correlation coefficient, ICC=0.80 to 0.95)[82]
	• Study looking at participation scores with older adults with functional limitations to ADLs and mobility (n=40) using short form of the LIFE-H; 5 to 10 days between evaluations[86]
	  ◦ *Excellent* total score (Interclass correlation coefficient, ICC=0.95)
	  ◦ *Excellent* sub-scores in all categories (ICC=0.83 to 0.97) except recreation (*adequate*, ICC=0.55), and fitness (*poor*=0.30)
	• Study looking at satisfaction scores with older adults with disabilities (n=30) using short form of the LIFE-H excluding the employment or education domains deemed irrelevant to population; 6 to 8 days between evaluations.[88]
	  ◦ *Excellent* total score (ICC=0.88)
	  ◦ *Excellent* domains of communication, leisure, interpersonal relationships, and responsibilities (ICC=0.80 to 0.88)
	  ◦ Adequate in all other domains (*adequate*, ICC=0.65 to 0.76)
	• Study looking at participation scores of adults with myotonic dystrophy (n=28) using short form of the LIFE-H; 2 weeks between evaluations.[84]
	  ◦ *Excellent* total score (ICC=0.86)
	  ◦ *Adequate to excellent* sub-scores in all categories (ICC=0.73 to 0.92) except in areas of fitness and communication (*poor*, ICC=0.12 to 0.20)

Inter-Rater	• Review of psychometric properties of LIFE-H in stroke rehabilitation found *adequate to excellent* inter-rater reliability (r=0.64 to 0.91) as well as agreement between patients with stroke and their proxies (ICC=0.73 to 0.82)[82]
	• Study with older adults with functional limitations to ADLs and mobility (n=44) using the short form of the LIFE-H[86]
	  ◦ *Excellent* total score (Interclass correlation coefficient, ICC=0.89)
	  ◦ *Adequate* sub-scores in all categories (ICC=0.55 to 0.72) except personal care (*excellent*, ICC=0.95), and fitness (*poor*=0.33)
	• Study looking at participation scores of adults with myotonic dystrophy (n=28) using short form of the LIFE-H[84]
	  ◦ *Excellent* total score (ICC=0.90)
	  ◦ *Excellent* in domains of personal care, mobility, interpersonal relationships, and community life (ICC=0.84 to 0.93)
	  ◦ *Adequate* in domains of housing, nutrition, responsibility and recreation (ICC=0.56 to 0.76)
	  ◦ *Poor* in areas of communication and fitness (ICC=0.21 to 0.47)
	• Study looking at the participation scores of children, aged 5 to 13 years old, with various impairments (n=94) using the children's version of the LIFE-H. Outcome measure was completed by the parents[87]
	  ◦ *Excellent* in all sub-domains (ICC=0.80 to 0.93) except
	  ◦ *Adequate* in areas of community life and interpersonal relationships (ICC=0.63 to 0.78)

Intra-Rater	• Study looking at the participation scores of children, aged 5 to 13 years old, with various impairments (n=94) using the children's version of the LIFE-H. Outcome measure was completed by the parents[87] ◦ *Excellent* in all sub-domains (ICC=0.83-0.95) except *adequate* in areas of community life and interpersonal relationships (ICC=0.58-78)

(continued)

Table 9-7 (continued)

ASSESSMENT OF LIFE HABITS SCALE (LIFE-H)

Validity	
Content	• Clear description of the aim of the measure, the concepts being measured, the method of item selection, and the involvement of experts • Items were developed from the 13 categories of life habits as classified by the Quebec Committee of the International Classification of Impairments, Disabilities, and Handicaps (QCICIDH). Twelve rehabilitation experts validated copies of the original instrument. Experts concluded that, generally, the items covered large parts of an individual's life habits.[83] • Established for the children's version through consultations with experts and parents (n=29); 90% of parents indicated item wording was easy to understand; 67% to 90% of experts judged the representativeness of items as adequate, while a higher percentage of parents did the same[87] • A meta-analysis evaluating the extent to which various instruments actually measure children's participation based on the definition by Coster and Khetani[6] found that only 33% of items found in the children's version of LIFE-H did this.[59]
Construct	• Correlation of children's version with the Pediatric Evaluation of Disability Inventory (PEDI) when used with children with disabilities (n=91)[87] ¤ Strong association between PEDI self-care and mobility dimensions with LIFE-H personal care and housing dimensions (Pearson correlation coefficient; $0.79 < r < 0.88$) ¤ Strong association between PEDI social function and LIFE-H communication and responsibility (r=0.80 to 0.81) ¤ Divergent validity found in associations between all PEDI dimensions with LIFE-H dimensions of interpersonal relationships and community life (r=0.44 to 0.66) • Correlation of children's version with the Functional Independence Measure for Children (WeeFIM) when used with children with disabilities (n=91) ¤ Strong association between WeeFIM self care and communication with LIFE-H housing, personal care and communication (r=0.89 to 0.94) ¤ Weaker associations found between WeeFIM communication and social cognition dimensions and LIFE-H motor dimensions (r=0.43 to 0.49)
Convergent	• Review of psychometric properties of LIFE-H in stroke rehabilitation found adequate to excellent convergent validity (r=0.57 to 0.91)[82]
Predictive	• According to a review of LIFE-H in stroke rehabilitation, no studies were reported on the predictive validity of LIFE-H with clients with stroke. Six studies examined the predictors of the LIFE-H score. After 6 months the best predictors were found to be: lower extremity coordination (R2=31%, length of stay (R2=3.0%), balance (R2=9.0%), age (R2=1.0%), and comorbidity (R2=1.0%). Two to 4 years post-stroke the best predictors were found to be age (R2=11.0%), comorbidity (R2=18.0%), motor coordination (R2 =15.0%), upper extremity disability (R2 =6.0%), and affect (R2=3.0%)[82]
Discriminant	• A meta-analysis of contemporary measures of participation including LIFE-H found that LIFE-H distinguishes people based on level and completeness of spinal cord injury, health status of older adults, and living situation of older adults.[85] • The same meta-analysis also found minimal floor effects and ceiling effects were found in some sub-scores.[85]
Responsiveness	• Has not been evaluated
Standardization	• Normative data is available for older adults (65+)[81] ******No manual was available; therefore, it could not be reviewed for standardization******

(continued)

Table 9-7 (continued)

Assessment of Life Habits Scale (LIFE-H)

Utility	
Research Programs	• Extensively used on populations with cerebral palsy, multiple sclerosis, older adults with disabilities, stroke, traumatic brain injury, spinal cord injury, pediatrics
Practice Settings	• Provides clinicians with useful information on perceived difficulties in participation, assistance required when participating, satisfaction in current activities and desire for change.
Strengths	• It is client-centered • Validated in adult and pediatric populations with a wide range of conditions • Can be used with proxies of clients who suffered from stroke • Comprehensive in its coverage of participation domains
Complexities	• Full version can take a long time • Response format can be complicated • Potential for recall bias for those with cognitive impairments

Table 9-8

London Handicap Scale

Source	Medical Outcomes Trust, 235 Wyman St. Suite 130, Waltham, MA, 02451; www.outcomes-trust.org
Key References	Kutlay et al[91]; Dubuc et al[92]; Lo et al[93]; Harwood and Ebrahim[94,95]; Jenkinson et al[96]
Purpose	• Measures the effects of disease or disability on participation. Serves as a general measure of disability.
Type of Client	• Adolescents and adults with and without disabilities.
Test Format	• Based on 6 dimensions of handicap identified in ICIDH. Respondents identify their perceived level of disadvantage in 6 dimensions: mobility, orientation, occupation, physical independence, social integration, and economic self-sufficiency. • Scoring: Each dimension has a 6-point rating scale, ranging from "none" (no disadvantage) to "extreme" (extreme disadvantage). A final score of 100 indicates no disadvantage, a score of 0 indicates maximum disadvantage. The authors of the instrument advise using a weighted system to calculate final scores; however, Jenkinson et al[96] found that scores could be accurately calculated without the weighted system, just by adding the respondent's raw scores.
Procedures	• Can be self-administered or via interview (with client or proxy).
Time Required	• Completion time 10 to 15 minutes.
Reliability	
Test-Retest	• Good to excellent. Studies found test-retest coefficient of 0.70 for 2 months and 0.91 for 2 weeks.
Internal Consistency	• Excellent. Cronbach's alpha has consistently scored at 0.80 or higher. Kutlay et al. (2011) found in the Turkish version, the Chronbach's alpha=.845, ICC=.845

(continued)

Table 9-8 (continued)

LONDON HANDICAP SCALE

Validity	
Content	• Based on ICIDH (1980).
Construct	• Good. Studies have found correlations between the LHS and age, impairment, motor disability, depression and anxiety, cognitive impairment, and life satisfaction.[92-96]
Convergent	• Good convergent validity. Studies have found strong correlations between LHS and other measures that examine similar constructs such as the Rankin and the Functional Abilities Index. Responsiveness was found to be more responsive to change than the Barthel Index in a day hospital program for individuals attending 10 or more sessions.[94,95]
Utility	
Research	• Designed as an epidemiological tool—particularly for randomized clinical trials.
Clinical	• Can also be used in cost analysis of different programs for health policy development. • Measure clinical outcomes and treatment effectiveness.
Strengths	• Although based on initial ICIDH framework, still conceptually linked to ICIDH-2. • Demonstrates strong psychometric properties thus far.
Complexities	• No inter-rater reliability studies completed. Therefore, it is difficult to comment on accuracy of proxy response. • Floor effects may exist in populations with mild to moderate level of disability (ie, they may have a score indicating no disadvantage, when in fact one exists.)

Table 9-9

PEDIATRIC ACTIVITY CARD SORT (PACS)

Source	Canadian Association of Occupational Therapists, CTTC Building, 3400-1125 Colonel By Drive, Ottawa, ON K1S 5R1
Key References	Calley et al[97]; Chien et al[59]; Taylor et al[98]
Purpose	• The PACS is an interview-style assessment that helps to determine children's level of occupational performance and engagement in typical activities of childhood. Seventy-five photographs are used to illicit information about a child's participation, level of participation, and/or reasons for lack of involvement. Information gathered through this interview can be used to develop an occupational profile for a child and to identify goals that can be used for therapeutic intervention.
Type of Client	• Children aged 5 to 14 years old ¤ Developmentally 4 years old ¤ Can respond to pictures and questions ¤ Can have any diagnosis
Test Format	• Consists of 83 cards: 8 blank cards and 75 photographs of children participating in typical activities that can be subdivided into 4 categories: self-care, school/productivity, hobbies/social activities, and sports.

(continued)

Table 9-9 (continued)

PEDIATRIC ACTIVITY CARD SORT (PACS)

Type of Client	
Procedures	• Children are meant to be interviewed, but parents can also be interviewed • The child is shown each of the photographs and asked if he or she has participated in the activities represented in the cards (yes or no). • The cards representing activities that the child does participate in are further sorted according to the frequency of their participation (daily, weekly, monthly, or yearly). • The child is then asked to select the 5 most important activities to them and the 5 that he or she would most like to do. • An occupational profile is developed from these results and includes the overall percentage of participation based on the number of current activities for that child and the total number of possible activities. A percentage of participation for each of the 4 categories can also be calculated.
Time Required	• 20 to 25 minutes to administer the measure
Reliability	• No studies reporting the reliability of the outcome measure has been identified
Validity	

Content	• No studies directly reporting the validity of the outcome measure has been identified. However, the measure has been used as an outcome measure in a study comparing the activity, participation, and quality of life for children with (n=19) and without (n= 19) spastic cerebral palsy (CP).[97]
	  ◦ Typically developing children were found to participate in more personal care activities than children with (CP) (t(36)=2.434, p=0.02).
	  ◦ No significant differences were found in the participation in the domains of school/productivity, hobbies/social activities, or sports
	  ◦ Weak correlation between domains of PACS and the Timed Up and Go (TUG) test with children with cerebral palsy (Pearson's r correlation coefficient, r2=-0.273 to -0.445)
	  ◦ Weak correlation between domains of PACS and 6-Minute Walk Test (6MWT) with children with cerebral palsy (Pearson's r correlation coefficient, r2=-0.133 to 0.447)
	• A meta-analysis evaluating the extent to which various instruments actually measure children's participation based on the definition by Coster and Khetani[6] found that only 27% of items found in the PACS measures participation.[59]

Standardization	****No access to the manual; therefore, standardization information could not be assessed****
Utility	
Research Settings	• Can be used to study patterns of activity for school-aged children with and without disabilities[98]
Practice Settings	• Provides useful information to a clinician about types and frequency of activity. • Can be used to identify goals for the therapeutic process • Can be used to assess the effectiveness of intervention on improving the activity of children.
Strengths	• Easy to use and administer • Client-centered approach in identifying goals because children are asked to identify the most important activities and which ones he or she would most like to be able to do • Can be enjoyable for clients to complete

(continued)

Table 9-9 (continued)

PEDIATRIC ACTIVITY CARD SORT (PACS)

Strengths	• Photographs allow assessment to be used when literacy is an issue • Based on the Activity Card Sort (ACS), which was designed for adults and has been shown to be valid and reliable through multiple studies.
Complexities	• Potential for recall bias from children • There are currently no normative data with which comparisons can be made. • Range and scope of activities may be limited due to cultural issues

Table 9-10

PERSONAL CARE PARTICIPATION ASSESSMENT AND RESOURCE TOOL (PC-PART), FORMERLY THE HART

Source	The PART Group, PO BOX 1039 G, Greythorn 3104, Australia PARTGroup@bigpond.com
Key References	Turner et al[99]; Darzins et al[100]; Vertesi et al[101]; Smith et al[102]; Darzins et al[103]; Darzins[104]; Barbara and Whiteford[105]
Purpose	• To assess what people can do alone, or get done for them, regarding personal care in their usual environments with the usual available help. • To comprehensively assess and record personal care participation—the minimum set of survival tasks for living in a given setting.
Type of Client	• Adults of any age, and also suitable for older youths. Can assess people with cognitive impairment or limited insight as well as the cognitively intact. Can assess people who cannot communicate.
Test Format	• The PC-PART consists of full color work sheets and a bi-fold summary sheet. • The worksheets guide the assessment and record the assessment. • The summary sheet gives an easily overviewed summary, risk assessment and plan. • Contains 43 items in 7 domains: clothing (5), hygiene (8), nutrition (8), mobility (9), safety (6), residence (5), and supports (2). Items are categorized as either "OK by self," OK with help," or "Not OK." • In addition the risk in each item is categorized as "high," "medium," or "low."
Procedures	• Administration: Each item is assessed by asking a single question of the person being assessed and, separately, of a key informant. If the given answers agree, the item can be scored. If the person being assessed and the key informant disagree, then the item is scored by either direct observation or from assessing a standard task (that is to be done with the usually available help). Key informants can be interviewed by telephone. • Self-administered for people who are motivated, cognitively intact, and who have good insight. This is only done at the clinician's discretion. There are no reliability studies of this. Self-administering the PC-PART can be used as screening checklist. • Scoring: The PC-PART does not provide an overall participation score. It lists personal care participation items and displays performance on these. This helps users to determine for which items or domains help is needed or is being provided. • Users can note change and infer improvement or deterioration. If users ignore the underlying construct of participation, they can simply treat the scores as continuous variables with interval characteristics—this crude summation is discouraged for individuals, but if appropriately interpreted, may be valid for aggregate data.

(continued)

Table 9-10 (continued)

Personal Care Participation Assessment and Resource Tool (PC-PART), Formerly the HART

Type of Client	
Time Required	• Initial assessments take about 40 minutes, including explanation, data collection, and documentation. Assessment of complex situations takes longer, especially if multiple key informants are needed. • Comprehensive assessment of personal care participation, including documentation of findings, using the PC-PART is faster than equivalent nonstructured assessment.
Reliability	
Test-Retest	• A prior version of the PC-PART (2000) showed good test-retest reliability, with kappa scores in each domain ranging from a low of 0.63 to 1.0.
Inter-Rater	• Comparison between 2 pairs of experienced occupational therapists—kappa scores ranged from 0.63 to 1.0. Inter-rater for people with variety of conditions by an interdisciplinary team was completed by Turner et al[99] with an overall Kappa value of .65 and Kappa values ranging from 0.15 to 0.78.
Internal Consistency	• No data available
Validity	
Content	• Items were created by a clinician-driven item-generation process, compared to an extensive literature review, reviewed by a group of experts, and then collated into an initial draft. Early drafts of the PC-PART were piloted with small samples. Subsequently, testing occurred with numerous samples, including developmentally disabled youths, adults with acquired brain injury, psychiatric hospital patients, and older adults. Testing has been done in urban and rural settings and in culturally and linguistically diverse groups. Testing was done in Canada and Australia.
Construct	• PC-PART data patterns matched clinical outcomes of rehabilitation and geriatric management and evaluation patients in consecutive case series in 2 units.
Criterion	• No data available
Standardization	• Manual provides comprehensive instructions—experienced clinicians can successfully use it without training or extensive reference to the manual.
Utility	
Research	• Can be used to examine and compare personal-care participation patterns of patients, including changes over time. • Can be used as an outcome measure for both inpatient and outpatient rehabilitation.
Clinical	• Provides useful information to clinicians and patients about the presence of personal care participation restrictions that threaten survival. • Can be used to assess the need for interventions, the effectiveness of interventions, and the efficiency of interventions. • Helps assessors to consider whether improvements in body structure or function or inactivity are likely to eliminate participation restriction and whether environmental modification will be required. • Found to be acceptable to clinicians. • Found to be superior to the SMAF in large scale testing in numerous rehabilitation and aged care services.

(continued)

Table 9-10 (continued)

Personal Care Participation Assessment and Resource Tool (PC-PART), Formerly the HART

Strengths	• Theoretically based on the WHO-ICIDH and subsequently on the WHO-ICF. • Measures just personal care participation—the tasks necessary for survival. • User-friendly for clinicians and time efficient. • Comprehensive; therefore, no critical survival items missed. • Written in common language; therefore, it is easy to administer. Wording deals well with potentially embarrassing items. Acceptable to patients. • Two instructional videos are available: "HART" and the "ICF," and "How to use the PC-PART in rehabilitation."
Complexities	• Looks longer and more daunting than it is. • Only measures one small component of health status. Users who do not appreciate this are disappointed by its narrow focus. • Additional psychometric testing is required to develop a valid approach to summation of scores within and across domains.

Table 9-11

Participation and Environment Measure for Children and Youth (PEM-CY)

Source	CanChild Centre for Childhood Disability Research, McMaster University, 1280 Main Street West, Hamilton ON, L8S 4L8 The PEM-CY is available for purchase for use in research or personal practice on the CanChild website (https://public.canchild.ca/inventory/readmore/e35f15ce-5dbe-4e09-a19b-8e2ba7f2e01d). For parents wishing to use a version of the PEM-CY for their own use, an electronic version is available for free on the CanChild website.
Key References	Bedell et al[106]; Coster et al[107-109]; Khetani et al[110]
Purpose	• The PEM-CY was created as a parent-report measure for use in large studies. It is designed to capture the participation of children and young people with and without disabilities across environments and also the extent to which environmental factors impact children's participation.[107] • The PEM-CY simultaneously measures 3 dimensions of participation and 2 dimensions of environmental factors across 3 settings: home, school, and community. The 3 dimensions of participation measured are 1) "frequency" of participation 2) "extent of involvement" in participation and 3) "desire for change in set of activities" available.[107(p 1030)] • It is a descriptive measure and will therefore be evaluated as such following the criteria established by Law[57] in this report.
Type of Client	• The PEM-CY was designed to be completed by the parents of all children and youth (ages 5 to 17 years), with or without a disability affecting the young person's physical, cognitive, social, or affective abilities.[107]
Test Format	• The PEM-CY was originally tested as an electronic survey.[107] • It is also available in paper format and has been used as such.[110]

(continued)

Table 9-11 (continued)

Participation and Environment Measure for Children and Youth (PEM-CY)

Type of Client	
Test Format	• The PEM-CY is subdivided into 3 sections based on setting: home (10 activity items, 8 environmental items), school (5 activity items, 12 environmental items), and community (10 activity items, 13 environmental items). For each activity item in each setting, the measure asks parents to identify how often over the past 4 months the child has participated (8-item ordinal scale from "daily" to "never"), the level of the child's involvement (5-point ordinal scale from "very involved" to "minimally involved"), and would the parents want to see the child's participation change (yes/no, then 5 options for type of change if parents answers "yes"). Each environmental item in each setting asks parents about specific feature of the setting (eg, physical layout) and its impact on the child's participation (4-point ordinal scale: "not an issue," "usually helps," "sometimes helps/sometimes makes harder," "usually makes harder"). In addition to the setting specific environmental questions, the measure asks parents about general resources' impact on their child's participation (eg, information, money, supplies) (4-point ordinal scale: "not needed," "mostly," "yes," "sometimes yes/sometimes no," "usually no").[107]
Procedures	• The administration and scoring instructions are clearly and comprehensively outlined in the PEM-CY's User's Guide.[109] • Parents or caregivers of children and young people with or without disabilities independently complete the PEM-CY by answering the questions and following the instructions that accompany the text • The PEM-CY produces the following summary scores, which are meant to describe attributes of the phenomenon under study (participation, the environment, and the interaction between the two): "participation: frequency," "participation: involvement," "participation: desire for change," "environment: supportiveness, total," "environment: supports," and "environment: resources." Each summary score is calculated as a straight percentage of a specific response or the "percent maximum possible."[107] • Users can then use the "frequency" summary score to "compare the intensity and diversity of participation in home, school, or community" between children with and without disabilities. The mean "involvement score" acts as a very general gauge of the extent to which a child is participating in each setting. The total number of activity items for which parents cite a "desire for change" indicates a setting where increasing supports may impact participation.[108] • The PEM-CY "community" section could be administered in isolation to aid with Health Impact Assessments (HIA).[110]
Time Required	• Respondents in one study took an average of 20 to 25 minutes to complete the PEM-CY.[107]
Reliability	
Test-Retest	• Coster et al[107] (n = 576) reports that the test-retest reliability of the PEM-CY is moderate for school setting (0.58) and good for home (0.84) and community (0.79) over a 1- to 4-week period. Assuming this statistic is the Chance-Corrected Kappa, the test-retest reliability of the school setting does not quite meet the 0.60 cut-off established by Law.[57] However, the authors note that this range is generally accepted for measures designed for population studies. Moreover, the PEM-CY is a very new measure and more psychometric testing is supported.

(continued)

Table 9-11 (continued)

Participation and Environment Measure for Children and Youth (PEM-CY)

Reliability	
Internal Consistency	• Coster et al[107] (n=576) reports that internal consistency for summary scores in each setting ranged from poor to excellent. For "participation frequency" in home, school, and the community, Cronbach's alpha measured 0.59, 0.61, and 0.70, respectively. For "participation: involvement" in home, school, and the community, Cronbach's alpha measured 0.83, 0.72, and 0.75, respectively. For all environmental summary scales, Cronbach's alpha was equal to or greater than 0.80 across all settings except for "Home—Supportiveness" (0.67) and "School—Resources" (0.73). Some of these statistics fall under the 0.70 cut-off established by Law[57] for internal consistency of descriptive instruments. However, the authors note that internal consistency would be moderate as multiple factors impact the attributes being measured by each summary scale.
Validity	
Content	• Scale construction is excellent. The PEM-CY was based on a comprehensive literature review plus the themes that emerged during focus-groups and interviews of parents with children with disabilities.[107,108] It was then reviewed by a panel that included parents, health care providers, and researchers.[107] • Chien et al[109] reviewed 16 instruments measuring children's participation and sought to determine the extent to which the measure captured participation. 82.9% of the participation items of the PEM-CY were found to capture participation.
Construct	• Coster et al[107] (n=576) report that the PEM-CY is able to discriminate between children with and without disabilities, finding a significant affect (effect size 0.51 to 1.86). Moreover, the instrument confirms the theoretical proposition that the more supportive an environment, the less the desire for environment change on the part of parents across all 3 settings (home: correlation coefficient -0.42; school: -0.59; community: -0.53). • Law et al[111] note the difference between children with and without disabilities is present even when controlling for child's age, gender, and/or annual household income. • Khetani et al[110] (n=89) report that the PEM-CY detected significant group differences in summary scores according to household income. Specifically, parents earning over $80,000/year reported their child participating in community activities more often ($t[77]= -.296$, $p=0.004$, $d=0.61$) and more environmental supports ($t[74]=-3.70$, $p<0.001$, $d=0.88$). Differences remained even after authors controlled for child's age and number of functional limitations. Their finding confirms current theory on socioeconomic status being positively correlated with participation. • Khetani et al[110] (n=89) compared the concurrent validity of the PEM-CY and the Craig Hospital Inventory of Environmental Factors for Children—Parent Version using Spearman Correlation Coefficients. They found moderate to strong associations between CHIEF-CP total CHIEF-CP product scores and 1) all PEM-CY Environmental supportiveness scores ($r=-0.49$ to -0.60, $p<0.05$ to 0.01), 2) PEM-CY total number of supports ($r=-.044$, $p<0.05$), and 3) PEM-CY total number of barriers ($r=0.58$, $p<0.01$). They also found moderate to strong associations between PEM-CY summary scores and CHIEF-CP total magnitude scores aside from "environment-supportiveness-school." In relation to specific settings, the CHIEF-CP total magnitude score was significantly associated with the PEM total "environment-supportiveness-home" ($r=-0.49$, $p<0.05$) and "environment-supportiveness-community" ($r=-0.46$, $p<0.05$). The CHIEF-CP total magnitude score was significantly associated with the PEM-CY total number of barriers score ($r=-0.52$, $p<0.05$) and the PEM-CY total number of supports score ($r=0.53$, $p<0.05$).
Standardization	• The PEM-CY is self-administered by parents or caregivers of children and young people with or without disabilities.

(continued)

Table 9-11 (continued)

Participation and Environment Measure for Children and Youth (PEM-CY)	
Utility	• Quick to administer which makes the measure well-suited for large research studies • Can be used for children and youth of various ages • The PEM-CY was used by a community service agency, Adaptive Recreation Opportunities (ARO), to assist with program development to encourage children's participation and staff reportedly found it a "detailed assessment process to identify individual and program-level needs" according to one Master's Thesis.[112(p ii)] However, the paper was not peer-reviewed and, therefore, results must viewed with caution. • Khetani et al[110] suggest the PEM-CY can be used by administrators of Health Impact Assessments (HIA's) to identify existing barriers in human-created environments that impact a child's participation and those results then used to guide practice and policy. • Although the measure has not yet been studied in this capacity, it could potentially be used by schools to assess accessibility of learning environments (ie, by comparing school summary scores of children with and without disabilities) and barriers to participation as perceived by parents • Potential uses of the PEM-CY identified by stakeholders include needs assessments by community service agencies to identify under-served populations, ongoing evaluation of the supports, and barriers to participation for children and youth who are the recipients of services through community agencies, follow-up surveys post-intervention, and for individual use by families so identify needs they would like to have addressed.[109]
Strengths	• Measure is relatively quick to administer and self-directed by the respondent (requires no special training) • Measure captures the interaction between participation and the environment rather than measuring the 2 dimensions in isolation • Measure perceives and measures participation both objectively (ie, frequency) and subjectively (ie, involvement) • Has been translated into eleven languages besides English with more translations forthcoming • Gender-neutral
Complexities	• The PEM-CY's psychometrics, as generated by the studies conducted thus far, do not yet meet the standards for an individual measure set out by Law[57] but are adequate for population-wise inquiries according to Coster et al.[107] More psychometric testing is therefore required to determine in which situations the PEM-CY's use is supported as it is a relatively new measure. • Measure is designed for parents and caregivers rather than children themselves; therefore, subjective measure of participation (ie, "child's involvement") may not measure the child's actual subjective experience of his or her participation • As the PEM-CY's User Guide makes clear, no normative data exist for researchers or administrators of the PEM-CY to make comparisons between scores. Those who interpret PEM-CY scores must therefore be cautious in drawing conclusions between groups or individuals as these differences result from personal preference as well as potential barriers to participation. • More study is required before cross-cultural validity is established: as Bedell et al[106] note, the majority of families studied were White, living the northeast United States or Ontario, and above the median income and education level of both countries.

Table 9-12

Reintegration to Normal Living Index (RNLI)

Source	Link to measure: http://www.strokengine.ca/pdf/rnli.pdf
Key References	Daneski et al[113]; Korner-Bitensky et al[114]; Stark et al[115]; Steiner et al[116]; Tooth et al[117]; Wood-Dauphinee et al[118]
Purpose	• To assess, quantitatively, the degree to which individuals who have experienced traumatic or incapacitating illness achieve reintegration into normal social activities such as recreation, movement in the community, and interaction in family or other relationships.
Type of Client	• Individuals with stroke, malignant tumors, degenerative heart disease, central nervous system disorders, arthritis, fractures and amputations, spinal cord injury, traumatic brain injury, rheumatoid arthritis, subarachnoid hemorrhage, hip fracture, physical disability, and community dwelling elderly persons.
Test Format	• Questionnaire
Procedures	• 11 declarative statements are presented to individuals—can be self-administered or interviewer-administered. Individuals rate each statement for how much it "describes their situation" anchored by "fully describes" or complete reintegration and "does not describe" or minimal integration with the aid of a visual scale. A 10-, 4-, and 3-point scale have all been used.
Time Required	• 10 minutes or less.
Standardization	• Item scores are summed to provide a total score out of 110 (which can proportionally converted to create a score out of 100). If using the 3-point scale, the scores are from 22 to 0 with a higher score indicating poorer integration.
Reliability	
Test-Retest	• Steiner et al[116] examined the test-retest for the 75 to 79 (r=0.82), 80 to 84 (r=0.93), and 85+ age group (r=0.76). • Korner-Bitensky et al[114] examined the test-retest agreement between the 2 modes of interview. However, for the self-respondents, poor community reintegration was reported more often during the home interview than the interview conducted over the telephone.
Internal Consistency	• Wood-Dauphinee et al[118] administered the RNLI to 3 samples of patients with varied diagnoses to determine internal consistency for patients, significant others, and health care professionals (alpha=0.90, 0.92, and 0.95, respectively). • Tooth et al[117] administered the RNLI to 57 pairs of patients and significant others 6 months after stroke rehabilitation. Cronbach's alphas were excellent for the total RNLI patient and significant other scores (alpha=0.80 and 0.81, respectively). • Stark et al[115] administered the RNLI to 604 people between the ages of 18 and 80 years who had a mobility limitation (including patients with spinal cord injury, multiple sclerosis, stroke, cerebral palsy, and polio), lived in the community, and had been discharged from rehabilitation for at least 1 year. The Cronbach's alpha for this sample was excellent (0.91).
Inter-Rater	• Wood-Dauphinee et al[118] analyzed the reliability of RNLI scores between patients and relatives and between patients and health professionals. Using Pearson's correlation coefficient to measure reliability they reported adequate significant other to patient correlations of r=0.62 and r=0.65 in 2 different patient/significant other samples. They also reported poor to adequate health professional to patient correlations of r=0.39 and r=0.43. Based on these results, the authors stated that patients or significant others could complete the RNLI, but that the use of health professionals as proxies should be avoided.

(continued)

Table 9-12 (continued)

Reintegration to Normal Living Index (RNLI)

Validity	
Content	• The RNLI was developed based on literature reviews, incorporation of experiences of investigators, and open- and closed-ended questionnaires given to patients with myocardial infarction, cancer, and other chronic diseases, health professionals (physicians, social workers, physical and occupational therapists, psychologists), significant others of patients; and clergy and other lay people.[118]
Construct	• Daneski et al[113] examined the construct validity of a postal version of the RNLI (RNLI-P) with other similar measures in 76 patients with stroke. Excellent correlations were found between the total score on the RNLI-P and the Frenchay Activities Index (FAI)[119] (r = 0.69), the Short Form 36 Health Survey (SF-36)
Utility	
Research Programs	• Can be used as an assessment with a wide range of patient- and community-dwelling populations.
Practice Settings	• Provides insight into the patient's perception of their daily life.
Strengths	• Short questionnaire that requires little to no training in order to be administered effectively
Complexities	• Simple to use.

Table 9-13

World Health Organization—Disability Schedule II (WHO-DAS II)

Source	WHO
Key References	Chisolm et al[120]; Luciano et al[121,122]; Pösl et al[123]; Garin et al[124]; Chwastiak and Von Korff[125]; WHO[5]
Purpose	• To assess a person's general level of disability, in accordance with the ICIDH-2.
Type of Client	• Adults aged 18 years and older, across a wide spectrum of cultures and diagnoses.
Test Format	• Reflects 6 domains of functioning in daily life: 1) communication, 2) physical mobility, 3) self-care, 4) interpersonal interactions, 5) domestic responsibilities and work, and 6) participation in society. • Scoring: Produces scores for each domain, as well as a total score. Scores range from 0 to 100, with higher scores reflecting greater disability.
Procedures	• Interview format. Can be administered in person or over the phone.
Time Required	• 12-item versions: 5 minutes; 36-item versions: 20 minutes
Reliability	
Test-Retest	• Not reported.
Internal Consistency	• Excellent. Cronbach's alpha = 0.95 for the total score and ranged from 0.65 (self- care) to 0.91 (work and household) for each domain. Chisolm et al[120] reported WHO-DAS II communication domain score was moderately and significant correlated with scores related to hearing (APHAB and HHIE). Luciano et al[121] found Chronbach's alpha = 0.89. Significantly associated with quality of life (EQ-5D) and depression severity (PHQ-9). Posl et al[123] used the 36-item version of WHO-DAS II and found Chronbach's alpha range from 0.70-0.97. ICC over .7 for all domains, Chronbach's alpha range from -.29 to -.65.[124]

(continued)

Table 9-13 (continued)

World Health Organization—Disability Schedule II (WHO-DAS II)

Validity	
Content	• Initial draft containing 89 items was site-tested in 19 countries. Measure was then decreased to 36 items based on the results of these studies, and a 12-item screening tool was developed.
Convergent	• In 2 samples (people with depression and people with low back pain) Total WHO-DAS II scores correlated moderately with composite scores from the SF-36 (r=-0.72). Strong correlations were found between WHO-DAS II subscales, and subscales of SF-36 that reflect the same ICIDH-2 dimensions for both the psychiatric condition and the physical condition. Luciano et al[121] conducted item response analyses that indicated the 12 items forming the WHO-DAS II perform very well.
Criterion	• Not reported
Standardization	• Has been translated into 15 languages
Utility	
Research	• Measure clinical outcomes and treatment effectiveness. • Identify level of disability in a sample.
Clinical	• Identify needs. • Development of treatment plans. • Track functioning over time. • Measure clinical outcomes and treatment effectiveness.
Strengths	• Conceptually linked to the ICIDH-2. • Cross-cultural measurement of disability. • Has been shown to be responsive to change. • Has been used in a variety of conditions and across multiple centers
Complexities	• Potential for ceiling effect limits responsiveness to change for people with mild to moderate impairments or disabilities.

Table 9-14

The Young Children's Participation and Environment Measure (YC-PEM)

Source	According to Khetani et al,[126] the assessment and user guide are currently being prepared for distribution. Limited information is available about the measure on the CanChild Centre website: http://participation-environment.canchild.ca/en/young_children_participation_environment.asp
Key References	Khetani et al[126]; Khetani[127]
Purpose	• The YC-PEM was designed as a caregiver report measure for use in large-sample research. It assesses features of young children's (0 to 5 years) participation and its relation to the children's environment. No such measure was previously available.[126] • It was adapted from the Participation and Environment Measure—Children and Youth. Conceptual mapping, parental input studies, and cognitive testing went into its creation.[126] • The YC-PEM contains 3 participation scales and 1 environment scale for 3 settings: home, daycare/preschool, and community. The 3 dimensions of participation measured are "frequency" of participation, "level of involvement" in participation, and "desire for change."[126] • It is a descriptive measure and will be evaluated as such following the criteria established by Law[57] in this report.

(continued)

Table 9-14 (continued)

The Young Children's Participation and Environment Measure (YC-PEM)

Type of Client

- The YC-PEM was designed to be completed by the caregivers of all young children (ages 0 to 5 years), with or without a disability.[126]

Test Format

- The YC-PEM was tested as an electronic survey.[126]
- The YC-PEM is subdivided into 3 sections based on setting: home (13 activity items, 13 environment items), daycare/preschool (3 activity items, 16 environment items), and community (12 activity items, 17 environment items). For each activity item in each setting, the measure asks parents to identify how often over the past 4 months the child has participated (8-item ordinal scale from "daily" to "never"), the level of the child's involvement (5-point ordinal scale from "very involved" to "minimally involved"), and would the parents want to see the child's participation change (yes/no; if "yes," then whether desired change was in frequency, involvement or broader range of offered activities; and lastly 3 strategies that caregivers had used to promote participation). For each environment item, the measure asks parents to identify whether environmental factors (eg, physical layout) impacted participation (3-point scale, "no impact," "usually helps," or "usually makes harder). Caregivers are then asked if environmental resources had an impact on participation (3-point scale, "not needed," "usually yes," "usually no"). Caregivers are then asked to describe up to 3 strategies they have used to promote participation in a particular setting.[126]

Procedures

Administration

- Procedures for administration are not yet available as the user guide is still being prepared.[126]

Scoring

- In terms of scoring, 4 YC-PEM scores can be calculated for each setting: 1) frequency as the average of all frequency ratings; 2) level of involvement as the average of all involvement ratings; 3) percent desired change, generated by dividing the sum of the number of items scored as "yes, change desired" by the total number of items and then multiplying by 100; and 4) environmental support generated by dividing the sum of responses from all environmental items for a setting by the sum by the maximum possible score and multiplying by 100.[126]

Time Required

- According to the recruitment flyer on the CanChild website, the YC-PEM takes 20 to 30 minutes to complete. Information is not available on the length of time the measure takes to score or report.

Reliability

Test-Retest

- Khetani et al[126] (n = 11-234) reports that the test-retest reliability of the YC-PEM is acceptable for some scales over a 2- to 4-week period. For the "Frequency," "Level of Involvement" and "Environmental Support" subscales for all 3 settings, interclass Correlations Coefficients range from poor to excellent (0.31 to 0.94). According to Law,[57] a measure is considered acceptable if ICC > 0.65, meaning that the test-retest reliability of "Daycare/preschool—frequency" (0.31) and "Community—frequency" (0.59) do not meet criterion. For the "Desire for Change" subscale, chance-corrected Kappa ranged from fair to good: home (0.57), daycare/preschool (0.59), and community (0.52). These statistics fall beneath the 0.60 cut-off established by Law.[57] However, as the YC-PEM is a very new measure, additional psychometric testing is required before a definitive answer can be given regarding the YC-PEM's test-retest reliability.

Internal Consistency

- Khetani et al[126] report that the internal consistency of participation scales for the 4 subscales across all 3 settings ranges from poor to excellent (Cronbach Alpha = 0.67-0.96). According to Law,[57] a measure is considered acceptable if alpha > 0.7, meaning that the internal consistency of "Daycare/preschool—change desired" (0.67) and "Community—Frequency" (0.68) fall slightly underneath this cut off. No age-related patterns were observed.

(continued)

Table 9-14 (continued)

The Young Children's Participation and Environment Measure (YC-PEM)

Validity	
Construct	• Khetani et al[126] found significant differences between children with disabilities and those without disabilities in all subscales in the daycare/preschool setting. For the other 2 settings (home and community), differences were found in level of involvement and environment scores. • Although previous studies suggest that young children's participation in the community changes as they age, Khetani et al[126] were unable to find this effect
Criterion	• Khetani[127] examined the environmental content of the YC-PEM compared to the Craig Hospital Inventory of Environmental Factors for Children—Parents Version (CHIEF-CP). Significant correlations between the 2 measures were found in 77% of the cases in which 2 measures were compared. For those cases when significant correlations were found, the strength of the correlations ranged from weak to moderate ($r=-0.13$ to -0.39).
Standardization	• The YC-PEM is self-administered by parents or caregivers of children and young people with disabilities.
Utility	• Quick to administer which makes the measure well-suited for large research studies
Strengths	• First measure of its kind according to the authors to measure participation and environment simultaneously for this age group in a manner that is appropriate for use in large-scale research studies • Measure is relatively quick to administer and can be self-directed by the respondent (if done via interview, administrators require no special training) • Measure captures the interaction between participation and the environment rather than measuring the 2 dimensions in isolation • Gender neutral
Complexities	• The YC-PEM's psychometrics, as generated by the studies conducted thus far, do not yet meet the standards for an individual measure set out by Law.[57] More psychometric testing is therefore required to determine in which situations the YC-PEM's use is supported. As things stand, it is a relatively new measure. • Studies with more diverse populations would establish the measure's cross-cultural validity: 81% of the families studied by by Khetani et al[126] were White. • The measure is designed for parents and caregivers rather than children themselves, therefore the subjective component of participation registered by the YC-PEM (ie, "child's involvement") may not measure the child's actual subjective experience of his or her participation. However, as the YC-PEM is designed for very young children, this limitation applies to many similar such measures. • No normative data available to provide comparisons. Those who interpret YC-PEM scores must therefore be cautious in drawing conclusions between groups or individuals as these differences naturally result from personal preference as well as potential barriers to participation.

References

1. Meyer A. The philosophy of occupation therapy. *Arch Occup Ther.* 1922;1(1):1-10.
2. Engelhardt HT. Defining occupational therapy: the meaning of therapy and the virtues of occupation. *Am J Occup Ther.* 1977;31(10):666-672.
3. Merriam-Webster online dictionary. http://www.m-w.com. Accessed June 29, 2015.
4. Free Dictionary online dictionary. http://www.thefreedictionary.com. Accessed June 18, 2016.
5. World Health Organization. *International Classification of Functioning, Disability and Health.* Geneva: WHO; 2001.

6. Coster WJ, Khetani MA. Measuring participation of children with disabilities: issues and challenges. *Disabil Rehabil.* 2008;30:639-648.
7. Baum C, Law M. Occupational therapy practice: focusing on occupational performance. *Am J Occup Ther.* 1997;51(4):277-288.
8. Law M, Baptiste S, Carswell A, McColl M, Polatajko H, Pollock N. *Canadian Occupational Performance Measure.* 5th ed. Ottawa, Canada: CAOT Publications; 2014.
9. Christiansen C, Baum C, Bass J. *Occupational Therapy: Performance, Participation, and Well-Being.* 3rd ed. Thorofare, NJ: SLACK Incorporated; 2004.
10. Townsend E, Polatajko H. *Enabling Occupation: An Occupational Therapy Perspective.* 2nd ed. Ottawa: CAOT Publications ACE; 2007.
11. American Occupational Therapy Association. *Occupational Therapy Practice Framework: Domain and Process.* 3rd ed. Rockville, MD: Author; 2014.
12. Freysinger VJ, Alessio H, Mehdizadeh S. Re-examining the morale-physical health-activity relationship: a longitudinal study of time changes and gender differences. *Activities, Adaptation and Aging.* 1993;17(4):25-41.
13. Larson RW, Verma S. How children and adolescents spend time across the world: work, play, and developmental opportunities. *Psychol Bull.* 1999;125(6):701-736.
14. Law M, Steinwender S, LeClair L. Occupation, health and well-being. *Can J Occup Ther.* 1998;65(2): 81-91.
15. Wilcock AA. Reflections on doing, being and becoming. *Can J Occup Ther.* 1998;65:248-257.
16. Menec VH, Chipperfield JG. Remaining active in later life. The role of locus of control in seniors' leisure activity participation, health, and life satisfaction. *J Aging Health.* 1997;9(1):105-125.
17. Statistics Canada. *Participation and Activity Limitation Survey: A Profile of Disability in Canada.* Ottawa: Author; 2002.
18. Stewart M, Reid G, Mangham C. Fostering children's resilience. *J Pediatr Nurs.* 1997;12(1):21-29.
19. Mahoney J, Schweder A, Stattin H. Structured after-school activities as a moderator of depressed mood for adolescents with detached relations to their parents. *J Community Psychol.* 2002;30(1):69-86.
20. Eccles J, Barber B, Stone M, Hunt J. Extracurricular activities and adolescent development. *J Soc Issues.* 2003;59(4):865-889.
21. Law M. Participation in the occupations of everyday life. *Am J Occup Ther.* 2002;56:640-649.
22. Sinclair R. Participation in practice: making it meaningful, effective and sustainable. *Children Society.* 2004;18(2):106-118.
23. Csikszentmihalyi M. *Flow: The Psychology of Optimal Experience.* New York: Harper and Row; 1990.
24. Whiteneck G, Dijkers MP. Difficult to measure constructs: conceptual and methodological issues concerning participation and environmental factors. *Arch Phys Med Rehabil.* 2009;90(11):S22-S35.
25. Baum CM, Edwards D. *Activity Card Sort.* 2nd ed. Bethesda, MD: American Occupational Therapy Association, Inc; 2008.
26. Baum CM, Edwards D. *Activity Card Sort.* St. Louis, MO: Washington University at St. Louis (Penultima Press); 2001.
27. Laver-Fawcett AJ, Mallinson SH. Development of the Activity Card Sort – United Kingdom version (ACS-UK). *OTJR.* 2013;33(3):134-145.
28. Hamed R, Holm MB. Psychometric properties of the Arab Heritage Activity Card Sort. *Occup Ther Int.* 2013;20(1):23-34.
29. Jong M, van Nes FA, Lindeboom R. The Dutch Activity Card Sort institutional version was reproducible, but biased against women. *Disabil Rehabil.* 2012;34(18):1550-1555.
30. Eriksson GM, Chung JCC, Beng LH, et al. Occupations of older adults: a cross cultural description. *OTJR.* 2011;31(4):182-192.
31. Packer TL, Boshoff K, DeJonge D. Development of the Activity Card Sort–Australia. *Aust Occup Ther J.* 2008;55(3):199-206.
32. Doney RM, Packer TL. Measuring changes in activity participation of older Australians: validation of the Activity Card Sort – Australia. *Australas J Ageing.* 2008;27(1):33-37.
33. Chan VW, Chung JC, Packer TL. Validity and reliability of the Activity Card Sort-Hong Kong version. *OTJR.* 2006;(26)4:152-158.
34. Katz N, Karpin H, Lak A, Furman T, Hartman-Maeir A. Participation in occupational performance: reliability and validity of the Activity Card Sort. *OTJR.* 2003;23(1):10-17.
35. Sachs D, Josman N. The Activity Card Sort: a factor analysis. *OTJR.* 2003;23(4):165-174.
36. Everard K, Lach H, Fisher E, Baum C. Relationship of activity and social support to the functional health of older adults. *J Gerontol Soc Sci.* 2000;55B(4):S208-S212.
37. Orellano E, Ito M, Dorne R, Irizarry D, Davila R. Occupational participation of older adults: reliability and validity of the activity card sort—Puerto Rican Version. *OTJR.* 2012;32(1):266-272.
38. Orellano E. Occupational participation of older Puerto Rican adults: reliability and validity of a Spanish version of the Activity Card Sort. PhD Dissertation, Nova Southeastern University; 2008; Montana.
39. Albert S, Bear-Lehman J, Burkhardt A. Lifestyle-adjusted function: variation beyond BADL and IADL competencies. *Gerontologist.* 2009; doi: 10.1093/geront/gnp064.
40. Baum CM. The contribution of occupation to function in persons with Alzheimer's disease. *J Occup Sci.* 1995;2(2):59-67.
41. Edwards DF, Hahn MG, Baum C, Perlmutter MS, Sheedy C, Dromerick AW. Undetected Impairment in Persons with Stroke: validation of the Post-Stroke Rehabilitation Guidelines. *Neurorehabil Neural Repair.* 2006;20:42-48.
42. Packer T, Girdler S, Boldy D, Dhaliwal S, Crowley M. Vision self-management for older adults: a pilot study. *Disabil Rehabil.* 2009;31(16):1353-1361.
43. Bult MK, Verschuren O, Kertoy MK, Lindeman E, Jongmans MJ, Ketelaar M. Psychometric evaluation of the dutch version of the assessment of preschool children's participation (APCP): construct validity and test-retest reliability. *Phys Occup Ther Pediatr.* 2013;33(4):372-383.
44. Chen CL, Chen CY, Shen IH, Liu IS, Kang LJ, Wu CY. Clinimetric properties of the Assessment of Preschool Children's Participation in children with cerebral palsy. *Res Dev Disabil.* 2013;34(5):1528-1535.

45. Law M, King G, Petrenchik T, Kertoy M, Anaby D. The assessment of preschool children's participation: internal consistency and construct validity. *Phys Occup Ther Pediatr.* 2012;32(3):272-287.
46. King G, Kertoy M, King S, Law M, Rosenbaum P, Hurley P. A measure of parents' and service providers' beliefs about participation in family-centered services. *Children's Health Care.* 2003;32(3):191-214.
47. Nina K, Sigrid Ø. A comparative ICF-CY–based analysis and cultural piloting of the Assessment of Preschool Children's Participation (APCP). *Phys Occup Therapy Pediatr.* 2015;35(1):54-72.
48. Killeen H, Shiel A, Law M, Segurado R, O'Donovan D. The impact of preterm birth on participation in childhood occupation. *Eur J Pediatr.* 2015;174(3):299-306.
49. Law M, King G, Petrenchik T, Kertoy M, Anaby D. The assessment of preschool children's participation: internal consistency and construct validity. *Phys Occup Therapy Pediatr.* 2012;32(3):272-287.
50. Wu KP, Chuang YF, Chen CL, Liu IS, Liu HT, Chen HC. Predictors of participation change in various areas for preschool children with cerebral palsy: a longitudinal study. *Res Development Disabil.* 2015;37:102-111.
51. Bedell G. *The Child and Adolescent Scale of Participation (CASP): Administration and Scoring Guidelines.* Boston, MA: Boston University; 2011. http://sites.tufts.edu/garybedell/files/2012/07/CASP-Administration-Scoring-Guidelines-8-19-11.pdf
52. Bedell G. Developing a follow-up survey focused on participation of children and youth with acquired brain injuries after discharge from inpatient rehabilitation. *NeuroRehabilitation.* 2004;19(3):191-205.
53. Bedell G. Further validation of the Child and Adolescent Scale of Participation (CASP). *Dev Neurorehabil.* 2009;12(5):342-351.
54. de Kloet AJ, Berger MAM, Bedell GM, Carsman-Berrevoets CE, van Markus-Doornborsch F, Vlieland TPV. Psychometric evaluation of the Dutch language version of the Child and Family Follow-up survey. *Dev Neurorehabil.* 2013;18(6):357-364.
55. Hwang AW, Liou TH, Bedell GM, et al. Psychometric properties of the child and adolescent scale of participation—traditional Chinese version. *Int J Rehabil Res.* 2013;36(3):211-220.
56. McDougall J, Bedell G, Wright V. The youth report version of the Child and Adolescence Scale of Participation (CASP): assessment of psychometric properties and comparison with parent report. *Child Care Health Dev.* 2013;39(4):512-522.
57. Law M. Measurement in occupational therapy: scientific criteria for evaluation. *Can J Occup Ther.* 1987;54(3):133-138.
58. Agnihotri S, Gray J, Colantonio A, et al. Arts-based social skills interventions for adolescents with acquired brain injuries: five case reports. *Dev Neurorehabil.* 2014;17(1):44-63.
59. Chien CW, Rodger S, Copley J, Skorka K. Comparative content review of children's participation measures using the International Classification of Functioning, Disability and Health—Children and Youth. *Arch Phys Med Rehabil.* 2014;95:141-152.
60. Anderson V, Beauchamp MH, Yeates KO, Crossley L, Hearps SJC, Catroppa C. Social competence at 6 months following childhood traumatic brain injury. *J Int Neuropsychol Soc.* 2013;19:539-550.
61. Badge H, Hancock J, Waugh MC. Evaluating pediatric brain injury services in NSW. *Child Care Health Develop.* 2009;36(1):54-62.
62. Zivani J, Desha L, Feeney R, Boyd R. Measures of participation outcomes and environmental considerations for children with acquired brain injury: a systematic review. *Brain Impair.* 2010;11(2):93-112.
63. Rainey L, van Nispen R, van der Zee C, van Rens G. Measurement properties of questionnaires assessing participation in children and adolescents with a disability: a systematic review. *Quality Life Res.* 2014;23:2793-2808.
64. Catroppa C, Crossley L, Hearps SJC, et al. Social and behavioral outcomes: pre-injury to six months following childhood traumatic brain injury. *J Neuotrauma.* 2015;32:109-115.
65. Tozato F, Tobimatsu Y, Wang CW, Iwaya T, Kumamoto K, Ushiyama T. Reliability and validity of the Craig Handicap Assessment and Reporting Technique for Japanese individuals with spinal cord injury. *Tohoku J Exp Med.* 2005;205(4):357-366.
66. Walker N, Melick D, Brooks CA, Whiteneck GG. Measuring participation across impairment groups using the craig handicap assessment reporting technique. *Am J Phys Med Rehabil.* 2003;82(12):936-941.
67. Dijkers M. Scoring CHART: survey and sensitivity analysis. *J Am Paraplegia Soc.* 1991;14:85-86.
68. Hall KM, Dijkers M, Whiteneck G, Brooks CA, Stuart Krause J. The Craig Handicap Assessment and Reporting Technique (CHART): metric properties and scoring. *Top Spinal Cord Inj Rehabil.* 1998;4(1):16-30.
69. Rintala D, Hart K, Fuhrer M. Handicap and spinal cord injury: levels and correlates of mobility, occupational, and social integration. Proceedings of American Spinal Injury Association Meeting; May 1993; San Diego, CA.
70. Whiteneck G. Outcome analysis in spinal cord injury rehabilitation. In Fuhrer M, ed. *Rehabilitation Outcomes: Analysis and Measurement.* Baltimore, MD: Paul H. Brooks; 1987.
71. Whiteneck G, Charlifue S, Gerhart K, Overholser D, Richardson G. Quantifying handicap: a new measure of long-term rehabilitation outcomes. *Arch Phys Med Rehabil.* 1992;73:519-526.
72. World Health Organization. *International Classification of Impairment, Disability and Handicap—ICIDH2.* Geneva, Switzerland: Author; 1998.
73. World Health Organization. *International Classification of Impairments, Disability and Handicap.* Geneva, Switzerland: Author; 1980.
74. Heinemann AW, Magasi S, Bode RK, et al. Measuring enfranchisement: importance of and control over participation by people with disabilities. *Arch Phys Med Rehabil.* 2013;94:2157-2165.
75. Heinemann AW, Lai JS, Magasi S, et al. Measuring participation enfranchisement. *Arch Phys Med Rehabil.* 2011;92:564-571.

76. Hammel J, Magasi S, Heinemann A, et al. What does participation mean? An insider perspective from people with disabilities. *Dis Rehabil.* 2008;30:1445-160.
77. Magasi S, Hammel J, Heinemann A, Whiteneck G, Bogner J. Participation: a comparative analysis of multiple rehabilitation stakeholders' perspectives. *J Rehabil Med.* 2009;41:936-944.
78. Cardol M, de Haan RJ, van den Bos GA, de Jong BA, de Groot IJ. The development of a handicap assessment questionnaire: the Impact on Participation and Autonomy (IPA). *Clin Rehabil.* 1999;13(5):411-419.
79. Cardol M, de Haan RJ, de Jong BA, van den Bos GA, de Groot IJ. Psychometric properties of the impact on Participation and Autonomy Questionnaire. *Arch Phys Med Rehabil.* 2001;82(2):210-216.
80. Cardol M, Beelen A, van den Bos GA, de Jong BA, de Groot IJ, de Haan RJ. Responsiveness of the impact on participation and autonomy questionnaire. *Arch Phys Med Rehabil.* 2002;83(11):1524-1529.
81. Desrosiers J, Robichaud L, Demers L, Gélinas I, Noreau L, Durand D. Comparison and correlates of participation in older adults without disabilities. *Arch Gerontol Geriatr.* 2009;49(3):397-403.
82. Figueiredo S, Korner-Bitensky N, Rochette A, Desrosiers J. Use of the LIFE-H in stroke rehabilitation: a structured review of its psychometric properties. *Disabil Rehabil.* 2010;32(9):705-712.
83. Fougeyrollas P, Noreau L, Bergeron H, et al. Social consequences of long-term impairments and disabilities: conceptual approach and assessment of handicap. *Int J Rehabil Res.* 1998;21(2):127-141.
84. Gagnon C, Mathieu J, Noreau L. Measurement of participation in myotonic dystrophy: reliability of the LIFE-H. *Neuromuscul Disord.* 2006;16(4):262-268.
85. Magasi S, Post MW. A comparative review of contemporary participation measures' psychometric properties and content coverage. *Arch Phys Med Rehabil.* 2010;91(9):S17-S28.
86. Noreau L, Desrosiers J, Robichaud L, et al. Measuring social participation: reliability of the LIFE-H in older adults with disabilities. *Disabil Rehabil.* 2004;26(6):346-352.
87. Noreau L, Lepage C, Boissiere L, et al. Measuring participation in children with disabilities using the Assessment of Life Habits. *Dev Med Child Neurol.* 2007;49(9):666-671.
88. Poulin V, Desrosiers J. Reliability of the LIFE-H satisfaction scale and relationship between participation and satisfaction of older adults with disabilities. *Disabil Rehabil.* 2009;31(16):1311-1317.
89. Roy-Bouthot K, Filiatrault P, Caron C, et al. Modification of the assessment of life habits (LIFE-Hm) to consider personalized satisfaction with participation in activities and roles: results from a construct validity study with older adults. *Disabil Rehabil.* 2013;36(9):737-743.
90. Sakzewski L, Boyd R, Ziviani J. Clinimetric properties of participation measures for 5- to 13-year-old children with cerebral palsy: a systematic review. *Dev Med Child Neurol.* 2007;49(3):232-240.
91. Kutlay S, Küçükdeveci AA, Yanık B, et al. The interval scaling properties of the London Handicap Scale: an example from the adaptation of the scale for use in Turkey. *Clin Rehabil.* 2011;25(3):248-255.
92. Dubuc N, Haley S, Ni P, Kooyoomjian J, Jette A. Function and disability in late life: comparison of the Late-Life Function and Disability Instrument to the Short-Form-36 and the London Handicap Scale. *Disabil Rehabil.* 2004;26(6):362-70.
93. Lo R, Harwood R, Woo J, Yeung F, Ebrahim S. Cross-cultural validation of the London Handicap Scale in Hong Kong Chinese. *Clin Rehabil.* 2001;15(2):177-185.
94. Harwood RH, Ebrahim S. Measuring the outcomes of day hospital attendance: a comparison of the Barthel Index and London Handicap Scale. *Clin Rehabil.* 2000;14(5):527-31.
95. Harwood RH, Ebrahim S. The London Handicap Scale. *J Neurol Neurosurg Psychiatry.* 2000;69(3):406.
96. Jenkinson C, Mant J, Carter J, Wade D, Winner S. The London handicap scale: a re-evaluation of its validity using standard scoring and simple summation [see comment]. *J Neurol Neurosurg Psychiatry.* 2000;68(3):365-367.
97. Calley A, Williams S, Reid S, et al. A comparison of activity, participation and quality of life in children with and without spastic diplegia cerebral palsy. *Disabil Rehabil.* 2012;34(15):1306-1310.
98. Taylor S, Fayed N, Mandich A. CO-OP intervention for young children with developmental coordination disorder. *OTJR.* 2007;27(4):124-130.
99. Turner C, Fricke J, Darzins P. Interrater reliability of the Personal Care Participation Assessment and Resource Tool (PC-PART) in a rehabilitation setting. *Aust Occup Ther J.* 2009;56(2):132-139.
100. Darzins S, Imms C, Di Stefano M. Measurement properties of the Personal Care Participation Assessment and Resource Tool: a systematic review. *Disabil Rehabil.* 2013;35(4):265-281.
101. Vertesi A, Darzins P, Edwards M, Lowe S, McEvoy E. Development of the Handicap Assessment and Resource Tool (HART). *Can J Occup Ther.* 2000;67:120-127.
102. Smith R, Darzins P, Steel C, Murray K, Osborne D, Gilsenan B. Outcome measures in rehabilitation. Report to the Department of Human Services. http://www.health.vic.gov.au/subacute/out-come_phase1.pdf. Accessed April 6, 2005.
103. Darzins P, Bremner F, Smith R. Outcome measures in rehabilitation phase 2. Report to the Department of Human Services. http://www.health.vic.gov.au/subacute/outcomefinal.pdf. Accessed April 6, 2005.
104. Darzins P. Section 10.8. The Handicap Assessment and Resource Tool (HART) and the ICF, in ICF Australian User Guide, Version 1.0. http://www.aihw.gov.au/publications/dis/icfaugv1/modules/ugmod_=108.pdf. Accessed April 6, 2005.
105. Barbara A, Whiteford G. The clinical utility of the Handicap Assessment and Resource Tool: an investigation of its use with the aged in hospital. *Aust Occup Ther J.* 2005;52:17–25.
106. Bedell G, Coster W, Law M, et al. Community participation, supports, and barriers of school-age children with and without disabilities. *Arch Phys Med Rehabil.* 2013;94:315-323.
107. Coster W, Bedell G, Law M, et al. Psychometric evaluation of the Participation and Environment Measure for Children and Youth. *Dev Med Child Neurol.* 2011;53(11):1030-1037.

108. Coster W, Law M, Bedell G, Khetani M, Cousins M, Teplicky R. Development of the participation and environmental measure for children and youth: conceptual basis. *Disabil Rehabil.* 2012;34(3):238-246.
109. Coster W, Law M, Bedell G, Anaby D, Khetani M, Teplicky R. *Participation and Environment Measure for Children and Youth (PEM-CY) User Guide.* Hamilton, ON: CanChild Centre for Disability Research; 2014.
110. Khetani M, Marley J, Baker M, et al. Validity of the Participation and Environment Measure for Children and Youth (PEM-CY) for Health Impact Assessment (HIA) in sustainable development projects. *Disabil Health J.* 2014;7:226-235.
111. Law M, Anaby D, Teplicky R, Khetani M, Coster W, Bedell G. Participation in the home environment among children and youth with and without disabilities. *Br J Occup Ther.* 2013;76(2):58-66.
112. Cliff AB. Utility of the participation and environment measure for children and youth (PEM-CY) for programmatic assessment and intervention planning: a mixed methods study (Master's dissertation). (Order No. 1544741). Available from ProQuest Dissertations & Theses A&I. (1438884798); 2013.
113. Daneski K, Coshall C, Tilling K, Wolfe CDA. Reliability and validity of a postal version of the Reintegration to Normal Living Index, modified for use with stroke patients. *Clin Rehabil.* 2003;17:835-839.
114. Korner-Bitensky N, Wood Dauphinee S, Shapiro S, Becker R. Eliciting health status information by telephone after discharge from hospital: Health professionals versus trained lay persons. *Can J Rehabil.* 1994;8(1):23-34.
115. Stark DL, Edwards DF, Hollingsworth H, Grey DB. Validation of the Reintegration to Normal Living Index in a population of community-dwelling people with mobility limitations. *Arch Phys Med Rehabil.* 2005;86(2):344-345.
116. Steiner A, Raube K, Stuck AE, et al. Measuring psychosocial aspects of well-being in older community residents: Performance of four short scales. *Gerontologist.* 1996;36(1):54-62.
117. Tooth LR, McKenna KT, Smith M, O'Rourke PK. Reliability of scores between stroke patients and significant others on the Reintegration to Normal Living (RNL) Index. *Disabil Rehabil.* 2003;25(9):433-440.
118. Wood-Dauphinee SL, Opzoomer MA, Williams JI, Marchand B, Spitzer WO. Assessment of global function: the Reintegration to Normal Living Index. *Arch Phys Med Rehabil.* 1988;69:583-590
119. Holbrook M, Skilbeck CE. An activities index for use with stroke patients. *Age Ageing.* 1983;12(2):166-170.
120. Chisolm TH, Abrams HB, McArdle R, Wilson RH, Doyle PJ. The WHO-DAS II: psychometric properties in the measurement of functional health status in adults with acquired hearing loss. *Trends Amplif.* 2005;9(3):111-126.
121. Luciano JV, Ayuso-Mateos JL, Fernández A, Serrano-Blanco A, Roca M, Haro JM. Psychometric properties of the twelve item World Health Organization Disability Assessment Schedule II (WHO-DAS II) in Spanish primary care patients with a first major depressive episode. *J Affect Disord.* 2010;121(1):52-58.
122. Luciano JV, Ayuso-Mateos JL, Aguado J, et al. The 12-item World Health Organization disability assessment schedule II (WHO-DAS II): a nonparametric item response analysis. *BMC Med Res Methodol.* 2010;10(1):45.
123. Pösl M, Cieza A, Stucki G. Psychometric properties of the WHODASII in rehabilitation patients. *Qual Life Res.* 2007;16(9):1521-1531.
124. Garin O, Ayuso-Mateos JL, Almansa J, et al. Research Validation of the" World Health Organization Disability Assessment Schedule, WHODAS-2" in patients with chronic diseases. *Health Qual Life Outcomes.* 2010;8:51.
125. Chwastiak LA, Von Korff M. Evaluation of the World Health Organization Disability Assessment Schedule (WHO-DAS II) in a primary care setting. *J Clin Epidemiol.* 2003;56(6):507-514.
126. Khetani MA, Graham JE, Davies PL, Law MC, Simeonsson RJ. Psychometric properties of the Young Children's Participation and Environment Measure. *Arch Phys Med Rehabil.* 2015;96(2):307-16.
127. Khetani MA. Validation of environmental content in the Young Children's Participation and Environment Measure. *Arch Phys Med Rehabil.* 2015;96(2):317-22.

Mine the Gold

The Person-Environment-Occupation (PEO) model supports comprehensive measurement of play/leisure occupations to inform individual- and community-level program development and to document the outcomes of therapy. This holistic model of occupational performance provides the rationale for "mining the gold" across the broad health and social sciences literature, in addition to that found in occupational therapy.

Become Systematic

Lack of consensus regarding definitions of play/leisure is problematic in terms of instrument development and usage in research and practice.

Use Evidence in Practice

Occupational therapists are committed to scientific rigor in the provision of high-quality evidence to improve individuals' play/leisure participation. Using evidence-based knowledge to strengthen practice is important as these occupational performance domains sometimes have not been given the same attention as other occupational performance domains.

Make Occupational Therapy Contributions Explicit

Occupational therapists have the skills necessary to promote and enhance play/leisure participation for all individuals throughout the lifespan. Practitioners, however, need to make occupational therapy contributions explicit by routinely measuring play/leisure participation and including goals for play/leisure within intervention programs.

Engage in Occupation-Based, Client-Centered Practice

Play and leisure are essential components of life that contribute to a person's health and well-being. Acknowledging the importance of these occupations as a source of personal meaning, with unique health and well-being implications for each client, has potential to improve a client's quality of life.

CHAPTER 10

Overview of Play and Leisure

Jenny Ziviani, PhD, BAppSc(OT), BA, MEd; Anne A. Poulsen, PhD, BOccThy (Hons); and Laura Miller, PhD, BSc(OT)(Hons), MHSM

Play and leisure are core occupations important to measure for practice and research. The motivational elements of these occupations are similar, with intrinsic motivation and self-determination characterizing both. As such, play and leisure represent important occupational performance domains, alongside work, self-care, and rest.[1]

Historically, research and clinical practice in the areas of play/leisure are less well represented in the literature than in areas of work/productivity and self-care.[2,3] Hence, there is a need to raise practitioners' awareness regarding the importance of systematic, routine measurement of play/leisure to inform interventions in these domains. Healthy leisure participation is an important social indicator of quality of life, contributing to physical and psychological well-being across an individual's lifespan.[4] For children, play is integral to the development of communication skills as well as cognitive, sensorimotor, and social-emotional capacities, and is recognized as an essential human right.[5] Social, physical, and mental participation in play/leisure can enhance subjective well-being, contribute to healthy living, and augment self-identity and development.[6]

Documenting the physical, social, and economic benefits of play/leisure in different contexts (eg, childcare centers, after-school care, asylum detention centers, impoverished home environments, aged care facilities) can inform strategies to improve health for potentially disadvantaged groups. From a health practitioner's perspective, the preventive effects of health-enhancing participation in play/leisure pursuits are frequently acknowledged but may be poorly attended to in many health implementation models.[3] The cultural bias toward seeking knowledge and understanding of occupations perceived to be more important in relation to economic standards of living may influence service delivery and research in this area. Educating service providers, addressing institutional cultures, and empowering and supporting practitioners regarding the need to measure outcomes of play/leisure therapeutic interventions are necessary. Developing workforce capacity and ensuring that there is adequate funding provision to enable routine measurement of play/leisure occupations in therapy requires endorsement by health, education, and disability government authorities. Practitioners may not fully embrace the importance of play/leisure and consumers also may not prioritize this aspect of professional service delivery.

Perhaps the very nature of play/leisure where engagement is seen as fun and discretionary has indirectly contributed to inconsistent attention and measurement of these important daily occupations. The lower prioritization of play/leisure over self-care/work occupations may also be an unconscious response to professional and institutional cultures where identity and status are preferentially linked to measurement of other occupations, or to reductionist performance component assessment and treatment approaches that are endorsed within many hospital settings.

There is a need to raise public awareness of the physical and mental health benefits of play/leisure because this is an important issue for public health. Overweight and obesity is an area where there is increasing public awareness of the health risks of sedentary lifestyles where individuals have low physically active leisure participation. Occupational therapy research has highlighted the need for practitioners to become involved in public health promotion and the design of community interventions regarding physically active play/leisure for children at risk of being overweight or obese.[7] This has continued more broadly to a call for diet-related interventions and obesity management, with measurement of outcomes required to build a strong evidence base supporting occupational therapy practice in this area.[8]

Law M, Baum C, Dunn W, eds. *Measuring Occupational Performance: Supporting Best Practice in Occupational Therapy, Third Edition (pp 153-199).*

A further example of occupational therapy contribution to broader public health is the provision of an informed health perspective in relation to playground design within schools and local communities.[9] Jarus and colleagues[10] suggested that understanding leisure participation from a broader occupational perspective (including diversity, intensity, with whom and where the activity occurs, and level of enjoyment) is useful for promoting healthy living more broadly. As Parnell and Wilding noted,[11] in this way, occupational therapy can address the challenges that plague contemporary life.

Evidence from large cross-sectional, time-series studies[12] suggests that reading books, listening to music, social visits, and participation in clubs/organizations is associated with fewer psychosomatic complaints, low likelihood of long-term illness, and high subjective well-being for children aged 2 to 17 years, pointing toward the impact of leisure on health and quality of life. During adolescence, extracurricular activity involvement provides opportunities to develop social connections outside of school and home. These enrichment activities can also extend an adolescent's learning opportunities for developing competencies beyond the classroom. Passmore[13] noted that, while adolescents who participate in social and achievement leisure had good mental health, youth who spent time in passive/time-out leisure had poor mental health. Active engagement is also considered elemental to the definition of an activity as play.[14] The absence of active engagement in either play or leisure is associated with passive states of boredom and inactivity.

Leisure participation patterns change with age in relation to diversity, intensity, and enjoyment. The health and well-being outcomes associated with participation in various leisure pursuits vary throughout the lifespan. For example, leisure participation may change after moving to an aged care facility because changes in mobility, cognition, or mental health status can significantly alter the quality, frequency, and type of leisure experiences. On the other hand, some older adults increase their participation after retirement because they have time to do things they have postponed because of work and family demands.

Positive psychological and physical effects of both active and less physically demanding forms of leisure, such as reading, attending theater, or contemplation, are well documented in the elderly population.[15] Because an engaged lifestyle is seen as an important component of successful aging, understanding the leisure interests and participation of older individuals in different environments (eg, community-dwelling, independent living facilities) is the focus of increased research attention. Rigorous baseline and outcome measurement of all aspects of play/leisure throughout the lifespan will support clinical practice and promote occupational therapy attendance to these occupations. Precise measurement is integral to the delivery and evaluation of play/leisure interventions, particularly if workplace or community cultural perceptions question the worth of these occupationally based interventions, either overtly or covertly.

Key Concepts

Play is internally regulated behavior involving participation in challenging, enjoyable pursuits.[16] Play activities are self-determined and personally valued rather than being externally regulated or controlled. Choice is often presented as a defining feature of play.[17] Salen and Zimmerman[18] argue that the essential characteristic of play is that it must be free and voluntary, for if one is forced to play, then it ceases to be called *play.* Bundy[19] describes play as a primary occupation, but one that is undervalued by society. Play captures children's attention, interest, and imagination.[20] During play, there is frequent, spontaneous engagement with objects, such as toys. The capacity for play to transcend reality as well as reflect reality differentiates play from many work experiences.[21]

Leisure is conceptually similar to play, sharing the same motivational features. Personally meaningful recreational activities that are voluntarily carried out during free time are regarded as *leisure occupations.* These activities do not involve obligatory work duties, assigned responsibilities, or the performance of other life-sustaining functions.[15] Freedom to choose what one would like to do, rather than feeling obligated to perform required tasks, differentiates many leisure activities from chores and work-related tasks. *Leisure* is defined as recreational activities voluntarily carried out during free time that does not involve obligatory work duties, assigned responsibilities, or the performance of other life-sustaining functions.[15]

The motivational aspects of play and leisure (eg, interest, enjoyment, and self-determination) are sometimes referred to as *subjective aspects.*[6] However, there can be a conceptual overlap between the subjective experiences of play/leisure and work experiences that occur when work is perceived to be self-directed, self-chosen, and enjoyable. This can occur in highly individualized professions where a person has freedom to determine goals and other elements of work, such as task difficulty and level of challenge. Historian John Hope Franklin is quoted as saying, "You could say that I worked every minute of my life, or you could say with equal justice that I never worked a day. I have always subscribed to the expression, 'Thank God it's Friday' because to me, Friday means I can work for the next 2 days without interruption."[22]

The etymological roots of the words provide a further basis to distinguish the core features of play/leisure from work. The Latin roots of leisure derive from *licére,* meaning "to be permitted." The origin of the word *play* is less clear. During the 13th century, the English adopted the Dutch word *pleien,* meaning to "dance, leap for joy, and rejoice" to describe the free and unimpeded movements, games, and sports of children. Conversely, the word *work,* which also entered the English language during the 13th century, describes actions involving effort or expending labor for remuneration or employment. In its original form, the Latin *laborem* (nom. *labor*) referred to "toil, pain, exertion, fatigue and work." The negative connotations associated with drudgery and energy depletion changed during late Middle English, when work became associated with the performance of good or moral deeds that contribute to feelings of satisfaction and pleasure. Nevertheless, even in more recent references to work compared to non-work time, there is the notion that leisure represents the antithesis of work because it is "private time" that allows for restoration of energy and freedom from the fatigue of work.[23]

The meta-theory of motivation, self-determination theory (SDT),[24] offers a lens to more fully understand the motivational elements of play/leisure and can help differentiate play/leisure from many work experiences. Using a motivational lens helps clarify an essential difference between these occupations. The SDT motivational continuum graphically depicts the interplay between external and internal regulatory influences on these occupations, and explains overlaps between self-determination (eg, level of choice) and self-direction. The Rocket Model of Motivation[25] diagrammatically depicts the increasing levels of internal regulation and decreasing extrinsic motivation until behavior is intrinsically motivated. For example, work can be described as "play-like" when there are elements of spontaneity, fun, self-direction, and perceived freedom to suspend reality during task performance. This occurs when there is low external control and high internal regulation. In the same way, play/leisure can sometimes be described as "work-like" when the activity is obligatory rather than optional, is effortful, and is controlled by others.

Play/leisure is frequently intrinsically motivated. Bundy[26] noted the importance of intrinsic motivation and internal control in her model of playfulness. Intrinsic motivation is the prototype of self-determined behavior, occurring when an individual engages in an activity for personal interest alone, and with a full sense of volition and choice, self-initiation, and self-direction. Similarly, informal/unstructured leisure (eg, creating a piece of art, reading a novel, or being immersed in listening to a piece of jazz music) is also self-determined with full or partial internal regulation. Individuals perform these activities because of intrinsic interest in the activity itself, and because of the pleasure and satisfaction inherently derived from participation.[24]

Intrinsic motivation propels an individual to engage and become fully absorbed in that activity. According to Vallerand and Ratelle,[27] there are 3 types of intrinsic motivation: intrinsic motivation to learn and know, intrinsic motivation to acquire expertise, and intrinsic motivation to experience sensory stimulation. Frequently, "flow"[28] is experienced during intrinsically motivated activities, such as play. Csikszentmihalyi[29] described flow as representing a metaphor for a water current/stream that carries individuals along while being engaged/immersed in a particular pasttime. Athletes might describe flow as a feeling of "being in the zone"; musicians might say, "I'm in the groove"; a game player might say, "I blink out"; and a scholar might question, "Where did the time go?" while fully attending to an absorbing research question.

Winnicott[30] described a child's intense preoccupation during play as being similar to the flow state. For instance, when a child is fully immersed in play and his or her focus is difficult to disrupt, Winnicott described this as akin to "near-withdrawal," where there is time transcendence (ie, time seems to stand still or pass quickly) accompanied by full, deep absorption. Other characteristics of flow include removal from awareness of the worries and frustrations of everyday life, so that considerations of self become irrelevant; a sense of implicit, personal control over actions that arises to meet the challenge of environmental demands; a lack of awareness of bodily needs (ie, the individual does not notice hunger or external distractions); and spontaneous joy and satisfaction. The activity itself provides sufficient internal rewards to preclude the need for external reward/feedback about behavior. Flow is described as the penultimate example of an intrinsically motivating, autotelic experience.[29]

During structured leisure, extrinsic motivation exerts an influence on participation (eg, organized sports, interest clubs, performance activities/lessons for dance, music or drama, religious service). Extrinsic motivation differs from intrinsic motivation because an individual engages in the activity as a means to an end rather than pursuing the activity for its own sake. When an individual participates in leisure pursuits that are enjoyable but require some form of commitment (eg, signing up to participate and meet certain rules and requirements, or attending practices in order to perform/play in a team competition), then those behaviors are considered to be extrinsically motivated to some extent. Internal regulation of behavior (eg, personal choice and decision making) may be accompanied by external control of behaviors (eg, needing permission from parents, paying fees to join a club, practicing to meet team/performance group stipulations), so that the behavior is not entirely intrinsically motivated. For example, a child who is learning to swim may have moments when he or she experiences sensory and aesthetic pleasure while gliding through the water, but may also experience times when the coach's instructions exert a strong influence on behaviors, thoughts, and/or feelings.

Intrinsic motivation and 2 types of extrinsic motivation (ie, integrated and identified regulation) are frequently experienced during self-chosen leisure pursuits. Integrated regulation is the motivational state that is closest to intrinsic motivation on the SDT continuum (Figure 10-1). The SDT continuum describes 4 different types of extrinsic motivation with varying degrees of influence over behavior: integrated regulation, identified regulation, introjected regulation, and external regulation.

Integrated regulation is a form of extrinsic motivation that occurs when external influences on patterns of behavior are acknowledged, but are fully integrated. For example, a young boy who is a passionate chess player might enjoy playing in the chess club at school as well as

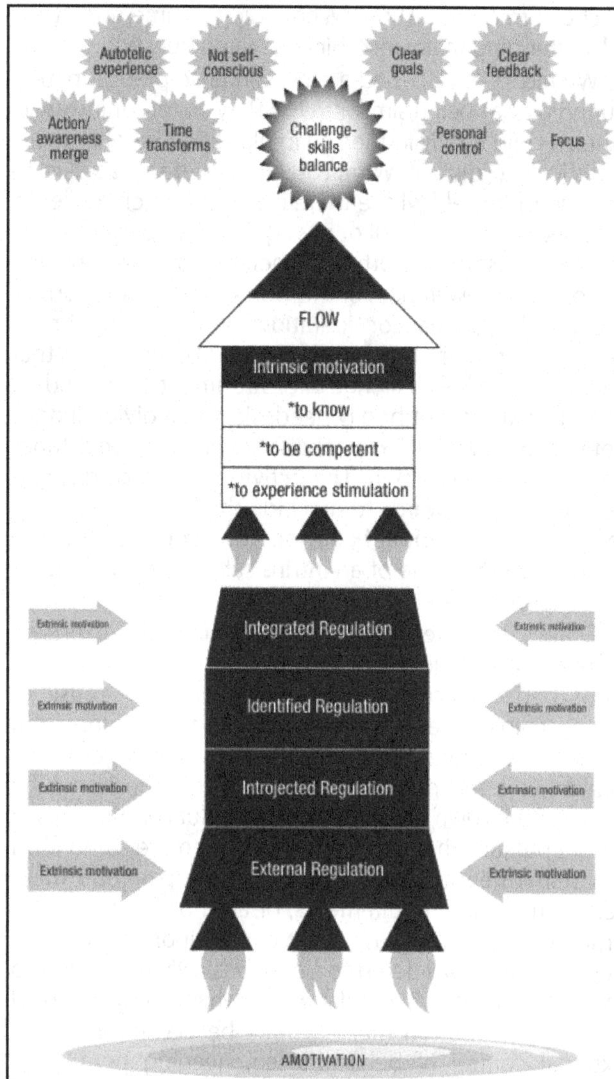

Figure 10-1. Rocket Motivation Model. (Reprinted with permission from Ziviani J, Poulsen AA, Cuskelly M, eds. *The Art and Science of Motivation: A Therapist's Guide to Working with Children.* London, UK: Jessica Kingsley Publications; 2013.)

at home with his father before going to bed each night. The child experiences inherent enjoyment and interest in chess playing, sees himself as a chess player for life, with visions firmly in place to represent his school during interschool competitions. In this example, we can see that there are strong intrinsic reasons for the boy's participation (ie, interest, enjoyment, and a vision of self as a competent chess player), but these are linked with reasons extrinsic to the self (ie, the elements of structured game playing that require adherence to the rules of the game and wanting to be a chess player like his father), and hence might be described as integrated regulation.

Identified regulation is another type of extrinsic motivation that is one step further removed from pure intrinsic motivation. There is well-internalized regulation and partially internalized external regulation. For example, in the chess-playing scenario, the child's instrumental reasons for continued participation might include having extrinsic aspirations to win accolades for the school and maybe win a trophy if the chess team is successful in the interschool competition. Higher levels of external influence and feedback represent progressively higher external regulatory influences on behavior.

External elements, such as rules and regulations, are key aspects of structured as opposed to unstructured leisure (eg, flying a kite in the park) or play (eg, building sandcastles at the beach). If an activity is personally endorsed, then higher levels of internal regulation will be evident in behaviors associated with participation in these activities. When external influences dictate participation (eg, a parent who encourages a child to sign up for a particular sport, or enrolls the child without the child's consent), this represents a strong extrinsic motivation for behavior initiation. These external influences may be internalized as the child experiences enjoyment, develops competence, and forms friendships. High external regulation can also occur during play experiences, such as when a child is either coerced into joining a game or feels a reluctant sense of duty to continue participating (eg, an unsupervised, free-for-all playground game of dodgeball for a child with developmental coordination difficulties).

Another difference between play and leisure is the intended target audience. For example, child leisure is less frequently used to describe the occupations of young children and babies. The term *leisure* is more commonly applied from adolescence onward to describe free time use during the out-of-work hours. Play is frequently used in reference to children. Adult play might be applied to highly engaging and enjoyable activities autonomously pursued by older individuals, but it would be rare to ask an adult, "What are you doing in your playtime today?" There may even be a potentially dismissive tone associated with the word *play* when applied to adult behavior, such as "it's as simple as child's play." Adult play might refer to unproductive or even guilty pleasures. On the other hand, there is a somewhat whimsical feeling associated with the phrase, "the lost art of play," and an individual might be admonished when being reminded that "all work and no play makes Jack a dull boy."

Although there are sometimes blurred boundaries between the experiences of play/leisure and work, economists differentiate these occupations using a straightforward time use perspective. For example, *leisure time* refers to discretionary out-of-school and out-of-work activity participation in recreational activities. This is sometimes referred to as *free time* and is likely to occur before or after regular weekday working hours or school hours, as well as on weekends and holidays. For younger children, playtime implies a period of time when children are free to go outside, abandon their chores and have fun with friends, or play with their toys.

A further distinction between play and leisure applies to the instruments or objects used as play or leisure props. Although toys are frequently mentioned as playthings, leisure objects tend to be called *equipment, materials,* or *tools*. This distinction, while not clear-cut, may reflect a perception that structured leisure is more serious than children's play. Belying this differential, the American occupational therapist Norma Alessandrini described play as "akin to a business or a career for children" in an *American Journal of Occupational Therapy* article published over 60 years ago.[31] This may reflect a culturally derived imperative at the time of writing to elevate the importance of play to a work-like status, and thus worthy of attention within the health arena. Alternatively, this view of play might imply a loss of free time, and a feeling that a child's play is primarily important for its purposive components rather than for the playful experiential element of play. These cultural perspectives are important to understand when considering play/leisure measurement and the real barriers to therapy service implementation with respect to these occupations.

Importance of Measurement in Play/Leisure

Play and leisure are consistently described as domains of primary concern for occupational therapy practitioners.[13] A key role for occupational therapists is to identify ways in which a person can fully participate in play/leisure activities that will lead to an enhanced quality of life. Measuring play and leisure experiences, participation patterns, and qualities of environments that support or hinder full participation has potential to enhance interventions aimed at improving mental and physical health of individuals referred to therapy. Understanding the qualities of environments that provide positive participatory and growth-enhancing experiences is important.

One reason for measuring play and leisure is to directly support evidence-based clinical practice. A second reason relates to health promotion. There is a growing need for occupational therapists to become involved in population-level preventive approaches using occupation-based knowledge about current play/leisure participation in order to develop broader strategies that will enhance opportunities for these to occur in the daily lives of all individuals. A third consideration involves building knowledge through research endeavors, to serve both aforementioned purposes. This research needs to focus on the development and testing of psychometrically sound measurement tools to provide baseline and discriminative individual- and community-level information about healthy play/leisure participation, as well as measure change following interventions.

Despite the occupational therapy profession's promotion of play as a centrally important occupational performance domain, and notwithstanding the steady increase in research attention directed toward play measurement and occupational experiences within the occupational therapy literature, occupational therapists do not regularly measure play in everyday practice.[3] Two surveys of pediatric American occupational therapists published 15 years apart[3,32] found few therapists focused on play as an outcome of importance for children aged 3 to 7 years. Practitioners who reported that they conducted play assessments (38%) did so primarily to obtain information about functioning in other areas, using assessments as part of a general developmental assessment.[3] Thus, play has sometimes been regarded as an activity base in assessing physical, cognitive, communication, social and emotional, and adaptive development, rather than being considered as a developmental domain in its own right.

The Revised Knox Preschool Play Scale[33] was selected by 4% of pediatric occupational therapists as the play instrument of choice in Kuhanek and colleagues' study.[3] The Test of Playfulness (ToP)[34] was selected by 3% of survey respondents. Similar results have been described in the United Kingdom[35] and Canada,[36] with therapists rarely setting goals for play in most pediatric therapy settings. In relation to setting play-related goals, only 4% of therapists surveyed by Kuhanek et al[3] reported that they focused on play as an outcome of their intervention.

Similar to play, leisure participation is an important occupational performance domain and is a recognized health domain in the World Health Organization's International Classification of Functioning Disability and Health (ICF)[37] and its extended version for children and youth (ICF-CY).[38] Despite consensus on the importance of leisure performance and participation, assessment tools for measuring leisure or its component elements are rarely used in school-based practices, with practitioners using interview methods more than standardized tools.[39] Healthy leisure participation also may be considered a core aspect of occupational therapy practice with adults, but in many settings, leisure assessments and interventions receive substantially less research attention than programs aimed at self-care.[2]

The inclusion of play and leisure participation within the ICF and ICF-CY[37,38] has increased health professionals' awareness of the need to evaluate participation levels, experiences, and competencies within these 2 occupational performance areas. There has also been a rapid increase in the number of participation-focused tools as practitioners use the ICF and ICF-Y frameworks to guide service delivery. Since the inception of the ICF and ICF-CY, health practitioners have adopted and operationalized participation elements in relation to health outcomes, with active development of participation-focused assessments that incorporate environmental factors. Qualifiers for involvement or subjective satisfaction with participation provide additional information within the ICF/ICF-CY. Further developments include the creation of linking rules to enable practitioners to categorize different activity participation as recreation/leisure or play when using the ICF and ICF-Y.[40] For example, engagement in games with rules (eg, playing card or board games) is considered recreation and leisure rather than play. In contrast, engaging with toys or building blocks is defined as *play* because there are no special, relatively consistent rules that provide structure and external regulation to this activity.[41]

The satisfactory use of leisure time is a major issue for many people with disabilities or mental/physical chronic ill health. Participation in leisure activities acts as an indicator of function and health that is correlated with quality of life and physical and emotional well-being.[42] Identifying constraints and affordances to participation is a key measurement focus. These elements inhibit or support leisure participation. They affect choice and participation and can be grouped using a Person-Environment-Occupation model (PEO)[43] as the following:

- Person-related factors (eg, meaning, commitment, skills, motivation)
- Occupation-level variables (eg, time requirements, grading)
- Environmental factors (eg, transport, physical and social features)

Reduced leisure engagement may constrain life participation more broadly.[2] There are 4 potential pathways where impoverished leisure participation can influence health-related quality of life. These include the following:

- Diminished subjective well-being (ie, life satisfaction and positive affect) when individuals are not able to pursue leisure interests
- Reduced social and cultural connectivity through play/leisure occupation
- Fewer opportunities to engage in leisure experiences that build positive identities and contribute to global self-concept
- Less access to leisure cognitive and physical development opportunities through leisure across the lifespan[44]

Practitioners need to measure engagement in culturally relevant and meaningful leisure opportunities for less privileged population groups. McKinstry and Fortune[45] advocate for the need for the occupational therapy profession to exert a clearer occupational presence beyond serving the needs of those with the most profound limitations, and expand practice into other sectors, such as primary health promotion. Although leisure participation has been acknowledged as an objective, tangible outcome that must be measured in rehabilitation and health programs,[42] evidence supporting the need to attend more broadly to leisure occupational deprivation in other groups must be drawn from the broader social science literature to expand occupational therapy-specific knowledge. There is limited community-based research investigating healthy communities, leisure, and lifestyle interventions, and some of the work has been conceptual in nature.[46] A range of potential topics has been identified for participatory and action-oriented research into integrated recreation for older adults; municipal policy and recreation for people with disabilities; community access to structured leisure and community development; and community reintegration of women in federal prisons through leisure participation.[47]

Understanding play and leisure participation, as well as the barriers to participation, are important considerations for occupational therapists. Barriers can include lack of access to a range of play/leisure alternatives, equipment, companions, cultural values, and habits. There may be restrictions on, and freedom around, outdoor play and safety in different public spaces; accessibility of buildings and types of building structure; access to public transportation and lack of ramps, elevators, and parking space for wheelchairs; concerns about crowds, terrain, and distance; and financial constraints. The weather, child and parental fears, and parental stresses associated with the age and gender of children can also represent constraints on play/leisure. Decreased opportunity for physically active play during school breaks is a specific environmental impediment to achieving adequate levels of daily physical activity for some children. Physical health problems, including pain, poor balance, fatigue, deconditioning and weakness, and social anxiety, can impede full leisure participation. Cognitive and behavioral difficulties are further obstacles to participation. Conversely, parental involvement, such as arranging play and vigilance, supervision and advocacy, and support of peers and classmates, represents social environmental opportunities or affordances.

Having choice of leisure activities and opportunities to experiment with different pursuits is associated with positive outcomes, such as leisure satisfaction, high self-esteem, and subjective quality of life.[48] Although there is increasing research into the benefits of leisure as an occupation, there is a need for further empirical work to specify the when, where, why, and how different leisure experiences can have positive effects for different populations. Researchers have found that play offers possibilities for developing creativity, persistence, and productivity, thus providing an adaptive mechanism promoting cognitive growth.[31] Play/leisure can provide opportunities for individuals to develop competence, express emotions, and connect with others.[16]

Measurement of play/leisure occupational performance represents a key aspect of therapy endeavors that is infrequently attended to despite explicit acknowledgement of the importance of these occupations for the health and well-being of clients. Measurement of motivational elements associated with occupational performance is considered important because this provides a unique perspective about factors influencing current participation (eg, engagement and persistence).

Factors to Remember

The ongoing tensions in establishing clear and consistent definitions for play and leisure have potentially compromised instrument development for measuring occupational performance in these domains.[15] From the viewpoint of traditional science, the absence of precise definitions lessens the likelihood of precise measurement.[31] Sound measurement is essential for design and evaluation of interventions and preventive approaches aimed at enhancing healthy play/leisure of all members of the population.

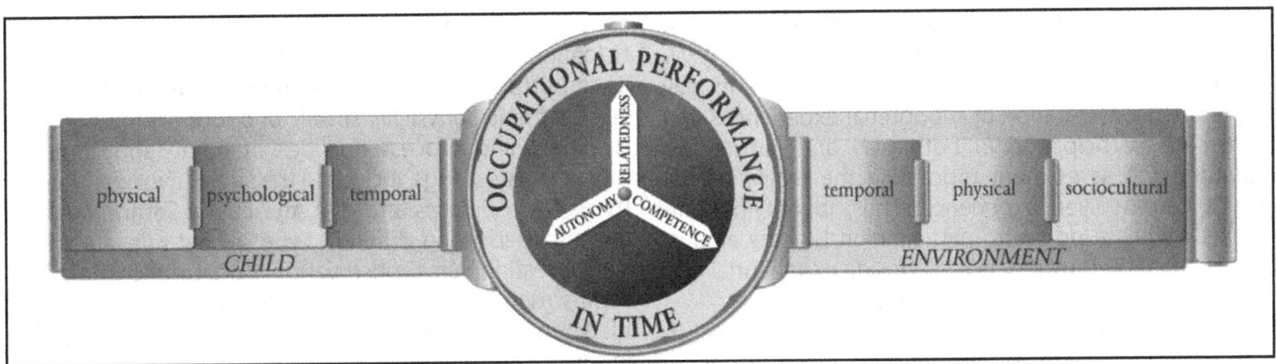

Figure 10-2. The SCOPE-IT Model. (Reprinted with permission from Ziviani J, Poulsen AA, Cuskelly M, eds. *The Art and Science of Motivation: A Therapist's Guide to Working with Children*. London, UK: Jessica Kingsley Publications; 2013.)

From a strengths-based perspective (ie, where strengths can include personal talents and competencies, or environmental supports and affordances) it could be argued that identifying leisure interest and leisure-time patterns before issues, problems, and barriers to participation are clarified represents a health, rather than disability/disease, orientation. This viewpoint supports an occupational health check approach whereby current capacity, supports, positive emotions, and experiences are appraised to identify motivation-related elements that can support growth. Thus, an occupational enrichment focus needs to be fostered, where the first point of measurement would be identifying play/leisure interests, satisfactions, and opportunities for self-actualization. This is not meant to discount the need to acquire information about the realities of current barriers and impediments to full participation. Understanding leisure constraints has been of interest to occupational therapists, particularly in relation to issues such as access and inclusion. A key role of practitioners has been to negotiate barriers that prevent full access and participation in leisure activities.[49]

A strength of occupational therapy is its comprehensive appreciation of client functioning from a PEO perspective.[43,50] Law and colleagues provided early, groundbreaking direction for health practitioners in the conceptualization of a PEO model that attends to intrinsic (or within-the-person) factors as well as contextual (or outside-the-individual) influences on occupational performance. Neither Law's PEO model nor the ICF[37,38] provides a quantitative means of predicting the magnitude or importance of PE and PEO variables on participation. Both frameworks attend to the importance of measuring PE elements to fully understand occupational experiences and effects associated with play/leisure participation.

The SCOPE-IT[51] model, which is based on PEO principles, considers the need to appraise and Synthesize Child Occupational Performance, Person and Environment—In Time factors as a basis for an occupational health check (Figure 10-2). Obtaining a broad overview of discretionary time use and occupational interests and experiences alongside environmental affordability and person-level factors (eg, the individual's ability to participate in desired leisure pursuits) has been described as creating an occupational profile.[52] Occupational therapy practitioners begin the evaluation process by creating an occupational profile that includes a focus on the meaning of leisure and social activities in the client's life with the aim of identifying enjoyable growth-enhancing play/leisure opportunities[53] (see Figure 10-2).

When conducting a play occupational performance profile, practitioners might focus on the identification of a child's play preferences and interests, favored play materials, and positive play-related social interactions before exploring concerns related to emotional and psychosocial experiences or barriers to participation. Kuhanek and colleagues[54] provided a detailed outline of the multiple aspects that need to be assessed during a comprehensive play evaluation, and a helpful grid for organizing this information. Examples of functional play-related goals that can be used to guide therapy and measure outcomes are provided by these occupational therapists.[3]

During a leisure evaluation, practitioners have historically used interest checklists, accompanied by interviewing and administration of standardized assessments, to fully understand the meaning and importance of these occupations for the individual. There is increasing use of validated instruments for the measurement of these variables rather than ad hoc questionnaires whose psychometric properties are not reported, but there is still much research needed to support evidence-based practice in the areas of play/leisure research and practice. Söderback and Hammarlund[55] outlined a useful framework for collecting and collating information about leisure participation and experiences that was described as the Occupational Therapy Assessment of Leisure Time.

The Neuropsychiatric Institute Interest Checklist (NPIIC),[56] developed almost 4 decades ago, has been extensively used in clinical practice as a starting point for leisure profiling. Occupational therapy scholars and clinicians have continued to develop and refine these historically important measures but have increasingly expanded practice and research into measurement of the experiential aspects of leisure. This is essential if the client's perspectives about meaningful leisure and optimal experiences are to be fully understood and pursued. There are many variants of the interest checklist that have been created for different cultural contexts, populations, and settings (eg, Japanese Interest Checklist for the Elderly[57]).

In contrast to measuring optimal performance in play and leisure, consideration of suboptimal experiences and barriers to participation in both play and leisure has grounded the assessment process in the reality of the client's current lived experience. Thus, identifying barriers as well as supports to participation is a key area of occupational therapy practice, alongside experiential and health-related benefits of participation.

The collection of ecologically relevant data about play/leisure behaviors ideally requires observations of play/leisure alongside interviews with family members and salient individuals. This has maximum potential for contributing relevant information to inform occupational therapy interventions.[58] Schneider and Rosenblum[59] emphasize the need to conduct narrative interviews with parents/caregivers to increase collaborative endeavors to discover the meaning of a child's play. The Play History,[60] a semi-structured interview conducted with a parent or other caregiver, provides rich information about a child's current and past play abilities and experiences, play materials, actions, people, and play settings. This historically important instrument was a starting point for many play assessments. However, concerns have been raised about the limited information on reliability and validity pertaining to the instrument and outdated information about some of the play developmental epochs described sensorimotor, symbolic and simple constructive, dramatic and complex constructive, games, and recreational.[19]

A 3-tiered model of service delivery[61] may help guide selection of appropriate measures by considering whether the information can be used at a Tier 1 level (ie, for promotion, prevention, and early intervention at the system and individual levels); Tier 2 (ie, for provision of targeted interventions for those at risk); and Tier 3 (ie, to measure change following intensive interventions). Documenting supports/barriers to play/leisure occupational performance for different target populations (eg, at risk of, or experiencing occupational deprivation) is a key role of occupational therapists at each level.[49] The selection of cost- and time-efficient measures that meet different needs for Tier 1, 2, and 3 services requires current knowledge of suitable instruments and approaches in a rapidly growing information space.

The selection and development of reliable and valid instrumentation to measure PEO elements and their interactive effects on health and participation will generate reliable evidence to support clinical practice and improve a person's health and quality of life.[62] A direct measure of PEO fit would provide useful information as a baseline approach to inform program development for each individual, and could also be used as an endpoint to document change. Currently, there is no single PEO-fit measure, although Venn diagrams plotting all possible logical relations between a finite collection of sets are a useful way of visualizing these relationships.[50] One proxy measure for indirectly gauging PEO fit is measurement of experiential elements associated with play/leisure participation. The evaluation of Activity Settings represents an important approach to the measurement of structural (ie, aesthetic, physical, social, and opportunity-related qualities), and process qualities of home and community activity settings, including the subjective experiences these environments afford.[63] An Activity Setting analysis is completed using different types of data (ie, standardized questionnaires, observations, photo-elicitation and semi-structured face-to-face interviews) to provide a multifaceted picture of activity setting experiences. Play and leisure instruments selected through a PEO approach can provide information not only about occupational performance behaviors and experiences, but also features of the occupational environment that influence occupational performance. Instruments such as the Measure of Environmental Qualities of Activity Settings (MEQAS),[64] in conjunction with its companion measure, Self-reported Experiences of Activity Settings (SEAS)[65] allow practitioners to obtain a deep understanding of real world leisure participation experiences, affordances, and barriers.[66] This information can provide directions to facilitate opportunities to enhance leisure participation in specific activity settings. The Home Observation for Measurement of the Environment (HOME),[67] which provides information about quality and type of environmental supports within family home as well as home-based childcare facilities for play participation, is another tool that practitioners can use to measure environmental factors. These measures, along with other assessments of environment, are reviewed in detail in Chapter 16.

Unfortunately, there are few available measures of motivational regulation that can determine where along the SDT continuum a child's motivation for play/leisure may lie. Preliminary evidence for the construct validity and internal consistency of behavioral regulation and need satisfaction scales has been satisfactory in measuring identified regulation and intrinsic motivation of physically active leisure participation among primary school-aged children.[68] There are several validated measures of self-determination theory constructs for use among adolescents and adults. The SDT website provides a detailed list of these measures with published data pertaining to their psychometrics (http://www.selfdeterminationtheory.org/).

Identifying optimal experiences, and in particular, intrinsically motivating play/leisure activities and experiences, is a challenging aspect of clinical practice to scientifically document. For adults, the Intrinsic Leisure Motivation Scale (ILM)[69] that uses the SDT framework to measure self-determination, competence/skill development, self-commitment, and challenge during leisure provides one option. The Leisure Diagnostic Battery[70] uses Attribution Theory[71] to measure an individual's perceived freedom in leisure by assessing 5 dimensions of self-perceiving competence, control, depth of involvement, leisure needs, and playfulness, as well as measuring barriers to leisure and frequency and type of leisure pursuits.

Playfulness is an important experiential element or quality of play, is a tapping intrinsic motivation, and can be evaluated for children using the ToP.[19] For older persons, the Adult Playfulness Trait Scale (P-APTS)[72] is one of several measures that use different conceptual models where playfulness is viewed as intrinsically motivating behavior or a personality style. The need for practitioners and researchers to select measures that have been developed with a guiding theoretical model is an important consideration when considering the many measures of playfulness that are available.

Flow, which is also regarded as an optimal experience during play/leisure, is another important experiential element for practitioners to evaluate and observe during therapy. Flow can be measured using ecological momentary assessment methods, such as the use of the Experience Sampling Form (ESF)[73] to evaluate near real-time motives for activity engagement. The costs and practical considerations of providing clients with a paging device (a pager, programmable watch, or handheld computer) that signals at preprogrammed times mean that this methodology has had limited use within clinical situations, and confined to use in research studies. With information technology advances (eg, smartphone technologies) application of ESF beyond the research arena is now a possibility.

A final challenge to measurement of play/leisure is how to best evaluate its characteristics and their "fit" with person and environment. Rigby and Huggins[74] have developed an observation guide that can be used for organizing PEO information regarding play experiences. The development of measures that incorporate person-, environment-, and occupation-level factors for investigating play/leisure engagement of individuals referred for occupational therapy is embryonic. One example of a measure specifically developed to reflect the PEO Model[43] is the My Child's Play Questionnaire (MCP).[59] The use of grids, such as that described by Kuhanek and colleagues[54] for measuring play, and the leisure assessment framework described by Söderback and Hammarlund[55] to organize information gathered from formal assessments, interviews, and observations, can be particularly helpful for collating multidimensional PEO information relating to these occupations.

Strategies for Selecting Measures for Play/Leisure

The different elements of play and leisure that practitioners will be interested in measuring can be grouped using a PEO classification scheme. The use of PEO models is increasingly embraced within the health sector and represents a powerful aspect of occupational therapy practice that can be used to facilitate decision making for measurement selection.[75] There is evidence that changes in participation experiences and outcomes are more likely when attention to both person and environmental factors are an integral part of assessment. For example, in a study investigating factors contributing to participation diversity for children with mild motor disabilities,[76] the total explained variance for participation diversity was more than doubled when social environmental variables were inserted into the regression model alongside child-level factors.

From an occupational therapy perspective, the comprehensive analysis of occupational performance analysis requires attention to all PEO aspects when choosing either an instrument or approach to collect data. Clinical decision making is inevitably required to select appropriate measures because of variation in individual and contextual conditions. Alongside the need to tailor measurements for individual client needs and different settings, there are other pragmatic considerations, such as time, cost, practitioner knowledge, familiarity and expertise with different media and methods, and considerations regarding whether measurement is conducted in situ (ie, within a naturalistic community setting) or through proxy reports. A feasibility study of simultaneously combining a number of diverse data collection methods found that an intensive amount of time was required for planning and supporting personnel to coordinate and collate data; hence, this process needs refinement.[66] Ideally, comprehensive measurement must also be brief and entail a low response burden for participants, but this may be difficult to achieve.

The basic elements within each PEO category that might be integrated within a comprehensive evaluation of play/leisure include the following:

- Person-level factors that are important to consider in relation to both play and leisure include the following:
    - Enjoyment and other affective experiences associated with participation: Note the quality or texture of the individual experience during play/leisure, such as emotions, thoughts, or images that influence a person's level of enjoyment of play/leisure
    - Interests: Identify liked and disliked activities, play/leisure interests, and skills and other motivational influences such as the unique personal meaning that influences initial decisions to engage, persist, and disengage from the play/leisure activity
    - Skills: Evaluate actual and perceived player/leisure participant competence and capacity
    - Person-level barriers and affordances to participation: Consider any attitudinal, cognitive, physical, developmental, age- and gender-related affordances/barriers that can change participation patterns and experiences
- Environment-level factors that support and cultivate engagement, as opposed to physical or social environmental barriers that preclude or hamper engagement, include the following:

    - Physical: Consider physical environments where play/leisure participation is supported, and note those settings where barriers and access to play/leisure engagement and persistence exist. Note other features of the physical environment that influence engagement (eg, seasonal and climatic aspects, equipment, and other contextual requirements of the play/leisure activity, such as costs or location)
    - Social: The attitudes and skills of parents/caregivers/coaches/teachers/leaders and other key individuals who are more proximal to the individual, such as siblings, leisure companions, and team members and their contributions in creating and fostering the play environment. Identify social companions for the play/leisure experience, the motivational climate, and availability of play/leisure companions
    - Societal: Consider the broader social, cultural, political, economic, and physical (eg, climatic) conditions that contribute to participation alongside those that contribute to disengagement, disinterest, or boredom
- Occupation-level factors include the following[6]:
    - Activity characteristics: Consider the elements of the play/leisure activity in terms of various dimensions (eg, active vs passive, structured/organized vs unstructured, social vs nonsocial, competitive vs noncompetitive recreational
    - Time sequences of activity participation: Are there relatively predictable sequences over time (eg, seasonal aspects, grading of participation level)?
    - Consider the sensory, motor, and cognitive elements of different activities (eg, challenges associated with participation, levels of difficulty, qualities of different play items, and experiences)

Criteria for choosing different measures vary according to the reasons for conducting the assessment and the level of investigation around key issues or concerns. Firstly, assessments might be selected because they can provide comprehensive or targeted baseline measurement of key variables that are important to document when making clinical decisions regarding program development. Objective measurement can supplement subjective clinical observations. Measures that provide information from different service recipients' perspectives can triangulate information from the client alone. Secondly, the purpose of measurement might be evaluative, with documentation of outcome achievement as the main purpose. This information may allow the practitioner to document progress during an intervention, or may act as an important means of providing feedback regarding service delivery for employers and funding bodies.

Different types of measures are applicable for both purposes, although there is some overlap and potential for more subjective instruments (eg, self-reports) to be used to measure change, as well as to inform program development. Self-report may be less reliable as an outcome measure for children under the age of 9 or 10 years[77] and therefore, reporting by parents alongside children (where possible) may be necessary.

Strategies for Reporting About Play/Leisure

The main aims of reporting are to provide information to document and enhance service delivery. The value of documenting the impact of programs has long been recognized in occupational therapy practice and is an integral component of outcome measurement aimed at monitoring, evaluating, and improving the quality of health care services.[2] Just as extensive testing is associated with high participant response burden, there are elements of reporting that can contribute to service delivery burden for health professionals. These include lengthy, imprecise reports that may be linked with measurement approaches and data analytical requirements that are arduous and time consuming.

Information dissemination strategies vary with the different tiers of practice.[61] Tier 1 level (ie, for promotion, prevention, and early intervention at the system and individual levels) requires systematic documentation of outcomes for reporting to funding agencies and community partners, as well as providing information for consumers that meets healthy literacy standards for the target population. Occupational therapy practitioners and researchers who work on play/leisure projects at the community level may need to record outputs from networking meetings using social media, publications, presentations, and other predetermined strategies that are identified during development of a program logic model.[78] Program logic models include methodology for planning and sharing of lessons learned, outcomes achieved, and how results of intended outcomes will be shared at different levels.

At Tier 2 and 3 levels, while it is the responsibility of individual practitioners to record outcomes empirically connected to target endpoints, the organizations for whom therapists work will have mandatory policies and procedures for information sharing. Regardless of tier level, the key starting point is always determining the purpose for describing, recording, and measuring. Implicit within this process is the need to consider client-centered reporting from a health literacy perspective.

Future Directions for Practice

It is imperative that researchers continue to develop conceptually and psychometrically sound measures to further occupational therapy understanding and optimization of play/leisure participation. Because there is still no consensus regarding a universal definition of play,[31] this represents a clear direction for future research. The defining elements of leisure also are inconsistently described.

Until clear, consistent definitions are available, a unified discourse on play/leisure, and play-/leisure-related occupational performance, is hampered.

Measuring the benefits of play/leisure program interventions for individuals who have disease or disability is necessary to inform future, evidence-based practice. Knowledge of these beneficial outcomes can build practitioner, consumer, and organizational service provider confidence and beliefs regarding the importance of routine play/leisure measurement in practice. The impediments to routine measurement of play/leisure occupational performance are well acknowledged, and building a sound knowledge base appears to be a strong way forward to increased clinical attention to these occupations.[3]

There is a need to increase the occupational therapy contribution to the measurement of play/leisure participation from a preventive health standpoint at the Tier 1 level. To do so, practitioners will require knowledge of methodologies that can provide understanding of population-level, universal health needs, and be able to identify where there are instances of occupational deprivation or alienation. In order for occupational therapists to act confidently as advocates for healthy play/leisure in the public health arena, there is the need to have a broader view of measurement beyond an individual level approach. Thus, an understanding of survey methods and other leisure surveillance tools can supplement instrument knowledge about how to measure the health impacts of play/leisure participation for different populations and in different contexts. Measuring outcomes of different leisure experiences, such as summer camps, is one example of such an approach where occupational therapy expertise can potentially enhance program development and provide a means for measuring outcomes of leisure participation.[79]

At all Tiers, occupational therapists need to select psychometrically sound measures that can provide PEO information regarding the quality, frequency, diversity, and motivational influences on play/leisure participation. Basic and translational research to inform and extend current practice about preventive health benefits associated with participation in play/leisure occupations must be provided for consumers, practitioners, organizations, and policy makers if the full potential of occupational enablement is to be realized. In this way, multilayered tiers of prevention and intervention strategies can be enacted. Approaches used to provide information for consultation and advocacy at a population level may include program logic evaluation and other methodologies that can inform multistrategy, cross-institutional, linked setting partnerships.[80]

Representation on relevant committees in governments, associations, and organizations and collaboration with key stakeholders is needed to ensure funding and legislative change that can support community uptake of healthy play/leisure actions. The application of a PEO model, such as SCOPE-IT[51] provides a framework for comprehensively appraising variables associated with health outcomes that reduce the burden of disability or illness, and it is a particular strength of the occupational therapy profession. Within the PEO framework, there is also allowance for consideration of obstacles to engagement in play/leisure pursuits that are personally meaningful and/or have health and well-being benefits. Occupational therapists have much to offer communities in terms of expertise in relation to identifying barriers and supports to play/leisure participation, prevent development of unhealthy lifestyles, and protect the vulnerable from being unable to fully engage in these valuable occupational performance areas. Ensuring that these aspects are well documented represents a future direction for measurement development.

Emerging areas of practice will require the identification and development of instrumentation to measure and document outcomes of play/leisure participation. One such area is leisure pursuits that offer "recovery-from-work" benefits for employees when allostatic load is reduced and chronic work-related stress is alleviated.[81] The much touted rise of a "leisure society," where leisure was believed to gradually replace work as the central motivating force in people's lives during the 20th and 21st centuries has not eventuated despite increasing labor-saving work mechanization and information technology expansion. Instead, an overworked and overcommitted culture of workers has emerged, along with a fall in every kind of leisure activity, from socializing to sports.[23] The potential for restorative leisure environments that are conceptually or physically different settings from work environments and that captivate the mind and foster exploration as mitigating the negative impact of stress on mental and physical health represents an area of research for occupational therapists. Despite increased measurement of the stress-alleviating effects of engaging in leisure pursuits, such as yoga and mindfulness meditation, walking in natural surroundings, engaging in after-work sports activities, taking vacations, having positive conversations with friends, and so on, there has been low uptake of self-care practices for many stressed workers.[82] Health practitioners themselves are unlikely to attend adequately to their own self-care needs, including participation in healthy leisure pursuits,[83] although this can change with early education about health promoting activity engagement during the student years.[84]

Although a leisure society has not emerged at a general population level, there is an increasing proportion of the community who will have more time for leisure pursuits following retirement from the workforce. There is a growing body of research into meaningful leisure participation for older individuals in terms of the health-enhancing nature of these pursuits. Measuring and promoting meaningful leisure participation throughout life and, in particular, during the later stages of life when leisure participation may overtake work-related tasks, is a growing area of practice.

From an occupational health perspective, exploring participation means not only exploring active participation, but also passive participation in play/leisure (eg, onlooker behavior, time-out/relaxation leisure). Thus, measuring outcomes that may be inversely as well as positively associated with different forms of leisure participation is necessary. An additional focus of client-centered occupational therapy is promoting healthy leisure through occupations. Measures such as the Health Promoting Activities Scale (HPAS)[85] provide practicing occupational therapists with a brief tool to assess current capacity and identify goals for participating in health-promoting leisure pursuits. This measure also reminds occupational therapists who work with families that caregiver health and well-being also are essential elements of family-centered practice.

Future directions for play/leisure scale development to further current knowledge and understanding of factors that characterize a child's play include the following:

- The development of appropriate, culturally sensitive evaluation tools with testing of validity and reliability for use in non-English as well as English speaking countries. The use of these measures will allow cross-cultural comparisons of children's participation in play/leisure. Over 90% of articles researching leisure measures are still focused on 10% of the world's population.[86] Consequently, knowledge about leisure in non-Western countries is very limited. Understanding the unique perspectives of individuals from different backgrounds and with varying health conditions in relation to play/leisure is of fundamental importance to inform quality interventions.
- Further clarification and well-defined descriptions of the different types of play/leisure and their social, physical, and cognitive underpinnings are necessary to precisely measure these play/leisure components. Leisure theory has been criticized for being weak, heterogeneous, and incoherent in relation to measuring some aspects of the leisure experience.[72] This weak theoretical base has, in some cases, contributed to the adoption bottom-up inductive approaches without a guiding theoretical model for measuring some aspects of play/leisure, such as adult playfulness.[72]
- Convergent and construct validity of many play/leisure tests is not always available and should be investigated in new research studies. Survey research and qualitative methods have dominated the research literature, with less attention to the development of psychometrically sound standardized tools.[86]
- Instrumentation to measure social and physical environmental influences on play/leisure is important. For play measures, it has been suggested that parents' engagement and influence on children's leisure should be evaluated as part of a comprehensive PEO assessment because this has been linked with beneficial health outcomes for children.[87] For example, a family-centered practice model also supports measurement of sibling support, and how shared leisure activities can facilitate and strengthen relationships between other family members and children. Other social environmental areas include motivational climate within clubs/teams/organized sports (ie, how the coach and other key individuals influence motivational elements such as whether activities are perceived to be competitive and/or learning opportunities). Because measurement of environmental factors is difficult, qualitative interviews with parents and children could help determine the environmental variables that are important to participation of children and families.
- A more comprehensive listing of possible activities is consistently suggested as one means of extending current measures, particularly those investigating frequency and enjoyment of leisure participation activities, interests, and participation. Longer measures containing a wider range of activities and exploring diverse participation contexts come at the cost of time, respondent burden, and ease of administration. Perhaps an interactive computer-based assessment would be more engaging? Some authors of these measures[88] have noted that the list of items of the California Older Person's Pleasant Experiences Scale (COPPES) can be changed (eg, if new information becomes available during interviews with individuals or their families).
- Understanding the quality of time spent in different play/leisure contexts from the client's perspective can be difficult in situations where an individual has limited communication skills. Assistive technology devices, such as augmentative and alternative communication (AAC), may be used to help an individual express interests and preferences, as well as observations about how they experience and evaluate their everyday activity settings. A future direction for research is to explore caregiver vs client perspectives using some of these AAC approaches and to apply and validate the use of these technologies to some of the measures used in practice.

Overview of Measures of Play/Leisure

The wide range of potential play/leisure measures for practitioner use in therapy settings means that no single measure of play/leisure can meet the broad needs of all therapists. An extensive array of potentially valuable instruments has been identified. These varied in terms of target population characteristics (eg, the age range of interest) and levels of specificity regarding elements of the play/leisure occupation for the target population (eg, play experiences, participation intensity, and diversity).

The information provided is not exhaustive regarding provision of a complete overview of measures for these areas of occupational performance. The measures allocated to exclusive tables are accompanied by specific information about their usage, psychometric data, and key features. Primary sources such as assessment manuals, research literature, and direct contact with authors were used to complete these tables.

Table 10-1

CHILD-INITIATED PRETEND PLAY ASSESSMENT (CHIPPA)

Source	Stagnitti[89]; www.assessmenttoolshop.com and www.therapybookshop.com
Key References	Stagnitti et al[90,91]; Stagnitti and Unsworth[92]; Uren and Stagnitti[93]; McAloney and Stagnitti[94]; Dender and Stagnitti[95]; Pfeiffer et al[96,97]; Fink et al[98]; Stagnitti and Lewis[99]; Stagnitti[100]; Reynolds et al[101]; O'Connor and Stagnitti[102]; Stagnitti[103]

(continued)

There were many other measures that were discussed within the text in terms of potential use for practitioners. In an effort to contain the number of tables, selection criteria for measures selected for separate review was necessarily very restrictive. The readers' attention is also directed to the previous edition of this book containing information regarding play/leisure measures in the field. Several measures have continued to be the subject of intense research attention, and as such, the information pertaining to developments since 2005 has been included in updated tables.

There were several criteria that guided the selection of instruments to be included within separate tables in this chapter. Firstly, psychometric data had to be published for each scale, even if limited. Additionally, it was decided that the instrument must provide a therapist, rather than a teacher or coach, with comprehensive information about play/leisure, not focus on one aspect of play/leisure alone, or be a proxy vehicle for evaluating other aspects of clinical concern. For example, while it was recognized that in some pediatric practice settings, play is an appropriate modality for engaging a child in assessment, this was not considered to be the prime purpose of a measurement focus on the occupation of play. Therefore, play-based assessments that provide alternatives to traditional standardized developmental assessments were not included. Although there are many sound developmental assessments that incorporate a play/leisure subscale as part of a broader assessment of development or participation, it was determined that the measure must be predominantly play/leisure-focused with an intended aim to enhance the provision of therapy services.

Fourteen measures have been included in 12 separate tables (Tables 10-1 through 10-12):

1. Child-initiated Pretend Play Assessment (ChIPPA) (Table 10-1)
2. Revised Knox Preschool Play Scale (RKPPS) (Table 10-2)
3. Play Observation Scale (POS) (Table 10-3)
4. Children's Leisure Assessment Scale (CLASS) (Table 10-4)
5. Test of Playfulness (ToP) Version 4.0 (Table 10-5)
6. Test of Environmental Supportiveness (TOES) Version 4.0 (Table 10-6)
7. Children's Assessment of Participation and Enjoyment (CAPE) and Preferences for Activities of Children (PAC) (Table 10-7)
8. McDonald Play Inventory (MPI) (Table 10-8)
9. Pediatric Interest Profiles (PIP) (Table 10-9)
10. Measure of Environmental Qualities of Activity Settings (MEQAS) (Table 10-10)
11. Self-Reported Experiences of Activity Settings (SEAS) (Table 10-11)
12. Activity Card Sort (ACS) (See Chapter 9)

Other measures, many of which would be beneficial for occupational therapists to consider for use when a more in-depth understanding of a particular aspect of play/leisure is needed for a target population, are included in combined tables (Tables 10-13 through 10-18). Despite being psychometrically sound and clinically relevant, the play/leisure component of some of these instruments was a subscale and, therefore, they have been included within a table that recognizes their importance as part of a broader measure. This chapter does not provide a comprehensive discussion of all of these formal assessments in play/leisure due to space limitations.

Since the inception of the ICF and ICF-CY,[37,38] there has been increasing attention to the development of measures for assessing play/leisure participation. Most participation measures encompass a broad overview of participation across several category domains, including activities of daily living, recreation, community mobility, and social activities, and these are described elsewhere in this text. The participation-oriented measures that contained a substantial element devoted to play/leisure are only briefly described within a combined table; however, they have much to offer practitioners and researchers when considering play/leisure in the context of other occupations, and in relation to health and well-being outcomes. Measuring leisure interests, leisure companionship, environmental affordance, and key experiences offers valuable insights into factors that may drive participation. Routine measurement of play/leisure participation and inclusion of goals for play/leisure within intervention programs is an important aim for both occupational therapy practitioners and researchers.

Table 10-1 (continued)

Child-Initiated Pretend Play Assessment (ChIPPA)

Purpose	• Assessment of quality of a child's ability to self-initiate pretend play.
Type of Client	• Children 3 to 7 years, 11 months with a range of disabilities (eg, developmental delay, cerebral palsy, autism spectrum, learning and emotional difficulties).
Test Format	• Observational measure
Procedures	• ChIPPA comprises 2 sessions using standard sets of toys: a conventional-imaginative session (eg, animals, trucks, people), and a symbolic play session (eg, unstructured objects such as boxes, tins) for the other. • Once materials are laid out, the child is invited to play, but no other directions are provided. At intervals, additional materials are introduced in a structured manner.
Time Required	• Training in the measure is recommended (www.karenstagnitti.com). For younger children (age 3 years), assessment can take approximately 18 minutes, and slightly longer (30 minutes) for older children. • Play behavior is scored according to percentage of elaborate play to total actions, object substitutions, and the child's imitation of the examiner in each session.
Standardization	• The first version of the ChIPPA was normed on 400 Australian children between the ages of 3 and 7 years.
Reliability	
Test-Retest	• Good to excellent test-retest reliability for elaborate play ability (ICC .73 to .84). A 63% to 84% agreement was found between 2 testing occasions. For object substitutions, the reliability was moderate (ICC .55 to .57).
Internal Consistency	• Cronbach alpha of .64[97]
Inter-Rater	• Inter-rater reliability was good to excellent with Swindells and Stagnitti[104] reporting .7 agreement using kappa. Stagnitti et al[91] reported excellent inter-rater (kappa .96 to 1.0) across all scores.
Validity	
Content	• Content validity established through an expert panel[89,105]
Construct	• Moderate correlations between elaborate play ability and social competence (rho = .35, $p < .05$), and between poor object substitution ability and social disruption (rho = -.32, $p < .05$) and social disconnection and poor elaborate play scores (rho = .35, $p < .05$)[93]
Criterion	• Stagnitti and Lewis[99] found quality of play scores on the ChIPPA predicted up to 20% of oral language ability in children 4 years later.
Utility	
Research Programs	• The ChIPPA has been used as an outcome measure for research into evidence on play-based curricula vs traditional curricula,[101] play-based intervention for children with IQ below 70.[102]
Practice Settings	• The ChIPPA has been used in research aimed to understand the play ability of children with cerebral palsy[96,97] and children with acquired brain injury.[98]
Strengths	• The ChIPPA assesses the quality of a child's ability to spontaneously initiate his or her own play in a nonobtrusive way within a clinically viable time frame.
Complexities	• The ChIPPA scoring needs practice. It is recommended that the first 10 children be videotaped when learning to score the ChIPPA.

Table 10-2

Revised Knox Preschool Play Scale (RKPPS)

Source	Knox[106]
Key References	Bledsoe and Shepherd[107]; Harrison and Kielhofner[108]; Knox[33,109]; Jankovich et al[110]; Lee and Hinojosa[111]; Pacciulo et al[112]; Kennedy-Behr et al[113]
Purpose	• Provides a developmental description of children's play behaviors.
Type of Client	• Infants and children aged up to 6 years.
Test Format	• Children should be observed both indoors and outdoors in a naturalistic or familiar environment, with peers present. • Children's play behaviors are observed across 4 play dimensions: space management, material management, pretense-symbolic, and participation.
Procedures	• Children play in natural settings (indoors and outdoors) with suitable toys and peers present. • Within each factor, observers score the child's play behavior on each descriptor, each time it is observed. Each factor is scored at the upper end of the age bracket (eg, ages 6 to 12 months is scored as 12 months). Dimension scores are determined by averaging the factor scores. An overall "play age" score is calculated by averaging dimension scores.
Time Required	• Two 30-minute observations, 1 indoors and 1 outdoors. • Children's play is described in 6-month increments for the first 3 years and in yearly increments for ages 4 through 6 years.
Standardization	• Children's play behaviors are observed as free as possible from adult intervention and direction.
Reliability	
Test-Retest	• Bledscoe and Shepherd[107] examined test-retest reliability of the Preschool Play Scale (PPS[33]) in 90 typically developing children. Correlation coefficients were high for dimension scores: Space Management (r=0.96); Material Management (r=0.94); Imitation (r=.86); Participation (r=0.92); and Overall Play Age (r=0.97). • Harrison and Kielhofner[108] reported correlation coefficients for PPS Dimensions and Play Age ranging from r=0.73 to 0.91 in 60 children with disabilities.
Internal Consistency	• Not reported
Inter-Rater	• Good inter-rater reliability with overall ICC values of 0.76 in 17 children with and without DCD[113]; 15 children with autism spectrum disorder (ICC=0.94)[114]; and percentage agreement between 81.8% and 100% for 38 young children.[110] • As reported by Knox,[106] Fallon[115] examined percentage agreement between 6 raters. For 4 of the cases the percent of agreement was 83%, and on the fifth case, agreement was 66%. The percent of agreement on the 12 categories ranged from 40% to 76%. • High inter-rater reliability of the PPS was identified by Bledscoe and Shepherd[107] in typically developing children (r=0.99) for overall play age. Category scores ranged from r=0.89 to r=0.98 and from r=0.86 to 0.96 for domain scores. • Inter-rater reliability for the PPS was high in children with disabilities (n=15; r=0.88) for overall play age. Category scores ranged from r=0.43 to r=0.91 and domain scores ranged from r=0.55 to r=0.91.[108]
Intra-Rater	• Pacciulio et al[112] examined intrarater and inter-rater reliability and repeatability of the Brazilian version for the RKPPS on 18 typically developing infants and children from 2 schools in Brazil. Inter-rater reliability was high for total and dimensions scores (r=0.78 to 0.99). • Pacciulio et al[112] reported a high intra-rater correlation coefficient in every dimension of the adapted RKPPS (Examiner 1 r=0.87 to 0.97; examiner 2 r=0.99 to 1.0).

(continued)

Table 10-2 (continued)

Revised Knox Preschool Play Scale (RKPPS)

Validity	
Content	• The RKPPS is based on a comprehensive review of play theory literature.[33,106,109]
Construct	• Kennedy-Behr et al[113] reported means of children in Developmental Coordination Disorder group (n = 32) were significantly lower than those of the typically developing children (n = 31) on all dimensions of the RKPPS (U = 223.00, z = -3.760, p = .000). • Jankovitch et al[110] reported play ages determined by raters matched the children's chronological ages for children in 36- to 47-month age range 57.1% of the time. Agreement was greater for the older age groups (48- to 59-month = 94.1%; 60- to 72-month = 100%). • Knox[106] reported on numerous studies utilizing the RKPPS to discriminate between different populations including typically developing children and children with Autistic Spectrum Disorder,[116] children from abusive backgrounds,[117] children with sensory integrative dysfunction,[118] children with juvenile rheumatoid arthritis.[119]
Criterion	• Lee and Hinojosa[111] examined concurrent validity between the RKPPS and the Vinelands Adaptive Behavior Scales (VABS[120]). The concurrent validity between the total score of the RKPPS and the total score of the VABS was equal r = 0.52 (n = 61). • Correlation coefficients of play age with Lunzer's Scale of Organization of Play Behavior in typically developing children and children with disabilities were r = 0.64 and r = 0.59, respectively.[107,121] Correlation scores of play age with Parten's Social Play Hierarchy[122] were r = 0.61 in typically developing children, and r = 0.60 in children with disabilities.[107,121] • Harrison and Kielhofner[108] reported significant correlations when comparing the Lunzer score with the category and dimension scores of the PPS (n = 60).
Utility	• The RKPPS has been translated into Spanish, German, Japanese, Korean, Norwegian, French, and Portuguese. • Does not require specialized toys or equipment and can be used to assess child play performance in natural settings.
Research Programs	• Used in a number of theses[115,123]; however, these remain unpublished. • Has been used as a measure of treatment effect (PPS); however, no recent studies on the updated version (RKPPS).
Practice Settings	• Used to assess play skills at baseline and measure play skills over time. • Used to identify play profiles of children, including their strengths and weaknesses, and play interest areas. • Used as a guide to the developmental aspects of play.
Strengths	• Useful to evaluate play skills of children whose underlying capacities cannot be evaluated easily with standardized testing. • Provides a structure to observe children's play. • Covers all areas of play development and reflects child's developmental status.
Complexities	• Not recommended as a sole measure of play. Should be used in conjunction with other measures such as play histories etc. • Measurements are in fairly large increments (6 months to 3 years and 4 to 6 years of age) and therefore are not sensitive to small changes. A child may make significant play gains but will not change levels due to these large increments. • The majority of validity data is based on studies conducted more than 10 years ago on the previous version (PPS).

Table 10-3

Play Observation Scale (POS)

Source	Rubin[124]
Key References	Kennedy-Behr et al[113]; Bar-Haim and Bart[125]; Coplan and Rubin[126]; Degnan et al[127]; Rubin and Krasnor[128]
Purpose	• The Play Observation Scale (POS)[124] records and categorizes a child's free-play behavior according to both social and cognitive domains.
Type of Client	• Children with and without disabilities.
Test Format	• Clinicians follow the norm-based time-sampling method as described by Rubin.[124] This involves observing a child engaged in play activities for at least 15 minutes and coding play behavior in 10-second intervals. Functional (sensorimotor), constructive, dramatic play, exploration, and games with rules are examined as they occur within the social participation categories of solitary, parallel, and group activity. In addition, aggressive behavior, rough-and-tumble play, and conversations with peers are coded.
Procedures	• Clinicians should observe a child for 30 seconds before beginning to record behaviors to familiarize themselves with the child's individual contextual cues and behaviors. The child is then observed for a 10-second interval. The predominant activity observed is then coded in the next 5 to 10 seconds (5 seconds preferably for length of coding time). The affect, that is, whether the interaction was positive (+), neutral (0), or negative (-), is also coded. Observations of raw frequencies for each child are then proportioned by dividing by the total number of coding intervals.
Time Required	• It is recommended a minimum of 15 minutes of POS data be gathered. By following the procedures outlined by Rubin[124] it will take 1.5 to 2 minutes to obtain 1 minute of recorded observations. It is recommend that only up to 5 minutes of the child's behavior be recorded on any given day in order to gather information regarding the child's general play styles over time.
Standardization	• Uses a norm-based time-sampling method as described by Rubin.[124] No further standardization; however, detailed instructions and coding is provided by Rubin.[124]
Reliability	
Test-Retest	• Rubin and Krasnor[128] conducted 5-way repeated measures ANOVA (age x sex x social play x cognitive play x time) for 20 3- to 4-year-old children over 4 time periods within 4 months. No significant time interactions were reported.
Internal Consistency	• Not reported
Inter-Rater	• Kennedy-Behr et al[113] reported good inter-rater reliability with overall ICC values of 0.65. • Degnan et al[127] reported high inter-rater reliability for 3 independent observers for each age (n total 153) with total variable matrix Cohen's kappas ranging from .71 to .86 at age 4 years and .84 to .88 at age 7 years. • Bar-Haim and Bart[125] reported high inter-rater reliability for 3 raters on a randomly selected set of coding intervals (20% of total). Percent agreement for the total variable matrix ranged between 93 to 96; Cohen's kappa ranged between 0.88 and 0.95. • Coplan and Rubin[126] reported inter-rater reliability data for 120 minutes of coding (20% of total data) was good with Cohen's Kappa was calculated at K=0.83.
Validity	
Content	• The Play Observational Scale (POS) is based on 2 long-standing play hierarchies: 1) social[122] and 2) cognitive[129]
Construct	• An extensive reference list of studies utilizing the POS to investigate children's play and social emotional development is provided at the end of the POS manual.[124]

(continued)

Table 10-3 (continued)

Play Observation Scale (POS)

Validity	
Construct	• More recently, Kennedy-Behr et al[113] reported good discriminative validity of the POS between children with and without motor difficulties. Children with (probable) DCD demonstrated less engagement in group play than children without motor difficulties (U=318.50, z=-2.441, p=.014), specifically group outdoor play (U=274.00, z=-3.055, p=.002). Children in the pDCD group were also more frequently involved in non-play behaviors.
Criterion	• Not reported
Utility	
Research Programs	• The POS has been used to determine (a) age and sex differences in children's play; (b) SES differences in play; (c) effects of ecological setting of play; (d) individual differences in play; (e) the social contexts within which the various forms of cognitive play are distributed; and (f) the associations between temperament and biological indices of emotion regulation and particular forms of POS-coded behaviors. • The POS has also been utilized in studies of behavior, attachment, temperament, parenting, and relationships.
Practice Settings	• The POS can be used to describe the play types, frequency, and social context of children with and without disabilities.
Strengths	• Provides descriptive data on the play behaviors of children with and without disabilities. • Although an observational assessment, the time taken to complete the assessment is acceptable
Complexities	• The majority of validity studies were conducted on earlier versions of the POS over 10 years ago. • Internal consistency of the measure is yet to be determined. • Manual is unpublished (but freely available online).

Table 10-4

Children's Leisure Assessment Scale (CLASS)

Source	Rosenblum et al[130]; http://chap.haifa.ac.il/
Key References	Schreuer et al[131]
Purpose	• The CLASS is a multidimensional scale to document children's perceptions concerning their time investment in leisure activities in terms of quantity and quality.
Type of Client	• The CLASS is suited for children and adolescents aged 10 to 18 years, developing typically or atypically.
Test Format	• It is a self-report questionnaire, comprising 40 leisure activities and open response option of "other activities."

(continued)

Table 10-4 (continued)

Children's Leisure Assessment Scale (CLASS)

Type of Client	
Procedures	• Children and adolescents are asked to complete the questionnaire according to instructions provided.
Time Required	• Administration requires 15 to 30 minutes. • The CLASS is scored on 5 dimensions of leisure participation: (1) Variety (which activities) sum of leisure activities; (2) Frequency (how often) 1=once every few months; 2=once a month; 3=twice a week; 4=every day; (3) Sociability (with whom) 1=alone; 2=with a relative (eg, parent, sibling); 3=with 1 friend; 4= with friends; (4) Preference (how much he or she likes the activity) 1 (do not like at all) to 10 (like very much); (5) Desired activities (activities desired, but not currently undertaken). • A mean score is computed for dimensions 2 to 4. • A mean score is computed for each of the CLASS factors: "instrumental indoor activities"; "outdoor activities usually performed with others"; "self-enrichment activities"; and "games and sports activities." • Reporting includes the child's participation levels in the 5 dimensions and 4 factors.
Standardization	• The CLASS was developed in Hebrew, culturally adapted, and translated to English and other languages in process.
Reliability	
Test-Retest	• Not reported
Internal Consistency	• Alpha coefficient (α=0.71) for the CLASS frequency dimension.[130] The 4 factors showed acceptable levels of internal reliability (Cronbach's alpha ranged from .57 to .83).
Inter-Rater	• Not reported
Validity	
Content	• CLASS items reviewed by experienced pediatric occupational therapists and parents.[130]
Construct	• Factor analysis revealed 4 factors explaining 32.73% of the total variance: (a) instrumental indoor activities; (b) outdoor activities usually performed with others; (c) self-enrichment activities; (d) games and sports activities.[130]
Criterion	• The CLASS was able to distinguish between participation of girls and boys[130] and children with typical development and physical disabilities.[131]
Utility	
Research Programs	• The CLASS can be used for research with children and young people with and without disabilities.
Practice Settings	• The CLASS may be useful for identifying children at risk of restricted leisure participation to inform intervention planning.
Strengths	• Provides children's perceptions of leisure activities in multiple dimensions.
Complexities	• Further studies with larger samples and varied cultural background are required.

Table 10-5

Test of Playfulness (ToP) Version 4.0

Source	Skard and Bundy[132]
Key References	Bundy et al[133-135]; Chang et al[136]; Cordier et al[137-139]; Okimoto et al[140]; Wilkes et al[141]; Wilkes-Gillan et al[142-144]
Purpose	• Assesses a child's approach to play (ie, playfulness). Items reflect 4 elements: intrinsic motivation, internal control, freedom from unnecessary constraints of reality, and "framing" (ie, giving and reading cues, maintaining a play theme)
Type of Client	• Young children through adolescents for whom play and playfulness may be of concern (eg, children with attention deficit disorder,[137-139] Autism, cerebral palsy[136])
Test Format	• An observation measure comprising 29 items
Procedures	• Unobtrusive observation of child in a free play situation in a familiar environment with one or more familiar playmates, preferably in more than one setting (indoor and outdoor). Observation period 15 minutes in each setting.
Time Required	• In addition to observation time, an additional 30 minutes is recommended for scoring, interpretation, and reporting.
Standardization	• The ToP has been standardized on children from 6 months to 18 years (commonly used with children 2 to 10 years of age)
Reliability	• Reliability data available for Versions 1 and 2 of ToP,[135] but only version 4 data are reported here.
Test-Retest	• Data from 96% of raters conform to the expectations of the Rasch model.[134] The ToP is designed for use in naturalistic environments so observations often differ between assessment occasions.[134] This is most influenced by presence of other children. When seeking to compare playfulness over time, social contexts should be similar.
Internal Consistency	• Point measure correlations range from .27 to .69 (M = .55; sd = .10) • The ToP was developed using Rasch analysis, which adjusts overall scores depending on rater severity.
Inter-Rater	• Not reported
Validity	
Content	• Developed in consultation with expert clinicians who operationalized the 4 elements contributing to playfulness.
Construct	• Goodness of fit statistics for 100% of items within the acceptable range: (MnSq range .6 to 1.4)
Criterion	• Saunders et al[145] found a significant relationship (r = .51, p = .02) between the ToP and the Coping Inventory[146] in preschoolers. Hess and Bundy[147] reported a significant correlation (r = .785; p < .01) in typically developing adolescents and adolescents with significant emotional disturbance.
Utility	
Research Programs	• Able to support investigation of playfulness as a construct in children's play.
Practice Settings	• Wide range of clinical and community settings.
Strengths	• Naturalistic observation of child playing in context that does not require special equipment. • Sensitive to change as result of intervention[141] • Supported by companion measure, Test of Environmental Supportiveness (TOES) (see Table 10-6).
Complexities	• Scores can be derived and compared with the overall sample on which the test was developed by using a keyform in Skard and Bundy.[132]

Table 10-6

TEST OF ENVIRONMENTAL SUPPORTIVENESS (TOES) VERSION 4.0

Source	Skard and Bundy[132]
Key References	Bronson and Bundy[148]; Bundy et al[149]
Purpose	• Best used as a basis for consultation with families, teachers and other professionals, paraprofessionals, and service providers seeking to establish an environment that is supportive of play. • Assesses the relative supportiveness of 4 elements of the environment to a child's play: caregivers, playmates (peer, younger, older), space, and playthings (eg, toys).
Type of Client	• Preschoolers and school-aged children and their caregivers.
Test Format	• An observation measure comprising 17 items.
Procedures	• The examiner establishes the child's motivations (ie, what the child is seeking in play), generally through observing. He or she then observes the play environment, asking the question, "to what extent do each of the elements support the child's motivations?" Observation period 15 minutes in each setting.
Time Required	• In addition to observation time, an additional 15 minutes is recommended for scoring, interpretation, and reporting.
Standardization	• The TOES has been standardized with children from ages 15 months to 6 years.
Reliability	
Test-Retest	• Not reported
Internal Consistency	• Not reported
Inter-Rater	• The TOES was developed using Rasch analysis, which adjusts overall scores depending on rater severity. Data from 100% of raters conformed to the expectations of the Rasch model.[148]
Validity	
Content	• Developed in consultation with a panel of expert clinicians who operationalized the 4 elements of a supportive environment.
Construct	• Goodness of fit statistics for 16/17 (94%) of items within the acceptable range: (MnSq range .6 to 1.4).
Criterion	• Not reported
Utility	
Research Programs	• Able to support investigation of playfulness as a construct in children's play.
Practice Settings	• Wide range of clinical and community settings.
Strengths	• Naturalistic observation of regular play environments. • Does not require special equipment.
Complexities	• While standard scores can be derived, these are far less meaningful than use of the items as the basis for consultation.

Table 10-7

Children's Assessment of Participation and Enjoyment (CAPE) and Preferences for Activities of Children (PAC)

Source	Psychological Corporation, Skill Builders Division, 555 Academic Court, San Antonio, TX, 78204
Key References	King et al[150-152]; Imms[153]; Bundy[19]
Purpose	• The CAPE measures 5 dimensions of participation in everyday activities outside of those mandated in school activities, including diversity (number of activities), intensity (frequency scale ranges from 0 to 7), with whom (7 possible responses), where (6 possible responses), and enjoyment (scale ranges from 0 to 5). • PAC addresses preferences for activities.
Type of Client	• Children and youth aged 6 to 21 years of age with sufficient ability to understand the task of sorting and categorizing activities.
Test Format	• Both measures include 55 informal and formal activities that can be organized into 5 activity types: recreational (12 items), active-physical (13 items), social (10 items), skill-based (10 items), and self-improvement (10 items). Activities are also categorized by 2 domains: formal and informal. Three levels of scoring are available: overall, activity domain, and activity type. If both CAPE and PAC are completed, participation scores for the following can be obtained: (1) overall; (2) 2 domains: informal and formal activities; and (3) activity types: recreational, physical, social, skill-based, and self-improvement activities.
Procedures	**CAPE** • Self-administered version: Children independently complete the CAPE by looking at drawings of children performing 55 different activities. Children indicate on a Likert-type scale if they have performed each activity in the last 4 months, how often, with whom they performed the activity, and their level of enjoyment. Children record their answers on the record form provided. • Interviewer-assisted version: Children complete a short questionnaire about whether they have performed each of the 55 activities in the past 4 months, and if so, how often. The interviewer then asks questions regarding each activity the child has performed, including who the activity was performed with, where the activity was performed, and how much enjoyment was experienced for each activity. • Scoring: The CAPE provides 3 levels of scoring including overall participation scores, scale scores, and domain scores. Complete scoring calculations are included in the manual. The CAPE Summary Score Sheet is used to calculate Overall Scores and allows simple transfer of the data from Record Form. Calculation of overall scores for the 6 participation dimensions is also possible. **PAC** • Self-administered version: Children record their preference for 55 different activities by circling 1 of 3 facial expressions that reflect their interest in the activity ("I would not like to do at all," "I would sort of like to do," "I would really like to do"). • Interviewer-assisted version: The child sorts the 55 drawings into 3 piles using the same response options as in the self-administered version. • The PAC Summary Score Sheet is used to calculate the Activity Type and Overall scores.
Time Required	• The manual reports that the CAPE takes 30 to 45 minutes to complete and the PAC 15 to 20 minutes.
Standardization	• The CAPE and PAC can be self-administered or interviewer-assisted. The manual provides comprehensive instructions and scoring assistance.

(continued)

Table 10-7 (continued)

Children's Assessment of Participation and Enjoyment (CAPE) and Preferences for Activities of Children (PAC)

Reliability	
Test-Retest	• King et al[150] reported adequate test–retest reliability for the CAPE by domain (n=48): overall participation (0.64 to 0.86); diversity (0.67 to 0.77); intensity (0.72 to 0.81); enjoyment (0.12 to 0.73). Enjoyment scores had low reliability, except for recreational activities. • Bult et al[154] reported good to excellent correlation coefficients for test-retest reliability of the CAPE Dutch version (0.61 and 0.78) in 232 children with (n=74) and without (n=158) disabilities.
Internal Consistency	• King et al[150] reports varied internal consistency of the CAPE by domain with Cronbach's alpha's ranging from poor to adequate: formal domain (0.35 to 0.42); informal domain (0.76 to 0.77); activity types (0.30 to 0.62) in a large sample size (n=427). Internal consistency for the PAC was adequate with Cronbach Alphas above 0.67: PAC domain=0.84 (informal); 0.76 to 0.78 (formal); PAC activity=0.67 to 0.77. • Anastasiadi and Tzetzis[155] report high consistency in PAC, but low consistency for the CAPE (Intensity): PAC α=0.92 (range 0.64 to 0.88); CAPE total α=0.64 (range 0.08 to 0.65). • Internal consistency for CAPE/PAC for the section on activity types was acceptable (0.60 to 0.79) for the Dutch version.[154] • Colon et al[156] reported the Puerto Rico version of the CAPE showed good internal consistency (0.92 overall scale; 0.90 formal domain and 0.70 informal domain scale).
Inter-Rater	• King et al[150] reports moderate to high consistency between the 2 formats of the CAPE: interviewer vs self-administration: intensity: 0.82 to 0.99; enjoyment: 0.47 to 0.78 (n=56).
Validity	
Content	• Development and item generation informed by comprehensive literature review, expert consultation, and pilot testing of research versions with children with and without disabilities.[150]
Construct	• King et al[150] reports the construct validity of the CAPE has been tested in a large sample of children (n=427) with small but significant correlations (r=-0.17 to 0.42) reported between domains, scale scores and measures of difference constructs obtained from a longitudinal study of predictors of children's participation. Principal component analysis of the PAC identified 5 factors. • Significant correlations reported between domains of the CAPE: recreational activities: social competence (r=0.18); active physical activities: athletic competence (r=0.15); social activities: social competence (r=0.22). • Correlations ranged from 0.22 to 0.61 for relationships between CAPE intensity and enjoyment scores and the Preferences for the Activities of Children (PAC). • The CAPE was shown to discriminate between boys and girls for intensity and enjoyment, children with and without disabilities, age groups for intensity, levels of severity in children with cerebral palsy, and different levels of impairment in body structure and function.[153,157] • Anastasiadi and Tzetzis[155] reported factor analysis for the Greek version (n typical=253; n disability=49) identified 55 items were loaded into 7 different categories of activities • Jarus et al[10] reported differences with moderate to high effect size in participation patterns across age. A decline in participation was detected in transition from childhood to adolescence. • Colon et al[156] report discriminant validity of the CAPE Puerto Rico version in a large sample (n=249). Children with disabilities showed significantly lower mean scores on the overall participation dimension scales of diversity (t=2.84; p=0.002), Intensity (t=1.75; p=0.041) and Where (t=1.75; p=0.041) in comparison with typically developing children.
Criterion	• Not reported

(continued)

Table 10-7 (continued)

Children's Assessment of Participation and Enjoyment (CAPE) and Preferences for Activities of Children (PAC)

Utility	
Research Programs	• Comprehensive in assessing participation patterns in children and youth with and without disabilities • Can evaluate changes in participation over time • Can measure the effectiveness of interventions and/or clinical trials over time • Appropriate for use in children over a wide age range—useful for longitudinal studies • Has also been used extensively in studies of typically developing children
Practice Settings	• Provides useful information to a clinician about the type, intensity, and enjoyment of activities their client has experienced. • Can assess the effectiveness of intervention focused on improving participation of children engaged in extracurricular activities.
Strengths	• Activities are substitutable—clinicians able to suggest suitable alternative activities that fit the child's preferences. • User-friendly for children and can capture both child and parent's perceptions of participation. • Culturally sensitive and gender neutral. • Accessible and engaging tool to use with children of wide age ranges and disability types. • Two options for administration: flexibility in clinical and research settings with individuals or groups.
Complexities	• Requires a solid understanding by the clinician prior to administration. • Potential for recall bias, both within the participant and proxy report. • Intellectual disability makes recall difficult. • Currently no normative data with which comparisons to nonclinical populations can be made. • Not appropriate for children who are unable to comprehend the task of recognizing and sorting activities or responding to questions. • If wishing to administer PAC, the CAPE should be conducted first as it was developed as an extension of the CAPE.

Table 10-8

McDonald Play Inventory (MPI)

Source	Dr. Ann E McDonald; Manual to be published.
Key References	McDonald and Vigen[158]
Purpose	• The MPI is divided into 2 parts: 1) McDonald Play Activity Inventory (MPAI) measures children's perceived frequency of engagement or participation in an activity (gross motor, fine motor, social group or solitary); and 2) McDonald Play Style Inventory (MPSI) elicits how the child feels, or the affective component of participation in 4 domains: physical coordination, cooperation, peer acceptance, and social participation.
Type of Client	• Children with and without disabilities; ages 7 to 11 years • High functioning Autism, learning disabilities, mild developmental delay, Down syndrome

(continued)

Table 10-8 (continued)

McDonald Play Inventory (MPI)

Type of Client	
Test Format	• The MPI is a 2-part, self-report inventory. • The MPAI comprises 4 mutually exclusive categories (10 activities in each). These categories form 4 subscales: fine motor, gross motor, social group, and solitary. • The MPSI comprises 24 play behavior items in 4 subscales (6 items in each), including both positive and negative items in 4 play-style categories. These include physical coordination vs incoordination, cooperation vs uncooperative behavior, social participation vs social isolation, and peer acceptance vs peer rejection.
Procedures	• MPAI: The child is asked to read each item and rate how frequently he or she participates in the activity by circling 1 of 5 Likert-scale responses (never, about once or twice per year, about once or twice per month, about once or twice per week, or almost every day). • MPSI: The same 5-point Likert scale is used for the response options (never, hardly ever, sometimes, a lot, always).
Time Required	• Approximately 15 minute for children requiring no assistance. Approximately 20 to 30 minutes for children requiring assistance.
Standardization	• Not reported • Instrument development procedures implemented for initial pilot test of MPI on 71 children (33 with learning disabilities [LD] and 38 non-LD) in 1987; updated and revised in 2010 on 124 children.
Reliability	• Reliability and validity studies[158] were conducted on 124 children, (n=89 typically developing children; n=35 children with disabilities – LD, Down syndrome, autism spectrum disorder, intellectual disability).
Test-Retest	• Pearson correlations were r=.69 for the MPAI and r=.82 for the MPSI in a small study sample (n=7). • Moderate correlations for inventory items were reported (r=0.27 to 0.75) with respective subscale scores. Moderate to strong correlations (r=0.47 to 0.81) were found between each subscale and total scale score. The total inventory score correlations (r=0.49), MPAI (r=0.84) and MPSI (0.79) were adequate.
Internal Consistency	• Not reported
Inter-Rater	• Low to moderate correlations are reported for parent-child agreement on the MPAI (r=0.04) and MPSI (r=0.49). Parents of children with disabilities agreed with child ratings on perceived play performance more often than parents of typical children.
Validity	
Content	• Play domains or categories were derived from the play literature and field studies.[158] MPAI and MPSI items were based on field studies, observations 1-day diary records, and the relevant play literature. • A panel of content experts (n=10 pediatric occupational therapists) placed the items in categories and recommended revisions. The final instrument was pilot tested on 10 children with and without disabilities.
Construct	• No statistically significant differences were found by gender or presence of disability on the self-reported play activities of the MPAI total inventory or subscale scores (n=124). • Significantly lower scores were found for children with disabilities on the total inventory score of the MPSI (p=.002) and all of the MPSI subscale scores (physical coordination; peer acceptance; social participation; and cooperation). Significant differences were identified between play of 10 and 11 year olds on MPSI (p=0.04).

(continued)

Table 10-8 (continued)

McDonald Play Inventory (MPI)

Validity	
Criterion	• Not reported
Utility	
Research Programs	• Further use in research studies has not yet been reported.
Practice Settings	• MPI can be used by clinicians wishing to evaluate the perceived performance in play during middle childhood.
Strengths	• Information from the MPI could contribute to the multidimensional assessment of play for children with a suspected play deficit. • Could use data to guide intervention programs. • Further research has recently been conducted and will be published shortly.
Complexities	• Not recommended as a sole measure of play. Should be used in conjunction with other measures such as play histories. • Further research is needed to gather normative data on children from diverse backgrounds and age ranges. • Further investigation of the psychometric properties of the measurement tool is warranted Reliability studies were conducted on small sample sizes and did not report on inter -or intrarater reliability. Further evidence of the validity of the measure is required.

Table 10-9

Pediatric Interest Profiles (PIP)

Source	Henry[159]
Key References	Henry[160]; Skar and Prellwitz[161]; Trottier et al[162]
Purpose	• Provide an easy way to gain a profile of the play interests of children and adolescents.
Type of Client	• Children and adolescents between 6 and 21 years of age without disabilities.
Test Format	• Composed of 3 assessments: the Kids Play Profile (KPP) (age 6 to 9 years), Pre-Teen Play Profile (PPP) (age 9 to 12 years), and Adolescent Leisure Interest Profile (ALIP) (age 12 to 21 years).
Procedures	• Paper-and-pencil checklist format. Children/adolescents respond to questions regarding interest, participation, and enjoyment in leisure/play activities typical of peers. Drawings are used in KPP and PPP to represent activities. • KPP: child answers up to 3 questions about 50 activity items regarding whether the child does and likes an activity and who the activity is done with. • PPP: child answers 5 questions for each of the 59 activity items (do they do activity, how often, do they like it, how good are they at it, and who is it done with). • ALIP: youth answer 5 questions about 83 activity items including how interested in activity, how often it is done, how well do they do it, how much it is enjoyed, and who it is done with. • Can be administered individually or in a small group (3 to 5 children).
Time Required	• Approximately 15 minutes (for KPP) to 30 minutes (for ALIP).

(continued)

Table 10-9 (continued)

PEDIATRIC INTEREST PROFILES (PIP)

Standardization	• Each test consists of standard choices to which the child/adolescent responds.
Reliability	
Test-Retest	• KPP: coefficients ranged from 0.45 to 0.91 for total scores (n=31 children without disabilities). • PPP: coefficients ranged from 0.51 to 0.75 for total scores (n=32 children without disabilities). • Henry[160] reported ALIP coefficients ranged from 0.61 to 0.85 for total scores (n=28 adolescents without disabilities). • Coefficients for adolescents with disabilities ranged from 0.62 to 0.78 for total scores (n=88).
Internal Consistency	• Henry[160] reported Cronbach's alpha for the ALIP ranged from 0.58 to 0.81 for subscale scores and was 0.92 for total scores for questions regarding level of interest in activities (n=88 adolescents with various disabilities). • Trottier et al[162] reported Cronbach's alpha for total scores of the "How interested?" and "How often?" questions were 0.93 and 0.87, respectively (n=37).
Inter-Rater	• Not reported
Validity	
Content	• Drawn from occupational perspective, particularly the Model of Human Occupation[163] • Items for all 3 versions developed from interviews and preliminary surveys of children or adolescents in the targeted age range.
Construct	• ALIP: question regarding level of enjoyment in activities was shown to discriminate among adolescents with and without disabilities. • Trottier et al[162] reported scores for concurrent validity with the Leisure Satisfaction Scale ranged from −0.43 to 0.68 indicating fairly poor correlations with the LSS.
Criterion	• Not reported
Utility	
Research Programs	• Can be used with large population to gain general understanding of leisure patterns of children and youth. • Easily used in most settings. • Can be used to establish treatment goals.
Practice Settings	• The only assessments specifically devoted to developing a profile of play interests from the perspective of children and adolescents. • Require minimal examiner training. • Facilitate conversation between clinician and child. • Designed to be easily understood by children within targeted age range.
Strengths	• Identify children and adolescents at risk of play-related problems • Identify activities used to engage child in therapeutic or educational interventions.
Complexities	• Reliability and validity studies are based on data from over 10 years ago. • Should not be used as a sole measure of leisure.

Table 10-10

Measure of Environmental Qualities of Activity Settings (MEQAS)

Source	https://flintbox.com/public/project/25723/
Key References	King et al[64]
Purpose	• To comprehensively assess place- and opportunity-related qualities of leisure activity settings for young people.
Type of Client	• The measure assesses environmental qualities rather than client-environment fit. It is relevant to activity settings for young people with and without disabilities.
Test Format	• An observer-rated measure comprising 32 items, containing the following scales: Opportunities for Social Activities, Opportunities for Physical Activities, Pleasant Physical Environment, Opportunities for Choice, Opportunities for Personal Growth, and Opportunities to Interact with Adults.
Procedures	• A trained rater observes and then rates the qualities of a youth activity setting.
Time Required	• Not reported
Standardization	N/A
Reliability	
Test-Retest	• Reported for sample of 8 activity settings. Range of 0.70 to 0.90 (M=0.84).
Internal Consistency	• Reported for sample of 80 MEQAS questionnaires. Cronbach's alpha coefficients for the scales range from 0.76 to 0.96 (M=0.88).
Inter-Rater	• Reported for a sample of 80 MEQAS questionnaires and rater pairs. Range from 0.60 to 0.93 (M=0.77).
Validity	
Content	• Items were generated based on a comprehensive review of the literature. The MEQAS content was reviewed by content experts and adults with disabilities.
Construct	• Examined through predictions involving different types of activity settings, including formal vs informal; group vs solitary; and active physical, passive recreational, and skill-based activities. The scales discriminated different types of settings and patterns of scale scores confirmed predictions, providing evidence of construct validity.
Criterion	N/A
Utility	
Research Programs	• The MEQAS allows researchers to comprehensively assess qualities and affordances of activity settings and can be used as a fidelity measure for contextual or participation-oriented interventions.
Practice Settings	• Can be used to design and assess environmental qualities of programs for young people.
Strengths	• A psychometrically sound, observer-rated measure of environmental qualities of youth activity settings.
Complexities	• The focus is on a specific activity setting. The MEQAS is not an aggregate of observations of an activity setting over time. Raters can find it difficult to not focus on an individual youth and instead direct attention to the properties/affordances of the environment.

Table 10-11

Self-Reported Experiences of Activity Settings (SEAS)

Source	https://flintbox.com/public/project/25724/
Key References	King et al[65,164]
Purpose	• To capture youth experiences of an activity setting. The measure assesses youth experiences in the following areas: personal growth, psychological engagement, social belonging, meaningful interactions, and choice and control
Type of Client	• Appropriate for youth with at least a Grade 3 level of language comprehension, including youth with different types of disabilities and those without disabilities. A version using picture communication symbols (SEAS-PCS) is available for youth who communicate using augmentative and alternative communication.
Test Format	• 22-item self-report questionnaire
Procedures	• To be given to a youth after participating in a specific activity for at least 15 minutes.
Time Required	• Administration time depends on capabilities of youth. Scoring can be done using SPSS syntax or an Excel file (currently in development).
Standardization	N/A
Reliability	
Test-Retest	• Reported for sample of 8 youth. Range of 0.51 to 0.94 (M = 0.68).
Internal Consistency	• Cronbach's alpha coefficients for the scales range from 0.71 to 0.88
Inter-Rater	N/A
Validity	• Developed from a comprehensive review of various literatures concerning youth experiences of activity settings.
Content	• A panel of experts reviewed the SEAS.
Construct	• The scales discriminated between different types of activity settings and patterns of scale scores confirmed predictions, providing evidence of construct validity.[65] Significant predicted differences were found between formal vs informal and group vs solitary activity settings, with large to medium effect sizes. Significant predicted differences were also found between 4 types of recreation and leisure activities, and as a function of people present (relatives, friends, no one).
Criterion	N/A
Utility	
Research Programs	• The SEAS can be used to gain greater understanding of situation-specific experiences of youth participating in various types of leisure activity settings.
Practice Settings	• Allows service providers to understand a youth's experience of an activity setting, and to modify programs based on young people's experiences.
Strengths	• Can be used with youth with disabilities, even severe disabilities, as well as youth without disabilities.
Complexities	• Items on social interaction are not applicable if youth are doing an activity by themselves with no one else around.

Table 10-12

Additional Play Measures Developed by Occupational Therapists

Name of Measure	My Child's Play (MCP)
Key Reference	Schneider and Rosenblum[59]
Information	MCP is a 50-item parent questionnaire designed to evaluate the play of children ages 3 to 9 years. There are 4 dimensions: (1) Executive Functions (ie, organization, concentration, attention control and persistence, sense of self- control); (2) Interpersonal Relationships and Social Participation; (3) Play choices and Preferences; (4) Opportunities in the Environment.
Name of Measure	The Play Skills Self Report Questionnaire (PSSRQ).
Key Reference	Sturgess[165]
Information	The PSSRQ is a 30-item child self-report of 29 current play skills for children aged 5 to 10 years. Self-perceptions of play skills are assessed in a range of contexts (home, school and community) with different companions and material resources. Available at http://www.playskillsselfreport.com/
Name of Measure	Play Assessment for Group Settings (PAGS)
Key Reference	Lautamo et al[166]
Information	The PAGS is a 38-item, occupation-based instrument for observing and scoring the frequency of specific play behaviors of 2- to 8-year-old children in natural group settings, such as day care. Play performance is conceptualized according to 6 elements: (1) child's spirit; (2) the child's skills; (3) the child's environment, 4) meaningful doing, (5) mindful doing, and (6) expression of mastery.
Name of Measure	Play History
Key Reference	Takata[60]
Information	The Play History provides rich qualitative information about play performance organized according to developmental epochs of play (i.e. sensorimotor, symbolic and simple constructive, dramatic and complex constructive and pre-game, games and recreational). Recent knowledge about the play epochs has not been updated and hence the content validity of some epochs may be in question.[19]

Table 10-13

Measures of Playfulness, Play-Related Affect, and Motivation

Name of Measure	Assessment of Ludic Behaviors (ALB)
Key Reference	Ferland[167]
Information	The ALB is a home-based observation and structured interview conducted with the parent/ principal caregiver. Five dimensions are measured: (1) General Interests; (2) Basic Ludic abilities and actions with regard to objects, space; (3) Ludic interests; (4) Ludic attitude (curiosity, initiative, sense of humor, pleasure, enjoyment of challenge and spontaneity); and (5) Communication.

(continued)

Table 10-13 (continued)

Measures of Playfulness, Play-Related Affect, and Motivation

Name of Measure	Child Behaviors Inventory of Playfulness (CBI)
Key Reference	Rogers et al[168]
Information	The CBI was developed for use with children from preschool to fourth grade to measure a child's internal predisposition to be playful. The 30-item caregiver questionnaire assesses 2 dimensions: (1) Overall playfulness (ie, orientation to a task, intrinsic motivation, nonlinearity; freedom from externally imposed rules, and active involvement during the task); and (2) Externality (ie, behaviors likely to reduce a child's ability to play).
Name of Measure	Children's Playfulness Scale (CPS)
Key Reference	Barnett[169]
Information	The CPS is a 30-item parent- or teacher-completed scale to measure playfulness as a trait characteristic of children from preschool. It was based on Lieberman's[170] model of playfulness with 5 dimensions: (1) Physical spontaneity; (2) Cognitive spontaneity; (3) Social spontaneity; (4) Manifest joy and (5) Sense of humor.
Name of Measure	Adult Playfulness Trait Scale (P-APTS)
Key Reference	Shen et al[72]
Information	The 19-item P-APTS measure playfulness as a personality trait in adults. Dimensions include: Fun belief, initiative, reactivity, uninhibitedness and spontaneity.
Name of Measure	Affect in Play Scale (APS)
Key Reference	Russ[171]
Information	The APS is a psychometrically sound measure that uses a set of 3 blocks and 2 puppets to assess affect and quality of fantasy expressed in play of children aged 6 to 10 years. Two dimensions are assessed: (1) Cognitive (ie, organization, imagination, comfort of play); and (2) Affective (ie, total affect, frequency and variety of positive and negative affect).

Table 10-14

Measures Focusing on Specific Types of Play (eg, Physical Activity, Pretend)

Name of Measure	Interactive Play Scenario
Key Reference	Frahsek et al[172]
Information	The interactive play scenario is used to examine pretend play of children aged 24 to 30 months. A semi-structured play sequence is used to explore various types of pretend play: (1) Self- and doll-directed pretence; (2) Object substitution; (3) Pretence with realistic objects; (4) Self-initiated pretend play; and (5) Understanding that an object has 2 identities.
Name of Measure	Children's Active Play Imagery Questionnaire (CAPIQ)
Key Reference	Cooke et al[173]
Information	The CAPIQ is a 16-item research-oriented instrument developed to measure 3 dimensions of play imagery related to physically active play: (1) Fun; (2) Social; and (3) Capability. The CAPIQ is a self-report tool used to explore children's reasons for participating in physically active play. The questionnaire is suitable for children aged 7 to 14 years.

(continued)

Table 10-14 (continued)

Measures Focusing on Specific Types of Play (eg, Physical Activity, Pretend)

Name of Measure	Westby Play Scale—Revised (WPS-R)
Key Reference	Westby[174]
Information	The WPS-R is an extension of the Westby Symbolic Play Scale originally published in 1980.[175] This checklist measures developmental stages of object play and the emergence of symbolic capacities during 5- to 10-minute free play. There are 13 core categories related to symbol comprehension and expression in play for children aged 9 months to 5 years.
Name of Measure	Penn Interactive Peer Play Scale (PIPPS)
Key Reference	Fantuzzo et al[176]
Information	The PIPPS is used to measure social components of preschooler play. There are 3 dimensions: (1) Play Interaction; (2) Play Disruption; and (3) Play Disconnection. Parent and teacher reports are used to evaluate social competence of preschoolers within concrete, observable contexts.
Name of Measure	Preschool Play Behavior Scale (PPBS)
Key Reference	Coplan and Rubin[126]
Information	This teacher rating scale focuses on the measurement of multiple forms of young children's solitary behavior. The PPBS was designed to assess preschoolers' free play behaviors and is coded using categories developed for Rubin's[177] Play Observation Scale (see Table 10-3).
Name of Measure	Children's Leisure Activities Study Survey (CLASS)
Key Reference	Telford et al[178]
Information	The Children's Leisure Activities Study Survey (CLASS) questionnaire was developed to assess the type, frequency, and duration of physical activity and sedentary behaviors of children. This tool and an adolescent version is available at http://www.acaorn.org.au/streams/activity/tools-validation/index.php
Name of Measure	Physical Activity Time Use Diaries
Key Reference	Lau et al[179]
Information	Traditionally, physical activity diaries in paper format have been used to examine leisure-time activity participation, but Lau and colleagues demonstrated how electronic activity diaries with data entered on smart phones have potential to reduce response burden.

Table 10-15

Play-Based Measures of Child Development

Name of Measure	Transdisciplinary Play-Based Assessment, Second Edition (TPBA-2)
Key Reference	Linder et al[180]
Information	The TPBA-2 uses a collaborative team approach between parents and early childhood service providers to collect information so that a developmental age score and a functionality score can be calculated for each of 4 developmental domains: (1) Cognitive; (2) Communication/language; (3) Motor; and (4) Social-emotional. The age range is 6 months to 6 years.

(continued)

Table 10-15 (continued)

Play-Based Measures of Child Development

Name of Measure	Play in Early Childhood Evaluation System (PIECES)
Key Reference	Kelly-Vance and Ryalls[181]
Information	PIECES is a transdisciplinary measure of cognitive development and social interaction of children under the age of 7. The child is observed while engaged in free play, and the assessment can be conducted in any setting with any set of toys as long as the toy set is large and varied enough to elicit a wide range of behaviors. Forms can be downloaded from: http://lkellyvance.wix.com/plais
Name of Measure	Play Assessment Scale (PAS)
Key Reference	Athanasiou[182]
Information	The Play Assessment Scale (PAS) evaluates play skills of children from 2 to 36 months. This 45-item scale is developmentally sequenced and is organized into 8 age ranges. Children are first observed in spontaneous play followed by a facilitated play session, with play behaviors coded to determine a composite play age.
Name of Measure	Mental Development Scales (MDS)
Key Reference	Wagner and Frost[183]
Information	The MDS is used to measure developmental status of infants and toddlers aged 3 years and younger. Structured, unstructured, and semi-structured play observations are conducted in group settings. There are 6 scales, each with 5 developmental levels: (1) Spontaneous Drawing; (2) Block Play; (3) Object Exploration; (4) Social Responsiveness and Discovery of Selfhood; (5) Communication; and (6) Symbolic Play.
Name of Measure	Developmental Play Assessment (DPA)
Key Reference	Lifter[184]
Information	The DPA is an assessment tool designed to identify developmentally relevant play activities in 15 categories. The DPA-Professional version was initially developed as a research tool for Project Play (https://www.northeastern.edu/projectplay/), and was subsequently found promising for identifying and working with children who have delays in play.

Table 10-16

Leisure Interest Inventories

Name of Measure	Neuropsychiatric Institute Interest Checklist (NPIIC)
Key Reference	Matsutsuyu[56]
Information	The NPIIC includes 80 items reflecting the intensity of a client's interest in 5 categories: ADL, manual skills, cultural/educational, physical sports, and social recreation.
Name of Measure	The Health Enhancement Lifestyle Profile–Screener (HELP-Screener)
Key Reference	Hwang[185]
Information	The HELP-Screener for older adults is a 15-item self-report questionnaire developed from the original 56-item HELP to measure various aspects of health-related lifestyle: (1) Exercise; (2) Diet; (3) Leisure; (4) Productive and Social Activities; (5) Activities of Daily Living (ADLs); (6) Stress Management and Spiritual Participation; and (7) Other Health Promotion and Risk Behaviors

(continued)

Table 10-16 (continued)

Leisure Interest Inventories

Name of Measure	Japanese Interest Checklist for the Elderly (JICE)
Key Reference	Nakamura-Thomas and Yamada[57]
Information	The JICE is a self-report instrument comprising 29 items reflecting activities common to Japanese older people. Participants indicate whether they have strong, casual, or no interest in different activities, such as pleasurable outings, cultural/educational activities, entertainment, nature-related activities and social activities.
Name of Measure	The Leisure Interest Questionnaire (LIQ)
Key Reference	Hansen and Scullard[186]
Information	The LIQ scales contain 250 leisure activities that the individual rates according to his/her level of interest in each pursuit using a 3-point scale (ie, like, indifferent, dislike). These include: (a) Athletic activities (eg, Adventure Sports, Team Sports, and Individual Sports); (b) Artistic activities (eg, Arts & Crafts, Writing & Literature, Cultural Arts, Dancing, and Culinary Pursuits); (c) Social activities (eg, Community Involvement, Socializing, and Partying); and (d) Outdoor activities.
Name of Measure	Change in Activities and Interests Checklist (CAIC)
Key Reference	Adams[187]
Information	The CAIC is a retrospective measure that examines changes in activity preference and involvement reported by older adults. There are 30 items measuring interests and investment in different social and leisure pursuits now, as compared with 10 years ago. There are 4 domains: active social, active instrumental, transcendent attitudes, and passive social/spiritual.
Name of Measure	Nottingham Leisure Questionnaire (NLQ)
Key Reference	Drummond et al[188]
Information	There is a long (38-item) and short (30-item) version of the NLQ that is used in research studies to measure frequency of engaging in specific leisure activities in rehabilitation settings. Additional space is provided at the end of the questionnaire for listing "other" leisure activities.
Name of Measure	Modified NPS Interest Checklist (MNPS)
Key Reference	Nilsson and Fisher[189]
Information	The MPNS has 4 dimensions of leisure: Interest, Performance, Motivation, and Well-being. It was developed from a Scandinavian survey of nondisabled people. Measures of validity and reliability were established. The 20 MNPS items in each dimension (interest, performance, motivation, and well-being) demonstrate uni-dimensionality (internal consistency)
Name of Measure	Pleasant Activities List (PAL)
Key Reference	Dijkstra and Roozen[190]
Information	The 139-item self-report PAL measures frequency and subjective pleasure of the engagement in activities. There are 7 factorially derived subscales: (1) Social Activities; (2) Sensation Seeking Activities; (3) Domestic Activities; (4) Activities on Culture/Science/Travelling; (5) Passive/Relaxing Activities; (6) Sport-related Activities; (7) Activities that involve Intimacy/Personal Attention; and (8) Miscellaneous Activities (MA).
Name of Measure	Leisure Activity Profile (LAP)
Key Reference	Mann and Talty[191]
Information	The 38-item LAP comprises 19 assumed to be associated with alcohol consumption and 19 not associated with alcohol consumption. Respondents rate the frequency and enjoyment of engaging in each activity, presence of social companions and alcohol consumption while engaging in each activity.

Table 10-17

Measures of Leisure Cognitions, Affect, and Motivation

Name of Measure	Leisure Boredom Scale (LBS)
Key Reference	Iso-Ahola and Weissinger[192]
Information	The LBS comprises 16 items measuring respondents' subjective perceptions of leisure. The LBS is scored on a 1- to 5-point Likert scale (1 = strongly disagree to 5 = strongly agree), with higher numbers indicating higher leisure boredom.
Name of Measure	Leisure Experience Battery for Adolescents (LEBA)
Key Reference	Caldwell et al[193]
Information	There are 4 subscales in this battery: boredom, challenge, awareness, and anxiety. No summative leisure experience total score is used. The authors indicated that leisure awareness related back to Iso-Ahola and Weissinger's[192] earlier research on the Leisure Boredom Scale.
Name of Measure	Leisure Diagnostic Battery (LDB)
Key Reference	Witt and Ellis[70]
Information	There are different batteries for different age groups (adolescent, adults and older individuals) with slight changes to item wording for each age group. There is a short (25-item) and long (95-item) version of each scale. The short versions contain items derived from 5 subscales that form Part I of the long version. The short forms are called Perceived Freedom in Leisure Scale – Short Form Version A or B (PFS). The 5 PFS subscales of the long version Part I include: (1) Competence; (2) Control; (3) Depth of Involvement; (4) Leisure Needs; and (5) Playfulness. The total score of the PFS represents a composite measure of perceived freedom in leisure and reflects the notion that helplessness and freedom occupy opposite ends of a continuum. The long version contains additional items to measure barriers to leisure and preferred leisure activities in Parts II and III.
Name of Measure	Personal Projects Analysis for Children (PPA-C)
Key Reference	Poulsen et al[194]
Information	PPA-C is an ipsative, ecologically sensitive tool completed by children aged 10 years and older. There are 2 modules in the child version of the PPA: (1) The child generates a list of personal leisure projects, goals or strivings, and describes where and with whom the project is carried out; and (2) Projects are then rated by the child on motivational and experiential elements.
Name of Measure	California Older Person's Pleasant Experiences Scale (COPPES; Spanish Version)
Key Reference	Rider et al[195]
Information	This measure taps an older person's thought processes about pleasant events in general. A large proportion of events relate to leisure experiences. The manual and scoring system are available online at http://oafc.stanford.edu/coppes.html There are 66 items that measure frequency of pleasant thought and enjoyment across 5 domains: (1) Socializing; (2) Relaxing; (3) Contemplating; (4) Being effective; and (5) Doing.
Name of Measure	Intrinsic Leisure Motivation Scale (ILM)
Key Reference	Weissinger and Bandalos[69]
Information	The ILM is a 24-item scale measuring the extent to which individuals perceive their personal needs are being met through leisure activities. There are 4 subscales: (1) Self-determination; (2) Competence/skill development; (3) Self-commitment; and (4) Challenge/adventure. Based on Self-Determination Theory.

(continued)

Table 10-17 (continued)

Measures of Leisure Cognitions, Affect, and Motivation

Name of Measure	Experience Sampling Methodology (ESM[196])
Key Reference	Chen et al[197]
Information	On a self-report form, participants respond to signals installed on an iPod touch or iPhone to report real-time actions, thoughts, and feelings in every-day settings, over time and across contexts. There is a free iPhone P.I.E.L. Application for iOS devices with accompanying manual that can be accessed at http://ses.library.usyd.edu.au//bitstream/2123/9490/2/PIEL_Survey_App_Manual.pdf
Name of Measure	Recreation Experiences Preference Scales (REP)
Key Reference	Manfredo et al[198]
Information	The REP scales contain 328 items but the entire list has never been used. Respondents rate their level of satisfaction and importance of reasons for participating in leisure using multiple domains: (1) Achievement; (2) Autonomy/Leadership; (3) Risk Taking; (4) Learning; (5) Meeting new people; (6) Being with similar people; (7) Family togetherness; (8) Enjoy nature; (9) Introspection; (10) Creativity; (11) Nostalgia; (12) Physical fitness; (13) Rest; (14) Escape; (15) Social security; (16) Teaching/leadership
Name of Measure	Leisure Competence Measure (LCM)[199,200]
Key Reference	Kloseck et al[199]
Information	The LCM comprises 8 domains: (1) Leisure Awareness; (2) Leisure Attitudes; (3) Leisure skills; (4) Social Appropriateness; (5) Group Interaction Skills; (6) Clinical Participation; (7) Social Contact; (8) Community Participation Has change and gain scores Eight subscales (leisure awareness, leisure attitude, leisure skills, cultural/social behaviors, interpersonal skills, community integration skills, social contact, community participation
Name of Measure	The Leisure Competence Scale (LCS)
Key Reference	Chang[201]
Information	The LCS comprises 6 items related to the perception of older adults regarding their ability to participate in leisure activities. The scale contains 6 5-point items related to older adults' perceived effectiveness of their ability to perform their leisure activities. The higher the scores, the stronger the leisure competence.
Name of Measure	Leisure Self-determination Scale[202] developed as part of a doctoral thesis cited in Craike et al[203]
Key Reference	Coleman and Iso-Ahola[204]
Information	The 24-item LSDS has 5 subscales: (1) Autonomous tendencies (self); (2) Fulfillment of personal values (personal values); (3) Perceived expectations of others (internalized others); (4) Deferment to others ideas and requests (valued others); and (5) Observations of environmental dominance (external control).
Name of Measure	Leisure Attitude Scale-Short Version (LAS-SV)
Key References	Teixeira and Freire[205]; Ragheb and Beard[206]
Information	18-item short version of the original LAS[206] has 3 dimensions: cognitive, affective, and behavioral/preferences. In the 1980s and early 1990s, Ragheb and Beard[206] developed several instruments measuring a range of leisure dimensions (eg, leisure attitude, leisure satisfaction, leisure interests, and leisure motivation) with varying psychometric data available for each measure. There are versions of these scales in several languages. A short version of the LAS has been developed.

(continued)

Table 10-17 (continued)

Measures of Leisure Cognitions, Affect, and Motivation

Name of Measure	Leisure Satisfaction Scale – Short Version (LSS-SV)
Key References	Di Bona[207]; Beard and Ragheb[208]
Information	The 51-item LSS measures the extent that an individual feels his or her needs are met as a result of participation in leisure activities. The LSS consists of 6 scales: (1) Psychological; (2) Educational; (3) Social; (4) Relaxation; (5) Physiological; and (6) Aesthetic on 5-point Likert scales. A short form has been developed.[207]
Name of Measure	Leisure Motivation Scale (LMS)
Key Reference	Beard and Ragheb[209]
Information	The 48-item LMS measures psychological and social reasons for participating in leisure activities on 4 12-item subscales: (1) Intellectual, (2) Social, (3) Competence-Mastery, and (4) Stimulus-Avoidance.
Name of Measure	Motivation for Leisure
Key Reference	Beiswenger and Grolnick[210]
Information	Motivation for Leisure[210] measures 4 types of motivation based on SDT: (1) Extrinsic motivation, or engaging in activities due to contingencies such as rewards or punishments; (2) Introjected motivation, related to the behavior of avoiding emotions perceived as negative such as guilt or anxiety; (3) Identified motivation, or engagement because of personal values or importance of activity; and (4) intrinsic motivation, doing activity for fun or pleasure.
Name of Measure	The Leisure Coping Scales (LCS)
Key Reference	Iwasaki and Mannell[211]
Information	Two versions of the LCS measure ways in which leisure helps people cope with stress. The Leisure Coping Belief Scale (LCBS) measures individuals' dispositional and relatively stable belief about gaining stress-coping benefits through leisure involvements, whereas the Leisure Coping Strategy Scale (LCSS) measures the extent to which leisure involvements help people cope with stress at the time of facing a stressful event in a specific situation.
Name of Measure	Leisure Meanings Gained Scale (LMGS)[212]
Key Reference	Porter et al[213]
Information	24 items with 5 dimensions: (1) Connection/belonging; (2) Identity; (3) Freedom/autonomy; (4) Power/control; and (5) Competence/mastery. This scale asks a person to list his or her most favorite leisure activities, and then rate the personal meaning of activity participation.
Name of Measure	Leisure Meanings Inventory (LMI)
Key Reference	Schulz and Watkins[214]
Information	The LMI comprises 27 items across 4 dimensions to measure subjective reasons for engaging in leisure: (1) Passing Time; (2) Exercising Choice; (3) Escaping Pressure; (4) Achieving Fulfillment.
Name of Measure	Modified Involvement Scale (MIS)
Key Reference	Kyle et al[215]
Information	The MIS is a child/adolescent self-report scale measuring 5 dimensions of involvement: (1) Attraction; (2) Centrality; (3) Social Bonding; (4) Identity Affirmation; and (5) Identity Expression. There is an adapted version for parent proxy report when child/adolescent self-report is not possible.

(continued)

Table 10-17 (continued)

Measures of Leisure Cognitions, Affect, and Motivation

Name of Measure	Leisure Time Satisfaction (LTS)
Key Reference	Stevens et al[216]
Information	The LTS was developed to address a need to understand the impact of caregiving on a caregiver's leisure participation. The 6-item LTS measures caregivers' satisfaction with their leisure experiences.
Name of Measure	Youth Outcomes Battery (YOB)
Key Reference	Sibthorp et al[79]
Information	There are 11 YOB constructs that have been used to measure the outcomes of youth camp experiences in relation to: Family Citizenship Behavior, Perceived Competence, Responsibility, Independence, Team Work, Problem-Solving Competence, Affinity for Nature, Affinity for Exploration, Camp Connectedness, Family Support, Spiritual Well-being.
Name of Measure	Self-Reported Experiences of Activity Settings (SEAS)
Key Reference	King et al[65]
Information	The SEAS measures key aspects of the experiences of youth with or without physical impairments in leisure activity settings at home and in the community. Experiences across activity settings (such as sports/active physical activities versus creative arts programs), as well as changes over time can be evaluated.

Table 10-18

Measures of Participation and Health-Related Lifestyle Behavior With Play/Leisure Subscales

Name of Measure	The Health Enhancement Lifestyle Profile (HELP)
Key Reference	Hwang[217]
Information	The HELP[217] is a self-report questionnaire about health-related lifestyle behaviors for older adults. There are 7 subscales: (1) Exercise; (2) Diet; (3) Work, Education, and Social Participation; (4) Leisure; (5) Activities of Daily Living; (6) Psychological Wellness and Spiritual Participation; and (7) Other Health Promotion and Risk Behaviors.
Name of Measure	Health Promoting Activities Scale to Measure Leisure Participation (HPAS)
Key Reference	Bourke-Taylor et al[85]
Information	The HPAS provides occupational therapists with a brief tool to measure the frequency with which mothers participate in self-selected leisure activities that promote health and well-being. The use of this instrument reminds occupational therapists to explore caregiver healthy leisure as well as child's leisure. Assists mothers in setting goals in relation to HPAS items and engaging in healthy lifestyle redesign of leisure pursuits.
Name of Measure	Measure of Environmental Qualities of Activity Settings (MEQAS)
Key Reference	King et al[64]
Information	The MEQAS provides a structured framework to observe real contexts in relation to activity participation. The 32 items are organized in 6 scales: (1) Opportunities for Social Activities; (2) Opportunities for Physical Activities; (3) Pleasant Physical Environment; (4) Opportunities for Choice; (5) Opportunities for Personal Growth; and (6) Opportunities to Interact with Adults.

(continued)

Table 10-18 (continued)

Measures of Participation and Health-Related Lifestyle Behavior With Play/Leisure Subscales

Name of Measure	Leisure Support Network Assessment Scale (LSNAS)
Key Reference	Iwasaki[218]
Information	The LSNAS assesses: (a) Size of support network; (b) Frequency, closeness, balance, complexity and nature of relationships; and (c) Levels of satisfaction with different aspects of social support (ie, emotional support, socializing, practical assistance, financial assistance, and advice/guide).
Name of Measure	Assistance to Participate Scale (APS)
Key Reference	Bourke-Taylor et al[219]
Information	The APS measures social rather than physical environmental supports. The amount of assistance needed by caregivers to enable child participation in play/leisure pursuits is evaluated in 8 scenarios (eg, watching TV, sharing time with a friend at home, and attending an organized recreational club) from the family's perspective.
Name of Measure	Participation and Environment Measure for Children and Youth (PEM-CY)
Key Reference	Khetani et al[220]
Information	The PEM-CY is a 25-item parent/caregiver report measuring a child's participation in different activities at home, school, and within the community. For each item on the PEM-CY, the caregiver reports: (1) Number of activities done at home; (2) Frequency of activities; (3) Level of involvement; (4) Number of activities in which change is desired; (5) Number of environmental supports; and (6) Number of environmental barriers.
Name of Measure	Craig Hospital Inventory of Environmental Factors (CHIEF)
Key Reference	Whiteneck et al[221]
Information	The CHIEF rates frequency and impact of 25 environmental elements that impede the participation of persons aged 16 to 95 years across 5 domains: (1) Policies; (2) Physical and Structural; (3) Work and School; (4) Attitudes and Support; (5) Services and Assistance.
Name of Measure	Your Ideas about Participation and Environment (YIPE)
Key Reference	Cheeseman et al[222]
Information	The YIPE is an 83-item self-report instrument that measures environmental facilitators and barriers to participation. The YIPE can help an individual set person-centered goals and identify supports. This tool is in the early stages of development and limited psychometric data is available.
Name of Measure	Assessment of Life Habits for Children (LIFE-H)
Key Reference	Noreau et al[223]
Information	The LIFE-H measures quality of social participation in 11 life habit categories, including leisure, in interviews with parents of children with disabilities aged 5 to 13 years. Level of difficulty and type of assistance required (technical assistance, physical arrangements, human help) is evaluated. There is a short and long version.

(continued)

Table 10-18 (continued)

MEASURES OF PARTICIPATION AND HEALTH-RELATED LIFESTYLE BEHAVIOR WITH PLAY/LEISURE SUBSCALES

Name of Measure	Child Participation Questionnaire (CPQ)
Key Reference	Rosenberg et al[224]
Information	The CPQ is a promising parent-completed questionnaire for assessing child participation across 6 occupational domains: Activities of Daily Living (eg, dressing), Instrumental Activities of Daily Living (eg, setting the table), Play (eg, imaginative play, computer games), Leisure (eg, bicycle riding, listening to a story), Social participation (eg, visiting a friend), and Education (eg, drawing and graphomotor exercises in preschool classroom). Parents rate 5 dimensions of participation: Intensity, Diversity, Independence, Child Enjoyment, and Parental Satisfaction.
Name of Measure	Assessment of Preschool Children's Participation (APCP)
Key Reference	Law et al[225]
Information	The APCP is a 45-item, parent-completed measure of frequency and diversity of a preschool child's participation in play, skill development, active physical recreation, and social activities during the past 4 months. The APCP used the same format as the CAPE and included many similar (n=15) or identical items (n=23) to the CAPE. Unlike the CAPE, the APCP does not collect information about where and with whom activities take place, and a child's rating of enjoyment.
Name of Measure	Lifestyle Assessment Questionnaire (LAQ)
Key Reference	Jessen et al[226]
Information	The LAQ is another parent-completed measure of a child's participation in 5 domains: communication, mobility, self-care, domestic Life, social and civic activities, and family impact for children.
Name of Measure	Child and Adolescent Scale of Participation (CASP; Bedell, 2009)
Key Reference	McDougall et al[227]
Information	The parent report version of the CASP measures children's extent of participation and restrictions in home, school and community life situations and activities compared with same age peers. The youth report version (11-17) measures activity and participation across all 9 ICF/ICF-CY chapters. They are very brief, relatively easy to complete tools that offers good global coverage of activity and participation.
Name of Measure	Home Observation for Measurement of the Environment (HOME)
Key Reference	Bradley et al[228]
Information	The HOME is a checklist comprising 45 items divided into 6 subscales that is completed following observation and interviews with the parent/caregiver. The different versions of the HOME can be used over a wide age span (birth to 15 years).

REFERENCES

1. Hammell K. Self-care, productivity, and leisure, or dimensions of occupational experience? Rethinking occupational "categories." *Can J Occup Ther.* 2009;76(2):107-114.
2. McColl MA, Law M. Interventions affecting self-care, productivity, and leisure among adults: a scoping review. *OTJR.* 2013;33(2):110-119.
3. Kuhanek HM, Tanta KJ, Coombs AK, Pannone H. A survey of pediatric occupational therapists' use of play. *J Occup Ther.* 2013;6(3):213-227.
4. Robertson T, Symonds M, Muehlenbein M, Robertson, C. Health, wellness and quality of life. In: Kassing G, ed. *Introduction to Recreation and Leisure.* 2nd ed. Champaign, IL: Human Kinetics; 2013.
5. Office of the United Nations High Commissioner for Human Rights. Convention on the Rights of the Child. General Assembly Resolution 44/25 of 20 November 1989. http://www.ohchr.org/en/professionalinterest/pages/crc.aspx. Accessed October 2, 2014.
6. Howell V. Leisure and play. In: Brown C, Stoffell VC, eds. *Occupational Therapy in Mental Health: A Vision for Participation.* Philadelphia, PA: F. A. Davis Co; 2011.

7. Poulsen AA, Ziviani J. Health-enhancing physical activity: factors influencing engagement patterns in children. *Aust Occup Ther J.* 2004;51:69-79.
8. Haracz K, Ryan S, Hazelton M, James, C. Occupational therapy and obesity: an integrative literature review. *Aust Occup Ther J.* 2013;60(5):356–365.
9. Bundy AC, Naughton G, Tranter P, et al. The Sydney playground project: popping the bubblewrap - unleashing the power of play: a cluster randomized controlled trial of a primary school playground-based intervention aiming to increase children's physical activity and social skills. *BMC Public Health.* 2011;11:680.
10. Jarus T, Anaby D, Bart O, Engel-Yeger B, Law M. Childhood participation in after-school activities: what is to be expected? *Br J Occup Ther.* 2010;73(8):344-350.
11. Parnell T, Wilding C. Where can an occupation-focused philosophy take occupational therapy? *Aust Occup Ther J.* 2010;57(5):345–348.
12. Berntsson LT, Ringsberg KC. Health and relationships with leisure time activities in Swedish children aged 2-17 years. *Scand J Caring Sci.* 2014;28(3):552-563.
13. Passmore A. The occupation of leisure: three typologies and their influence on mental health in adolescence. *OTJR.* 2003;23(2):76-83.
14. Rubin KH, Fein GG, Vandenberg B. Play. In: Mussen PH, ed. *Handbook of Child Psychology.* Vol. 4. New York: John Wiley and Sons; 1983.
15. Leitner MJ, Leitner SF. *Leisure in Later Life.* New York: The Haworth Press; 2012.
16. Deci EL, Moller AC. The concept of competence: a starting place for understanding intrinsic motivation and self-determined extrinsic motivation. In: Elliot AJ, Dweck CS, eds. *Handbook of Competence and Motivation.* New York: The Guilford Press; 2005:579-597.
17. King P, Howard J. Children's perceptions of choice in relation to their play at home, in the school playground and at The Out-of-School Club. *Children Soc.* 2014;28(2):116-127.
18. Salen K, Zimmerman E. *The Game Design Reader: A Rules of Play Anthology.* Cambridge, MA: The MIT Press; 2006.
19. Bundy AC. Measuring play performance. In: Baum C, Dunn W, Law M, eds. *Measuring Occupational Performance.* Thorofare, NJ: SLACK Incorporated; 2005:129-153.
20. Lifter K, Foster-Sanda S, Arzamarski C, Briesch J, McClure E. Overview of play: its uses and importance in early intervention/early childhood. *Infants & Young Children.* 2011;24(3):225-245.
21. Stagnitti K, Cooper R. *Play as Therapy: Assessment and Therapeutic Interventions.* Philadelphia: Jessica Kingsley Publishers; 2009.
22. Seligman MEP. *Authentic Happiness: Using the New Positive Psychology to Realize Your Potential for Lasting Fulfillment.* New York: Free Press; 2002.
23. Veal AJ. *The Elusive Leisure Society.* 3rd ed. School of Leisure, Sport and Tourism Working Paper 9. Sydney: University of Technology; 2009.
24. Deci EL, Ryan RM. The "what" and the "why" of goal pursuits: human needs and the self-determination of behavior. *Psychological Inquiry.* 2000;11(4):227-268.
25. Poulsen AA, Rodger S, Ziviani J. Understanding children's motivation from a self-determination theoretical perspective: implications for practice. *Aust Occup Ther J.* 2006;53(2):78-86.
26. Bundy A. Play and playfulness: what to look for. In: Parham LD, Fazio LS, eds. *Play In Occupational Therapy for Children.* St. Louis, MO: Mosby; 1997:52-66.
27. Vallerand RJ, Ratelle CF. Intrinsic and extrinsic motivation: a hierarchical model. In: Deci EL, Ryan RM, eds. *The Motivation and Self-determination of Behavior: Theoretical and Applied Issues.* Rochester, NY: University of Rochester Press; 2002.
28. Engeser S. *Advances in Flow Research.* New York, NY: Springer; 2012.
29. Csikszentmihalyi M. *Flow: The Classic Work on How to Achieve Happiness.* London, UK: Rider; 2002.
30. Winnicott DW. *Playing and Reality.* New York: Basic Books; 1971.
31. Parham LD. Play and occupational therapy. In: Parham LD, Fazio LS, eds. *Play in Occupational Therapy for Children.* 2nd ed. St. Louis: Mosby; 2008:3-39.
32. Couch K, Dietz J, Kanny E. The role of play in pediatric occupational therapy. *Am J Occup Ther.* 1998;52(2):111-117.
33. Knox SH. A play scale. In: Reilly M, ed. *Play as Exploratory Learning: Studies of Curiosity Behavior.* Beverly Hills, CA: Sage Publications; 1974:247-266.
34. Bundy A. *Test of Playfulness (ToP).* Version 4.0. Sydney: University of Sydney; 2004.
35. Howard L. A survey of pediatric occupational therapists in the United Kingdom. *Occup Ther Int.* 2002;9(4):326-343.
36. Saleh MN, Komer-Bitensky N, Snider L, et al. Actual vs best practices for young children with cerebral palsy: a survey of pediatric occupational therapists and physical therapists in Quebec, Canada. *Dev Neurorehabil.* 2008;11(1):60-80.
37. World Health Organization. *International Classification of Functioning, Disability and Health.* Geneva: WHO; 2001.
38. World Health Organization. *International Classification of Functioning, Disability and Health: Version for Children and Youth.* Geneva: WHO; 2007.
39. Burtner PA, McMain MP, Crowe TK. Survey of occupational therapy practitioners in southwestern schools: assessments used and preparation of students for school-based practice. *Phys Occup Ther Pediatr.* 2002;22(1):25-39.
40. Adolfsson M, Malmqvist J, Pless M, Granuld M. Identifying child functioning from an ICF-CY perspective: everyday life situations explored in measures of participation. *Disabil Rehabil.* 2011;33(13-14):1230-1244.
41. Chien C-W, Rodger S, Copley J, Skorka K. Comparative content review of children's participation measures using the International Classification of Functioning, Disability and Health-Children and Youth. *Arch Phys Med Rehab.* 2014;95(1):141-152.
42. Shikako-Thomas K, Dahan-Oliel N, Shevell M, et al. Play and be happy? Leisure participation and quality of life among school aged children with cerebral palsy. *Int J Pediatr.* 2012;2012:387280.
43. Law M, Cooper B, Strong S, Stewart D, Rigby P, Letts, L. The Person-Environment-Occupation Model: a transactive approach to occupational performance. *Can J Occup Ther.* 1996;63(1):9-23.

44. Iwasaki Y. Leisure and quality of life in an international and multicultural context: what are major pathways linking leisure to quality of life? *Social Indicators Research.* 2007;82(2): 233-264.
45. McKinstry C, Fortune T. Realising our social and occupational value: could a graduate over-supply push occupational therapy in the right direction? *Aust Occup Ther J.* 2014;61(4):284-286.
46. Poulsen AA, Bush R, Tirendi J, et al. Research around practice partnerships: an example of building partnerships to address overweight and obesity in children. *Aust J Primary Health.* 2009;15(4):285-293.
47. Hutchison P, Lord J. Community-based research and leisure scholarship: a discernment process. *Leisure/Loisir.* 2012;36(1):65-83.
48. Mitchell EJ, Veitch C, Passey M. Efficacy of leisure intervention groups in rehabilitation of people with an acquired brain injury. *Disabil Rehabil.* 2014;36(17):1474-1482.
49. Connolly K, Law M, MacGuire B. Measuring leisure performance. In: Baum C, Dunn W, Law M, eds. *Measuring Occupational Performance.* Thorofare, NJ: SLACK Incorporated; 2005:249-272.
50. Law M, Dunbar SB. Person-Environment-Occupation Model. In: Dunbar SB, ed. *Occupational Therapy Models for Intervention with Children and Families.* Thorofare, NJ: SLACK Incorporated; 2007.
51. Poulsen AA, Ziviani J, Cuskelly M. Understanding motivation in the context of engaging children in therapy. In: Ziviani J, Poulsen AA, Cuskelly M, eds. *The Art and Science of Motivation: A Therapist's Guide to Working with Children.* London, UK: Jessica Kingsley Publications; 2013.
52. Park S, Byers-Connon S. Promoting engagement in leisure and social participation. In: Early MB, ed. *Physical Dysfunction Practice Skills for the Occupational Therapy Assistant.* 3rd ed. St. Louis, MO: Mosby Elsevier; 2013.
53. Majnemer A. Promoting participation in leisure activities: expanding role for pediatric therapists. *Phys Occup Ther Pediatr.* 2009;29(1):1-5.
54. Kuhanek HM, Spitzer SL, Miller E. *Activity Analysis, Creativity and Playfulness in Pediatric Occupational Therapy: Making Play Just Right.* Sudbury, MA: Jones & Bartlett Publ; 2010.
55. Söderback I, Hammarlund C. A leisure-time frame of reference based on a literature analysis. *Occup Ther Health Care.* 1993;8(4):105-133.
56. Matsutsuyu JS. The Interest Checklist. *Am J Occup Ther.* 1969;23(4):323-328.
57. Nakamura-Thomas H, Yamada T. A factor analytic study of the Japanese Interest Checklist for the Elderly. *Br J Occup Ther.* 2011;74(2):86-91.
58. Burke JP, Schaaf RC, Hall TBL. Family narratives and play assessment. In: Parham LD, Fazio LS, eds. *Play in Occupational Therapy for Children.* 2nd ed. St Louis, MO: Mosby Elsevier; 2008:195-215.
59. Schneider E, Rosenblum S. Development, reliability, and validity of the My Child's Play (MCP) questionnaire. *Am J Occup Ther.* 2014;268(3):277-285.
60. Takata N. Play as a prescription. In: Reilly M, ed. *Play as Exploratory Learning: Studies in Curiosity Behavior.* Beverly Hills, CA: Sage Publishing; 1974:209-246.
61. Bazyk S. *Promoting Mental Health and Social Participation in Children and Youth: An AOTA Self-Paced Clinical Course.* Bethesda, MD: American Occupational Therapy Association Press; 2011.
62. Hilton CL, Goloff SE, Altaras O, Josman N. Review of instrument development and testing studies for children and youth. *Am J Occup Ther.* 2013;67(3):30-54.
63. King G, Rigby P, Batorwicz B. Conceptualizing participation in context for children and youth with disabilities: an activity setting perspective. *Disabil Rehabil.* 2013;35(18):1578–1585.
64. King G, Rigby P, Batorowicz B, et al. Development of a direct observation Measure of Environmental Qualities of Activity Settings. *Developmental Medicine & Child Neurolology.* 2014;56(8):763-769.
65. King G, Batorowicz B, Rigby P, McMain-Klein M, Thompson L, Pinto, M. Development of a measure to assess youth Self-reported Experiences of Activity Settings (SEAS). *International Journal of Disability, Development and Education.* 2014;61(1):44-66.
66. Gibson BE, King G, Kushki A, et al. A multi-method approach to studying activity setting participation: integrating standardized questionnaires, qualitative methods and physiological measures. *Disabil Rehabil.* 2013;36(19):1652-1660.
67. Bradley RH, Caldwell BM, Corwyn RF. The Child Care HOME Inventories: assessing the quality of family child care homes. *Early Child Res Q.* 2003;18(3):294-309.
68. Seibre SJ, Jago R, Fox KR, Edwards MJ, Thompson JL. Testing a self-determination theory model of children's physical activity motivation: a cross-sectional study. *Int J Behav Nutr Phys Act.* 2013;10:111.
69. Weissinger E, Bandalos D. Development, reliability and validity of a scale to measure intrinsic motivation in leisure. *Journal of Leisure Research.* 1995;27(4):379-400.
70. Witt P, Ellis, G. The Leisure Diagnostic Battery User's Manual. State College, PA: Venture Publishing; 1989.
71. Weiner B, Frieze I, Kukla A, Reed L, Rest S, Rosenbaum R. *Perceiving the Causes of Success and Failure.* Morristown, NJ: General Learning Press; 1971.
72. Shen XS, Chick G, Zinn H. Playfulness in adulthood as a personality trait: a reconceptualization and a new measurement. *Journal of Leisure Research.* 2014;46(1):58-83.
73. Hektner JM, Schmidt JA, Csikszentmihalyi M. *Experience Sampling Method: Measuring the Quality of Everyday Life.* Thousand Oaks, CA: Sage; 2007.
74. Rigby P, Huggins L. Enabling young children to play by creating supportive environments. In: Letts L, Stewart D, eds. *Using Environments to Enable Occupational Performance.* Thorofare, NJ: SLACK Incorporated; 2003:17-31.
75. Doucet BM, Gutman SA. From the Desk of the Editor and Associate Editor—Quantifying function: the rest of the measurement story. *Am J Occup Ther.* 2013;67(1):7-9.
76. Soref B, Ratzon NZ, Rosenberg L, Leitner Y, Jarus T, Bart O. Personal and environmental pathways to participation in young children with and without mild motor disabilities. *Child: Care, Health & Development.* 2011;38(4):561–571.
77. Dwyer G, Baur L, Higgs J, Hardy L. Promoting children's health and well-being: broadening the therapy perspective. *Phys Occup Ther Pediatr.* 2009;29(1):27-43.

78. Funnell S. Developing and using a program theory matrix for scheme evaluation and performance monitoring. In: Rogers P, Hacsi T, Petrosino A, Huebner A, eds. *Program Theory in Evaluation: Challenges and Opportunities, New Directions for Evaluation.* San Francisco, CA: Jossey-Bass Publishers; 2000:91-101.
79. Sibthorp J, Bialeschki MD, Morgan C, Browne L. Validating, norming, and utility of a Youth Outcomes Battery for recreation programs and camps. *Journal of Leisure Research.* 2013;45(4):514-536.
80. Fielden SJ, Rusch ML, Masinda MT, Sands J, Frankish J, Evoy B. Key considerations for logic model development in research partnerships: a Canadian case study. *Eval Program Plann.* 2007;30(2):115-124.
81. Sonnentag S. Psychological detachment from work during leisure time: the benefits of mentally disengaging from work. *Current Directions in Psychological Science.* 2012;21(2): 114-118.
82. Poulsen AA. Avoiding burnout and promoting work engagement: coaching as a resource for occupational therapists. In Pentland W, Heinz A, Gash J, Isaacs-Young J, eds. *Coaching in Occupational Therapy Practice.* (in press)
83. Tsai Y-C, Liu C-H. Factors and symptoms associated with work stress and health-promoting lifestyles among hospital staff: a pilot study in Taiwan. *BMC Health Services Research.* 2012;12:199.
84. Stark MA, Hoekstra T, Hazel DL, Barton B. Caring for self and others: increasing health care students' healthy behaviors. *Work.* 2012;42(3):393-401.
85. Bourke-Taylor H, Law M, Howie L, Pallant JF. Initial development of the health promoting activities scale to measure the leisure participation of mothers of children with disabilities. *Am J Occup Ther.* 2012;66(1):e1-e10.
86. Ito E, Walker GJ, Liang H. A systematic review of non-western and cross-cultural/national leisure research. *J Leisure Res.* 2014;46(2):226-239.
87. Zaborakis A, Zemaitiene N, Borup I, Kuntsch E, Moreno C. Family joint activities in a cross-national perspective. *BMC Public Health.* 2007;7:94.
88. Beukelman DR, Mirenda P, eds. *Augmentative and Alternative Communication: Supporting Children and Adults with Complex Communication Needs.* 3rd ed. Baltimore, MD: Paul H.Brookes Publishing Co; 2013.
89. Stagnitti K. *Child-Initiated Pretend Play Assessment (ChIPPA): Manual and Kit.* Melbourne, Australia: Co-ordinates Publications; 2007.
90. Stagnitti K, Rodger S, Clarke J. Determining gender-neutral toys for play assessment with preschool children. *Aust Occup Ther J.* 1997;44(3):119-131.
91. Stagnitti K, Unsworth CA, Rodger S. Development of an assessment to identify play behaviours that discriminate between the play of typical preschoolers and preschoolers with pre-academic problems. *Can J Occup Ther.* 2000;67(5):291-303.
92. Stagnitti K, Unsworth C. The test-retest reliability of the Child-Initiated Pretend Play Assessment. *Am J Occup Ther.* 2004;58(1):93-99.
93. Uren N, Stagnitti K. Pretend play, social competence and learning in preschool children. *Aust Occup Ther J.* 2009;56(1):33-40.
94. McAloney K, Stagnitti K. Pretend play and social play: the concurrent validity of the Child-Initiated Pretend Play Assessment. *Int J Play Therapy.* 2009;18(2):99-113.
95. Dender A, Stagnitti K. Development of the indigenous Child-Initiated Play Assessment: selection of play materials and administration. *Aust Occup Ther J.* 2011:58(1):34-42.
96. Pfeifer LI, Queiroz MA, Santos JLF, Stagnitti K. Cross-cultural adaptation and reliability of the Child-Initiated Play Assessment (ChIPPA). *Can J Occup Ther.* 2011;78(3):187-195.
97. Pfeifer L, Pacciulio AM, Abrão dos Santos C, Licio dos Santos J, Stagnitti K. Pretend play of children with cerebral palsy. *Phys Occup Ther Pediatr.* 2011;31(4):390-402.
98. Fink N, Stagnitti K, Galvin J. Pretend play of children with acquired brain injury: an exploratory study. *Dev Neurorehabil.* 2012;15(5):336-342.
99. Stagnitti K, Lewis F. Quality of preschool children's pretend play and subsequent development of semantic organization and narrative re-telling skills. *Int J Speech Lang Pathol.* 2015;17(2):148-158.
100. Stagnitti K. Pretend play assessment. In: Stagnitti K, Cooper R, eds. *Play as Therapy: Assessment and Therapeutic Interventions.* London: Jessica Kingsley Publishers; 2009:87-101.
101. Reynolds E, Stagnitti K, Kidd E. Play, language and social skills of children aged 4 to 6 years attending a play based curriculum school and a traditionally structured classroom curriculum school in low socio-economic areas. *Aust J Early Childhood.* 2011;36(4):120-130.
102. O'Connor C, Stagnitti K. Play, behaviour, language and social skills: the comparison of a play and a non-play intervention within a specialist school setting. *Res Dev Disabil.* 2011;32(3):1205-1211.
103. Stagnitti K. The use of psychometric play-based assessment to inform research-supported treatment of children with autism. In: Green E, Myrick A, eds. *Play Therapy with Vulnerable Populations: No Child Forgotten.* Washington DC: Rowman & Littlefield Publishers; 2014.
104. Swindells D, Stagnitti K. Pretend play and parents' view of social competence: the construct validity of the Child-Initiated Pretend Play Assessment. *Aust Occ Ther J.* 2006:53(4):314-324.
105. Stagnitti K. *The Development of a Child-Initiated Assessment of Pretend Play. Volumes 1 & 2.* Unpublished Thesis. Melbourne, Australia: LaTrobe Uni; 2002.
106. Knox S. Development and current use of the Revised Knox Preschool Play Scale. In: Parham LD, Fazio LS, eds. *Play in Occupational Therapy for Children.* 2nd ed. St Louis: Mosby Elsevier; 2008:55-70.
107. Bledsoe NP, Shepherd J. A study of reliability and validity of a Preschool Play Scale. *Am J Occup Ther.* 1982;36(12):783-788.
108. Harrison H, Kielhofner G. Examining the reliability and validity of the Preschool Play Scale with handicapped children. *Am J Occup Ther.* 1986;40(3):167-173.
109. Knox S. Development and current use of the Knox Preschool Play Scale. In: Parham LD, Fazio LS, eds. *Play in Occupational Therapy for Children.* St. Louis: Mosby; 1997:35-51.
110. Jankovich M, Mullen J, Rinear E, Tanta K, Deitz J. Revised Knox Preschool Play Scale: Inter-rater agreement and construct validity. *Am J Occup Ther.* 2008;62(2):221-227.

111. Lee SC, Hinojosa J. Interrater reliability and concurrent validity of the Preschool Play Scale with preschool children with Autism Spectrum Disorders. *J Occup Ther, Schools, Early Intervention.* 2010:3(2):154-167.
112. Pacciulo AM, Pfeifer LI, Santos JLF. Preliminary reliability and repeatability of the Brazilian version of the Revised Knox Preschool Play Scale. *Occup Ther Int.* 2010;17(2):74-80.
113. Kennedy-Behr A, Rodger S, Mickan S. A comparison of the play skills of preschool children with and without developmental coordinator disorder. *OTJR.* 2013;33(4):198-208.
114. Lee S. Reliability and validity of the Preschool Play Scale (revised) of Preschool Children With Autism. Paper presented at the annual conference of the AOTA; St. Louis, MO; April 23, 2007.
115. Fallon J. An exploratory study of the free play of children with intellectual disabilities Unpublished Thesis. Dublin, Ireland: Trinity College; 2006.
116. Restall G, Magill-Evans J. Play and preschool children with autism. *Am J Occup Ther.* 1994;48(2):113-120.
117. Howard A. Developmental play ages of physically abused and non-abused children. *Am J Occup Ther.* 1986;40(10):691-695.
118. Bundy A. A comparison of the play skills of normal boys with sensory integrative dysfunction. *Occup Ther J Res.* 1989;9(2):84-100.
119. Morrison C, Bundy A, Fisher A. The contribution of motor skills and playfulness to the play performance of preschoolers. *Am J Occup Ther.* 1991;45(8):687-694.
120. Sparrow S, Balla D, Cicchetti D. *Vineland Adaptive Behavior Scales.* Circle Pines, MN: American Guidance Service; 1984.
121. Hulme I, Lunzer EA. Play, language and reasoning in subnormal children. *J Child Psychol Psychiat.* 1986;7(2):107-123.
122. Parten M. Social play among pre-school children. *J Abn Soc Psychol.* 1933;28(2):136-147.
123. Tanta K. The effect of peer-play level on the behavior of preschool children with delayed play skills. Unpublished Doctoral Dissertation. Seattle, WA: University of Washington; 2002.
124. Rubin KH. *The Play Observation Scale (POS).* College Park, MD: University of Maryland; 2001. http://www.rubin-lab.umd.edu/CodingSchemes/POS%20Coding%20Scheme%202001.pdf
125. Bar-Haim Y, Bart O. Motor function and social par¬ticipation in kindergarten children. *Social Devel.* 2006;15(2):296-310.
126. Coplan RJ, Rubin KH. Exploring and assessing non-social play in the preschool: the development and validation of the Preschool Play Behavior Scale. *Social Devel.* 1998;7(1):72-91.
127. Degnan KA, Henderson HA, Fox NA, Rubin KH. Predicting social wariness in middle childhood: the moderating roles of child care history, maternal personality and maternal behavior. *Social Devel.* 2008;17(3):471-487.
128. Rubin KH, Krasnor LR. Changes in the play behaviors of preschoolers: a short-term longitudinal investigation. *Can J Behav Sci.* 1980;12(3):278-282.
129. Piaget J. *Play, Dreams and Imitation in Childhood.* New York, NY: Norton; 1962.
130. Rosenblum S, Sachs D, Schreuer N. Reliability and validity of the Children's Leisure Assessment Scale. *Am J Occup Ther.* 2010;64(4):633-641.
131. Schreuer N, Sachs D, Rosenblum S. Participation in leisure activities: differences between children with and without physical disabilities. *Res Dev Disabil.* 2014;35(1):223-233.
132. Skard G, Bundy AC. The Test of Playfulness. In: Parham LD, Fazio LS, eds. *Play in Occupational Therapy for Children.* 2nd ed. St. Louis, MO: Mosby; 2008:71-93.
133. Bundy AC, Luckett T, Naughton GA, et al. Playful interactions: occupational therapy for all children on the school playground. *Am J Occup Ther.* 2008;62(5):522-527.
134. Brentnall AC, Bundy AC, Kay FCS. The effect of the length of observation on Test of Playfulness Scores. *OTJR.* 2008;28(3):133-140.
135. Bundy AC, Nelson L, Metzger M, Bingaman K. Reliability and validity of a test of playfulness. *OTJR.* 2001;21(4):276-292.
136. Chang H-J, Chiarello LA, Palisano RJ, et al. The determinants of self-determined behaviors of young children with cerebral palsy. *Res Dev Disabil.* 2014;35(1):99-109.
137. Cordier R, Bundy AC, Hocking C, Einfeld S. Playing with a child with ADHD: a focus on the playmates. *Scand J Occup Ther.* 2010;17(3):191-199.
138. Cordier R, Bundy AC, Hocking C, Einfeld S. Empathy in the play of children with ADHD. *OTJR.* 2010;30(3):122-132.
139. Cordier R, Bundy A, Hocking C, Einfeld S. Comparison of the play of children with attention deficit hyperactivity disorder by subtypes. *Aust Occup Ther J.* 2010;57(2):137-145.
140. Okimoto AM, Bundy AC, Hanzlik JR. Playfulness in children with and without disability: measurement and intervention. *Am J Occup Ther.* 2000;54(1):73-82.
141. Wilkes S, Cordier R, Bundy A, Docking K, Munro N. A play-based intervention for children with ADHD: a pilot study. *Aust Occup Ther J.* 2011;58(4):231-240.
142. Wilkes-Gillan S, Bundy A, Cordier R, Lincoln M. Child outcomes of a pilot parent-delivered intervention for improving the social play skills of children with ADHD and their playmates. *Dev Neurorehabil.* 2015 Aug 24:1-8 [Epub ahead of print].
143. Wilkes-Gillan S, Bundy A, Cordier R, Lincoln M. Eighteen month follow-up of a play-based intervention to improve the social play skills of children with ADHD. *Austr Occup Ther J.* 2014;61(5):299-307.
144. Wilkes-Gillan S, Bundy A, Cordier R, Lincoln M. Evaluating a pilot parent-delivered play-based intervention for children with ADHD. *Am J Occup Ther.* 2014;68(6):700-709.
145. Saunders I, Sayer M, Goodale A. The relationship between playfulness and coping in preschool children: a pilot study. *Am J Occup Ther.* 1999;53(2):221-226.
146. Zeitlin S. *Coping Inventory.* Bensonville, IL: Scholastic Testing Service; 1986.
147. Hess L, Bundy A. The association between playfulness and coping in adolescents. *Phys Occup Ther Ped.* 2003;23(2):5-7.
148. Bronson M, Bundy AC. A correlational study of the Test of Playfulness and the Test of Environmental Supportiveness. *OTJR.* 2001;21(4):241-259.
149. Bundy AC, Waugh K, Brentnall J. Developing assessments that account for the role of the environment: an example using the Test of Playfulness and Test of Environmental Supportiveness. *OTJR.* 2009;29(3):135-143.
150. King G, Law M, King S, et al. *Children's Assessment of Participation and Enjoyment (CAPE) and Preferences for Activities of Children (PAC).* San Antonio, TX: Pearson; 2004.

151. King GA, Law M, King S, et al. Measuring children's participation in recreation and leisure activities: construct validation of the CAPE and PAC. *Child Care Health Dev.* 2007;33(1):28-39.
152. King G, Law M, King S, Rosenbaum P, Kertoy M, Young NL. A conceptual model of the factors affecting the recreation and leisure participation of children with disabilities. *Phys Occup Ther Pediatr.* 2003;23(1):63-90.
153. Imms C. Review of the Children's Assessment of Participation and Enjoyment and the Preference for Activity of Children. *Phys Occup Ther Pediatr.* 2008;28(4):389-404.
154. Bult MK, Verschuren O, Gorter JW, Jongmans MJ, Piskur B, Ketelaar M. Cross-cultural validation and psychometric evaluation of the dutch language version of the children's assessment of participation and enjoyment (CAPE) in children with and without physical disabilities. *Clin Rehab.* 2010:24(9):843-853.
155. Anastasiadi I, Tzetzis G. Construct validation of the Greek version of the Children's Assessment of Participation and Enjoyment (CAPE) and Preferences for Activities of Children (PAC). *J Phys Act Health.* 2013;10(4):523-532.
156. Colon WI, Rodiguez C, Ito M, Reed CN. Psychometric evaluation of the Spanish version of the Children's Assessment of Participation and Enjoyment and Preferences for Activities of Children. *Occup Ther Int.* 2008;15(2):100-113.
157. Majnemer A, Shevell M, Law M, et al. Participation and enjoyment of leisure activities in school aged children with cerebral palsy. *Dev Med Child Neurol.* 2008;50(10):751-758.
158. McDonald AE, Vigen C. Reliability and validity of the McDonald Play Inventory. *Am J Occup Ther.* 2012;66(4):e52-e60.
159. Henry AD. Assessment of play and leisure in children and adolescents. In Parham LD, Fazio LS, eds. *Play in Occupational Therapy for Children.* St Louis, MO: Mosby Elsevier; 2008:95-125.
160. Henry AD. Development of a measure of adolescent leisure interests. *Am J Occup Ther.* 1998;52(7):531-539.
161. Skar L, Prellwitz M. Participation in play activities: a single-case study focusing on a child with obesity experiences. *Scand J Caring Sci.* 2008;22(2):211-219.
162. Trottier AN, Nrown GT, Hobson SJG, Miller W. Reliability and validity of the Leisure Satisfaction Scale (LSS –short form) and the Adolescent Leisure Interest Profile (ALIP). *Occup Ther Int.* 2002;9(2):131-144.
163. Kielhofner G. *A Model of Human Occupation: Theory and Application.* 2nd ed. Baltimore: Williams & Wilkins; 1995.
164. King G, Batorowicz B, Rigby P, Pinto M, Thompson L, Goh F. The leisure activity settings and experiences of youth with severe disabilities. *Dev Neurorehabil.* 2014;17:259-269.
165. Sturgess JA. A model describing play as a child-chosen activity- is this still valid in contemporary Australia? *Aust Occup Ther J.* 2003;50(2):104-108.
166. Lautamo T, Laakso ML, Aro T, Ahonen T, Törmäkangas K. Validity of the play assessment for group settings: an evaluation of differential item functioning between children with specific language impairment and typically developing peers. *Aust Occup Ther J.* 2011;58(4):222-230.
167. Ferland F. *Play, Children With Physical Disabilities and Occupational Therapy: The Ludic Model.* Ottawa, ON: University of Ottawa Press; 1997. http://www.caot.ca/
168. Rogers CS, Impara JC, Frary RB, et al. Measuring playfulness: development of the Child Behavior Inventory of Playfulness. In: Duncan M, Chick G, Aycock A, eds. *Play and Cultural Studies.* Greenwich, CT: Ablex Publishing; 1998:121-135.
169. Barnett LA. The playful child: measurement of a disposition to play. *Play Culture.* 1991;4(1):51-74.
170. Lieberman JN. Playfulness and divergent thinking: an investigation of their relationship at the kindergarten level. *J Gen Psychol.* 1965;107:209-224.
171. Russ SW. *Play in Child Development and Psychotherapy: Toward Empirically Supported Practice.* Mahwah, NJ: Lawrence Erlbaum Associates Publishers; 2004.
172. Frahsek S, Mack W, Mack C, Pfalz-Blezinger C, Knopf M. Assessing different aspects of pretend play within a play setting: towards a standardized assessment of pretend play in young children. *Br J Dev Psychol.* 2010;28(2):331-345.
173. Cooke L, Munroe-Chandler K, Hall C, Tobin D, Guerrero M. Development of the children's active play imagery questionnaire. *J Sports Sci.* 2014;32(9):860-869.
174. Westby C. A scale for assessing children's play. In: Gitlin-Weiner K, Sandgrund A, Schaefer CE, eds. *Play Diagnosis and Assessment.* 2nd ed. Hoboken, NJ: John Wiley & Sons; 2000:15-57.
175. Westby CE. Assessment of cognitive and language abilities through play. *Lang Speech Hear Serv in Schools.* 1980;11:154-168.
176. Fantuzzo J, Sutton-Smith B, Coolahan KC, Manz PH, Canning S, Debnam D. Assessment of preschool play interaction behaviors in young low-income children: Penn Interactive Peer Play Scale. *Early Childhood Research Quarterly.* 1995;10:105-120.
177. Rubin KH. *The Play Observation Scale (POS).* Maryland, MD: University of Maryland, Center for Children, Relationships, and Culture; 2001.
178. Telford A, Salmon J, Jolley D, Crawford D. Reliability and validity of physical activity questionnaires for children: the children's leisure activities study survey (CLASS). *Pediatr Exerc Sci.* 2004;16(1):64-78.
179. Lau J, Engelen L, Bundy A. Parents' perceptions of children's physical activity compared on two electronic diaries. *Pediatr Exerc Sci.* 2013;25(1):124-137.
180. Linder TW, Anthony TL, Bundy AD, et al. *Transdisciplinary Play-Based Assessment (TPBA2).* 2nd ed. Baltimore, MD: Paul H. Brookes Co; 2008.
181. Kelly-Vance L, Ryalls BO. A systematic, reliable approach to play assessment in preschoolers. *School Psychol Int.* 2005;26(4):398-412.
182. Athanasiou MS. Play-based approaches to preschool assessment. In: Bracken BA, Nagle RJ, eds. *The Psychoeducational Assessment of Preschool Children.* 4th ed. Mahwah, NJ: Lawrence Erlbaum Associates; 2007:219-238.
183. Wagner BS, Frost JL. Assessing play and exploratory behaviors of infants and toddlers. *J Res Child Edu.* 1986;1(1):27-36.
184. Lifter K. Linking assessment to intervention for children with developmental disabilities or at-risk for developmental delay: The Developmental Play Assessment (DPA) instrument. In: Gitlin-Wiener K, Sangrund A, Schaefer C, eds. *Play Diagnosis and Assessment.* New York: John Wiley & Sons, Inc; 2000:228-261.

185. Hwang JE. Validity of the Health Enhancement Lifestyle Profile–Screener (HELP-Screener). *OTJR.* 2012;32(4):135-141.
186. Hansen JIC, Scullard MG. Psychometric evidence for the Leisure Interest Questionnaire and analyses of the structure of leisure interests. *J Couns Psychol.* 2002;49(3):331-341.
187. Adams KB. Changing investment in activities and interests in elders' lives: theory and measurement. *Int J Aging Hum Dev.* 2004;58(2):87-108.
188. Drummond A, Parker C, Gladman J, Logan P. Development and validation of the Nottingham Leisure Questionnaire (NLQ). *Clin Rehabil.* 2001;15(6):647-656.
189. Nilsson I, Fisher AG. Evaluating leisure activities in the oldest old. *Scand J Occup Ther.* 2006;13(1):31-37.
190. Dijkstra BAG, Roozen HG. Patients' improvements measured with the pleasant activities list and the community reinforcement approach happiness scale: preliminary results. *Addictive Disorders & Their Treatments.* 2012;11(1):6-13.
191. Mann WC, Talty P. Leisure Activity Profile: Measuring use of leisure time by persons with alcoholism. *Occup Ther Ment Health.* 1990;10(4):31-41.
192. Iso-Ahola SE, Weissinger E. Perceptions of boredom in leisure: conceptualization, reliability, and validity of the leisure boredom scale. *J Leisure Res.* 1990;22(1):1-17.
193. Caldwell LL, Smith EA, Weissinger E. Development of a Leisure Experience Battery for Adolescents: parsimony, stability, and validity. *J Leisure Res.* 1992;24(4):361-376.
194. Poulsen AA, Barker FM, Ziviani J. Personal projects of boys with developmental coordination disorder. *OTJR.* 2011;31(3):108-117.
195. Rider K, Gallagher-Thompson D, Thompson L. *California Older Person's Pleasant Events Schedule.* Palo Alto, CA: Stanford School of Medicine, Older Adult and Family Center; 2004.
196. Ellis, GD, Voelkl JE, Morris C. Measurement and analysis issues with explanation of variance in daily experience using the flow model. *J Leisure Res.* 1994;26(4):337-356.
197. Chen Y, Bundy A, Cordier R, Einfeld S. Feasibility and usability of experience sampling methodology for capturing everyday experiences of individuals with autism spectrum disorders. *Disabil Health J.* 2014;7:361-366.
198. Manfredo M, Driver BL, Tarrant MA. Measuring leisure motivation: a meta-analysis of the recreation experience preference scales. *J Leisure Res.* 1996;28(3):188-213.
199. Kloseck M, Crilly RG, Ellis GD, Lammers E. Leisure Competence Measure: development and reliability of a scale to measure functional outcomes in therapeutic recreation. *Therapeutic Recreation J.* 1996;30(1):13-26.
200. Kloseck M, Crilly RG, Hutchinson-Troyer L. Measuring therapeutic recreation outcomes in rehabilitation: further testing of the Leisure Competence Measure. *Ther Rec J.* 2001;35(1):31-42.
201. Chang L. An interaction effect of leisure self-determination and leisure competence on older adults' self-rated health. *J Health Psychol.* 2012;17(3):324-332.
202. Coleman DJ. The ability of selected leisure based factors to reduce the detrimental impact of stress on health. Unpublished doctoral thesis. Brisbane, Australia: Griffith University; 1999.
203. Craike M, Coleman DJ. Buffering effect of leisure self-determination on the mental health of older adults. *Leisure.* 2005;29(2):301-328.
204. Coleman D, Iso-Ahola S. Leisure and health: the role of social support and self-determination. *J Leisure Res.* 1993;25(2):111-128.
205. Teixeira A, Freire T. The Leisure Attitude Scale: psychometrics properties of a short version for adolescents and young adults. *Leisure/Loisir.* 2013;37(1):57-67.
206. Ragheb MG, Beard JG. Measuring leisure attitude. *J Leisure Res.* 1982;14(2):155-167.
207. Di Bona L. What are the benefits of leisure? An exploration using the Leisure Satisfaction Scale. *Br J Occup Ther.* 2000;63(2):50-58.
208. Beard J, Ragheb M. Measuring leisure satisfaction. *J Leisure Res.* 1980;12:20-33.
209. Beard JS, Ragheb MG. Measuring leisure motivation. *J Leisure Res.* 1983;15:219-228.
210. Beiswenger KL, Grolnick WS. Interpersonal and intrapersonal factors associated with autonomous motivation in adolescents' after-school activities. *J Early Adolesc.* 2010;30(3):369-394.
211. Iwasaki Y, Mannell RC. Hierarchical dimensions of leisure stress coping. *Leisure Sciences.* 2000;22:163-181.
212. Porter HR. Developing a Leisure Meanings Gained and Outcomes Scale (LMGOS) and exploring associations of leisure meanings to leisure time physical activity (LTPA) adherence among adults with type 2 diabetes. *Dissertation Abstracts Int.* 2009;70(6):3469.
213. Porter H, Iwasaki Y, Shank J. Conceptualizing meaning-making through leisure experiences. *Society Leisure/Loisir et Societe,* 2011;33:167-194.
214. Schulz J, Watkins M. The development of the Leisure Meanings Inventory. *J Leisure Res.* 2007;39(3):477-497.
215. Kyle GT, Absher J, Norman W, Hammitt W, Jodice L. A Modified Involvement Scale. *Leisure Studies.* 2007;26(4):399-427.
216. Stevens Director AB, Coon D, Wisniewski S, et al. Measurement of leisure time satisfaction in family caregivers. *Aging Ment Health.* 2004;8(5):450-459.
217. Hwang JE. Promoting healthy lifestyles with aging: development and validation of the Health Enhancement Lifestyle Profile (HELP) using the Rasch measurement model. *Am J Occup Ther.* 2010;64:786-795.
218. Iwasaki, Y. Testing an optimal matching hypothesis of stress, coping and health: leisure and general coping. *Loisir et Societe/Society Leisure.* 2001;24(1):163-203.
219. Bourke-Taylor HM, Law M, Howie L, Pallant JF. Development of the Assistance to Participate Scale (APS) for children's play and leisure activities. *Child Care Health Dev.* 2009;35(5):738-745.
220. Khetani M, Marley J, Baker M, et al. Validity of the Participation and Environment Measure for Children and Youth (PEM-CY) for Health Impact Assessment (HIA) in sustainable development projects. *Disabil Health J.* 2014;7(2):226-235.
221. Whiteneck GG, Gerhart KA, Cusick CP. Identifying environmental factors that influence the outcomes of people with traumatic brain injury. *J Head Trauma Rehabil.* 2004;19(3):191-204.

222. Cheeseman D, Madden R, Bundy A. Your Ideas About Participation and Environment: A new self-report instrument. *Disabil Rehabil.* 2013;35(22):1903-1908.

223. Noreau L, Desrosiers J, Robichaud L, Fougeyrollas P, Rochette A, Viscogliosi C. Measuring social participation: reliability of the LIFE-H in older adults with disabilities. Disabil Rehabil. 2004;26(6):346-352.

224. Rosenberg L, Jarus T, Bart O. Development and initial validation of the Child Participation Questionnaire, CPQ. Disabil Rehabil. 2010;32:1633-1644.

225. Law M, King G, Petrenchik T, Kertoy M, Anaby D. The assessment of preschool children's participation: internal consistency and construct validity. Phys Occup Ther Pediatr. 2012;32(3):272-287.

226. Jessen C, Colver AF, Mackie PC, Jarvis SN. Development and validation of a tool to measure the impact of childhood disabilities on the lives of children and their families. Child Care Health Dev. 2003;29:21-34.

227. McDougall J, Bedell G, Wright V. Youth report version of the Child and Adolescent Scale of Participation (CASP): assessment of psychometric properties and comparison with parent report. Child Care Health Dev. 2013;39(4):512-522.

228. Bradley RH, Caldwell BM, Corwyn RF. The Child Care HOME Inventories: assessing the quality of family child care homes. Early Child Res Q. 2003;18(3):294-309.

CHAPTER 11

Measuring Work Performance

Vicki Kaskutas, OTD, OTR/L, FAOTA

Work is a central construct underlying productivity, and one of the key domains of occupational therapy practice. Although individuals engage with their world in many different ways, it is through work that much of life's meaning is actualized. Therefore, a professional and practice imperative for occupational therapists is to embrace a client-centered, systematic way with which to approach the measurement and analysis of client skills and abilities to engage in work roles. Work is one of the emerging areas of practice for occupational therapy[1] and 1 of the 8 areas of occupation of our profession.[2] The Occupational Therapy Practice Framework defines 7 activities of work: employment interests and pursuits, employment seeking, employment acquisition, job performance, retirement preparation and adjustment, volunteer exploration, and volunteer participation.[2] As the workforce ages and the need to continue to work well past the traditional retirement age increases, there is a growing need for work evaluation and rehabilitation services. For the purposes of this chapter, *work* is defined as the occupations in which individuals engage in order to participate in their communities, and for which they are remunerated or rewarded in some way. Remuneration or reward can be in the form of payment, as in paid work, or in satisfaction or sense of achievement, as in voluntary occupations.

We will use the Person-Environment-Occupation-Performance (PEOP) model to examine the assessment of work participation (Figure 11-1). This client-centered model considers the Person's abilities and skills, the tasks and roles performed for the Occupation, and the work Environment and context for work Performance. Examining the workers' abilities without a context represents an incomplete approach to assessment and treatment in occupational therapy. Understanding the job and the work environment is essential in the area of work practice—the requirements of people's work tasks have a much greater variance than the requirements for other areas of occupation, such as activities of daily living (ADL) and education. The PEOP model allows us to define the "client" as one worker, a work group or organization, or the population or community, which has routinely been embraced in the area of work practice and is becoming central to most other areas of occupational therapy practice.

Who Are the Clients?

Work is an important part of most people's lives, whether a college student with a sports-related concussion who works a part-time pizza delivery job; a 32-year-old computer scientist with multiple sclerosis; a 45-year-old construction worker with a work-related back injury; a 61-year-old office worker with carpal tunnel syndrome and depression; or a 75-year-old seamstress with a history of knee replacements, stroke, and arthritis. Work provides meaning, routine, self-esteem, quality of life, energy expenditure,[3] and social interaction. Return to work has been shown to improve many aspects of personal health, including subjective well-being, life satisfaction,[4] physical well-being,[5] and memory in some populations.[6] Additionally, shorter sick leave and/or the time required to return to work is often correlated with decreased medical costs and increased occupational income during follow-up.

Besides preventing financial problems, work has been associated with prevention of depression,[7] psychological distress,[8] weight gain,[9] and physical deconditioning.[10] Clients who are recovering from conditions that prevent them from working for an extended period of time may begin to see themselves as "patients" whose role is to rest and take medication vs "workers" who are off work for several weeks or months to get back into shape for the workplace. If an individual has been in the patient role for

Law M, Baum C, Dunn W, eds. *Measuring Occupational Performance: Supporting Best Practice in Occupational Therapy, Third Edition (pp 201-237).*

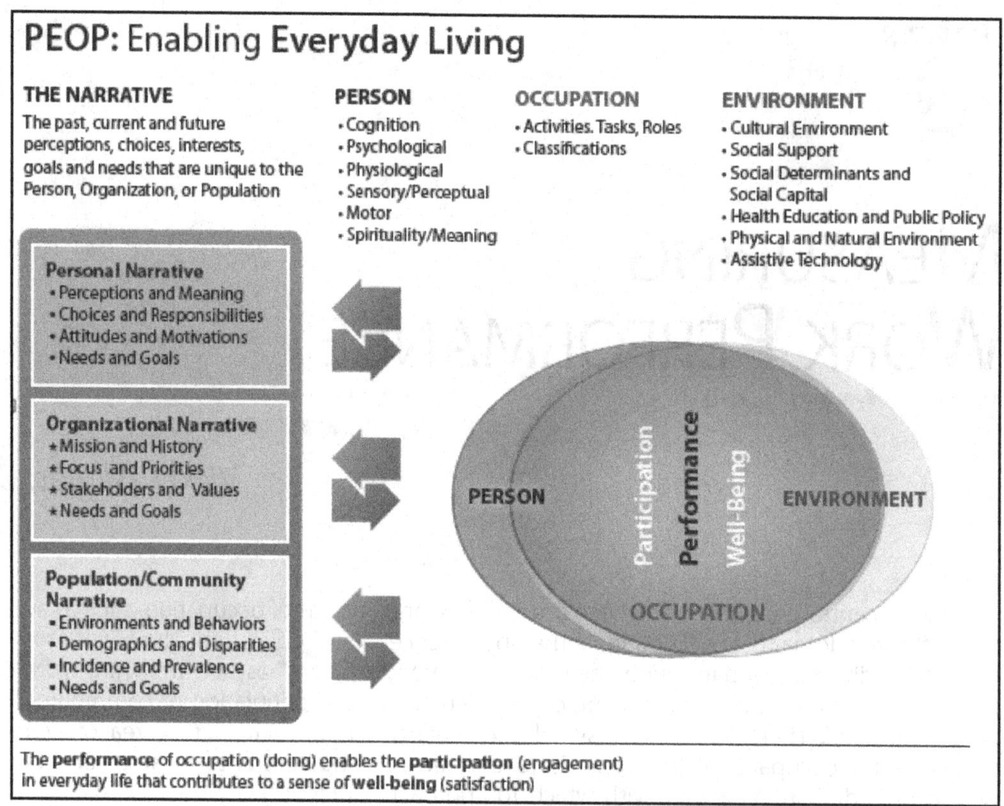

Figure 11-1. PEOP.

an extended period of time, he or she may have difficulty integrating work back into daily life. The occupational therapist can help an individual make the paradigm shift from patient to worker. Occupational therapists working with clients with a new injury/illness or clients with progression of an existing health condition can prevent them from losing touch with their worker role by addressing work during the initial evaluation and weaving work performance throughout treatment. Work can be a powerful motivator for many people, and lack of work can trigger a stream of negative consequences, resulting in occupational deprivation and poor quality of life.

Many aging Americans are choosing to work long past the traditional retirement age of 65 years. The labor force participation rate of people ages 65 to 74 years increased from 16.3 in 1992 to 26.8 in 2012, and it is projected to increase to 31.9 by 2022.[11] Participation of people over age 75 in the labor force is expected to rise to 10.5% in 2022. Remaining in the workforce is often a financial decision fueled by the increased retirement age for social security, the need for health insurance, financial stressors due to the recent economic recession, and decreased prevalence of retirement pensions through employers. However, many people are choosing to work longer in order to maintain occupational engagement and well-being.

Occupational therapists will encounter clients who aspire to return to work in most treatment and community settings, including hospitals, schools, outpatient rehabilitation centers, day programs, day treatment centers, community programs, or the workplace. Unemployment is nearly twice as high for individuals with disabilities compared with those without disabilities (http://www.dol.gov/odep/), which can result in poverty, a poor living situation, and lack of health care. When clients identify work as a meaningful occupation in which they want to participate, it is important to expand the evaluation beyond traditional assessment measures in the facility's protocol. Helping a client return to work is part of community reintegration, a service provided by occupational therapists in a wide array of treatment settings. In order to deliver client-centered care, we must focus on the occupations of primary importance to our clients, which may not necessarily be those occupations that are the traditional focus of the facilities where we encounter our clients. All occupational therapists have been prepared to address the occupation of work with their clients.

Understanding the Narrative and the Person

Understanding a client's narrative begins with the occupational profile. When assessing work performance, the occupational profile also focuses on education and training, work history, work capabilities and limitations prior to injury/illness, and the client's return-to-work goal. As with all initial evaluations, the therapist must understand the client's diagnoses, medical treatment, and physician-imposed restrictions prior to the assessment. The therapist must be familiar with the client's medical history, including current conditions for which the client is being treated, pre-existing conditions, and other concomitant health conditions. This information can be gathered from the medical record if available; otherwise, a standardized checklist of health history should be completed. The therapist must know medications that the client is taking and understand the general purpose of each medication, including prescription and nonprescription drugs. It is also essential to understand the required job tasks, the employer's performance expectations, the work environment, and workplace routines; therefore, a job evaluation is always included in the initial assessment, which is discussed in detail in this chapter. It is important to consider other factors about the individual and his or her life when making work decisions, such as other required life roles and the importance of work to the client. This information is an important part of the occupational profile that must be considered.

A good match between the individual and the workplace is the first step to optimal work performance. Individuals must be able to perform the job in a safe manner, day after day, and at a level competitive for the workforce. The consequences of returning to work too early are numerous: the health condition or other conditions can escalate, the individual or a coworker can suffer a work injury or illness, or the individual can lose his or her job. There are also many legal and financial ramifications associated with work and the consequences of returning to work without possessing the ability to meet requirements of the workplace. The occupational therapist should perform a comprehensive assessment of the wide range of factors affecting work performance and closely collaborate with the client, medical team, and employer when helping to make return-to-work decisions.

Important Issues to Consider When Assessing Work Performance

The assessment battery used to help the client make decisions regarding work must: 1) be *safe*, 2) provide accurate and *reliable* results, 3) be a *valid* representation of the actual work performed, and 4) be *practical* (NIOSH). Safety is always the first criteria that must be considered when administering any assessment; safety should never be compromised for the sake of reliability or validity. For example, prior to asking a client to lift the actual object he or she moves from floor to overhead level at work, it is important to know whether the client can assume the required positions, maintain balance, grip in the manner necessary to hold the object, and understand the directions. These basic functions should be screened prior to performing any lifting assessment. A lift test that has been proven to be safe and reliable should also be administered before job-specific lifting is assessed. Safety should be closely monitored throughout the assessment, including vital signs, ratings of perceived exertion, fatigue, frustration, body mechanics and pace, and observing for signs of distress or maximum tolerance.

As noted in previous chapters, there are many factors affecting the reliability of an assessment: the evaluator's ability to consistently following the administration protocol, the consistency of the client's effort throughout the assessment, and the accuracy and precision of the assessment protocol. The therapist is responsible for choosing reliable assessment measures, administering the assessment reliably, and ensuring that the client understands assessment directions and procedures so that he or she provides reliable effort; however, the client ultimately controls the consistency of his or her effort. If the injury or illness is work related, there may be a push from the worker's compensation carrier for the therapist to focus heavily on the client's reliability, often termed *sincerity of effort* or *validity indicators.*

There are many reasons that the work assessment results of a client recuperating from an injury, illness, surgery, and/or extended time away from work may not be reliable. These include pain, fear, fatigue, medications, weight gain, muscle loss, cardiopulmonary deconditioning, decreased agility, and lack of understanding of the testing goal and/or procedure. As a result, it is best to ensure that the client understands the importance of consistent effort during the assessment, to closely monitor and record the client's response to each subtest and the reason for stopping (including behaviors, statements, vital signs, grimaces, rubbing, pain ratings, and perceived exertion ratings), and to help keep the client on track to consistent performance whenever possible, remembering that safety is always more important than reliability. Symptom magnification, "a self-destructive, socially reinforced behavioral response pattern consisting of reports or displays of symptoms that function to control the life circumstances of the sufferer,"[12(p 43)] can exist in people with injuries and/or illness. It is very different from malingering, which is willful exaggeration of symptoms and disabilities. Good therapeutic use of self can help the therapist deal with a client who is not demonstrating reliable results due to symptom magnification.

Establishing the validity of work assessments is more challenging than most other areas of occupation because the requirements of the many jobs performed by people vary significantly. Therapist-designed job-simulated assessments will have content validity, but the therapist may not be evaluating the actual construct that he or she set out to assess. For example, when designing a standardized assessment of lift capacity, firefighters were asked to lift a plastic crate with increasing weights until they reached their limit. This appeared to be a good measure of lift capacity; however, when the firefighters were asked why they discontinued the assessment, it was due to discomfort from the heavily loaded plastic crate cutting into their hands (oral communication, Leonard Matheson, 1999). The test measured hand pain, not lift capacity. Most people perform their work for an entire work shift (whether it is 6, 8, or 12 hours in length) as well as travel to the workplace several days in a row (normally 5 days per week). This complicates the task of performing a work assessment. If a client can perform simulated work for 1 hour during the therapy session that occurs 3 times per week, does that mean that he or she can work five 8-hour shifts as is required by the job? In order for the work assessment to be valid, it must predict actual work performance, which is difficult to achieve. It took Leonard Matheson over 20 years to validate the lift assessment described here, which has progressed significantly from the early editions.[13]

Because work assessment can be considered an employment test, therapists who make employment decisions must comply with laws enforced by the Equal Employment Opportunity Commission; these laws prevent discrimination due to race, national origin, religion, sex, age, or disability. The assessment protocol and each assessment measure used must not discriminate in any way. For example, a lifting assessment cannot require a woman to advance 5 pounds per lift while a man advances 10 pounds per lift because the woman would have to perform 10 lifts to get to 50 pounds, whereas the man would only have to perform 5 lifts. Individuals over 40 years of age are protected against age discrimination, so the testing protocol must proceed similarly for a worker who is 20, 40, or 60 years of age. Obviously, the testing protocol must have safety guidelines built into it that allow for adequate rest and recovery. This is not to say that there are not physiological changes that occur with aging that affect strength, agility, cardiopulmonary function, and sensory functions, just that assessments utilized to make work decisions must not discriminate against older people. There are also guidelines from several professional associations that can guide the therapist performing work assessments, including the American Association of Psychologists, the American College of Sports Medicine, the American Physical Therapy Association, and the Academy of Physical Medicine and Rehabilitation.

Understanding the Job and the Work Environment

Occupational therapists understand the requirements and routinely assess clients' ADL, instrumental ADL, and education-related occupations. There is not a huge amount of variation in the requirements and methods used to get dressed; after clothing is chosen, it is stepped into, pulled over, or wrapped around the person and any closures are fastened. With over 840 detailed occupations in the United States economy,[14] there is a large amount of variation in what people do at work. Clinicians may have an elementary understanding of what a carpenter does at work, but the duties of a carpenter installing cubicle workstations in an office building is very different from a carpenter constructing a bridge. The therapist must have a good understanding of the job in order to develop an assessment battery that provides enough detailed information to know whether the client can safely and reliably perform the job. The clinician must understand the tasks performed and the tools and equipment used at work, in addition to the level of skill, ability, and knowledge required to perform this job. The therapist must understand the environmental conditions encountered in the workplace and the employer policies.

It is important to understand the fit between the person, the job, and the workplace prior to the injury or illness. The therapist begins by asking the client to talk about his or her job satisfaction, relationships with supervisor and coworkers, perceived match between the employer's policies and the client's life, and goals for returning to this job. During a conversation with the employer, the therapist attempts to get a feel for the employer's perceptions of what type of a worker the client was and how willing the employer is to collaborate to transition the client back to work. The therapist also discusses the job requirements, tools and technologies utilized, work schedule, and work environment, including the physical, policy, and cultural environment. Job information can be gathered from the employer through a written job description, verbal discussion, and/or onsite job analysis. As is always the case, the therapist cannot reveal protected health information per the Health Insurance Portability and Accountability Act (HIPAA), including the client's past, present, or future physical or mental health/condition, evaluation results, and health care services provided.[15] If the clinician anticipates that any protected health information will be disclosed during an interaction with the employer, such as the diagnosis or impairments that the client is demonstrating, written permission from the client must be secured prior to disclosure.

Therapists can consult the Occupational Information Network (O*NET) (http://www.onetonline.org/) for useful generic job information that can guide the work assessment. O*NET is the US Department of Labor's (DOL) system for describing characteristics of the job, worker, and work environment for every job in the US economy. O*NET replaced the Dictionary of Occupational Titles (DOT) in 1998. O*NET identifies the work tasks required for each job and ranks these tasks by level of importance and relevance. Requisite knowledge, skills, abilities, and work activities are identified and ranked for importance and level of function. Other work interests, work styles, and work values associated with the job are identified, as well as work context, tools and technology, and educational/vocational preparation. Wages, employment trends, and job openings by state are included, as are videotapes about the job and other related jobs. O*NET has a wealth of information about job requirements, and even more can be found by looking at the additional resources on their website. This includes level ratings on a 7-point behavioral anchored scale and a 5-level importance rating scale After understanding this generic information, the clinician can work with the client and his or her employer to understand the requirements of the client's actual job. Several studies have found that the O*NET data are fairly reliable with observed requirements from job analysis and self-report on standardized measures.[16] Table 11-1 describes the categories within O*NET and lists examples of elements within each category. Table 11-2 described 5 generic physical demand levels of work based on the frequency and amount of weight lifted and typical energy requirements.

The Job Performance Measure (JPM) (Appendix A) is an assessment developed at Washington University School of Medicine that uses the O*NET system to identify the client's job tasks and frequency of task performance. After identifying the job title(s) that most closely match the client's job, the clinician consults O*NET to identify tasks that are commonly performed by people who hold this specific job title. This task list serves as a starting point for understanding the specific tasks that are required of the job, rather than asking a client to identify the work tasks performed without any organizing criteria. Tasks identified by O*NET are reviewed with the client; tasks that are required of the client's job are recorded on the JPM, task descriptions are modified for tasks that are not worded exactly as required, and additional tasks that were not identified are described on the JPM form. It may be necessary to search for other job titles if the client's job does not neatly fit into one job on O*NET. This may be the case for a maintenance person at an apartment complex. This person may be required to perform laborer, locksmith, heating and cooling, and carpentry duties during the course of a work week. The next step is to converse with the client about each task to identify the manner in which it is performed and tools or equipment needed to perform these tasks. An Internet search can reveal pictures of the tasks and tools; even the size and dimensions can be identified. Next, the frequency of performing each task is reported by the client on a 7-point DOL rating scale. This scale ranges from once or less each year to every hour or more. The JPM has a second purpose, which is to identify the client's perceptions of his or her ability to perform each job task. This purpose will be described in detail in the following section.

Assessing the Client's Work Abilities and Limitations

There is a wide range of constructs that will potentially need to be assessed when addressing return-to-work with a client with injury, illness, or chronic conditions, including factors that are intrinsic to the client and extrinsic factors that involve the work environment, employer, and industry. The occupation of work engages individuals in a series of tasks and activities that vary widely; however, each job requires a basic level of intrinsic abilities in order to perform it safely. It is important to perform a screening test of sensory, motor, emotional, and cognitive factors prior to initiating job-specific performance-based testing. For example, the ability to follow written directions is essential for many assessments administered to measure work performance, not to mention upon return to work. Adequate balance and strength are requisite for many climbing and lifting tasks that may be performed during the assessment. Table 11-3 lists Person-level functions that should be screened and provides suggestions for assessments that can be used to screen these Person-level constructs. The reader is referred to www.rehabmeasures.org for more information about standardized assessments listed in Table 11-3.

When evaluating physical capacities necessary for work, such as lifting, carrying, and other material handling tasks, there are several methods to decide the endpoints for the testing. When an individual is performing at his or her maximum level, it is normal to see changes in movement patterns, body mechanics, pace of movement, heart and respiratory rate, blood pressure, and perspiration. Biomechanical, otherwise known as *kinesiophysical endpoints*, have been suggested by some authors,[17] including use of unsafe body mechanics (such as hyperextending or twisting the back), abnormal pace (such as jerking or throwing the load to maintain momentum), or losing control of the load. Cardiac endpoints are also suggested, such as keeping heart rate below 85% of the predicted maximum. Psychophysical endpoints have some usefulness, such as ratings of perceived exertion. Symptoms such as pain and fatigue can serve as another endpoint, along with the client's request to stop the test. An approach that uses a combination of all of these approaches is recommended, with the therapist's top priority being maintenance of the client's safety throughout the assessment.

If a therapist is not observing any of the changes described previously that suggest a client is providing maximal effort, the therapist should discuss his or her observations with the client and re-explain the need for full effort during the assessment. It is novel for a client who is recovering from a long-standing illness or injury that required him or her to rest, limit movement, and avoid pain to now be participating in an assessment that requires his or her maximal effort. It is important for the client to feel safe throughout the assessment, which is the therapist's responsibility. If the client is unable to provide maximum effort, this should be discussed with the client and the referring physician. Results of the assessment should not be reported as representing full effort, with the therapist avoiding making any assumptions regarding the reason behind the client's behaviors. The therapist needs to maintain a client-centered approach throughout testing and reporting.

Pain should be monitored throughout the work assessment in all clients, especially those who present with pain. Pain is normal for up to 3 days after increased activity, but the symptoms normally subside after 24 hours and disappear within 5 to 7 days.[18] After participating in a functional capacity evaluation, 82% of individuals without a diagnosis or condition noted pain, including 51% in the thigh, 38% in the low back, 37% in the shoulders, and 36% in the upper arms.[19] Symptoms decreased to pre-evaluation levels in an average of 3 days. The intensity and duration of the pain response of healthy subjects is not significantly different from the response of patients with chronic low back pain. It is important to understand baseline symptoms, measure symptoms after each activity, and observe for painful behaviors throughout, such as grimacing, posture or movement pattern changes, stretching, rubbing, and change of pace. The therapist should compare symptoms and observations to baseline, self-reports, and health conditions/diagnoses to understand if the symptoms are normal activity-related or if they may suggest an advancement of a health condition. Symptoms that appear to be nonpathological responses to tasks should not be criteria to stop the test unless the client requests to discontinue testing. Symptoms are closely monitored during and after the assessment. If new symptoms that indicate pathological responses occur, the test is stopped and progression/regression of symptoms is monitored. The use of ice and analgesics may be indicated. Clients who experience significant persistent symptoms during or for a prolonged period after the initial evaluation may not be competitive in the workplace. In addition to causing physical changes, pain can impede ability to cognitively process and make good decisions, which can affect safety in the workplace.

There is also a role for nonstandardized screening measures to assess select Person-level functions. Let's say that the therapist observes the client sitting for 15 minutes to independently complete the initial evaluation packet (sign consent forms, record health history, complete standardized written surveys, and diagram painful symptoms) and these materials are accurately completed. The therapist knows that sitting tolerance and attention span are at least 15 minutes, visual acuity is functional, the client can read and write, and ability to organize and manipulate lightweight objects is fairly good. Results of all Person-level function screening tests, whether using standardized measures or not, should be documented. This is especially important when addressing work performance because work tasks and simulations have greater exposures than most ADL, education, and IADL tasks that are performed during an initial evaluation. In addition, there is a high rate of litigation in the worker's compensation arena.

There is also a role for nonstandardized assessment when addressing ability to work. Job simulations are especially useful; however, the clinician must ensure that the methods used are safe and reproducible (ie, reliable). Job simulations may inherently have validity; however, they may not be practical due to the equipment, space, and time required. When designing a nonstandardized assessment using job simulations, the clinician begins by identifying construct(s) that need to be measured, designing a simulation that mimics that job task, acquiring tools and supplies necessary for the simulation, deciding the measurement methods that will be used (eg, time, repetitions, number of items dropped, weight lifted), and setting up the environment to match the work environment the client appears able to tolerate (eg, physical environment, coworker interaction, noise level). Prior to performing job simulation testing, it is important to screen the client's ability to perform skills embedded in simulation (eg, standing, balance, ambulation, and vision should be assessed before asking a client to perform a job-simulated climbing task). The client should be involved in planning the work simulation in order to make testing as realistic as possible, and he or she should understand mock-ups prior to testing, such as using soft theraputty to simulate ground meat for a chef. During the simulated nonstandardized assessment, the therapist observes for each construct that is being measured, recording behaviors, methods, and ability to self-manage pain, fatigue, or other symptoms. Standardized measures of work performance that can be tiered over these nonstandardized assessments are discussed next.

Prior to work-specific testing, the may have already administered standardized assessments measuring the intrinsic body functions (such as sensation, strength, memory, and executive function), or other areas of occupation, such as ADL and IADL. The results of these same assessments can serve as the screen for the assessment of work performance. The therapist should not assume a level of work ability based on a cognitive or motor screen or an assessment of ADL or IADL performance. A woman who can independently run a household may not be able to perform her job as a nurse, while a young man who requires assistance to get dressed may be able to perform his job as a packer in a factory. Therapists who are helping make return-to-work decisions or assessing for work disability must make decisions based on assessment information that is at the occupational performance level, not the person, environment, or occupation level only. Work motivates some people to utilize every resource within their body and environment to perform. What becomes tricky is when therapists are asked to make predictions regarding long-term work ability. Will the client who is using every resource possible be able to work at a competitive level without tearing down his or her body in the future? Therapists do not have crystal balls that allow them to make these types of decisions.

Assessment Measures of Work Performance

There are many standardized assessments to measure a client's work ability and limitations, as well as workplace exposures, social climate, and work policies. According to Innes and Straker,[20] work-related assessments should be safe, accurate, comprehensive, credible, objective, useful, valid, measurable, relevant, practical, reproducible, specific, structured, flexible, and generalizable. This list is daunting, but there are many standardized and nonstandardized assessments that can be used (Table 11-4).

The Assessment of Work Performance (AWP) is a standardized assessment by Jan Sandqvist that assesses 14 skills while a client performs a work activity, including 5 motor skills (posture, mobility, coordination, strength, physical energy), 5 process skills (mental energy, knowledge, adaptation, organization of space/objects and time), and 4 communication/interaction skills (physicality, language, relations, information exchange). The clinician rates the client's performance on a 4-point ordinal rating scale (1=incompetent performance, 2=limited performance, 3=unsure performance, and 4=competent performance). Tiering the AWP over a job-simulated nonstandardized assessment allows the therapist to gather objective data that can be used to measure changes over time. The AWP does not result in an overall rating of the client's ability to perform the simulated work activity; however, the clinician can comment on the overall performance in order to be at an occupational performance level.

The Work Ability Index (WAI) is a self-report measure of work ability used in health assessments, workplace surveys, and outcome research.[21] The index considers the physical and mental demands of work and the worker's health status and resources. Constructs measured include number of diagnosed health conditions, amount of sick leave during the past year, estimation of work impairment, work ability compared to life and lifetime best, prognosis of work ability in 2 years, and mental resources. Work ability is categorized as poor, fair, moderate, good, or excellent. The WAI can help to identify supports needed to continue work and predict threats of work disability.

When assessing work performance, it is also important to consider other areas of occupation that are important for work. Individuals must be clean and dressed to be employed competitively at most jobs; individuals do not need to perform these tasks independently in order to work, but they must be performed by someone. While at the workplace, individuals must be able to don/doff coat and toilet (toileting is most likely required during a traditional-length work shift). Although clients do not need to perform these tasks independently, arrangements must be made for them to be performed while at work. Similarly, individuals must be able to mobilize around the workplace and community to work, whether it requires assistive devices or alternative methods of transportation. Most importantly, individuals must be able to manage their health while at the workplace, including nutrition, medication, skin care, rest, or safety.

There are several work performance assessment protocols that cluster standardized and nonstandardized assessments into a battery that has standardized administration procedures and has been validated; however, many of these require certification or are fee-based. As always, when utilizing a standardized assessment or battery of assessment, it is critical to abide by the directions in the manual and/or protocol. It is important to utilize both qualitative and quantitative approaches when performing an assessment of work ability, with the client's beliefs and concerns about work ascertained and strongly considered. Use of audit trails, detailed descriptions, member checking, debriefing, triangulation of data, and persistent observation is suggested until saturation of data has been achieved.[20]

Several nonstandardized assessments (denoted by an asterisk in Table 11-4) are very useful when assessing work performance. In addition to being used for job analysis, the JPM is useful to measure the client's perceptions of his or her ability to perform the tasks required of his or her job. After experiencing a new injury or illness, the client may not have an accurate perception of his or her ability to perform the job-required duties, but it is prudent to understand the client's beliefs about his or her capabilities prior to performing the actual work tasks. There is evidence suggesting that self-reported abilities do correlate with actual performance, and understanding the client's perspective is always useful. The client is asked to identify his or her current ability to perform each job task identified from the O*NET on a 10-point scale, ranging from not able to extremely well. This rating scale was borrowed from the Canadian Occupational Performance Measure (with approval from the authors), so it has been widely researched. The JPM has been used clinically with hundreds of work rehabilitation clients in several research studies. Although the psychometric properties have not been formally measured, the JPM was the best predictor of return to work success in clients with mild to moderate stroke.[22]

The Feasibility Evaluation Checklist (FEC) (Table 11-13) is a client self-report and clinician observational tool that rates 23 items in 3 areas: 1) general productivity (quantity and quality of work, attendance, and workplace endurance), 2) safety (ability to follow safety rules), and 3) interpersonal behaviour (ability to work and get along with coworkers and accept supervision) (available at http://www.epicrehab.com/products/index.php?main_page=product_info&cPath=14&products_id=88). The client performs a real or simulated work task and rates his or her performance for each item on a 4-point scale (poor, fair, good, or excellent) and rates the amount of potential for improvement (uncertain, low, moderate, or high). The client's rating can be compared to the clinician's ratings for the same 23 items; however, the 4-point observer's ratings include independent, minimal assistance, moderate assistance, and not employable. The self-report and observer rating forms and the administration manual are available for free from the Employment Potential Improvement Center (http://www.epicrehab.com/free_resources). The FEC has been widely used for over 30 years; however, the psychometric properties have not been examined.

After administering standardized assessments, testing using work simulations that are similar to the work requirements can be performed, ensuring that safety is always maintained. The client must be a close partner with the clinician, advising the clinician when the simulation is as realistic as possible. In order to be able to know work tolerances and track progress, work simulations should include objective measurements, whether it is tracking repetitions, timing tolerance, counting number of errors, describing prehension patterns, observing nonverbal communication skills, or ability to manage frustration. Because these assessments are being administered in order to make a return to work decision, Title 1 of the Americans with Disability Act applies both in the workplace and in the therapy clinic. Clients with qualified disabilities who request reasonable accommodations should be provided with these *during* the assessment. Testing protocols, equipment, environments, and facilities used in the rehabilitation setting should not discriminate against individuals with disabilities.[23]

Models of Practice Useful in Work Assessment and Rehabilitation

The wide array of theoretical approaches and models of practice with which most occupational therapists are familiar are appropriate for work assessment and intervention. Central to the care of all clients is a model of occupational performance, such as the Person-Environment-Occupation-Performance model, the Model of Human Occupation, the Canadian Model of Occupational Performance, and the Kawa River Model. Motor learning theories (Schmidt's Schema Theory, Ecological Theory, Fitts and Posner Three-Stage Model, and the Systems Three-Stage Model) and biomechanical approaches may be helpful when clients are acquiring movements, whether it is moving an extremity affected by stroke or learning to move the body using good body mechanics. Developmental theories can help guide work assessment and treatment (Havighurst Developmental Tasks, Erikson Psychosocial Development Crises, Lifespan Development theory, Self-determination theory, Baltes Theory, and the transition support model), as can emotional/affective theories (James-Lange Theory, Cannon-Bard Theory, Singer-Schachter/Two-factor theory), cognitive theories (cognitive-behavioral theory, cognitive disability model, dynamic interactional model of cognition), the transtheoretical model, and the psychiatric rehabilitation model. An environmental theory or model can be extremely useful when helping clients return to work, such as Bronfenbrenner Ecological Systems Theory, Lawton & Nahemow's Ecological Model. The taxonomies such as the Occupational Therapy Practice Framework: Domain and Process and the International Classification of Functioning, Disability, and Health can help to conceptualize and classify the myriad supports and barriers to consider when addressing work performance.

Theories and models that are more specific to work performance have roots in vocational rehabilitation. According to Braveman,[24] early vocational theories focused on the content of career choice, later theories focused more on the process and stages of career development and exploration, and the more recent constructivist perspective emphasizes context, cultural diversity, and self-construction. Several of the popular vocational theories were developed in the 1950s, including Super's Theory on Vocational Development; Ginzberg, Ginzburg, Axelrad, and Herma's Developmental Theory; and Holland's Career Typology. These early theorists stressed the relationship between self-concept and career choice, individuals' values as they relate to work, and the interaction between the individual and the work environment. Despite not representing the changing demographics of the workforce (women, older workers, racial and ethnic groups, disabled), societal changes, new professions and technology, and economic globalization, these theories continue to drive vocational development.[25] Lent, Brown, and Hackett's[26] social cognitive career theory extends social cognitive theory to career choice, proposing that career choice is influenced by beliefs developed through personal performance accomplishments, vicarious learning, social persuasion, and physiological states and reactions. This theory focuses on the individual's beliefs and the influence of social and economic context on vocational choice. The more recent systems theory framework of career development focuses on intrapersonal and contextual factors and the interaction between these 2 factors that occurs over time.[25] It is more in line with current theoretical approaches, models of practice, and organizational taxonomies.

The Model of Work Performance[22,23] is based on the Person-Environment-Occupation-Performance model, Lawton's Ecological Model, and Kurt Lewin's Field Theory, which views behavior as a mathematical expression of the person and the environment (B=f (P x E)). This model for rehabilitation of the injured worker depicts work performance as the result of the interaction between the personal competence of the individual and the environmental affordances of the environment. In this model, work performance is defined as the ability to perform the tasks and routines of the job within the context of the workplace. Personal competence is defined as how well an individual integrates the intrinsic factors to successfully perform a task or role. Environmental affordances are defined as what the environment provides or invites that allows an individual to perform a task or role. Job demands are the variety and demands of job tasks and work environments and the level of demand required of the job. The job demands, personal competence, and environmental affordances are assessed and depicted by vectors, with the length of the vector representative of the amount or degree of the construct (Figure 11-2). A job with few work tasks with a low-demand level will have a smaller vector than a job with a wide variety of tasks that

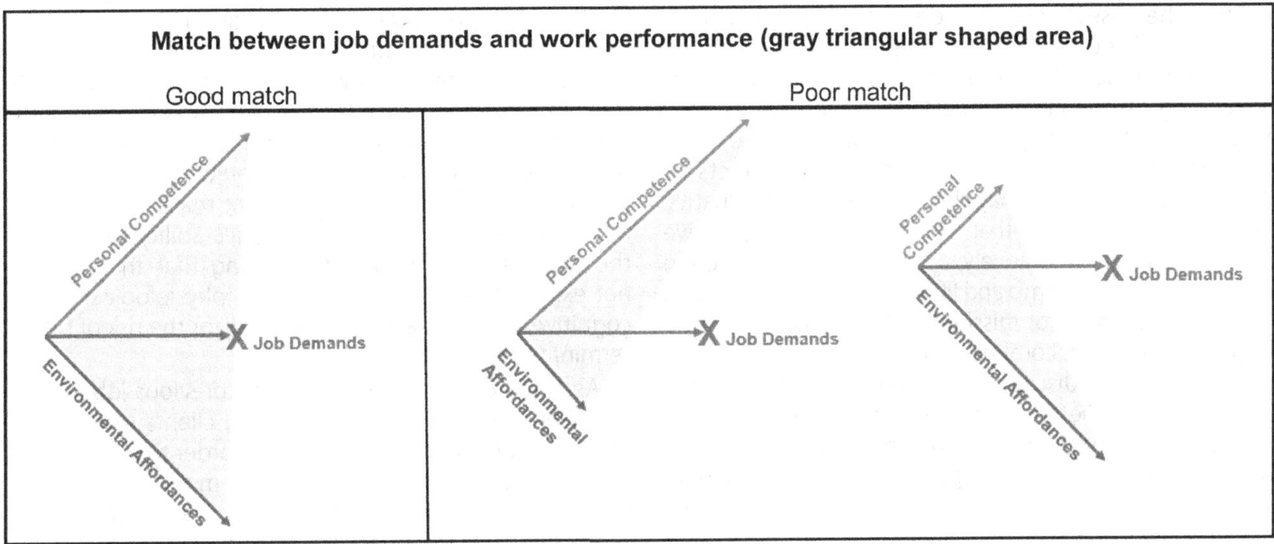

Figure 11-2. Kaskutas Model of Work Performance.

requires a high level of performance. The same is true for personal competence and environmental affordances; the vectors representing limited function and few environmental affordance will be short, whereas high personal competence and environmental affordances are denoted by long vectors.

In this model, work performance is represented by the region in the triangle formed by the personal competence and environmental affordances vectors (see Figure 11-2). If the head of the vector representing the job demands lies within the work performance region, the client should be able to return to work (diagram 1 in Figure 11-2). If the head of the vector extends past the job demands, the client will not be able to perform the job as defined by the job demands (diagrams 1 and 2 in Figure 11-2). Interventions can be directed to decreasing the job demands (the type and level of tasks required of the job), increasing personal competence, or increasing the environmental affordances. This leads the therapist to different models of practice and intervention approaches, whether it is modifying the job requirements or work schedule, introducing technology or equipment to compensate, modifying the environment or using public policies, restoring impaired body functions, or learning self-management techniques.

The Model of Work Performance provides a theoretical basis for rehabilitation of individuals with work injuries. The model visually demonstrates how manipulation of the person, environment, and occupation can result in enhanced work performance. The pictorial representation is easy for the client, employer, physician, and case manager to understand. Treatment approaches to restore, compensate, modify, and prevent are utilized within this model, such as biomechanical, motor learning, cognitive behavioral, rehabilitation, environmental, and acquisitional. The model is designed for assessment and intervention of common work injuries; however, it may be useful for prevention of work injuries and outcome measurement. Further research to validate the model is needed.

After the Assessment

If the client does not possess the ability return to work after the assessment but wants to return to work and there is potential to do so, a treatment plan can be initiated. The profession of occupational therapy defines the occupation of work as employment interests and pursuits, employment seeking and acquisition, job performance, retirement preparation and adjustment, volunteer exploration, and volunteer participation.[2] Much of the work rehabilitation that has occurred in the professions of occupational and physical therapy over the past 25 years has been directed at returning people with work-related musculoskeletal disorders to their jobs through services such as work hardening, work conditioning, and post-offer pre-employment testing. Historically, people who have strokes are at or above working age, so return to work has not been a major focus of treatment. Some individuals who experience a stroke may be focused on returning to their previous job; however, others will need to identify residual abilities and seek new employment, others will choose to pursue volunteer work experiences, and others will decide to retire. It is important to understand that rehabilitation to address work can focus on one or more of these levels of participation. For example, the initial focus may be on returning to the previous job (ie, job performance); however, if that does not appear to be realistic, the client may choose to seek alternative employment, pursue volunteer work, or retire from the workforce. The intervention plan should address work as defined by the client at the time/point that he or she is involved in rehabilitation.

After the assessment, if there is a major mismatch between a client's abilities and the requirements of the job, return to the previous job is most likely not possible. Depending on the client's goals, treatment may or may not be warranted. For example, a client with major expressive communication deficits who negotiated contracts for a Fortune 500 company may choose to explore alternative careers at the company that do not hinge on expressive communication. Alternatively, a 60-year-old construction worker who cannot climb and lift may choose to retire and focus on his passion for mission work. When a client is no longer able to work competitively, the financial ramifications need to be discussed. The occupational therapist should refer the client to a social service agency regarding both finances and health insurance. In some cases, the occupational therapist's documentation regarding limitations in the client's work abilities may be used to help the client qualify for long-term disability.

If the client demonstrates the ability to safely perform the job demands at a competitive level and appears capable of tolerating the work schedule and environmental demands, discussions with the employer are recommended. A work trial may be warranted prior to a full return to work. The occupational therapist can be involved in negotiating this and can even go to work with the client on the first day to observe the client's performance in context. It is important to ascertain that the client is able to perform at the required level of performance for the entire work shift, and that this can be performed dependably on a regular basis. A client may be able to perform most of the job functions, nearly meet the productivity requirements, or fall just short of tolerating the required work schedule. In these cases, the therapist will work with the client and the employer to identify the best course of action to address the shortcomings, whether it is treatment to restore lost functions, compensatory strategies, or providing accommodations at the workplace, or a combination of these. Some employers may consider a graduated work schedule to manage fatigue, whereas others will require that the client return to the customary work schedule. As with other areas of practice, the occupational therapist addressing return to work must be a creative problem solver who is capable of negotiating innovative solutions.

When assisting a person with return to work, the client must follow certain procedures, beginning with disclosure of the disability. The client must be able to perform the essential functions of the job with reasonable accommodations, which must be specifically requested from the employer. It is important for the clinician to address all of these areas with the client prior to recommending that the client return to work. The Job Accommodations Network (JAN) (http://askjan.org/) is an online resource that provides free, expert, and confidential guidance on workplace accommodations and disability employment issues, including determining whether a client has a disability under the Americans with Disabilities Act (ADA). JAN consultants provide individual online and phone guidance for workplace accommodations, and the website provides accommodations for various disabilities. Clinicians can refer employers to JAN to learn about their role in providing reasonable accommodations. Often, employers are willing to allow the client a work trial at the workplace; it is important to protect client, employer, and yourself when performing work trials. The clinician must have a good feel for the client's ability to re-enter the workplace environment, ensuring that the client is not exposed to injurious conditions, physiological stress, cognitive overload, emotional turmoil, or the risk of being terminated from work.

Assisting clients to return to their previous job can be a challenging task; however, helping clients understand their work abilities and limitations in order to identify and search for a new position is often a more difficult task. Clients who attempt to return to their same job at the same employer are usually the most successful. The client can draw on knowledge, skills, relationships, workplace norms, routines, and other familiar environmental characteristics when returning to the same job with the same employer. The employer is also familiar with the employee, his or her work behaviors and prior performance; however, if changes in the client's skills, executive functions, workplace tolerances, stamina, interaction abilities, affect, and/or work ability have occurred, these will most likely be evident to an employer who knows the client. Nearly half of the individuals who returned to work after mild stroke reported that they were performing at 75% or less of their pre-stroke work abilities and nearly one-third were not satisfied with their initial post-stroke work performance.[27] Often, people are able to return to work with accommodations, but changes from a client's premorbid status may impact success in the workplace. Reduced work speed, organization and concentration problems, and fatigue were reported 6 months after return to work after stroke.[27] Clinicians need to be sure that clients are not only able to return to work, but they are able to stay at work. Staying at work involves going to work day after day and tolerating the required work duties on a dependable basis without causing any harm to the client, his or her coworkers, or property and/or products in the workplace. Although returning to the prior job is preferred, some employers will offer a new or modified position to workers who have been exceptional employees in the past. This may be preferred over seeking new employment, but if the client can perform duties of his or her previous job, performing the same job title with a different employer is a viable option. Changing to a different job title with a new employer is commonly the most difficult thing to do. Relationships may be an important driver behind this phenomenon.

It has been established that the requirements of each client's job vary significantly; however, there are some requirements of working that are generic to all workplaces and jobs. Many of these issues are temporal in nature: workers must arrive to work on time, consistently work

Table 11-1

O*NET Categories for Work

	Definition	*Groupings*
Abilities	Enduring attributes of the individual that influence performance	*Cognitive abilities*: 21 abilities, such as deductive reasoning, oral comprehension, visualization, memorization, problem sensitivity *Physical abilities*: 9 abilities, such as dynamic flexibility, stamina, static strength *Psychomotor abilities*: 10 abilities, such as finger dexterity, reaction time, speed of limb movement *Sensory abilities*: 12 abilities, such as far vision, sound localization, auditory attention
Knowledge	Organized sets of principles and facts in general domains	*Subject categories*: 33 categories, such as fine arts, clerical, mathematics, mechanical, psychology, sales/marketing, education, administration, design, accounting, building
Skills	Developed capacities that facilitate learning or the more rapid acquisition of knowledge	*Basic skills*: 10 skills, such as active listening, critical thinking, learning strategies, writing *Complex problem solving skills*: identifying complex problems and reviewing related information to develop and evaluate options and implement solutions *Resource management skills* *Social skills*: coordination, persuasion, negotiation, instructing, service orientation, social perceptiveness *Systems skills*: judgment/decision making, systems analysis, systems evaluation *Technical skills*: 11 skills, such as installation, programming, repairing, troubleshooting, technology design
Work Activities	General types of job behaviors occurring on multiple jobs	*Information input*: 5 activities, such as getting information, monitor processes/materials/surroundings *Interacting with others* *Mental processes* *Work output*
Work Context	Physical and social factors that influence the nature of work	*Interpersonal relationships* *Physical work conditions* *Structural job characteristics*
Work Values	Global aspects of work that are important to a person's satisfaction	*Achievement* *Independence* *Recognition* *Relationships* *Support* *Working conditions*

their required schedule, perform assigned work tasks for a specified period of time, take and return from work breaks on time, and tolerate working the number of hours they are scheduled to work. Workers must sustain required productivity levels and/or complete all assigned work. Work must be performed accurately and the quality of the output must be acceptable. In most work settings, workers must have good hygiene, be well groomed, and wear clothing and personal protection equipment that is required of the workplace. Workers must be able to accept direction from their supervisors, modify behaviors based on feedback, interact with coworkers in an acceptable manner, and maintain socially appropriate behaviors in the workplace. It is important for the occupational therapist to address these generic work requirements in addition to the specific abilities required to perform required job tasks.

Table 11-2

Physical Demand Characteristics of Work

	Occasional 0% to 33%	*Frequent 34% to 66%*	*Constant 67% to 100%*	*Energy Requirement*
Sedentary	10 lbs	Negligible	Negligible	1.5 to 2.1 mets
Light	20 lbs	10 lbs	Negligible	2.2 to 3.5 mets
Medium	20 to 50 lbs	10 to 25 lbs	10 lbs	3.6 to 6.3 mets
Heavy	50 to 100 lbs	25 to 50 lbs	10 to 20 lbs	6.4 to 7.5 mets
Very heavy	Over 100 lbs	Over 50 lbs	Over 20 lbs	Over 7.5 mets

Reprinted with permission from Matheson L, Matheson M, Grant J. Development of a measure of perceived functional ability. *J Occup Rehabil.* 1993;3(1):15-30.

Table 11-3

Assessment Method/Measures of Person-Level Functions

Person-Level Functions	*Assessment Method/Measure*
Cognition	Montreal Cognitive Assessment
Executive function	Executive Function Performance Test, Test of Everyday Attention
Self-awareness	Patient Competency Rating Scale, Awareness Questionnaire, Self-Awareness of Deficits Interview, Gage Self-efficacy Scale
Motor	
Strength/endurance	Grip/pinch, manual muscle testing, isokinetic testing, muscle endurance test
Flexibility	Gross body screen, goniometry, inclinometry, sit and reach test, estimation
Manual material handling	EPIC Lift Capacity Test, Gibson Approach
Positional tolerance	Gross Screen of job specific positional tolerance testing
Manipulation/coordination	Crawford Small Parts, Minnesota Rate of Manipulation, 9-hole, Jebsen Hand Function, Purdue Pegboard, O'Connell Finger Dexterity
Physiology	
Resting/exercise vital signs	Blood pressure, heart rate, respiration rate, oxygen saturation
Cardiopulmonary endurance	Rockport Walking test, 6-minute walk test, YMCA 3-minute step test
Perceived exertion	Borg's perceived rate of exertion scale, talk test
Fatigue	Multidimensional Assessment of Fatigue Scale
Psychological/Emotional	
Depression	Beck Depression, Center for Epidemiologic Studies Depression Scale
Fear avoidance	Fear Avoidance Beliefs Questionnaire
Anxiety	Hopkin's Symptom Check List, State-Trait Anxiety Inventory
Sensory	
Pain	University of Alabama Pain Behavior Scale, Brief Pain Inventory, Ransford Pain diagram, Visual analogue scale, Roland Morris Disability Questionnaire, Dallas Pain Questionnaire, McGill Pain Questionnaire, Pain Disability Index

(continued)

Table 11-3 (continued)

ASSESSMENT METHOD/MEASURES OF PERSON-LEVEL FUNCTIONS

Person-Level Functions	*Assessment Method/Measure*
Sensory	
Touch Sensation	Light touch, Semmes-Weinstein Monofilaments, Moberg pickup test, vibrometry threshold tests, touch pressure, pain, temperature, static and moving 2-point discrimination, proprioception
Vision	Acuity, visual field, eye dominance, scanning, color vision, depth perception
Audition	Ability to follow directions and answers interview questions
Balance	Berg Balance Test, Get up and go, Tinetti Balance Screen
Olfaction	Scratch and Sniff test, job-related smell test

Table 11-4

ASSESSMENTS FOR WORK PERFORMANCE AT THE ENVIRONMENT AND OCCUPATIONAL LEVEL

Environment Level Measures

- Work Environment Impact Scale
- Job Content Questionnaire
- Job Requirements and Physical Demands Survey
- American Conference of Governmental Industrial Hygienists' Threshold Limit Value for Hand-Activity Level
- Work Organization Assessment Questionnaire
- Work Organization Assessment Tool
- Moos Work Environment Scale
- Physical measures (force gauge, tape measure, scale)*

Occupation Level Measures

- Assessment of Work Performance
- Canadian Occupational Performance Measure
- Career Assessment Inventory
- Dialogue About Ability Related to Work
- Disability Arm Shoulder Hand Work Module
- Functional Abilities Confidence Scale
- Feasibility Evaluation Checklist*
- Job Content Questionnaire
- Job Performance Measure*
- Need for Recovery After Work
- Occupational Questionnaire
- Occupational Performance History Interview
- Occupational Role Questionnaire
- Occupational Self-Assessment
- Personnel Test for Industry—Oral Directions Test
- Roland Morris Disability Questionnaire
- Self-Directed Search
- Spinal Function Sort
- Valpar Work Samples
- Vermont Disability Question
- Wonderlic Personnel Test
- Work Ability Index
- Work Confidence Measure*
- Work Instability Scale
- Work Limitations Questionnaire
- Work Productivity and Impairment Questionnaire
- Worker Role Interview

*Non-standardized assessment

Table 11-5

Assessments for Work Performance at the Environment and Occupational Level

Productivity

- Quality of productivity
- Quantity of productivity
- Attendance
- Timeliness
- Workplace tolerance
- Workplace instructability
- Workplace memory
- Follow through with accepted direction
- Concentration

Safety

- Timeliness
- Workplace instructability
- Adherence to safety rules
- Use of proper body mechanics
- Workplace safety—audition
- Workplace safety—vision
- Workplace safety—sensation
- Workplace safety—balance
- Use of protective behavior

Interpersonal Behavior

- Accept direction from supervisor
- General worker attitude
- Follows dress code
- Adjusts to different supervisors or supervisory styles
- Response to fellow workers
- Response to customers
- Response to change

Table 11-6

Constructs and Assessment for Work

Person-Level Functions	*Assessment Method/Measure*
Cognition	Montreal Cognitive Assessment
Executive function	Executive Function Performance Test, Test of Everyday Attention
Self-awareness	Patient Competency Rating Scale, Awareness Questionnaire, Self-Awareness of Deficits Interview, Gage Self-efficacy Scale
Motor	
Strength/endurance	Grip/pinch, manual muscle testing, muscle endurance test
Flexibility	Gross total body screen, goniometry for select joints
Manual material handling	EPIC Lift Capacity Test, Gibson Approach
Positional tolerance	Gross screen of job specific positional tolerance testing
Manipulation/coordination	Crawford Small Parts, Minnesota Rate of Manipulation
Physiology	
Resting/exercise vital signs	Blood pressure, heart rate, respiration rate, oxygen saturation
Cardiopulmonary endurance	Rockport Walking test, 6-minute walk test, YMCA 3-minute step test
Perceived exertion	Borg's perceived rate of exertion scale, talk test
Fatigue	Need for Recovery After Work Instrument

(continued)

Table 11-6 (continued)

Constructs and Assessment for Work

Person-Level Functions	*Assessment Method/Measure*
Psychological/Emotional	
Depression	Beck Depression, Center for Epidemiologic Studies Depression Scale
Fear avoidance	Fear Avoidance Beliefs Questionnaire
Anxiety	Hopkin's Symptom Check List, State-Trait Anxiety Inventory
Sensory	
Pain	University of Alabama Pain Behavior Scale, Brief Pain Inventory, Pain diagram, 0 to 10 rating scale, Visual analogue scale, Roland Morris Disability Questionnaire, Dallas Pain Questionnaire
Touch Sensation	Light touch, Semmes-Weinstein Monofilaments, Moberg pickup test, vibrometry threshold tests, touch pressure, pain, temperature, static and moving 2-point discrimination, proprioception
Vision	Visual acuity (Snellen), visual field testing, eye dominance, visual scanning
Audition	Ability to follow directions and answers interview questions
Balance	Berg Balance Test, Get up and go, Tinetti Balance Screen
Olfaction	Scratch and Sniff test, job-related smell test
Spirituality	Hope Questions, FICA Spiritual Assessment Tool, Spiritual Well-Being Scale
Social Capital	Life Stressors and Social Resources Inventory, Kouvonen's measure
Social Support	Social Support Inventory for People with Disabilities
Work Requirements	Job Content Questionnaire, Work Environment Scale
Physical Environment	Observational Checklist during Onsite Job Analysis, OSHA tool, NIOSH Revised Lift Equation, Rapid Upper Limb Assessment, Rapid Entire Body Assessment, Job Strain Index

Table 11-7

Occupation Level Work Assessment Tables in Chapter

Occupation Level Measures

- Assessment of Work Performance
- Career Assessment Inventory
- Dialogue About Ability Related to Work-DOA
- Disability Arm Shoulder Hand Work Module
- Functional Abilities Confidence Scale
- Feasibility Evaluation Checklist
- Job Content Questionnaire
- Need for Recovery After Work
- Occupational Questionnaire
- Occupational Performance History
- Interview
- Occupational Role Questionnaire
- Occupational Self-Assessment
- Personnel Test for Industry-Oral Directions Test
- Roland Morris Disability Questionnaire
- Self-Directed Search
- Spinal Function Sort
- Valpar Work Samples
- Vermont Disability Question
- Wonderlic Personnel Test
- Work Ability Index
- Work Instability Scale
- Work Limitations Questionnaire
- Work Productivity and Impairment Questionnaire
- Worker Role Interview

Table 11-8

Assessment of Work Performance

Source	Sandqvist[28]
Key References	Sandqvist and Henriksson[29]; Sandqvist et al[30]; Kielhofner[31]
Purpose	• Assesses individual's observable working skills • Provides information regarding how efficiently and appropriately the client performs a work activity.
Type of Client	• Individual with various kinds of working clients. It is not limited to any particular diagnosis or deficits, nor does it target any specific tasks or contexts.
Test Format	• Observation instrument where the client plays an active role in selecting work tasks and work environment to evaluate the client's performance.
Procedures	• The assessor observes the client perform a work task. The assessor makes notes regarding the client's performance on 14 different skills and ranks the performance on a 4-point ordinal rating scale (1 = incompetent performance; 4 = competent performance).
Time Required	• May be used by occupational therapists or other professionals familiar with assessing work functioning. • Testing time may vary from a few hours to weeks, depending on client's work demands.
Standardization	• Administration manual available for $40.00. Assessor needs to have experience examining work performance.
Reliability	• Not reported
Validity	• Questionnaire was answered by 67 respondents who had previously used the AWP in work rehabilitation settings in Sweden. The majority of respondents (63%) believed that the AWP examined all potential working skills "to a great extent."[30]

Table 11-9

Career Assessment Inventory

Source	http://www.pearsonclinical.com/psychology/products/100000574/career-assessment-inventory-the-enhanced-version-cai.html
Key References	Johansson[32]
Purpose	• Occupational interest inventory for college-bound or non-college-bound individuals
Type of Client	• 15 years of age or older; 8th grade reading level or above.
Test Format	• Paper and pencil or computer based administration.
Procedures	• Each individual is given test booklet and data collection form. The test is not timed and there are 370 items. All questions on 5-point rating scale. Non-completion of up to 25 items will have little impact on overall patterns or results.
Time Required	• No specific training required, but must be familiar with administration manual. • 35 to 40 minutes to complete.
Standardization	• Standardization of scales was developed through mailing 900 representatives from various occupational groups. These scales have been standardized and updated.
Reliability	• Test-retest reliability ranged from 0.91 to 0.96 for general theme scales, 0.88 to 0.95 for basic interest scale, 0.81 to 0.96 for the occupational scales.
Validity	• Internal consistency coefficient between 0.89 and 0.92.

Table 11-10

DIALOGUE ABOUT ABILITY RELATED TO WORK

Source	Linddahl et al[33]
Key References	Linddahl[34]; Norrby and Linddahl[35]
Purpose	• The purpose is to provide support for both the client and therapist in assessing the client's ability to work and rehabilitate. Follows the Model of Human Occupation.
Type of Client	• Working age individuals involved in both paid and unpaid activities.
Test Format	• Two sections: Client self-assessment and professional's objective assessment focusing on the individual's working ability. • Followed by a dialogue to distinguish goals related to the return-to-work process based on client's preference.
Procedures	• Client assesses self, therapist assesses client, then discussion occurs between client and therapist about therapist's interpretation of the client's ability.
Time Required	• Not noted
Standardization	• Has been studied widely in the US and Sweden.
Reliability	• Spearman Rank Correlation test for most items $r = 0.51$ to 0.75. Percentage of agreement 93.1% to 96.5%[35]
Validity	• 29 of 34 items showed acceptable goodness-of-fit statistic MnSq values from >0.6 to <1.4 in association with Z values from –2 to 2. Five items that did not fit well were revised.[33]

Table 11-11

DISABILITIES OF THE ARM, SHOULDER, AND HAND (DASH): WORK MODULE

Source	Solway et al[36]; For full DASH assessment and scoring instructions: http://dash.iwh.on.ca/
Key References	Hudak et al[37]; Marx et al[38]; Beaton et al[39,40]; Kennedy et al[41]; Hunsaker et al[42]
Purpose	• Assesses the impact of upper extremity disorders on work performance • The Work DASH is an optional module of the full DASH (30 items)
Type of Client	• Individuals with upper extremity disorders who are currently employed or for whom the worker role is important
Test Format	• 4-item questionnaire self-report survey based on a 1-week recall period. (Psychometrics not tested for test administration by proxy or telephone.)
Procedures	• Client is provided a paper version of the survey; there is no time limit. The questionnaire should be completed with no assistance from others (family, friends, or clinicians).
Time Required	• 4 questions, 1 to 2 minutes to complete. Proctors should be familiar with testing procedure specified in user manual.
Standardization	• The user manual describes procedures for proctoring and scoring exam. The administration procedures were jointly developed by the Institute for Work and Health, Ontario Canada and the American Academy of Orthopedic Surgeons, Rosemont Illinois.
Reliability	• Internal Consistency: Cronbach Alpha = 0.89[43]

(continued)

Table 11-11 (continued)

Disabilities of the Arm, Shoulder, and Hand (DASH): Work Module

Validity	• Spearman correlation coefficients when compared to similar measures • Work Instability Scale for Rheumatoid Arthritis (RA-WIS): 0.52 • Work Limitations Questionnaire (WLQ-16): -0.59 • Stanford Presenteeism Scale (SPS): -0.34[43]
Strengths	• Widely used in research and clinical practice • Established norms • Quickly and easily administered • Short completion time • No formal training required
Weaknesses	• Little psychometric testing done on the Work DASH alone • Assessment is self-report

Table 11-12

Functional Abilities Confidence Scale

Source	http://www.cptrehab.com/agencyforms/CPT%20forms/Functional_abilities_confidence_scale.pdf
Key References	Williams et al[44,45]
Purpose	• To measure the degree of self-efficacy or confidence a patient exhibits with various movements or postures
Type of Client	• Client able to complete questionnaire.
Test Format	• Pen/paper
Time Required	• 15 questions, 10 minutes to complete
Standardization	• Standardization performed with group of 20 subjects to measure test-retest reliability and to 94 subjects for validity testing
Reliability	• ICC = .94
Validity	• Discriminant: baseline scores and 3-week scores judged by clinicians demonstrated ability to discriminate ability to work • Responsiveness to change: able to detect gains in all aspects of physical conditioning over 3-week program. Strong within-group change for subjects with and without back injuries, effect size of .49 was positive and in direction and moderate in magnitude (change of 13 units on 100-point scale represents clinically important differences) • Convergent validity: moderate positive correlations with Resumption of Activities of Daily Living Scale and inversely with Roland-Morris scale score, slight relationship with Physical Self-Efficacy Scale[44]
Strengths	• Strong psychometric properties. Systematic review of self-report health-related work outcome measures for patients with musculoskeletal disorders gave the FAC the highest quality ratings of all measures identified (6 constructs reviewed were content and construct validity, internal consistency, test-retest reliability, responsiveness, and ease of scoring)[45]
Weaknesses	• Only available in English. Focuses on confidence in physical abilities only, not social, cognitive, or self-management abilities

Table 11-13

Feasibility Evaluation Checklist (FEC)

Source	Program in Occupational Therapy, Washington University School of Medicine, 4444 Forest Park, St. Louis, 63108
Key References	Matheson et al[46]
Purpose	• Designed to evaluate the presence of behavioral requirements all employers in the competitive labor market have of any employee. These include attendance, timeliness, workplace tolerance, and ability to accept supervision.
Type of Client	• Adolescents and adults for whom the worker role is pertinent.
Test Format	• 21-item behavior rating scale. Each item is briefly described on the scale.
Procedures	• 21 factors in the FEC are measured by observation of the evaluee in an actual or simulated work environment, often in a sheltered workshop or at a therapeutic workstation. The work environment must be structured to approximate the temporal demands of work, requiring regular daily attendance and adherence to a set schedule.
Time Required	• 5 to 10 minutes
Standardization	• The administration procedures were developed at the Work Preparation Center at Rancho Los Amigos Hospital in Downey, California.
Reliability	• Matheson[47] used a simple scoring system to identify the number of items that were rated "non-feasible" with 43 industrial rehabilitation clients. Over a 24-hour interval, the FEC demonstrated a reliability coefficient of 0.78.
Validity	• The items for the FEC were identified by employers and rehabilitation placement specialists in a survey conducted at Rancho as those that most often cause a return to work attempt by a disabled client to result in failure. Altogether, 53 items were identified. These were grouped and items that overlapped were consolidated to provide the current set of 21 items.
Strengths	• Has been used in a wide variety of rehabilitation settings since its introduction. • Can be used by professional raters, paraprofessional raters, and for self-rating by clients.
Weaknesses	• Need to observe client for a full workday over multiple days in work environment or simulated work environment.
Final Word	• Can be used to evaluate first steps in the return to work process. Requires more validity testing.

Table 11-14

Job Content Questionnaire (JCQ)

Source	Karasek[48]
Key References	Cheng et al[49]; Ostry et al[50]; Karasek et al[51,52]; Storms et al[53]
Purpose	• Measure perceptions of social and psychological characteristics of jobs for assessments of work quality at both the level of the individual and system or organizational level.
Type of Client	• Individual workers and work organizations.
Test Format	• Self-report instrument of 49 questions organized along 5 scales: 1) decision latitude, 2) psychological demands, 3) social support, 4) physical demands, 5) job insecurity

(continued)

Table 11-14 (continued)

Job Content Questionnaire (JCQ)

Type of Client	
Procedures	• Rate statements about their jobs using a 4-point scale (1 = fully agree/very unlikely; 4 = fully disagree/very likely). Scores are summed within 5 scales and are often collapsed into dichotomous scores for interpretation of high and low. Scores can be compared to national scale scores or norms from US and Sweden by sex, occupation, and industry (eg, compare findings in a plant to national averages).
Time Required	• JCQ takes 15 minutes to complete.
Standardization	• JCQ has a manual with norms and has been translated in over 12 languages. International board of researchers decides on policy and developmental issues. It has short direct-questioning format (subscales condensed into 1 question) and validated in Holland as a potential screening tool.
Reliability	• Cronbach's alpha were 0.71 and 0.76, with one notable item-to-total Pearson correlation of 0.21 for control subscale "repetitive work." Psychological Demands scale has consistently scored lower than other scales (ie, 0.57 to 0.67 in 4 different samples).
Validity	• Scales are based on Karasek's demand/control model of job strain development. Items derived statistically from survey data collected for the US Department of Labor. Core set of 27 questions developed on a pooled sample of 4,900 respondents. To increase efficiency, utility, and applicability, test has had multiple revisions. For criterion validity, individual subscales of the Dutch version correlated significantly with 7 criterion variables, including a General Health Questionnaire. • For construct validity, Karasek et al[52] established cross-national validity in United States, Canada, Netherlands, and Japan across wide occupational spectrum (16,601 participants) and ages; conditions in modern industrial nations are more consistent across national boundaries than across occupational groups; consistent ability to discriminate occupation. Scores predictive of job-related illness development (eg, psychological distress, coronary heart disease, musculoskeletal disease, reproductive disorders) in several countries[52] and confirmed constructs of Karasek's demand/control model.[51]
Strengths	• Well standardized for multiple cultures • Can be self-administered with minimal assistance • Has theoretical basis that allows application in social policy and organizational change. • Used broadly in many different settings both to analyze effect of job characteristics on individual's relative risk of job-related illness development, and testing of social policy effect on worker group's activation, motivation, and job satisfaction.
Weaknesses	• For comprehensive assessment of stress, would need to add measure of non–job-related stress. • For coping with stress, would need to add personality scales. • Demand/control model does not account for cognitive appraisal of events. • Psychological Demands subscale consistently performs weaker than other subscales. • Organizational-level job factors not included. • Usage fee required in some instances. The JCQ is provided with research documentation to most users free of charge, but commercial use and large research studies pay a usage fee. Approval required from author prior to using; contact JCQ Center at http://www.jcqcenter.org.
Final Word	• Well-standardized tool with broad application and use.

Table 11-15

Need for Recovery After Work (NFR)

Source	van Veldhoven[54]
Key References	Sluiter et al[55]; van Veldhoven and Broersen[56]
Purpose	• Need for recovery after work is based upon the Effort-Recovery Model.[57] Job demands produce load effects (emotional, cognitive, and behavioral) that are reversed when work stops. The NFR is the English version of the Dutch Questionnaire on the Experience and Assessment of Work.
Type of Client	• Any worker
Test Format	• 11-item dichotomous self-report scale that measures severity and duration of symptoms indicating that the respondent is not fully recovered from work effort
Procedures	• Evaluee completes the 11 yes/no questions
Time Required	• 5 minutes
Standardization	• The Dutch version has been widely studied, but the English version is less researched
Reliability	• Rho=.87.[58] Cronbach's alpha=.88.[56] Test-retest reliability=.55 to .69 in truck drivers and .48 to .80 in nurses.[59]
Validity	• Correlates with the Utrecht Burnout Scale at .84 in occupational physicians[60] and .75 in policemen.[60] Prospective correlation with accidents found a RR=2.28 for workers in the highest tertile on NFR compared to those in the lowest tertile (95% CI=1.4 to 3.66).[61] High baseline NFR scores were associated with an increased risk for subsequent sickness absence (OR=2.19, 95% CI 1.13 to 4.24) after adjustment for age, previous sickness absence, marital status, educational level, and company size.[62]
Strengths	• Simple scale that is quick and easy to administer and score • Widely researched
Weaknesses	• Does not measure fatigue at work • Not widely researched in the US

Table 11-16

Occupational Performance History Interview II (OPHI-II)

Source	Kielhofner et al[63]
Key References	Kielhofner et al[64,65]; Mallinson et al[66]
Purpose	• Designed to assess 3 constructs of occupational adaptation: occupational identity, occupational competence, and the impact of occupation behavior settings
Type of Client	• Occupational therapy clients who are capable of responding to an in-depth interview
Test Format	• Semi-structured interview. Focuses on the following thematic areas: occupational roles, daily routine, activity/occupational choices, critical life events, and occupational behavior settings
Procedures	• Interview administered by occupational therapist. It consists of 3 rating scales (Occupational Identity, Occupational Competence, and Occupational Behavior Settings) and the Life History Narrative (qualitative data from interview)
Time Required	• OPHI-II takes approximately 1 hour

(continued)

Table 11-16 (continued)

Occupational Performance History Interview II (OPHI-II)

Standardization	• Manual available from AOTA provides rating scales and suggests possible sequence and format of questions
Reliability	• Rater separation statistics indicated that raters have the same degree of severity and leniency • Test-retest validity was not reported; however, data for original OPHI showed poor to adequate test-retest reliability (r=0.31 to 0.68)
Validity	• For content validity, using RASCH analysis methods, strong evidence that test items captured underlying traits. Low percentage of misfit statistics (8% to 9%) indicate validity across different subjects. For construct validity, separation statistics indicate OPHI-II can detect meaningful differences between persons and levels of competence.
Strengths	• OPHI-II can be readily learned through the manual and used with a wide variety of clients. • Validity evidence is stronger than the original OPHI • Based on well-known theory • Intervention plan can be developed from assessment results
Weaknesses	• Therapist, rather than client, assigns the scores • Presumes therapist familiarity with Model of Human Occupation • Administration may be time consuming
Final Word	• Client-centered assessment for establishment of clinical goals. Most appropriate when therapy can be structured to maximize knowledge of client's life history

Table 11-17

Occupational Role Questionnaire

Source	Kopec and Esdaile[67]
Key References	Amick et al[68]
Purpose	• To study chronic condition effects on occupational role, specifically in the workplace
Type of Client	• 18 years old and older
Test Format	• 8-item self-report questionnaire
Procedures	• 2 subscales with 4 items in each scale. One scale is the productivity/job performance scale; the other is a satisfaction with work scale. Scales are aggregated into a single summary scale
Time Required	• 10 minutes
Standardization	• The scales have sound psychometric support. Available in both French and English
Reliability	• Internal consistency, alpha=0.88), test-retest reliability (0.91), and correlates with pain (r5)
Validity	• The items have face validity; identifies 2 distinct factors

Table 11-18

Occupational Self Assessment (OSA)

Source	Baron et al[69]
Key References	Taylor et al[70]; Kielhofner et al[71]; Keller et al[72]
Purpose	• Outcome measure intended to be assessed at initial evaluation and follow-up to create a client-centered therapy plan • Designed to capture clients' perceptions of their own occupational competence and of the occupations they consider important • Used to plan and establish priorities for occupational goals • Assess client progress and program effectiveness
Type of Client	• Ability to self-reflect and have a higher level of functioning and some insight. OSA requires basic reading skills and the ability to collaborate in goal-setting tasks. There are no cultural background limitations. Designed for individuals over the age of 12 years; however, the COSA (children's version) is available for ages 12 years and younger.
Test Format	• OSA has 2-part self-rating form and 3 content areas with the following subcontent areas: 1) Skills/Occupational Performance; 2) Habituation—Habits, Roles; 3) Volition—Personal Causation, Values, Interests. There are 8 steps: create appropriate context for administration, communicate intent of the OSA to the client and explain instructions, have client self-administer and complete the rating forms, review OSA with client, collaborate to identify therapy goals and strategies, complete planning, implement occupational therapy services form with client, and complete OSA key forms. For comparison of progress, have client complete OSA follow-up form.
Procedures	• The preferred setting is client-based. If clients will do better and be able to reflect on their answers, assigning it as "homework" may suit the client. If the client would do better given time during therapy so the client can ask questions then that can be done as well. It is important that the client has sufficient time to reflect in a quiet, private area.
Time Required	• 10 minutes for client to fill out. Approximately an additional 15 minutes for the therapist to discuss possible goals • Manual for training/administration: $40.00
Standardization	• OSA user's manual

Table 11-19

Personnel Tests for Industry: Oral Directions Test (ODT)

Source	Langmuir[73]
Key References	Angoff and Thorndike[74]; Doppelt and Seashore[75]; Wolfe and Davis[76]
Purpose	• Assess an individual's ability to follow oral directions.
Type of Client	• Designed for selection of applicants, adolescent or adults. It is especially effective in identifying more able individuals in low educational levels
Test Format	• Paper and pencil test
Procedures	• The ODT is a recorded test. Proctors should provide answer sheets and pencils, and ensure that volume is loud enough for participants.
Time Required	• Proctors should be familiar with test and procedures, which are explained in the manual. • Test lasts 15 minutes.

(continued)

Table 11-19 (continued)

Personnel Tests for Industry: Oral Directions Test (ODT)

Standardization	• Administration manual describes procedures for proctoring and scoring exam.
Reliability	• For internal consistency, split half reliability ranged from .73 to .86. • Between the first and second testing, test-retest reliability ranged from .79 to .93. Test-retest reliability for 1160 participants from the Dayton VA Center Domiciliary was .88
Validity	• For construct validity, ODT had a correlation of .70 Wechsler Adult Intelligence Scale (WAIS) for various groups of prison inmates and vocational rehabilitation clients. For concurrent validity, the correlation between ODT and Short Employment tests ranged from .30 to .49. Wolfe and Davis[76] found that the ODT and Wesman had a correlation coefficient of .67, while the ODT and WAIS full-scale IQ had a correlation coefficient of .86 and Wesman Verbal Test.

Table 11-20

Roland Morris Disability Questionnaire (RDQ)

Source	Roland and Fairbank[77]
Key References	Stratford et al[78]; Smeets et al[79]; Artus et al[80]; Wilkens et al[81]; Lamb et al[82]; Hay et al[83]; Mannion et al[84]
Purpose	• Assesses physical disability due to low back pain (LBP)
Type of Client	• Client presenting with low back pain
Test Format	• Self-report with 24 questions
Procedures	• Indicate whether the statement related to back pain is true to you during that day. Scores range from 0 (no disability) to 24 (maximal disability). Lower scores indicate less disability, whereas higher scores represent greater disability.
Time Required	• 5 minutes
Standardization	• Translations are available in Arabic (Egyptian), Bulgarian, Chinese, Croatian, Czech, Danish, Dutch, English (Canadian, US, Australian), Flemish, French, German, Greek, Hungarian, Icelandic, Iranian, Italian, Japanese, Korean, Norwegian, Polish, Portuguese, Brazilian Portuguese, Moroccan, Romanian, Russian, Spanish, Argentinean, Columbian, Mexican, Puerto Rican, Venezuelan, Swedish, Thai, Tunisian, and Turkish, as well as for India (Hindi, Kannada, Marathi, Tamil, Telugu, Urdu). Several of these versions have not been validated.
Reliability	• For internal consistency, r = .84 to .96.[77] For test-retest, r = .83 to .91.[77] Pearson's correlation coefficients for test–retest in patients with acute/subacute LBP are 0.91 for the same day, 0.88 for 1 week, and 0.83 for 3 weeks. In patients with chronic LBP, a correlation coefficient of 0.72 (interval 2 days to 6 months) was found.[77]

(continued)

Table 11-20 (continued)

Roland Morris Disability Questionnaire (RDQ)

Validity	• For construct validity, RDQ scores correlate moderately to strongly with other self-reported disability measures: Quebec Back Pain Disability Scale (r=0.60), Back Pain Functional Scale(r=0.79) , Aberdeen Back Pain Scale (r=0.68), Isernhagen Works Systems Functional Capacity (r=0.20), EuroQol (r=0.50).[85-87]
Strengths	• The RDQ is the most comprehensively validated measure in low back pain. • It is short, simple to complete, and readily understood by patients and clinicians. • Psychometric properties are acceptable to good and the RDQ is available in many language versions. It can be used in patients with acute, subacute, and chronic LBP, and has been translated and validated in multiple languages.
Weaknesses	• There is some evidence that the RDQ does not provide a sufficient spread of items representing activities on a continuum from easy to hard. • The poor fit of some items to the factor "disability" needs further attention. None of the versions have sufficient items of higher difficulty to assess persons with low levels of disability, making it inadequate for assessing function in patients with little disability
Final Word	• The administrative and respondent burden is very low. RDQ scores and changes scores must be interpreted with caution due to poor-fitting items and the fact that the RDQ does not appear to have interval-level properties. It is inadequate for use in patients with little disability.

Table 11-21

Self-Directed Search (SDS)

Source	PAR (Psychological Assessment Resources, Inc), PO Box 998, Odessa, Florida, USA, 33556
Key References	SDS[88]
Purpose	• Designed to help individuals discover and evaluate potential career interests and future planning for education (eg, college, training)
Type of Client	• Clients who are capable of completing an in-depth inventory. High school/college students, adults, and those with a fourth grade reading level or above
Test Format	• Self-administered questionnaire; computerized administration available, can be administered individually or in groups
Procedures	• Each individual is given test booklet and self-completes it
Time Required	• No specific training required, but must be familiar with administration manual • 25 to 35 minutes to complete • 20 minutes to complete online
Standardization	• Standardized using a sample of 1739 people
Reliability	• Internal consistency coefficients for Activities, Competencies, and Occupation scales ranged from 0.72 to 0.93. Test-retest reliability ranged from 0.78 to 0.98
Validity	• SDS results have been supported by over 500 research studies • Concurrent validity was 54.7%, higher than the average range found in interest inventories

Table 11-22

Spinal Function Sort

Source	Employment Potential Improvement Corporation, P.O. Box 3897, Ballwin, MO.
Key References	Gibson and Strong[89]; Matheson et al[90-92]; Robinson et al[93]; Sufka et al[94]
Purpose	• To evaluate self-perceived ability to perform frequently encountered physical work tasks • To compare the evaluee's perception of ability to perform these tasks with his or her perception of the tasks and demand levels that are required in his or her occupational role
Type of Client	• Adolescents and adults for whom the worker role is pertinent
Test Format	• 50-item instrument organized in a test booklet, each item composed of a drawing of an adult of working age performing a work task. Two of the items have matched pairs in the instrument to allow checks on internal consistency.
Procedures	• Each evaluee is provided a test booklet, response sheet, and a pencil. The evaluee describes his or her ability to perform the task along a 5-point scale from "able" to "unable." The test is administered on an untimed basis.
Time Required	• 6 to 12 minutes
Standardization	• Administration procedures were developed in 6 industrial rehabilitation clinics with 180 subjects. Each drawing is accompanied by a simple task description presented in English, French, German, or Spanish. A tape recording of the task descriptions is provided for evaluees who are not functionally literate.
Reliability	• Matheson et al[91] reported that the split-half reliability of the Spinal Function Sort was evaluated through a comparison of odd and even items, yielding a Spearman-Brown correlation of 0.983. Gibson and Strong[89] reported a Cronbach's alpha of 0.98. Matheson et al[91] performed separate studies for men and women based on the "Rating of Perceived Capacity." Pearson coefficients for a 3-day interval were 0.85 for 126 adult males and 0.82 for 84 adult females. Similar coefficients have been reported in other studies.
Validity	• Correlated with the Pain Self-Efficacy Questionnaire (.78), Pain Disability Index (-.64), and Work Reentry Questionnaire (.67) with $p < .001$.[89]

Table 11-23

VALPAR Component Work Samples (VCWS)

Source	VALPAR International Corporation, PO Box 5767, Tucson, Arizona, USA, 85745
Key References	VALPAR[95]
Purpose	• Developed in order to assess task performance on simulated work tasks. The tasks have all been analyzed according to the Dictionary of Occupational Titles.
Type of Client	• Adolescents and adults for whom the worker role is pertinent
Test Format	• 50-item instrument organized in a test booklet, each item composed of a drawing of an adult of working age performing a work task. Two of the items have matched pairs in the instrument to allow checks on internal consistency.
Procedures	• Consists of individual work samples that simulate task performance, eg, for repetitive assembly work. For each task, there is a complete analysis of the skills and attitudes required for worker to complete that task. The client is instructed to perform each task according to a standard procedure, and then scored on timing and other characteristics.

(continued)

Table 11-23 (continued)

VALPAR Component Work Samples (VCWS)

Type of Client	
Time Required	• Tasks range from completion time of 20 to 90 minutes
Standardization	• The VALPAR is a complete standardized measure with specific manuals, instructions, and scoring directions for each work sample. Methods-Time-Measurement (MTM) methodology provides a time standard for the completion of the work sample. (MTM is standard representative of the time it would take for a well-trained worker to perform the task in a typical industrial setting in an 8-hour workday). MTM has also been used to establish normative data for the VALPAR Work samples related to Time percentiles and Time percent.
Reliability	• Test-retest reliability values of 0.70 to 0.99
Validity	• For content validity, many studies have been completed demonstrating high correspondence between items on the VALPAR Work Samples and required worker characteristics in the Dictionary of Occupational Titles. For construct validity, the VALPAR Work Samples are able to discriminate between workers employed or not employed in specific jobs.
Strengths	• Provides a comprehensive assessment of simulated job tasks • The samples have been well tested and scoring information for normative comparison is extensive
Weaknesses	• Requires more psychometric testing for predictive validity of return to work • Not readily available at this time
Final Word	• Useful for assessment of person and occupation, but does not take into account unique environmental demands with each job

Table 11-24

Vermont Disability Prediction Questionnaire

Source	Hazard et al[96]
Key References	Hazard et al[97]; Cats-Baril and Frymoyer[98]; Gray et al[99]
Purpose	• To predict chronic disability after occupational low back injury
Type of Client	• Clients who injured their back on the job
Test Format	• 11 self-report questions including physical and psychosocial factors on disability
Procedures	• Consists of individual work samples that simulate task performance (eg, for repetitive assembly work). For each task, there is a complete analysis of the skills and attitudes required for the worker to complete that task. The client is instructed to perform each task according to a standard procedure, and then scored on timing and other characteristics.
Time Required	• 5 minutes
Standardization	• No published information regarding translations
Reliability	• Not available

(continued)

Table 11-24 (continued)

Vermont Disability Prediction Questionnaire

Validity	• Good face and content validity. All items with Kappa > .1. Predicative Validity: RTW Kappa .048 and .36 (both at 3 months). Time Interval sensitivity: 0.94 and 0.75 (both at 3 months).[99]
Strengths	• Free and quick completion time • Assesses both psychosocial and physical factors • Useful scoring template and is able to be administered by telephone.
Weaknesses	• Psychometrics are only established from original authors in 2 studies • Not widely used
Final Word	• Useful instrument to use for workers who have injured their backs while at work and make recommendations for intervention to avoid long-term sick leave or chronic disability

Table 11-25

Wonderlic Personnel Test (WPT)

Source	*Wonderlic Personnel Test*[100]
Key References	Dodrill[101]; Dodrill and Warner[102]; McKelvie[103]; Wonderlic and Hovland[104]
Purpose	• Tests general cognitive ability and gauges the level at which an individual learns, understands instructions, and problem solves. • Provides quantitative insight to how easily an individual can be trained, adjust, and solve problems on the job.
Type of Client	• Primarily used by organizations examining job applicants
Test Format	• 50-item questionnaire that can be filled out in a test booklet or administered through a computer program.
Procedures	• Applicant is provided a test booklet and an exam proctor times the testing session for exactly 12 minutes. Proctors cannot answer questions. • Proctors of exam should be familiar with testing procedure specified in manual
Time Required	• Test must be completed in 12 minutes
Standardization	• Administration manual describes procedures for proctoring and scoring exam.
Reliability	• For English versions, internal consistency was .87.[103] Dodrill[101] found that short-term test-retest reliability ranged from .82 to .94, whereas long-term test-retest reliability was .94.
Validity	• For content validity, Hunter[105] determined that the WPT includes the same verbal, quantitative, and spatial items recognized as assessing general cognitive ability. For predictive validity, Schmidt and Hunter[106] found that predictive validity for ability was .63, college grades, biodata, education, reference checks, interests, interview, and age ranged from -.02 to .33. For construct validity, Dodrill and Warner[102] WPT and Wechsler Adult Intelligence Scale (WAIS) had a .92 correlation.

Table 11-26

Work Ability Index

Source	Tuomi et al[107]
Key References	DeZwart et al[108]; Kujala et al[109]; Ahlstrom et al[110]; Radkiewich and Widerszal-Bazyl[111]
Purpose	• Measures an individual's capacity to work. Physical and mental demands of work taken into account.
Type of Client	• Individual workers.
Test Format	• Self-report 10 questions on 7 dimensions: 1) current work ability compared with lifetime best; 2) work ability in relation to the demands of the job; 3) number of current diseases diagnosed by a physician; 4) estimated work impairment due to diseases; 5) sick leave during the past year; (6) own prognosis of work ability 2 years from now; 7) mental resources
Procedures	• Clients rate aspects of their job based on Likert scale. A work ability score is calculated. Scores range from 7 to 49 and are grouped and classified as poor, moderate, good, and excellent in regards to work ability. Norms can be found in the manual.
Time Required	• 10 minutes
Reliability	• Test-retest is acceptable with 66% agreement on 4-week interval.[108] For internal consistency: Iranian version found Chronbach's alpha = 0.79.[112]
Validity	• For criterion validity, Brazilian and Iranian versions found that the WAI was significantly correlated with the SF-36. The Brazilian and Iranian versions found the WAI to be explained by 3 components: mental resources (20.6% total variance), perception of work ability (18.9% total variance), and presence of diseases (18.4% of total variance).[112,113]
Strengths	• Widely used • Established norms • Easily administered
Weaknesses	• May need further probing to learn more about job demands • Not performance based
Final Word	• The work ability index is useful in the occupational health field to gain an overall assessment of a worker's work ability and also provides information regarding whether additional testing should be performed for the mental or physical demands of their work.

Table 11-27

Work Instability Scale

Source	Gilworth et al[114]
Key References	Beaton et al[115]; Tang et al[116,117]
Purpose	• Measures the extent of work instability (WI), which is defined as "a state in which the consequences of a mismatch between an individual's functional abilities and the demands of his or her job can threaten continuing employment if not resolved." • Originally developed specifically for rheumatoid arthritis (RA).
Type of Client	• Working clients with arthritis.
Test Format	• 23 questions, self-report.

(continued)

Table 11-27 (continued)

Work Instability Scale

Type of Client	
Procedures	• Yes/no response categories recalling information pertaining to that moment in time. Scores range from 0 to 23 and then categorized into low, moderate, or high work instability.
Time Required	• 5 minutes
Standardization	• Available in 18 languages. Adaptation of the scale requires explicit permission from Galen Research in Manchester. Cross-cultural validity of the RA-WIS has been shown for English, Dutch, German, and French.[118]
Reliability	• Gilworth et al[114] reported a test-retest correlation of r=0.89 (n=51); in a sample of 250 workers with RA or OA. Kuder-Richardson Formula-20 (KR-20) for the RA-WIS was 0.91 and item-total correlation ranged from 0.34 to 0.71. KR-20 was 0.93 for 130 patients with OA within this sample.
Validity	• For construct validity, r=.54 to .74.[116] For concurrent validity, Workplace Activity Limitations Scale (r=0.77), 6-item Stanford Presenteeism Scale (r=0.69), Endicott Work Productivity Scale (r=0.64), and Work Limitations Questionnaire Index (r=0.61), and correlated moderately with the HAQ (r=0.66), self-rated arthritis severity (r=0.62), and pain intensity (r=0.67).[114]
Strengths	• Quick and easy • Free • Solid psychometric properties
Weaknesses	• Limited population • Further questions may be needed to understand impact on work instability because recall is only in that day • Limited response categories
Final Word	• The RA-WIS is feasible and is a measure that has been well received by patients with arthritis or other musculoskeletal conditions. It has potential for clinical use for risk prognostication of adverse future work outcomes.

Table 11-28

Work Limitations Questionnaire (WLQ)

Source	Lerner et al[119]
Key References	Amick et al[68]; Noben et al[120]; Munir[121]; Prasad et al[122]
Purpose	• Assesses the degree to which health problems interfere with specific aspects of job performance and the consequent productivity impact of the work limitations.
Type of Client	• Individuals who are employed and experiencing limitations on the job due to health-related problems.
Test Format	• Paper and pencil, telephone, and online versions. • There are 2 versions of this test (25-item questionnaire, 8-item questionnaire) • An additional questionnaire was developed, WL-26 (particularly used by facilities evaluating musculoskeletal disorders).
Procedures	• WLQ is self-administered with instructions found within the questionnaire.

(continued)

Table 11-28 (continued)

WORK LIMITATIONS QUESTIONNAIRE

Type of Client	
Time Required	• No training is required and questionnaire takes 5 to 10 minutes to complete for either the short or long form.
Standardization	• Manual with scoring information. • Has been translated in over 30 languages for the telephone version.
Validity	• For construct validity, in a cross-sectional mail study, the relationship for each WQL scale was compared to the SF-36 Role/Physical scale and the Role/Emotional scale. Each WQL scale explained a significant portion of the variance in the SF-36 Role/Physical scale, and 3 WLQ scales explained a significant amount of the variation in the SF-36 Role/Emotional scale.[119] • For relative validity, each of the WLQ scales were compared to self-reported work productivity, compared to percent of time absent because of health, effectiveness of on symptom days, and the SF 36- Role Limitation scales. It was found that the WLQ Output Demands was the best predictor of productivity loss. The WLQ Mental-Interpersonal Demands and the SF-36 Role Limitation scales each exhibited half of the predictive power of the Output Demand scale. The remaining measures had poorer predictive Power.[119] • For criterion validity, there is conflicting evidence regarding criterion validity because in the 3 studies examining criterion validity, 1 study is in poor, 1 study is in fair, and 1 study is in good methodical quality.[120]

Table 11-29

WORK PRODUCTIVITY AND IMPAIRMENT QUESTIONNAIRE (WPAI)

Source	http://www.reillyassociates.net/WPAI_General.html
Key References	Reilly et al[123]; Wahlqvist et al[124]
Purpose	• The WPAI was designed to assess the amount of both absenteeism and presenteeism due to health problems
Type of Client	• Clients able to complete questionnaire, it cannot be modified, but it can be adapted to various specific diseases or health problems
Test Format	• Pen/paper • Online
Procedures	• The evaluee completes the survey with pen or online
Time Required	• No training required, questionnaire can be found on website for various conditions and in various languages
Standardization	• Reliability and validity vary depending on condition adaptation • Studies and information can be found on their website: http://www.reillyassociates.net/WPAI_References5.html

Table 11-30

Worker Role Interview (WRI)

Source	Velozo et al[125]; AOTA Products, PO Box 3800, Forrester Center, WV, 25438, (887) 404-AOTA
Key References	Biernacki[126]; Ekbladh et al[127]; Gern[128]; Lin[129]; Velozo et al[130]
Purpose	• Identify the psychosocial and environmental variables influencing a worker returning to work • Intended to be used during initial assessment as part of a physical and/or work capacity assessment • Facilitate rehabilitation planning by offering worker's perceptions and information about worker's ability to adjust habits and routines, commitment to the worker role
Type of Client	• Injured workers in vocational assessment/rehabilitation.
Test Format	• The WRI has 6 content areas with the following subcontent areas or rated factors: 1) Personal Causation—personal assessment of abilities & limitations, expectations of job success, takes responsibility; 2) Values—commitment to work, work-related goals; 3) Interests—enjoys work, pursues interests consistent with work; 4) Roles—identifies with being a worker, appraises work expect expectations, influence of other roles; 5) Habits—work habits, daily routine, adapts routine to minimize difficulties; 6) Environment—physical setting, perception of family and peers, perception of boss, perception of coworkers.
Procedures	• Five steps: interview preparation, semi-structured interview (at start of initial assessment), the usual physical/work capacity assessment procedures used by the organization, scoring the WRI Rating Form (following initial assessment), rescoring WRI Rating Form (at discharge from treatment). Therapist rates each subcontent area on a scale of 1 (strongly interferes with returning to job) to 4 (strongly supports client returning to job) giving brief comments in the margin to support each rating.
Time Required	• 30 to 45 minutes for interview, plus observation of work capacity assessment
Standardization	• WRI user's manual and videotape of interview administration available.
Reliability	• For internal consistency, Velozo et al[130] used Rasch Analysis to determine person separation reliability (analogous to Cronbach's alpha). They found that the WRI reliably differentiated injured workers based on ability levels. For inter-rater reliability, Biernacki[126] computed for 3 raters (n=30 adults in rehab for upper extremity injury): ICCs of 6 content areas ranged from 0.46 to 0.92. Test-retest reliability was high; ICCs ranged from 0.86 to 0.94 with total value of 0.95.
Validity	• For content validity, items are based on the Model of Human Occupation[131] and review of literature of factors impacting return to work. For criterion validity, there was evidence that the WRI discriminated between clients on psychosocial capacity for work. Velozo et al[130] studied work-injured claimants and found that the WRI did not predict return to work. Ekbladh et al[127] found that only 5 of 17 items predicted return to work for 48 injured workers; content area Personal Causation had the best predictive validity, while content areas values, interests and habits demonstrated no predictive validity. For construct validity, Velozo et al[130] conducted 2 studies with injured workers that found the WRI measures a unidimensional construct.
Strengths	• Has a theoretical basis • Provides descriptive information about how a worker views self as a worker and work environment • Facilitates understanding potential barriers to return to work and thereby facilitates rehab planning
Weaknesses	• Suggested questions require reorganization for better flow and rephrasing to reduce reactivity • Needs to be more broadly applied and tested in a variety of settings, therapists, and populations before used as an outcome measure
Final Word	• One of the few tools available to assess psychosocial and environmental variables influencing a worker returning to work

Appendix A: Job Performance Measure

I need to understand the job task you do at work and how well you think you can currently do these tasks. Here is a list of the job tasks for your job title. How often do you do each of these tasks?

If you had to do the task right now, how well do you think you would be able to do it?

- Transfer core task descriptions for client's job from O*NET website to form.
- Review task descriptions with client; modify descriptions to accurately reflect the client's job duties.
- If client performs additional work tasks on a daily basis that are not recorded, add these tasks to form.
- Record client's frequency ratings for each task using 1 to 7 scale.
- Record client's perception of current ability to perform the job task ratings on 1 to 10 scale.
- Total performance ratings and divide by number of tasks rated.

Frequency Rating 1 to 7	*O*NET Task Description*	*Performance Rating 1 to 10*

Performance Score = Total of all performance ratings __ / Total # of items rated __ =

Frequency		*Performance*
every hour or more	(7)	
several times a day	(6)	
daily	(5)	1 2 3 4 5 6 7 8 9 10
more than once a week	(4)	not able to do it — do it extremely well
more than once a month	(3)	
more than once a year	(2)	
once a year or less	(1)	

References

1. American Occupational Therapy Association. AOTA's centennial vision and executive summary. *Am J Occup Ther.* 2007;61:613-614.
2. American Occupational Therapy Association. Occupational therapy practice framework: Domain and process. 3rd ed. *Am J Occup Ther.* 2014;68:S1-S48.
3. Ruiz-Quintanilla S, England G. How working is defined: structure and stability. *J Organizational Behavior.* 1996;17:515-540.
4. Passier PE, Visser-Meily JM, Rinkel GJ, Lindeman E, Post MW. Life satisfaction and return to work after aneurysmal subarachnoid hemorrhage. *J Stroke Cerebrovasc Dis.* 2011;20(4):324-329
5. Baker NA, Jacobs, K. The nature of working in the United States: an occupational therapy perspective. *Work.* 2003;20(1):53-61.
6. Vestling M, Tufvesson B, Iwarsson S. Indicators for return to work after and the importance of work for subjective well-being and life satisfaction. *J Rehabil Med.* 2003;35:127-131.
7. Keogh J, Nnuwayhid I, Gordon J, Gucer P. The impact of occupational injury on injured workers and family: outcomes of upper extremity cumulative trauma disorders in Maryland workers. *Am J Ind Med.* 2000;39:4998-5061.
8. Turner J, Franklin G, Fulton-Kehow D, et al. Early predictors of chronic work disability associated with carpal tunnel syndrome: a longitudinal workers' compensation cohort study. *Am J Ind Med.* 2007;50:498-506.
9. Cawley J. An instrumental variables approach to measuring the effect of body weight on employment disability. *Health Serv Res.* 2000;35:1159-1179.
10. Musich S, Napier D, Edington DW. The association of health risks with workers' compensation costs. *J Occup Environ Med.* 2001;43(6):534-541.
11. Bureau of Labor Statistics. *Employment Projections: Civilian Labor Force Participation Rates By Age, Sex, Race and Ethnicity.* http://www.bls.gov/emp/ep_table_303.htm. Accessed September 30, 2014.
12. Matheson L. Symptom magnification syndrome structured interview: rationale and procedure. *J Occup Rehabil.* 1991;1(1):43-56.
13. Matheson LN, Verna J, Dreisinger TE, Leggett S, Mayer J. Age and gender normative data for lift capacity. *Work.* 2014;49(2):257-269.
14. Bureau of Labor Statistics. Occupational Classifications. http://www.bls.gov/soc/. Accessed September 30, 2014.
15. US Congress. Health Insurance Portability and Accountability Act of 1996, Public Law 104-191. Washington, DC: US Government Printing Office; 1996. https://www.gpo.gov/fdsys/pkg/PLAW-104publ191/html/PLAW-104publ191.htm. Accessed September 29, 2016.
16. Dale AM, Gardner BT, Zeringue A, et al. Self-reported physical work exposures and incident carpal tunnel syndrome. *Am J Ind Med.* 2014;57(11):1246-1254.
17. Isernhagen SJ. Functional capacity evaluation: rationale, procedure, utility of the kinesiophysical approach. *J Occup Rehabil.* 1992;2(3):157-168.
18. Cheung K, Hume P, Maxwell L. Delayed onset muscle soreness: treatment strategies and performance factors. *Sports Med.* 2003;33(2):145-164.
19. Soer R, Groothoff JW, Geertzen JH, van der Schans CP, Reesink DD, Reneman MF. Pain response of healthy workers following a functional capacity evaluation and implications for clinical interpretation. *J Occup Rehabil.* 2008;18(3):290-298.

20. Innes E, Straker L. Strategies used when conducting work-related assessments. *Work.* 2002;19(2):149-165.
21. Tuomi K, Järvinen E, Eskelinen L, Ilmarinen J, Klockars, M. Effect of retirement on health and work ability among municipal employees. *Scand J Work Environ Health.* 1991;17(Suppl 1):75-81.
22. Kaskutas V. The Job Performance Measure. Presented at 2008 American Occupational Therapy Association Annual Conference, Long Beach, CA.
23. Kaskutas V. Work incentives and policies in the United States and around the world. In: Braveman BH, Page JJ, eds. *Work: Promoting Participation & Productivity through Occupational Therapy.* Philadelphia: F.A. Davis Co; 2012:347-364.
24. Braveman BH, Page JJ. *Work: Promoting Participation & Productivity through Occupational Therapy.* Philadelphia: F.A. Davis Co; 2012:28-48.
25. Patton W, McMahon M. *Career Development and Systems Theory: Connecting Theory and Practice.* 2nd ed. Rotterdam: Sense Publishers; 2006:49-75.
26. Lent RW, Brown SD, Hackett G. Social cognitive career theory. *Career Choice Develop.* 2002;4:255-311.
27. O'Brien AN, Wolf TJ. Determining work outcomes in mild to moderate stroke survivors. *Work.* 2010;36(4):441-447.
28. Sandqvist J. *Assessment of Work Performance.* Norrkoping, Sweden: Linkoping University; 2009.
29. Sandqvist JL, Henriksson CM. Work functioning: a conceptual framework. *Work.* 2004;23(2):147-157.
30. Sandqvist JL, Gullberg MT, Henriksson CM, Gerdle BU. Content validity and utility of the Assessment of Work Performance (AWP). *Work.* 2008;30(4):441-450.
31. Kielhofner G. *Model of Human Occupation: Theory and Application.* 4th ed. Baltimore, MD: Lippincott Williams & Wilkins; 2008.
32. Johansson CB. *Career Assessment Inventory: The Enhanced Version.* Minnetonka, MN: National Computer Systems, Inc; 1986.
33. Linddahl I, Norrby E, Bellner AL. Construct validity of the instrument DOA: a dialogue about ability related to work. *Work.* 2002;20(3):215-224.
34. Linddahl I. *Validity and Reliability of the Instrument: A Dialogue About Working Ability.* Jönköping: Hälsohögskolan; 2007:50.
35. Norrby E, Linddahl I. Reliability of the instrument DOA: dialogue about ability related to work. *Work.* 2005;26(2):131-139.
36. Solway S, Beaton DE, McConnell S, Bombardier C. *The DASH Outcome Measure User's Manual.* Toronto, Ontario: Institute for Work & Health: 2002:5.
37. Hudak P, Amadio PC, Bombardier C. Development of an upper extremity outcome measure: the DASH (disabilities of the arm, shoulder, and hand). *Am J Ind Med.* 1996;29:602-608.
38. Marx RG, Bombardier C, Hogg-Johnson S, Wright JG. Clinimetric and psychometric strategies for development of a health measurement scale. *J Clin Epidemiol.* 1999;52(2):105-111.
39. Beaton DE, Davis AM, Hudak P, McConnell S. The DASH (disabilities of the arm, shoulder and hand) outcome measure: what do we know about it now? *J Hand Ther.* 2001;6(4):109-118.
40. Beaton DE, Eerd D, Smith P, et al. Minimal change is sensitive, less specific, to recovery: a diagnostic testing approach to interpretability. *J Clin Epidemiol.* 2011;64(5):487-496.
41. Kennedy CA, Beaton DE, Solway S, McConnell S, Bombardier C. *The DASH and QuickDASH Outcome Measure User's Manual.* 3rd ed. Toronto, Ontario: Institute for Work & Health; 2011.
42. Hunsaker FG, Cioffi DA, Amadio PC, Wright JG, Caughlin B. The American Academy of Orthopaedic Surgeons outcomes instruments – normative values from the general population. *J Bone Joint Surg Am.* 2002;84-A(2):208-215.
43. Tang K, Pitts S, Solway S, Beaton D. Comparison of the psychometric properties of four at-work disability measures in workers with shoulder or elbow disorders. *J Occup Rehabil.* 2009;19(2):142-154.
44. Williams R, Myers A. Functional Abilities Confidence Scale: a clinical measure for injured worker with acute low back pain. *Phys Ther.* 1998;78(6):624-634.
45. Williams RM, Schmuck G, Allwood S, Sanchez M, Shea R, Wark G. Psychometric evaluation of health-related work outcome measures for musculoskeletal disorders: a systematic review. *J Occup Rehabil.* 2007;17(3):504-521.
46. Matheson L, Ogden L, Violette K, Schultz K. Work hardening: occupational therapy in industrial rehabilitation. *Am J Occup Ther.* 1985;39(5):314-321.
47. Matheson LN. *Feasibility Evaluation Checklist: A Measure of Vocational Readiness.* St. Charles, MO: EpicRehab, LLC; 2011.
48. Karasek RA. *Job Content Questionnaire and User's Guide.* Lowell: University of Massachusetts Lowell, Department of Work Environment; 1985.
49. Cheng Y, Luh W, Guo, Y. Reliability and validity of the Chinese version of the Job Content Questionnaire in Taiwanese workers. *Int J Behav Med.* 2003;10(1):15-30.
50. Ostry AS, Marion SA, Demers PA, et al. Measuring psychosocial job strain with the Job Content Questionnaire using experienced job evaluators. *Am J Industr Med.* 2001;39(4):397-401.
51. Karasek RA, Theorell T. *Healthy Work: Stress, Productivity and the Reconstruction of Working Life.* New York: Basic Books; 1990.
52. Karasek R, Brisson C, Kawakami N, Houtman I, Bongers P, Amick B. The Job Content Questionnaire (JCQ): an instrument for internationally comparative assessments of psychosocial job characteristics. *J Occup Health Psychol.* 1998;3(4):322-355.
53. Storms G, Casaer S, De Wit R, Van den Bergh O, Moens G. A psychometric evaluation of a Dutch version of the Job Content Questionnaire and of a short direct questioning procedure. *Work & Stress.* 2001;15(2):131-143.
54. van Veldhoven MJPM. Need for recovery after work: an overview of construct, measurement and research. In: Houdmont J, Leka S, eds. *Occupational Health Psychology: European Perspectives on Research, Education and Practice.* Nottingham: Nottingham University Press; 2008:1-25
55. Sluiter JK, Van der Beek AJ, Frings-Dresen MHW. The influence of work characteristics on the need for recovery and experienced health: a study on coach drivers. *Ergonomics.* 1999;42:573-583.

56. van Veldhoven MJPM, Broersen S. Measurement quality and validity of the need for recovery scale. *Occup Environ Med.* 2003;60 Suppl:i3-i9.
57. Meijman TF. [Effort and recovery: a conceptual framework for psychological research of workload]. In: Meijman TF, ed. [*Mental Workload and Job Stress: A Work Psychological Approach*]. Assen, Netherlands: Van Gorcum; 1989:5-20.
58. Veldhoven MJPMV. *Psychosociale arbeidsbelasting en werkstress.* Doctoral dissertation. Groningen, Netherlands: University of Groningen; 1996.
59. de Croon EM, Sluiter JK, Frings-Dresen MH. Psychometric properties of the Need for Recovery after work scale: test-retest reliability and sensitivity to detect change. *Occup Environ Med.* 2006;63(3):202-206.
60. Schaufeli WB, van Dierendonck D. *UBOS Utrechtse Burnout Schaal: Handleiding.* Amsterdam, Netherlands: Swets Test Publishers; 2000.
61. Swaen GMH, Van Amelsvoort LGPM, Bültmann U, Kant IJ. Fatigue as a risk factor for being injured in an occupational accident: results from the Maastricht Cohort Study. *Occup Environ Med.* 2003;60(suppl 1):i88-i92.
62. de Croon EM, Sluiter JK, Frings-Dresen MH. Need for recovery after work predicts sickness absence: a 2-year prospective cohort study in truck drivers. *J Psychosom Res.* 2003;55(4):331-339.
63. Kielhofner G, Mallinson T, Crawford C, et al. *The Occupational Performance History Interview (Version 2.0) OPHI-II.* Chicago, IL: Model of Human Occupation Clearinghouse; 1998.
64. Kielhofner G, Henry A. Development and investigation of the Occupational Performance History Interview. *Am J Occup Ther.* 1988;42(8):489-498.
65. Kielhofner G, Mallinson T, Forsyth K, Lai JS. Psychometric properties of the second version of the Occupational Performance History Interview (OPHI-II). *Am J Occup Ther.* 2001;55(3):260-267.
66. Mallinson T, Mahaffey L, Kielhofner G. The Occupational Performance History Interview: evidence for three underlying constructs of occupational adaptation. *Can J Occup Ther.* 1998;65(4):219-228.
67. Kopec JA, Esdaile JM. Occupational role performance in persons with back pain. *Disabil Rehabil.* 1998;20(10):373-379.
68. Amick BC 3rd, Lerner D, Rogers WH, Rooney T, Katz JN. A review of health-related work outcome measures and their uses, and recommended measures. *Spine.* 2000;25(24):3152-3160.
69. Baron K, Kielhofner G, Iyenger A, Goldhammer V, Wolenski J. *A User's Manual for the Occupational Self-Assessment (OSA)(Version 2.2).* Chicago: Model of Human Occupational Clearinghouse; 2006.
70. Taylor R, Lee SW, Kramer J, Shirashi Y, Kielhofner G. Psychometric study of the Occupational Self-Assessment with adolescents after infectious mononucleosis. *Am J Occup Ther.* 2011;65:e20–e28.
71. Kielhofner G, Forsyth K, Kramer J, Iyenger A. Developing the Occupational Self-Assessment: the use of Rasch analysis to assure internal validity, sensitivity and reliability. *Br J Occup Ther.* 2009;72(3):94-104.
72. Keller J, Kafkes A, Kielhofner G. Psychometric characteristics of the Child Occupational Self-Assessment (COSA), part one: an initial examination of psychometric properties. *Scand J Occup Ther.* 2005;12(3):118-127.
73. Langmuir CR. *Personnel Tests for Industry: Oral Directions Test.* New York: Psychological Corporation; 1974.
74. Angoff W, Thorndike R. Scales, norms, and equivalent scores. In: *Educational Measurement.* Washington DC: American Council on Education; 1971:508-600.
75. Doppelt J, Seashore H. Psychological testing in correctional institutions. *J Couns Psychol.* 1959;6:81-92.
76. Wolfe R, Davis J. Use of the Oral Directions Test in a domiciliary setting. *J Gerontol.* 1964;19:349-351.
77. Roland M, Fairbank J. The Roland Morris Disability Questionnaire and the Oswestry Disability Questionnaire. *Spine.* 2000;25(4):3115-3124.
78. Stratford PW, Binkley J, Solomon P, et al. Defining the minimum level of detectable change for the Roland-Morris Questionnaire. *Phys Ther.* 1996;76:359-365.
79. Smeets RJ, Vlaeyen JW, Hidding A, Kester AD, Van Der Heijden GJ, Knottnerus JA. Chronic low back pain: physical training, graded activity with problem solving training, or both? The one-year post-treatment results of a randomized controlled trial. *Pain.* 2008;134:263-276.
80. Artus M, van der Windt DA, Jordan KP, Hay EM. Low back pain symptoms show a similar pattern of improvement following a wide range of primary care treatments: a systematic review of randomized clinical trials. *Rheumatology (Oxford).* 2010;49:2346-2356.
81. Wilkens P, Scheel IB, Grundnes O, Hellum C, Storheim K. Effect of glucosamine on pain-related disability in patients with chronic low back pain and degenerative lumbar osteoarthritis: a randomized controlled trial. *JAMA.* 2010;304:45-52.
82. Lamb SE, Hansen Z, Lall R, et al. Group cognitive behavioural treatment for low-back pain in primary care: a randomised controlled trial and cost-effectiveness analysis. *Lancet.* 2010;375:916-923.
83. Hay EM, Mullis R, Lewis M, et al. Comparison of physical treatments versus a brief pain-management programme for back pain in primary care: a randomised clinical trial in physiotherapy practice. *Lancet.* 2005;365:2024-2030.
84. Mannion AF, Muntener M, Taimela S, Dvorak J. A randomized clinical trial of three active therapies for chronic low back pain. *Spine (Phila Pa 1976).* 1999;24(23):2435-2448.
85. Reneman MF, Jorritsma W, Schellekens JM, Göeken LN. Concurrent validity of questionnaire and performance-based disability measurements in patients with chronic non-specific low back pain. *J Occup Rehabil.* 2002;12(3):119-129.
86. Kopec JA, Esdaile JM. Functional disability scales for back pain. *Spine.* 1995;20(17):1943-1949.
87. Garratt AM, Moffett JK, Farrin AJ. Responsiveness of generic and specific measures of health outcome in low back pain. *Spine.* 2001;26(1):71-77.
88. Holland JL, Fritzsche BA, Powell AB. *SDS Self-Directed Search Technical Manual.* Odessa, FL: Psychological Assessment Resources, Inc; 1994.
89. Gibson L, Strong J. The reliability and validity of a measure of perceived functional capacity for work in chronic back pain. *J Occup Rehab.* 1996;6(3):159-175.
90. Matheson L, Matheson, M. *PACT Spinal Function Sort.* Wildwood, MO: Employment Potential Improvement Corporation; 1989.
91. Matheson L, Matheson M, Grant J. Development of a measure of perceived functional ability. *J Occup Rehabil.* 1993;3(1):15-30.

92. Matheson L, Mooney V, Grant J, Leggett S, Kenny K. Standardized evaluation of work capacity. *J Back Musculoskel Rehabil.* 1996;6(3):249-264.
93. Robinson RC, Kishino N, Matheson L, et al. Improvement in postoperative and nonoperative spinal patients on a self-report measure of disability: the Spinal Function Sort (SFS). *J Occup Rehabil.* 2003;13(2),107-113.
94. Sufka A, Hauger B, Trenary M, et al. Centralization of low back pain and perceived functional outcome. *J Ortho Sports Phys Ther.* 1998;27(3):205-212.
95. *VALPAR Component Work Samples (VCWS) Manuals.* Tucson, AZ: VALPAR International Corporation; 1986.
96. Hazard RG, Haugh LD, Reid S, et al. Early prediction of chronic disability after occupational low back injury. *Spine.* 1996;21:945-951.
97. Hazard RG, Haugh LD, Reid S, McFarlane G, MacDonald L. Early physician notification of patient disability risk and clinical guidelines after low back injury: a randomized, controlled trial. *Spine.* 1997;22(24):2951-2958.
98. Cats-Baril WL, Frymoyer JW. Identifying patients at risk of becoming disabled because of low-back pain. *Spine.* 1991;16(6):605-607.
99. Gray H, Adefolarin AT, Howe TE. A systematic review of instruments for the assessment of work-related psychosocial factors in individuals with non-specific low back pain. *Manual Therapy.* 2011;16(6):531-543.
100. Wonderlic EF. *Wonderlic Personnel Test & Scholastic Level Exam: User's Manual.* Vernon Hills, IL: Wonderlic, Inc; 2002.
101. Dodrill C. Long-term reliability of the Wonderlic Personnel Test. *J Consult Clin Psychol.* 1983;51(2):316-317.
102. Dodrill C, Warner M. Further studies of the Wonderlic Personnel Test as a brief measure of intelligence. *J Consult Clin Psychol.* 1988;56:145-147.
103. McKelvie SJ. The Wonderlic Personnel Test: reliability and validity in an academic setting. *Psychol Rep.* 1989;65:161-162.
104. Wonderlic EF, Hovland CI. The Personnel Test: restandardized abridgement of the Otis-S-A Test for business and industrial use. *Psychol Rep.* 1939;62:131-134.
105. Hunter JE. *The Wonderlic Personnel Test As a Predictor of Training Success and Job Performance.* Vernon Hills, IL: Wonderlic, Inc; 1989.
106. Schmidt FL, Hunter JE. A within setting empirical test of the situational specificity hypothesis in personnel selection. *Personnel Psychol.* 1984;37(2):317-326.
107. Tuomi K, Ilmarinen J, Jahkola A, Katajarinne L, Tulkki A. *Work Ability Index.* 2nd ed. Helsinki: Finnish Institute of Occupational Health; 2006.
108. DeZwart BC, Frings-Dresen MH, Van Duivenbooden JC. Test-retest reliability of the Work Ability Index questionnaire. *Occup Med (Lond).* 2002;52(4):177-181.
109. Kujala V, Tammelin T, Remes J, Vammavaara E, Ek E, Laitinen J. Work Ability Index of young employees and their sickness absence during the following year. *Scand J Work Environ Health.* 2006;32(1):75-84.
110. Ahlstrom L, Grimby-Ekman A, Hagberg M, Dellve L. The Work Ability Index and single-item question: associations with sick leave, symptoms, and health--a prospective study of women on long-term sick leave. *Scand J Work Environ Health.* 2010;36(5):404-12.
111. Radkiewich P, Widerszal-Bazyl M. Psychometric properties of Work Ability Index in the light of comparative survey study. In: *Assessment and Promotion of Work Ability, Health and Well-being of Ageing Workers.* Proceedings of 2nd International Symposium on Work Ability. International Congress Series 1280. The Netherlands: Elsevier; 2005:304-309.
112. Abdolalizadeh M, Arastoo AA, Ghsemzadeh R, Montazeri A, Ahmadi K, Azizi A. The psychometric properties of an Iranian translation of the Work Ability Index (WAI) questionnaire. *J Occup Rehabil.* 2012;22(3):401-408.
113. Martinez MC, Latorre M do RD de O, Fischer FM. Validade e confiabilidade da versão brasileira do Índice de Capacidade para o Trabalho. *Rev Saúde Pública.* 2009;43:525-32.
114. Gilworth G, Chamberlain MA, Harvey A, et al. Development of a work instability scale for rheumatoid arthritis. *Arthritis Rheum.* 2003;49:349-354.
115. Beaton DE, Tang K, Gignac MA, et al. Reliability, validity, and responsiveness of five at-work productivity measures in patients with rheumatoid arthritis or osteoarthritis. *Arthritis Care Res (Hoboken).* 2010;62:28-37.
116. Tang K, Beaton DE, Lacaille D, et al. The Work Instability Scale for Rheumatoid Arthritis (RA-WIS): does it work in osteoarthritis? *Qual Life Res.* 2010;19:1057-1068.
117. Tang K, Beaton DE, Boonen A, Gignac MA, Bombardier C. Measures of work disability and productivity: Rheumatoid Arthritis Specific Work Productivity Survey (WPS-RA), Workplace Activity Limitations Scale (WALS), Work Instability Scale for Rheumatoid Arthritis (RA-WIS), Work Limitations Questionnaire (WLQ), and Work Productivity and Activity Impairment Questionnaire (WPAI). *Arthritis Care Res (Hoboken).* 2011;Suppl 11:S337-S49.
118. Gilworth G, Emery P, Barkham N, Smyth MG, Helliwell P, Tennant A. Reducing work disability in Ankylosing Spondylitis–development of a work instability scale for AS. *BMC Musculoskelet Disord.* 2009;10(1):1.
119. Lerner DJ, Amick BC III, Roger WH, Malspels S, Bugay K. The Work Limitations Questionnaire: A self-administered instrument for assessing on-the-job work disability. *Medical Care.* 2001:39(1):72-85.
120. Noben C, Evers S, Nijhuis F, de Rijk E. Quality appraisal of generic self-reported instruments measuring health-related productivity changes: a systematic review. *BMC Public Health.* 2014;14(115):1-21.
121. Munir F. The Work Limitations Questionnaire. *Occup Med.* 2008;58(4):310-311.
122. Prasad M, Wahlqvist P, Shikiar R, Tina Shih YC. Review of self-report instruments measuring health-related work productivity. *PharmacoEconomics.* 2004;22(4):225-244.
123. Reilly M, Bracco A, Ricci JF, Santoro J, Stevens T. The validity and accuracy of the work productivity and activity impairment questionnaire—irritable bowel syndrom version (WPAI:IBS). *Aliment Pharmacol Ther.* 2004;20(4):459-467.
124. Wahlqvist P, Carlsson J, Stalhammar NO, Wiklunch I. Validity of a work productivity and activity impairment questionnaire for patients with symptoms of gastro-esophageal reflux disease (WPAI-GERD): results from a cross-sectional study. *Value Health.* 2002;106-113.

125. Velozo CA, Kielhofner G, Fisher, G. *A User's Guide to the Worker Role Interview (Version 9.0).* Chicago: Model of Human Occupation Clearing House; 1998.
126. Biernacki SD. Reliability of the Worker Role Interview. *Am J Occup Ther.* 1993;47:797-803.
127. Ekbladh E, Haglund L, Thorell, L. The Worker Role Interview: preliminary data on the predictive validity of return to work of clients after an insurance medicine investigation. *J Occup Rehabil.* 2004;14(2):131-141.
128. Gern A. *Validity of the Worker Role Interview.* Unpublished master's thesis, University of Illinois at Chicago; 1993.
129. Lin FL. *The Worker Role Interview: Construct Validity Across Diagnoses.* Unpublished master's thesis, University of Illinois at Chicago; 1994.
130. Velozo CA, Kielhofner G, Gern A, et al. Worker Role Interview: Validation of a psychosocial work-related measure. *J Occup Rehabil.* 1999;9(3):153-168.
131. Keilhofner G. *A Model of Human Occupation: Theory and Application.* Baltimore, MD: Williams & Wilkins; 1995.

Mine the Gold

The United States Federal Legislation that supports education includes occupational therapy as a vital member of the team (see Legislative Resources at the end of this chapter). In other countries, occupational therapy services in education are also growing. Both occupational therapy and interprofessional evidence point out the important contributions that related service professionals make to learning outcomes. Our support of teachers, students, and families builds their capacity to support their children's learning as well.

Become Systematic

By using measures that inform the team (including family) of our interest in children's engagement in the school day, we teach them that our focus is on participation. We link our skilled observations to the teacher's comments and test data to create a complete picture of the student in the context of school. We set education outcomes with the team and take responsibility for these outcomes, trusting that our expertise will support common goals.

Use Evidence in Practice

Interprofessional literature indicates that embedding professional expertise into the student's and teachers' authentic settings and routines supports both teacher competence and positive learning outcomes for students. Education literature suggests that teachers improve their use of evidence-based practices when they have follow-along support within their teaching routines to implement those practices; as related service professionals, occupational therapists are in a unique position to provide this ongoing support for more effective teachers and classrooms.

Make Occupational Therapy Contributions Explicit

When occupational therapists spend time in classrooms, hallways, or lunchrooms, we send the message that how the students operate within all learning contexts matters to our work. When we ask teachers about their priorities, what they see as supports and barriers, and how they organize the school day, we let them know that how they perceive and structure learning matters to our work. When our reflective listening informs the teacher's problem-solving process, we communicate our confidence in the teacher's ability to fulfill the educator role.

Engage in Occupation-Based, Client-Centered Practice

At school, children's participation centers around learning, taking care of personal needs throughout the day, and engaging with others, including peers and adults in areas of interest. When school-based occupational therapy practice remains focused on these educationally relevant goals, we fulfill our roles as related service professionals (ie, we relate our expertise to the role of student learning and engagement). Educators set the context for learning and engagement; we support their way of inviting children to learn and interact with others. By supporting the educators, we support their participation as teachers.

CHAPTER 12

Measuring Participation at School

Winnie Dunn, PhD, OTR, FAOTA; Becky Nicholson, OTD, OTR/L; and Lauren Foster, OTD, OTR/L

Occupational therapy practice in schools is an essential part of the overall demographics of our profession in the United States and other countries around the world. As we collaborate to implement education mandates, we must also be mindful of our unique contribution as occupational therapists and as related service providers to contribute to the educational outcomes for students. As part of this milieu, our measurements must reflect our core values while being educationally relevant.

Overview of School Performance

Key Concepts

School-based practice in the United States has developed immensely in the last 4 decades. The advent of federal legislation about every child's right to a "free and appropriate public education" included occupational therapy as a needed service; this legislation and subsequent updates defined our role in schools (see Legislation Resources at the end of this chapter). Likewise, school-based practice has grown significantly in other countries around the world. For example, in Canada, innovative models of school-based practice are being developed and tested.[1] Occupational therapy emphasizes supporting people in their authentic contexts, so including services in school-based practices is consistent with our values. Schools are a unique context; "student" is a specific role in young people's lives. Most importantly, occupational therapy has distinct contributions to make to support successful and satisfying participation at school.

Furthermore, the enactment of No Child Left Behind (NCLB) in the US requires that schools show that all students (including those with disabilities) show learning progress. Because occupational therapists are part of an interprofessional team that is required to measure student learning, we can also contribute to overall assessment in schools, not limiting ourselves to children who have particular needs. With this additional responsibility on the team, it is vital that occupational therapists employ participation-focused measures to illustrate our commitment to outcomes that matter at school.

One of the biggest challenges occupational therapy faced when entering public education was figuring out how to be relevant to the needs of students and teachers at school. Initially, we tried to import our classically medical model approaches into the schools; we set up clinical areas to provide segregated intervention. However, the evidence began to suggest that there were 2 challenges with a segregated approach. First, the students were not generalizing use of skills learned in a segregated way to the everyday routines in the classroom. For example, a student working on balance with the therapist might not transfer that skill to the balance needed for getting on the bus. Secondly, the time spent in therapy reduced the time spent in the education milieu, which was the children's primary reason for being at school. Students who needed more support for learning were getting less time in classroom activities.

Returning to our core principles, we began to ask ourselves how to be relevant to this setting (school), these activities (learning), and the priorities of these people (students, teachers, families). What has emerged is a contextually relevant approach to school practice. We use assessment strategies that are synchronous with priorities at school. In collaboration with the team, we plan interventions based on the teacher's, student's, and families' main interests. Finally, we recognize how to support the education process with our distinct point of view and expertise.

Law M, Baum C, Dunn W, eds. *Measuring Occupational Performance: Supporting Best Practice in Occupational Therapy, Third Edition (pp 239-266).*

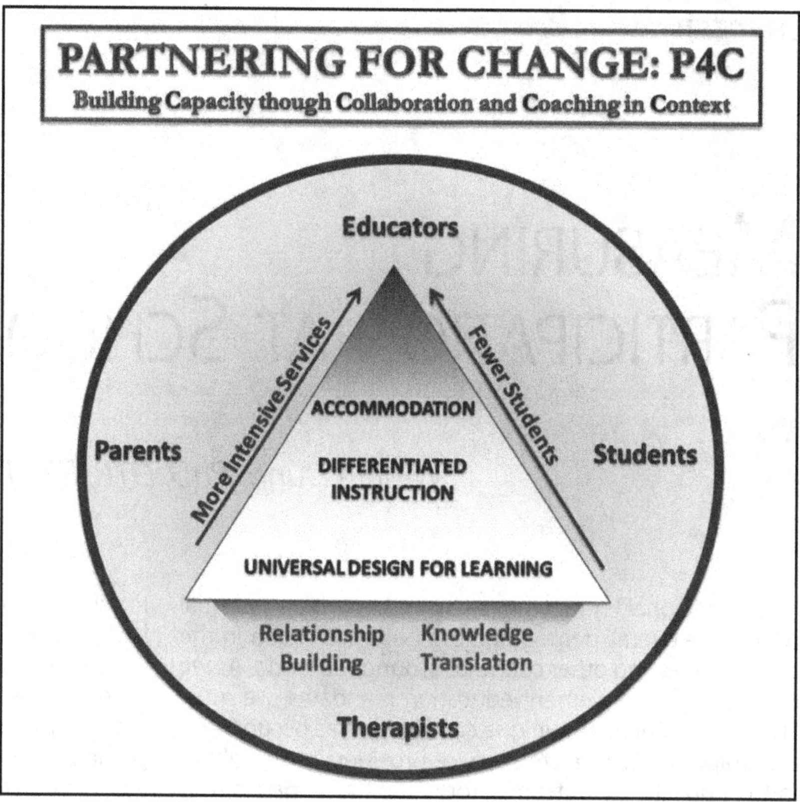

Figure 12-1. Partnering for Change: P4C. (Reprinted with permission from Missiuna C, Pollock N, Campbell W, Levac D, Whalen S. *Partnering for Change Model.* Hamilton, ON: *CanChild*, McMaster University; 2016.

Importance of Measurement of School Performance

Our measurement strategies have developed along with our evolution within the school setting. Early in the process, educators and therapists were concerned about identification and eligibility for special education services. With the enactment of NCLB in 2002, the requirements now focus on learning progress for all students, so eligibility is less important. Furthermore, we consider all aspects of a student's participation at school, including recess, lunchtime, and extracurriculars, and how we can inform the teaching/learning process to achieve and document successful and satisfying outcomes in any of these areas. Being comprehensive within the school experience means that we must be aware of many ways to gather data to generate hypotheses, implement interventions, and evaluate process and outcomes. For some students, the focus is on curricular and cognitive aspects of learning needed to advance knowledge. For other students, the focus is on functional living skills needed for self-determination, while for others, addressing social emotional features of school life is most important. Occupational therapy at school requires nimble thinking and an arsenal of measurement methods to support every student and teacher. When we direct our attention to the student's occupational performance at school, we also inform the team how we can contribute to educational outcomes. Because the context of school is so central to school-based practices, the Ecology of Human Performance (EHP) provides a useful structure for organizing our planning and interventions. Figure 12-1 provides examples of school practice within the Person-Environment-Occupation (PEO) model. All of the assessments are coded by these categories (see Chapter 2 for explanation).

Factors to Remember

There are 4 factors that drive relevant occupational therapy practice in schools. First, we must adopt a strengths-based perspective when working in schools. Second, we must understand the "Response to Intervention" model in schools so that we can situate our work within this educational framework. Third, we must embrace the collaborative team approach to assessment, planning, and implementation and understand how "related service professionals" fit into that structure. Fourth, we must employ data from interprofessional assessments as part of our interpretation and planning processes. Let's consider each of these factors in more detail.

Employ a Strengths-Based Perspective

There is a groundswell of both public opinion and evidence that supports strengths-based approaches. Scholars from Positive Psychology, Social Welfare, and Nutrition have shown that people have the resources to manage their own lives.[2-4] Dunn et al[5,6] summarize the strengths perspective and illustrate how it might be applied to occupational therapy. If we are going to be evidence-based providers at school, we need to embrace the concept that all students have strengths and that, as we support participation, we foster those strengths within the daily routines. Hansen and Philo[7] suggest we change our thinking from asking students to "do things normally" (the expected way from our knowledge of human development), to considering the "normality of doing things differently," embracing all the ways a student might participate successfully. Occupational therapists are key team members that implement this way of thinking.

Understand Response to Intervention

In the United States, the NCLB initiative mandates that schools have evidence-based methods to mechanisms in place to identify and evaluate students who may be eligible for special education services. A prominent mechanism in recent educational research and practice is called *Response to Intervention* (RtI), which is an evidence-based 3-tiered model aimed at supporting students with learning needs within their classrooms.[8] RtI emphasizes prevention rather than remediation. Tier 1 (primary prevention) approaches address all students to make the learning environment useful to a wider range of learners. For example, after observing in a classroom, an occupational therapist might notice that the teacher's movement around the room during direct instruction makes it challenging for the students to follow her directions. The occupational therapist might propose that the teacher select a more defined area for moving during direct instruction to keep the class engaged during these group instructional moments. Tier 1 interventions include all aspects of Universal Design[9] and Universal Design for Learning, making occupational therapists key members of the RtI teams at the classroom level rather than reserving occupational therapists for individual student interventions.

Tier 2 (secondary prevention) approaches address students who appear to be at risk for success within the learning environment. For example, if some students are distracted by the teacher's small group instruction, the occupational therapist and teacher might plan new furniture arrangements to create some separation between seatwork and small group work to facilitate task completion. Occupational therapists are skilled at making adjustments to increase effectiveness in the learning environment. The Social Skills Improvement System (SSIS) Performance Screening Guide and the Social Profile are examples of Tier 2 assessments (see Tables 12-7 and 12-10). The SSIS Performance Screening Guide is a measure that assesses social behaviors among all students in a classroom, whereas the Social Profile is a measure that helps assess performance in groups.

Tier 3 (tertiary prevention) approaches involve individualized interventions to provide additional support for students for whom secondary prevention was unsuccessful. For example, after rearranging the furniture, perhaps one student still is not completing seatwork. The occupational therapist hypothesizes from assessment data (including observations) that this student is more distracted by the visual environment. This student sits right in front of the window that looks out on a busy street. After collaborating with the teacher, the occupational therapist and teacher decide to move this student's seat to face a divider to reduce the visual distraction during seatwork. Many of the assessments presented in this chapter are Tier 3 assessments; they help team members identify specific strengths and area of growth for specific students. Frequently, Tier 3 assessment data leads to development of an Individualized Educational Plan (IEP).

Occupational therapists use skills in occupational analysis along with formal assessments outlined in this chapter to determine whether students would benefit from more individualized support. For example, occupational therapists might analyze the cafeteria environment to determine how environmental and personal factors impact the lunchtime routine. Occupational therapists then work with educators and staff to adjust the cafeteria experience so students can navigate and participate successfully.[10]

Partnering for Change: An Evidence-Based Service Delivery Model

Models of service delivery based on RtI principles are increasingly being used by Canadian school health occupational therapists. Partnering for Change (P4C) is an innovative, evidence-informed model for delivery of rehabilitation services to children in schools.[11] The goals of P4C include early identification of children with special needs, promoting everyday functioning and participation in school, preventing secondary consequences, and building capacity within schools and families.

The P4C service model supports capacity building by fostering active collaboration between health professionals and educators, with coaching of educators taking place in the school context. Strategies that enable children to be successful are identified through observation of the child at school, are trialled to ensure they facilitate increased participation, and then are shared with educators so they understand why particular strategies help. In the Tier 1 example mentioned previously, the occupational therapist might have observed that children with attentional difficulties or central auditory processing issues are particularly affected by not being able to see the teacher's face when she is giving instruction. Coaching the teacher about children's increased ability to focus when they can see her mouth moving builds capacity because the teacher is highly likely to use the strategy of facing the class directly, a strategy that is "good for all but essential for some."

Tier 2 in P4C involves differentiating instruction for children who are having difficulty performing grade-level activities, despite exposure to the class-wide strategies used in Tier 1. At this tier, the P4C occupational therapist and educator collaborate to try different ways of addressing the students' needs. For example, the occupational therapist may determine whether students are experiencing difficulties due to a lack of experience or because of more specific developmental needs. The therapist conducts observational assessments in context, whether in the classroom, playground, lunchroom, or gym, and uses a process called *dynamic performance analysis* to implement specific strategies in response to what is observed. Dynamic performance analysis involves the therapist altering the task or environment, monitoring the child's response, and, if the strategy was not successful, introducing an alternate strategy. Throughout this process, the P4C occupational therapist communicates with the educator to explain why the various strategies are tried to enable increased capacity. Examples of this might include a child using visual cues to support sequencing of classroom tasks or dressing to go outside. The therapist may also try strategies such as encouraging children with low tone and postural instability to lean against a wall during circle time rather than leaning on peers.

P4C services are provided within a tiered RtI pyramid that allows provision of services based on need; students with higher needs receive increasingly intense levels of support. Students' response to services is monitored regularly and adjusted as environmental or occupational demands change. At a Tier 3 level, the P4C occupational therapist always seeks consent from families to suggest very specific strategies for one child. While still emphasizing knowledge translation to the teacher about why that strategy is needed, the occupational therapist also shares the strategy with families and talks to them about how this may support the child at home.

P4C is being evaluated in more than 60 schools in Ontario, Canada. Early results have shown that this model requires additional training and mentoring of occupational therapists; however, it has eliminated wait lists for occupational therapy services and has reached far more children at different levels of the Tiers than the traditional 1:1 service.

Embrace Role in Collaborative School Teams

School-based practice is built on legislation that mandates an interprofessional team serve students. Our role as a related service professional mandates that we support student education and learning. Therefore, we partner with students and their teachers and parents to design solutions to learning challenges. There is no work in public schools without other disciplines. The planning and IEP teams are by nature interprofessional as well. That is why our measures must not only gather information about the student, but also convey a sense of our focus on participation.

Employ Interprofessional Assessment Data

It is important for occupational therapists to review the most common assessments from other disciplines so that occupational therapists can link reports from other disciplines to occupational therapy findings. The Disability Rights Education and Defense Fund, Inc. provides a summary for parents explaining the most common assessments in educational testing and their purpose (see http://dredf.org/special_education/Assesments_chart.pdf)

For example, on the Woodcock-Johnson IV Test of Achievement,[12] there are "oral expression" and "listening comprehension" subtests that examine these skills in standardized items. Occupational therapists consider functional use of language in skilled observations, and could offer insights about how the student uses oral expression and listening comprehension in the classroom.

Strategies for Selecting Measures for School Performance

The most critical measurement skill for school-based practice is one's ability to conduct skilled observation. The insights we gain from skilled observation direct our attention to what other assessments might be needed, situate the participation and behavior of interest in the proper context, and provide a way to communicate using relevant examples when planning with teachers and other team members.

With skilled observation in mind, we selected measures for this chapter by considering all of the areas of participation that are the focus at school. This includes academic performance, social-emotional engagement with peers and adults, navigating within the various school contexts, and managing one's self during the day. School practice requires interprofessional assessment, so we must not only understand occupational therapy's contribution, we also must recognize how to create an interface with other discipline assessments so that a comprehensive plan is possible.

Strategies for Reporting About School Performance

In the past, it was common for each discipline to write their own reports and plans for students at school, even though the federal mandates specified there should be a single plan. School-based teams are now recognizing the importance of collaborating to create integrated plans for entire districts, schools (see SWIFT reference in Legislation Resources), classrooms, and individual students. Occupational therapists as related service providers contribute to these integrated plans.

With more work occurring at building and classroom levels, occupational therapy documentation becomes part of the documents the teams produce, with all team members signing these integrated documents. Even when a student has an IEP, the goals on that IEP reflect that student's participation in the learning environment effectively; the team members take responsibility for that participation outcome together. Subsequently, teams use their collective expertise to design interventions that reflect everyone's wisdom to meet the goals.

Occupational therapists may also document their reflections, observations, and insights that contribute to the team's plans as background documentation for the record. We may contribute a brief (1 to 2 pages) summary of assessments as background documentation as well, but these do not replace the integrated documentation that serves as the working document for everyone.

Future Directions for Practice and Research in School Performance

For practice in schools, occupational therapists must recalibrate away from skills assessment and development toward supporting participation in authentic contexts. The assessments we review in this chapter provide a strong basis for shifting this focus because they evaluate students as they engage in relevant educational activities. By design, these assessments also inform families and school professionals what occupational therapists care about at the big picture level. When we emphasize our core values in assessment, we increase our opportunities to use our expertise for maximum benefit and provide leadership for the overall educational endeavor.

For research about school practice, we need to gather more evidence about our impact on educationally relevant outcomes. Research designs need to address our impact on participation that matters to teachers, students, and families. We need to test our outcomes within authentic activities and settings. Evidence across disciplines does not support the effectiveness of skills-based training on generalized use of skills during authentic opportunities. With our philosophical emphasis on effective and satisfying lives, we can lead teams in evaluating relevant outcomes at school.

Overview of Measures of School Performance

Selection Criteria for Review

List of Measures of School Participation Reviewed in This Chapter

There are 4 categories of assessments that we are going to present in this chapter. First, we provide a list of appropriate school-based assessments that are reviewed in other chapters of this book (see Table 12-1). We want to make sure you know about them for your practice, and there is no need to repeat the complete reviews here. Secondly, we provide a review table for a number of appropriate School-based Practice Assessments. Third, we provide an overview and brief examples of appropriate school-based assessments that are embedded within the school routines. Finally, we provide a list of web-based resources for emergent assessment methods that may be appropriate for your particular practice (see Table 12-2).

Measures Reviewed in This Chapter

This list and subsequent tables summarize the characteristics and evidence of the following School-based Assessments. Please note that some of these assessments are developed by and for occupational therapists, while others derive from the educational literature. Because we are in an interprofessional environment, employing interprofessional assessments is important to our role as related service professionals.

- Adaptive Behavior Assessment System, 2nd edition (Table 12-3)
- Behavior Assessment Scale for Children (BASC) School [and home] (Table 12-4)
- Early Coping Inventory (Table 12-5)
- Evaluation of Social Interaction (ESI) (Table 12-6)
- Functional Behavior Assessment (Table 12-7)
- Pediatric Evaluation of Disability Inventory—Computer Adaptive Test (PEDI-CAT) (Table 12-8)
- Scale for the Assessment of Teacher's Impressions of Routines and Engagement (SAT-IRE) (Table 12-9)
- School AMPS (Table 12-10)
- Short Children Occupational Performance Evaluation (SCOPE) (Table 12-11)
- School Function Assessment (Table 12-12)
- Social Profile (Table 12-13)
- Social Skills Improvement System, School [and home] (Table 12-14)
- Sensory Profile 2 [infant, toddler, child, school companion, short] (Tables 12-15 and 12-16)
- Vineland Adaptive Behavior Scales (Table 12-17)

Assessment Methods That Are Embedded Within the School Routines

Another very important assessment feature in school-based practice involves evaluating the student's participation within the authentic routines. Skilled observation occurs regularly and the methods we illustrate next provide scaffolding for documenting your observations within these routines. We summarize and illustrate 4 methods here:

1. Functional behavioral assessment
2. Occupational analysis
3. Goal attainment scaling
4. Ecological inventories.

Functional Behavioral Assessment

Functional Behavioral Assessments (FBAs) provide a structure for determining the cause or function of a behavior. Specialists believe that we can design more effective interventions when we understand a student's behavior. Positive Behavior Support or Positive Behavior Intervention Supports (PBIS) refer to interventions that promote positive behavior and prevent behaviors that impair learning. PBIS is mandated by public school legislation. Typically, school personnel collaborate to determine the "function" of a student's behaviors with interviews, observations, rating scales, and trial interventions. Direct skilled observation or reviewing video of a selected circumstance is the most direct way to see what triggers, supports, or diminishes both desirable and undesirable behaviors. The biggest categories for the function of challenging behaviors are attention getting, escape/avoidance, or gaining pleasure. Occupational therapists are trained to look at all aspects of the environment, person, and tasks, making us well qualified to perform FBAs. More information on FBAs and PBIS can be found in the following locations:

- The Center for Effective Collaboration and Practice provides a summary of practice (http://cecp.air.org/fba/)
- This source includes a special education perspective (www.specialeducationguide.com/pre-k-12/behavior-and-classroom-management/functional-behavior-assessment-and-behavior-intervention-plans/)
- Multimodal provides forms and examples (http://mfba.net/forms.html)

Occupational Analysis

In all settings, therapists must balance the need to complete an occupational profile and occupational analysis that reflect performance issues while remaining focused on the impact on the occupation of daily life at school. This can be particularly challenging when, as related service professionals, we must contribute to the development of the IEP while remaining true to the concept of occupation-based practice. Too often, the educational team relies on deficit-identifying information to guide intervention.

In an attempt to bridge the gap between occupation-based practice and school priorities, Coster et al[13] developed the School Function Assessment (SFA), which emphasizes the top-down approach to assessment and intervention. The SFA provides occupational therapists with a way to examine students in the context of school while obtaining participation supports and barriers, which we need for planning interventions within the school routines.

Additionally, in a study examining the use of assessment tools in occupational therapy practice, therapists ranked the Sensory Profile[14] as the most used assessment tool in pediatric practice.[15] With the publication of the Sensory Profile 2 (SP2),[16] which includes a teacher version (School Companion Sensory Profile 2) and a parent version (Child Sensory Profile 2), there is current standardization data available for school practice. Colleagues in school practice have come to rely on occupational therapists to contribute expertise about the contribution of sensory processing patterns to students' ability to engage in classroom learning. The SP2 battery, particularly the teacher form, also bridges the gap between occupation-based practice and school priorities. Using teachers' insights to inform our knowledge about a student's sensory processing patterns in that classroom, occupational therapists can support the teacher and student in their respective occupations throughout the day.

Therapists may find the information from the SFA and the SP2 helpful in identifying school-specific ideas to contribute to team planning from an occupational perspective. These assessments communicate the occupational therapy perspective and therefore foster use of occupational therapists in a more global way rather than thinking that occupational therapists only address skill development (eg, fine motor development).

Goal Attainment Scaling

Goal Attainment Scaling (GAS) is a tool that measures behavioral changes in small increments. It is a useful tool for school measurement because many students have conditions that make standardized assessment challenging and inaccurate. GAS can be developed by whomever wants to measure goal achievement (teachers, paras, therapists). Because GAS is specific to the person's goals, the GAS developer must be precise in observations and interviews to gather the appropriate information for creating a GAS. When the course of expected development is altered, we must have sensitive ways to document legitimate changes in function and participation.[17] GAS provides that method by creating an accurate and reliable marker of outcomes that matter to the teacher, parents, team, and student. GAS can also be a helpful way to measure a student's IEP progress. Cusik and colleagues[18] reported that both the GAS and the COPM were sensitive to change in a pediatric population, and that they measured different aspects of change in participation. McLaren and Rodger[17] provide an overview of the history and procedures of GAS along with examples for children.

Ecological Inventory

An Ecological Inventory is a method for documenting routines, expectations, and current performance that sets the stage for team-based embedded intervention planning. Ecological inventories are typically worksheets with several columns for the team to complete. First, the team documents what happens in the classroom routine and how a typical student would engage in that activity. Then, a team member, such as an occupational therapist, observes and records what a target student does in this same routine, looking for parts that work and parts that are not currently effective. The teacher and occupational therapist then discuss ways to accommodate, adapt, or support the student in parts that are not effective as a means for increasing successful participation. Ecological Inventories situate your planning within the authentic activities that matter to the student and teacher, and it is easy to see the effectiveness of the intervention plans. There are several sources that provide examples of Ecological Inventories, including Dunn.[19]

Table 12-1

Appropriate School-Based Assessments Reviewed in Other Chapters of This Book

Assessment	*Chapter reviewed in*
Activities Scales for Kids (ASK)	13
Affect in Play Scale (APS)	10
Assessment of Life Habits for Children (LIFE-H)	9
Assessment of Preschool Children's Participation	9
Beery VMI	5
Canadian Occupational Performance Measure	7
Child and Adolescent Scale of Participation (CASP)	9
Child Behavior Checklist (CBCL)	5
Child Behaviors Inventory of Playfulness (CBI)	10
Child Occupational Self-Assessment (COSA)	7
Child Participation Questionnaire (CPQ)	10
Child-Initiated pretend Play Assessment (ChIPPA)	10
Children's Active Play Imagery Questionnaire (CAPIQ)	10
Children's Assessment of Participation Enjoyment (CAPE)	9
Children's Leisure Activities Study Survey (CLASS)	10
Children's Leisure Assessment Scale (CLAS)	10
Children's Playfulness Scale (CPS)	10
Developmental Play Assessment (DPA)	10
My Child's Play Questionnaire (MCP)	10
Peabody Developmental Motor Scales-2 (PDMS-2)	5
Pediatric Activity Card Sort (PACS)	9
Pediatric Interest Profile	10
Play Assessment for Group Settings (PAGS)	10
Play Assessment Scale (PAS)	10
Play History	10
Play in Early Childhood Evaluation System (PIECES)	10
Play Observation Scale (POS)	10
Play Skills Self Report Questionnaire (PSSRQ)	10
Preschool Play Behavior Scale (PPBS)	10
Test of Playfulness (ToP)	10
Weschler Abbreviated/ scale of intelligence (WASI)	5
Young Children's Participation and Environment Measure (YC-PEM)	9
Youth Outcomes Battery (YOB)	10

Web-Based Resources for Emergent Assessment Approaches

There are also some emergent resources for school-based assessment that are available from online sources. These materials meet specific school-based practice needs, so we wanted to make sure you had them available. Table 12-2 summarizes these additional resources.

Table 12-2

Additional Resources for School-Based Assessments

CSEA free	https://sites.google.com/site/cseafree/ 160 items that remind you what to consider in a student's school context from a sensory point of view
Interest Survey/ Careers	http://dlr.sd.gov/lmic/pdfs_and_other_files/cwonders_interest_survey.pdf Focuses on what a student is good at for career consideration
Collaborative for Academic and Social Emotional Learning	www.casel.org Provides resources about social emotional learning and assessments
Strengths Based Assessment of Social Emotional Learning	http://www.centerforresilientchildren.org/school-age/assessments-resources/the-devereux-student-strengths-assessment-dessa-kit/ Provides both individual and whole classroom assessments about social emotional factors and resilience
Every Moment Counts initiative in Ohio Schools	www.everymomentcounts.org Enjoyment of participation in cafeteria and recess, friendliness of peers, supervisors, pre and post-test measures that show initial validity for detecting changes

Table 12-3

The Adaptive Behavior Assessment System, Second Edition (ABAS-II)

Source	http://www.pearsonclinical.com/psychology/products/100000449/adaptive-behavior-assessment-system-second-edition-abas-second-edition.html
Key References	Wei et al[20]; Rust and Wallace[21]
Purpose	• Identify strengths and challenges in adaptive behavior skills and provide information regarding progress in skill acquisition over time. • The Adaptive Behavior System, Second Edition (ABAS-II) is a norm-referenced assessment that examines the adaptive behavior skills of individuals from birth to 89 years of age. The ABAS-II is designed to evaluate specific areas of adaptive behavior identified by the American Psychological Association (APA)[22] and the American Association on Mental Retardation (AAMR)[23,24] and the *Diagnostic and Statistical Manual of Mental Disorders, Fourth Edition—Text Revision* (DSM-IV-TR). Professionals working in school settings must include measurement of adaptive behavior performance as part of the comprehensive assessment of children. The ABAS-II provides the opportunity for multiple respondents to contribute to the evaluation process providing information regarding the child's performance across environments.

(continued)

Table 12-3 (continued)

The Adaptive Behavior Assessment System, Second Edition (ABAS-II)

Type of Client	• Individuals/students with adaptive behavior concerns
Test Format	• Parent/caregiver, teacher/daycare provider rating forms
Procedures	• Teacher/daycare provider and parent/primary caregiver completes the rating form on the following areas: communication, community use, functional pre-academics, school/home living, health and safety, leisure, self-care, self-direction, social, motor.
Time Required	• Approximately 20 minutes to complete the rating form and 5 to 10 minutes to score • Computerized scoring software is available
Reliability	
Test-Retest	• Test-retest reliabilities by age group were generally above or near .90 for teacher, parent, and adult form. Sample sizes ranged from 30 to 207.[21]
Internal Consistency	• Internal consistency coefficient for the standardization sample's GAC ranged from .97 to .99.
Inter-Rater	• Inter-rater reliability for sample's GAC ranged from .82 to .93
Validity	• The ABAS and the Vineland Adaptive Behavior Scales (VABS-Classroom Edition) high correlation supports the validity of the ABAS with correlations ranging from. 70 to .84.
Content	• The ABAS and the Behavior Assessment Scale for Children demonstrated a negative correlation as behavior problem increased, adaptive behavior scales decreased.
Construct	• The ABAS correlations between several measures of intelligence ranged from .40 to .50 supporting previously reported research indicating that adaptive behavior skills are related to intelligence but are distinct constructs.
Standardization	• The standardization sample for the school-aged and adult form was collected by 139 independent examiners from 107 cities in the United States. The standardization data for the infant-preschool forms were collected by 214 independent examiners in 184 cities in the United states. Total number of Preschool Teacher/Daycare Provider forms = 750, Parent Primary Caregiver = 1350, Teacher = 1690, and Parent = 1670 • The clinical cases for the ABAS included biological risk factors, language disorders, PDD-NOS developmental delay motor impairment, ADHD, Alzheimer's disease, autistic disorder, behavior disorder, emotional disturbance, hearing impaired, learning disability, mental retardation, Parkinson's disease, speech impairment, stroke, brain injury , and visual impairment.
Utility	
Research Programs	• Test reviewers indicate that ABAS is a useful tool for a wide range of populations. • Used widely in research
Practice Settings	• Schools, residential treatment programs, community-based programs
Strengths	• Provides information from multiple sources across environments • Sensitive enough to measure change over time • The adult version can be completed by the respondent or individual familiar with the adult • Theoretically and technical sound instrument
Complexities	• Record forms are well written and easy to use • The updated version provides expanded age range covered

Table 12-4

Behavior Assessment System for Children, Second Edition (BASC-2)

Source	http://www.pearsonclinical.com/psychology/products/100000658/behavior-assessment-system-for-children-second-edition-basc-2.html
Key References	Reynolds and Kamphaus[25]; Volker[26]; Mahan[27]; Titus[28]
Purpose	• The BASC-2 evaluates children's behaviors (home and school) and self-perceptions. It rates adaptive and maladaptive behaviors on multiple scales.
Type of Client	• All students at home and at school
Test Format	• Questionnaire
Procedures	• The parent, teacher and/or student complete the appropriate questionnaire.
Time Required	• Approximately 30 minutes to complete the instrument
Reliability	
Test-Retest	• Test retest reliability: .78 to .91 across scales
Internal Consistency	• Some scales are low (e.g., .19) due to variability of settings (e.g., day care, school)
Inter-Rater	• Inter-rater reliability: .53-.65
Validity	
Content	• With Connors Teacher Rating Scale: .75-.85
Construct	• With first edition of the BASC: .83 or higher
Criterion	• They tested children with various conditions: ADHD, Bipolar disorder, depression, emotional/ behavioral conditions, hearing impairment, learning disability, mental retardation, developmental delay, motor impairments, PDD, speech/ language conditions. In each case, children in these groups had differences from peers without these conditions on the BASC-2. The differences were individualized for each group rather than a 'disability' profile.
Standardization	• 13,000 children ages 3-18; 375 sites in 40 states • Other measures: educational professionals, parents, and adolescents served as informants • Scales include activities of daily living, adaptability, aggression, anxiety, attention problems, atypicality, conduct problems, depression, functional communication, hyperactivity, leadership, learning problems, social skills, somatization, study skills, and withdrawal • Summary scores: externalizing problems, internalizing problems, school problems, adaptive skills, and behavioral symptoms index
Utility	
Research Programs	• Used widely in research
Practice Settings	• Used by School Psychologists in practice
Strengths	• Used widely across disciplines • Can be used as pre-/post-test measure • Multiple raters available • Profiles of scores are specific to particular groups [see above]
Complexities	• Must be 'familiar' with students before administering • Uses clinical language , e.g., 'maladaptive' which may overly pathologize children's behaviors

Table 12-5

Early Coping Inventory

Source	Scholastic Testing Service, Inc, Bensenville, IL 60106-8056
Key References	Zeitlin et al[29]
Purpose	• The Early Coping Inventory is a criterion referenced observation instrument that is designed to evaluate the coping related behavior of children 4 to 36 months of age or older children who function developmentally within this age range[29(p 35)]
Type of Client	• Children 4 to 36 months, or developmentally this age.
Test Format	• Observation measure
Procedures	• Any appropriate care provider
Time Required	• Approximately 20 minutes to complete the instrument
Reliability	
Test-Retest	• Videotape analysis of children's behavior. Manual provides exact observations of raters (.33 to .51)
Internal Consistency	• Item reliability .41 to .52
Inter-Rater	• Test-retest reliability performed; statistics provided in manual but no reliability index
Validity	
Content	• Developed definitions and items from other prominent coping works of the time: ◻ Considered relevance of behavior for adaptive coping ◻ Consistency with theoretical framework of coping ◻ Documentation in professional literature ◻ Clinical experience
Construct	• Six judges reviewed the items and provided critical feedback
Criterion	• Factor analysis yielded patterns that led to the organizational structure of the measure: ◻ Sensorimotor organization ◻ Self-initiated behavior ◻ Reactive behavior
Standardization	• 1440 children from various incomes and with various conditions
Utility	
Research Programs	• Used in practice with families and children
Practice Settings	• Sometimes used in conjunction with the Coping Inventory
Strengths	• One of the few ways to evaluate coping in young children
Complexities	• Older measure, so some statistics are outdated

Table 12-6

Evaluation of Social Interaction (ESI)

Source	http://www.innovativeotsolutions.com/content/esi/
Key References	Simmons et al[30]; Søndergaard and Fisher[31]
Purpose	• To assess the "quality" of a person's social interaction in natural contexts • Tests 27 different performance skills
Type of Client	• Individuals over the age of 2.5 years with social interaction/communication concerns
Test Format	• Interview and observation • Criterion referenced
Procedures	• Therapist completes interview to determine the client's goals, then the therapist observes the client in a naturally occurring social situation. If occupational therapy is indicated, the therapist provides occupation-based and client-directed interventions. The ESI can then be used to re-evaluate.
Time Required	• Approximately 10 to 20 minutes following interview
Reliability	
Test-Retest	• 96.1% of 511 raters demonstrated reliability (18 of 511 raters did not show goodness of fit in the many faceted Rasch Model or MFR Model)
Internal Consistency	• Standard Error = p < .15 means that this test is sensitive to a person's change in social interaction
Inter-Rater	• Parallel forms reliability coefficient was r = .84, meaning the test is good at determining a person's social exchange from one setting to the next • Rasch equivalent of Cronbach's alpha was r = .94, which supports high reliability
Validity	• Sensitive to differences in age and disability
Content	• Criterion referenced
Construct	• 25 of 27 items demonstrated goodness of fit within the many faceted Rasch (MFR) model
Criterion	• Person separation reliability .89 means that this test accurately discriminates between high and low performers on this test • The item separation reliability .98 indicates that the test accurately appraises social interaction items from easiest to more difficult using MFR. The pilot study indicates the ESI is effective in measuring a wide range of social interaction skills
Standardization	• Standardization sample: 6552 (6254 following 377 omitted for errors)
Utility	
Research Programs	• Used to assess social interactions across contexts; the assessment has been validated to test the quality of social interactions across settings
Practice Settings	
Strengths	• Collaboration between therapist and student helps determine accommodations • Measures occupational performance, not underlying deficits
Complexities	• Cannot be used on individuals who do not communicate • Does not assess environmental factors that impact social participation • Requires 3-day training course to demonstrate valid and reliable scoring

Table 12-7

FUNCTIONAL BEHAVIOR ASSESSMENT (FBA)

Source	N/A
Key References	Dunn-Buron and Wolfberg[32]; DuPaul et al[33]; Kamps et al[34]
Purpose	• A FBA is a comprehensive, multi-disciplinary assessment that examines a child's behavior and the influences of the contextual environment on disruptive behavior. It is "a method of identifying the underlying cause of a behavior by analyzing the behavior's antecedents and consequences."[32(p 370)] IDEA mandates that schools complete a functional behavior assessment when challenging behaviors interfere with the child's ability to participate in his or her education. FBAs are conducted by a multidisciplinary team, which can include an occupational therapist.
Type of Client	• School-aged children
Test Format	• FBA is done using interview, checklists, or direct interaction with the child within the natural environment
Procedures	• Members of a multidisciplinary team gather information from interviews with teachers and service providers in the educational setting. Evaluators may implement checklists to assess specific skills. In addition, information comes from direct interaction with the child or observations within the natural environment.
Time Required	• Not provided
Reliability	• No information available
Validity	• No information available
Utility	
Practice Settings	• The format and content of the functional behavior assessment is determined by each multidisciplinary team. See references for templates, case studies, and guidance for implementation.
Strengths	• The development of an FBA creates the foundation for individualized assessment of behavioral challenges and abilities of children in their specific educational setting. Input from a variety of disciplines facilitates the development of interventions that can be carried out by all disciplines and tailored to the child's needs.
Complexities	• The usefulness of the measure is dependent on the skills of interviewer, observational skills, and the effectiveness of collaboration of team members.

Table 12-8

PEDIATRIC EVALUATION OF DISABILITY INVENTORY—COMPUTER ADAPTIVE TEST (PEDI-CAT)

Source	http://pedicat.com/category/ordering/
Key References	Dumas et al[35,36]; Haley et al[37,38]; Kao et al[39]
Purpose	• The PEDI-CAT is intended to provide a description of a child's functional status or progress in the ability to perform functional skills in everyday life.
Type of Client	• The measure is designed for children from birth to 20 years of age with any diagnosis in any setting.
Test Format	• Caregiver or professional report on 276 functional activities in the domains of (1) Daily Activities; (2) Mobility; (3) Social/Cognitive; and (4) Responsibility.

(continued)

Table 12-8 (continued)

PEDIATRIC EVALUATION OF DISABILITY INVENTORY—COMPUTER ADAPTIVE TEST (PEDI-CAT)	
Type of Client	
Procedures	• Does not require any special environment, materials, or activities to administer. The measure utilizes computerized scoring requiring the CAT software. The PEDI-CAT can be completed independently by the child's caregiver(s), through structured interview, or by professional judgment. The measure provides information regarding current, typical performance on functional tasks in daily life. Respondents must know the child well. The PEDI-CAT can be completed on multiple occasions for the same child (eg, intake, interim assessment, discharge, and follow-up) and there is no minimum time that must pass between assessments.
Time Required	• Speedy ("Precision") CAT: 5 to 15 items per domain. • The score report for the Speedy CAT includes a percentile score, a T-score, a scaled score on a 20 to 80 metric scale, and a list of the answers to all PEDI-CAT items administered. Fastest method to obtain an estimate of performance. • Content-Balanced ("Comprehensive") CAT: Approximately 30 items per domain. The score report for the Comprehensive CAT includes a percentile score, a T-score, and a scaled score on a 20 to 80 metric scale. This measure is most useful for individual program planning.
Reliability	
Test-Retest	• Test-retest reliability ranged from 0.958 to 0.997 for all 4 domains.
Internal Consistency	• Item-specific reliability was rated good to excellent on items in the mobility domain
Inter-Rater	
Validity	
Content	• Differences between the normative and the disability groups were significant at $p < .05$ in 22/24 comparisons.
Construct	
Standardization	• Data for the normative sample were derived from a sample of 2205 parents. Within each age group, efforts were made to ensure that groups were representative of Year 2000 Census Bureau data in terms of gender, race, and ethnic distribution in the US. • Data were collected from a sample of 617 parents of children with disabilities from the same Polimetrix sample source. An additional 86 respondents were recruited from the Minneapolis and Boston areas in order to increase the sample size.
Utility	• The PEDI-CAT terminology is consistent with the framework of the WHO's International Classification of Functioning, Disability and Health (ICF) and the version for children and youth, ICF-CY. The manual is robust and provides comprehensive information for administration, interpretation, and psychometric properties. Illustrations are provided for daily activities and mobility items to facilitate understanding.
Strengths	• Can be used with a wide variety of children regardless of physical or intellectual challenges. • The revised PEDI has expanded age range to 20 years allowing for ongoing comparisons of performance. • Theoretically and technically sound instrument. • Provides comprehensive information for program planning. • Examines functional performance in daily life.
Complexities	• Comprehensive measure can be time consuming and requires that the respondent is very familiar with the child.

Table 12-9

The Scale for the Assessment of Teachers' Impressions of Routines and Engagement (SATIRE)

Source	http://www.siskin.org/downloads/SATIRE.pdf
Key References	N/A
Purpose	• Provides functional information regarding a child's abilities and needs in daily classroom routines • The Scale for the Assessment of Teachers' Impressions of Routines and Engagement (SATIRE) is designed to evaluate how a child functions during daily classroom routines. This instrument is intended to be used in conjunction with the Routines-Based Interview (RBI) of the family.
Type of Client	• Children attending preschool or childcare programs
Test Format	• Interview, observation, and rating of child's performance
Procedures	• Professionals interview teachers in preschool settings or caregivers in childcare settings to obtain information about performance during daily routines. Professionals are encouraged to observe the child's level of engagement (attention, participation, and goal-directed behavior), in addition to level of independence and social relationships with adults and children during each routine.
Time Required	• Not provided
Reliability	• No information available
Validity	• No information available
Utility	
Practice Settings	• This tool is designed to give immediate information regarding the child's performance in preschool classroom tasks. This tool is intended to guide professionals through the assessment process and determine how well the child functions during daily routines.
Strengths	• This tool allows for multiple disciplines to be involved in the analysis of daily routines and provide guidance in making informed decisions regarding interventions. This tool is intended to be used in conjunction with the RBI of the family, thus providing a more comprehensive examination of the child's performance in a variety of contexts.
Complexities	• The usefulness of the measure is dependent on the skills of the interviewer to synthesize the information provided by the teacher with observations of the child in natural contexts.

Table 12-10

School Version of the AMPS (School AMPS)

Source	http://www.innovativeotsolutions.com/content/school-amps/
Key References	Munkholm et al[40]; Fingerhut et al[41]; Atchison et al[42]; Fisher et al[43]
Purpose	• To assess the "quality" of a student's performance in academic tasks • Tests 36 different performance skills.

(continued)

Table 12-10 (continued)

School Version of the AMPS (School AMPS)

Type of Client	• Students ages 3 to 15 years (norms available up to age 13 years)
Test Format	• Interview and observation • Criterion- and norm-referenced
Procedures	• The occupational therapist interviews the client (student, teacher and parent, if appropriate). • The occupational therapist then determines with what school tasks the student is struggling. • The occupational therapist observes the student perform the task(s). • Using the scoring form, the occupational therapist scores the student on his or her performance according to performance (there are 16 motor performance items and 20 process items). • The occupational therapist enters the raw score into the School AMPS software to generate the report.
Time Required	• 1 hour
Reliability	
Test-Retest	• The reliability coefficients for school motor and process is > 0.70, and all but one is > 0.80.
Internal Consistency	
Inter-Rater	• Inter-rater reliability = 1.0[42]
Validity	
Content	• The School AMPS was compared to the Peabody Developmental Motor Scale (PDMS); the School AMPS Motor section had a r = .45 correlation with the PDMS-FM, whereas the School AMPS process section had a r = .35 correlation. This suggests that the School AMPS motor section has a moderate correlation with the PDMS. It also suggests that the motor and process sections of the School AMPS measure different constructs.
Construct	
Criterion	• Scale validity, person response validity, and intrarater reliability all demonstrated "acceptable" goodness of fit within the many faceted Rasch model (MFR).
Standardization	• Standardization Sample: 6552 (6254 following 377 omitted for errors).
Utility	• School
Strengths	• Can be used for healthy students as well as students who are suspected of having performance barriers. • Occupation-based
Complexities	• Requires a 5-day course for therapists to demonstrate reliability • Norms are available up to age 13 years.

Table 12-11

Short Children Occupational Performance Evaluation (SCOPE)

Source	http://www.cade.uic.edu/moho/productDetails.aspx?aid=9
Key References	Bowyer et al[44]; Kielhofner[45]
Purpose	• "Provides overview of child's occupational functioning" • "Evaluates how the child's environment supports or detracts from occupational participation"[44(p 1)] • Concepts and constructs based on MOHO • Screens children for the need to further assess occupational performance
Type of Client	• Any child
Test Format	• Observation (primary) with therapist using other sources of information (reports, interviews) to assess
Procedures	• Complete formal and informal assessment of child • Complete rating forms
Time Required	• Between 20 to 40 minutes to complete the form, based on therapist's experience
Reliability	N/A
Validity	N/A
Standardization	N/A
Utility	• Community and clinical
Strengths	• Occupation-based • Pulls information from multiple sources • Guides therapists in intervention planning • Can be used to retest
Complexities	• No validity/reliability scores

Table 12-12

The School Function Assessment (SFA)

Source	Psychological Corporation, Skill Builders Division, 555 Academic Court, San Antonio, TX, 78204
Key References	Sakzewski et al[46]; AOTA[47]; Coster[48]
Purpose	• The School Function Assessment is used to measure a student's performance of functional tasks that support his or her participation in the academic and social aspects of an elementary school program. It was designed to facilitate collaborative program planning for students with a variety of disabling conditions.
Type of Client	• Children enrolled in elementary school.
Test Format	• Rating scales are administered to respondents who are familiar with the student's typical performance. Teachers, occupational therapists, physical therapists, and speech language pathologists as well as classroom and therapy assistants may serve as respondents. • The rating form has 26 scales; each scale is scored using a 4- or 6-level rating, depending on the item. For example, functional activities ratings range from 1 (does not perform) to 4 (consistent performance)

(continued)

Table 12-12 (continued)

THE SCHOOL FUNCTION ASSESSMENT (SFA)

Type of Client	
Procedures	• The assessment is completed by the team, either under the supervision of a coordinator who contacts individual team members and records their scores or by the team collaboratively completing the assignment together.
Time Required	• Not provided
Reliability	
Test-Retest	• Test-retest studies were conducted using intervals ranging from 2 to 4 weeks. Reliability coefficients (both Pearson's r's and intraclass coefficients) ranged from 0.80 to 0.99. The lowest coefficients were on the task support items.
Internal Consistency	• Coefficient alpha's ranged from 0.92 to 0.98. Fit statistics in Item Response Theory methods were also computed. The fit statistics confirmed the coherence of the items within each scale.
Validity	
Content	• Two content validity studies were completed. The first used a sample of 30 content experts who were asked to rate the comprehensiveness and relevance of the items. A second study involved a field trial of the SFA with 40 students. Related service professionals assessed students and then provided an evaluation of the relevance, comprehensiveness, and usefulness of the items and ratings scales.
Construct	• A series of Rasch, multiple regression, and Item Response Theory analyses tested each aspect of construct validity. The scales were found to have excellent predictive and discriminative power.
Utility	• The SFA was carefully developed and appears to be a very practical and empirically robust measure. The scale was designed to reflect current models of function and special education legislation. It will help organize the input from a number of different sources into an assessment used to plan and evaluate interventions for school-aged children. The manual is informative and easy to read.
Strengths	• This tool is very comprehensive and is sensitive to incremental improvements in nonacademic tasks in an elementary school setting. This tool gives clear information regarding participation and identifies the need for adaptations when high levels of assistance are required for tasks in school. This tool may be particularly useful to novice therapists when prioritizing interventions for complex children. Because this tool is based on respondents' interpretations, it enables objective evaluation for children that may be impossible to evaluate using traditional measures.
Complexities	• The child must be in the setting for a minimum of 1 month. It is important to utilize the rating scale guide to ensure that the distinctions between the rating scales are clear. Completion requires coordination of a variety of team members and requires practice in scoring items.

Table 12-13

The Social Profile (SP)

Source	http://myaota.aota.org/shop_aota/prodview.aspx?TYPE=D&PID=160964175&SKU=1244
Key References	Donohue[49,50]
Purpose	• The Social Profile is an observational assessment intended to measure the level of cooperation within a group engaged in an activity or the performance of an individual within a group. The child version assesses parallel, associative, and basic cooperation levels of social interaction. The adult version assesses supportive cooperative and mature types of social participation in addition to the 3 basic levels assessed in the child version during a single session or over an extended period of time.
Type of Client	• The child version was designed for teachers, therapists, and team leaders to assess social participation in children ages 18 months to 11 years. The adult version is intended to be used to evaluate social participation in individuals 12 years of age or older.
Test Format	• Observation forms and Likert rating scales for child and adult populations.
Procedures	• Therapists, teachers, or group leaders complete rating forms following observation of a group activity of at least 30 minutes in duration. Raters may score whole group or individual performance. Individuals with adequate intellectual functioning may complete self-assessment of performance. In addition, the group may collaborate to assess social participation following the group activity. • The SP is divided into 3 sections identifying group cooperation: 1. Activity participation: How do the activities influence group interaction? 2. Social interaction: How do group members interact with each other? 3. Group membership and roles: Do members feel they belong to the group? • Each of the sections are then divided into the 5 different levels of social participation: Parallel, Associative, Basic Cooperation, Supportive Cooperation, and Mature[51,52]
Time Required	• Requires observation of a group activity of 30 minutes or more • Observation of 3 separate session of 30 minutes or more. Time to complete rating scales is not provided.
Reliability	
Test-Retest	• Test-retest reliability correlation of .75
Internal Consistency	• ICC statistical test[53] revealed reliability for preschool and senior center groups a .8813 and for psychiatric groups a .8028
Inter-Rater	• Additional reliability information for the preschool population: ¤ Inter-rater reliability for parallel level scores range from .71 to .90 ¤ Inter-rater reliability for cooperative groups ranged from .59 to .79 **Authors hypothesized that lower rates of reliability may be related to the fact that cooperative groups include a wider range of behaviors and are not as discrete as behaviors in the parallel level.
Validity	
Content	• Research found good content and construct validity based on ratings by an expert panel of judges, cluster analysis, and factor analysis. See test manual for descriptions for each area across groups.
Construct	• Parallel behaviors ranged from .78 to .90 • Supportive cooperative from .84 to .93 • Associative behaviors from .77 to 94 • Basic cooperative from .64 to .75

(continued)

Table 12-13 (continued)

THE SOCIAL PROFILE (SP)

Validity	
Criterion	• Criterion validity reported .85 for preschool level when compared to Parten[52]
Standardization	• 187 typically developing children in 3 daycare and preschool programs in Manhattan.
Utility	
Research Programs	• Studies reveal potential for SP as a tool to identify social participation of children participating in group activities.
Practice Settings	• The SP may be particularly useful in developing observational skills in therapy students and novice therapists assessing group performance. • Academics report utility in training students in observational skills and conducting research in social participation. • Schools, clinics, residential treatment programs, and community-based programs
Strengths	• The shortened version is efficient and may expand the clinical utility of the instrument. It is useful as a descriptive measure rather than an evaluative measure of change over time.
Complexities	• Reliability of rating is dependent on observer's clear understanding of the various levels of social participation. Training in the distinction between the different levels is recommended.

Table 12-14

SOCIAL SKILLS IMPROVEMENT SYSTEM (TIERS 2 AND 3) (SSIS)

Source	http://www.pearsonclinical.com/education/RelatedInfo/ssis-overview.html
Key References	Gresham and Elliot[54]
Purpose	• SSIS, Performance Screening Guide: Screens the whole classroom for prosocial behaviors • SSIS, Rating Scales: Assesses individual student social behavior
Type of Client	• All students
Test Format	• Questionnaire
Procedures	• SSIS, Performance Screening Guide: Teacher completes instrument on entire classroom • SSIS, Rating Skills: Teacher, parent, and/or student completes instrument on individual student
Time Required	• Approximately 20 minutes to complete the instrument
Reliability *Test-Retest* *Internal Consistency* *Inter-Rater*	• Rating scales ▫ Teacher forms: Coefficients range from .68 to .86 with median adjusted reliability coefficient of .81 ▫ Parent: Subscales in .70s with median adjusted reliability coefficient of subscales at .80 ▫ Students: Range between .59 to .81 with median adjusted reliability coefficient of .71 • Performance screening guide ▫ Preschool test-retest was moderate (.53 to .62) ▫ Elementary and secondary test-retest were upper .60s and low .70s, which were "substantial." According to the manual, these can be considered "moderate-strong" test-retest reliability ▫ Inter-rater: overall mean is similar across groups included in the standardization.

(continued)

Table 12-14

Social Skills Improvement System (Tiers 2 and 3) (SSIS)

Validity *Content* *Construct* *Criterion*	• Teacher Forms (Preschool, Elementary, Secondary) .62 to .79 coefficients for Social Skills; .70 to .85 for Problem Behaviors; .87 to .89 for Academic Competence. • Parent Form: .69 to .75 for Social Skills; .65 to .77 for Problem Behaviors • Student Form: .36 to .64 Social Skills (Problem Behaviors not reported) • Valid in reporting differences among students with various disabilities (eg, ADHD, ASD, emotional/behavioral conditions, gifted/talented, intellectual disability, speech language impairment).
Standardization	• 4700 children ages 3 to 18; 115 sites in 36 states • Other measures: ¤ Behavior Assessment System for Children (BASC), Vineland-II Adaptive Behavior Scales, Walker-McConnell Scale of Social Competence and School Adjustment, Home and Community Social Behavior Scales • Other groups: ¤ Autism, ADHD, developmental delay, emotional/behavioral disturbance, gifted/talented, intellectual disability, specific learning disability, speech/language impairment
Utility *Research Programs* *Practice Settings*	 • Used widely in research • Used by school psychologists in practice
Strengths	• Used widely across disciplines • Can be used as pre-/post-test measure • Multiple raters
Complexities	• Must be familiar with students before administering

Table 12-15

Child Sensory Profile 2 (CSP2)

Source	www.sensoryprofile.com
Key References	Dunn[16] Sample evidence from first edition: Engel-Yeger et al[55]; Naish and Harris[56]; Ohl et al[57]; Perez Robles et al[58]; Reynolds et al[59]; Shea and Wu[60]
Purpose	• The purpose of the Child Sensory Profile 2 is to provide a standardized way to document children's sensory processing patterns.
Type of Client *Test Format* *Procedures* *Time Required*	• Children 3 years to 14 years, 11 months. • The CSP2 is a caregiver questionnaire. • There are 86 items that caregivers rate on a 5-point Likert scale from 1 (almost never) to 5 (almost always). Caregivers complete the questionnaire on their own. • Paper/pencil and web-based options are available, including a standardized reporting system. • It takes 15 minutes to complete the CSP2. • It takes 30 minutes to score and report about the findings.

(continued)

Table 12-15 (continued)

Child Sensory Profile 2 (CSP2)

Reliability	
Test-Retest	• Test-retest correlation coefficients for the CSP2 are .87 to .97.
Internal Consistency	• Internal consistency for the CSP2 is generally .80 to .90; visual processing is .60.
Inter-Rater	• Inter-rater reliability occurred between 2 caregivers; correlation coefficients ranged from .73 to .89, generally. Visual (.49) and Touch (.55) processing were lower.
Validity	
Content	• The author reports that content validity was established through examinations of available evidence, expert reviews, and pilot studies.
Construct	• The CSP2 correlates with the Sensory Profile First Edition .67 to .87. • There are many studies that provided evidence for the first edition of the Sensory Profile. These studies verify that there are specific patterns of sensory processing for children who have various conditions, including autism and ADHD and several others. The following articles provide some recent examples: Abele-Webster et al[61]; Davis et al[62]; Fox et al[63]; Hildenbrand and Smith[64]; Jewers et al[65]; Riby et al[66]; Shahar et al[67]; Van der Linde et al[68]; Taal et al[69]
Criterion	• For the CSP2, the manual contains comparisons between the CSP2 and several other measures. Generally, when children have higher frequency sensory processing patterns, they are less adaptable; lower frequency sensory processing patterns are correlated with higher adaptability scores. • Behavior Assessment System for Children, 2nd ed [home] • Social Skills Improvement System [parent] • Vineland II Adaptive Behavior Scale [parent] • Sensory Profile [first edition] • Examples of criterion validity reported in other studies: Dar et al[70]; Gouze et al[71]; Lidstone et al[72]; O'Donnell et al[73]
Standardization	• The CSP2 was standardized across the United States with 697 children (caregivers completed the form). Ten percent of the standardization sample represented children with various disabilities; the overall sample was stratified based on the population distribution.
Utility	
Research Programs	• The authors created the Short Sensory Profile 2 (SSP2) for use in research programs. The SSP2 contains 34 items selected from the CSP2 as highly discriminating items. The SSP2 is brief enough to be either a central or an ancillary measure for research protocols. It provides data on the child's sensory processing patterns, and so provides an additional perspective about the child's participation.
Practice Settings	• The CSP2 can be used in screening programs to determine which children might need additional consideration related to how sensory processing affects participation. • The CSP2 is specifically designed for practice, so it is very relevant to children's participation in home and community. Having the caregiver's perspective about how a child interacts based on sensory patterns is quite useful as the team makes recommendations.
Strengths	• The CSP2 is easy to administer and score. It is based on Dunn's Sensory Processing Framework[16] so has a theoretical foundation based on research from the first editions of the Sensory Profile tests. Validity and reliability are strong for the second edition.

(continued)

Table 12-15 (continued)

Child Sensory Profile 2 (CSP2)

Strengths	• The CSP2 contains items that are familiar behaviors for caregivers, making this assessment relevant to everyday life. Scores for sensory, behavioral and patterns are consistent with the school version, making it easy to compare across settings.
Complexities	• Online report generation requires that you collect additional information about the child's interests, the family priorities, and goals so that participation outcomes can be linked to sensory processing patterns identified during the assessment. • The CSP2 is based on strengths perspectives; professionals may have to recalibrate their ways of characterizing findings. The CSP2 is not designed to find things that are wrong or need to be fixed, but rather focuses on differences and similarities to the standardization sample. The impact of sensory patterns can only be determined in the context of the particular child's/family's life.

Table 12-16

School Companion Sensory Profile 2 (SCSP2)

Source	www.sensoryprofile.com
Key References	Dunn[16] Sample evidence from first edition: Brown and Dunn[74]; Buitendag and Aronstam[75,76]; Dunn[77]
Purpose	• The purpose of the School Companion Sensory Profile 2 is to provide a standardized way to document children's sensory processing patterns at school.
Type of Client	• Students 3 years to 14 years, 11 months old
Test Format	• The SCSP2 is a teacher questionnaire.
Procedures	• There are 44 items that teachers rate on a 5-point Likert scale from 1 (almost never) to 5 (almost always). Teachers complete the questionnaire on their own. • Paper/pencil and web-based options are available, including a standardized reporting system.
Time Required	• It takes 10 to 15 minutes to complete the SCSP2. • It takes 30 minutes to score and report about the findings.
Reliability	
Test-Retest	• Test-retest correlation coefficients for the SCSP2 are .66 to .93.
Internal Consistency	• Internal consistency for the SCSP2 is .81 to .92.
Inter-Rater	• Inter-rater reliability occurred between the student's primary teacher and another educator selected by that teacher; ratings generally ranged from . 76 to .90. Registration (.56) and Visual processing (.53) were lower.
Validity	
Content	• The author reports that content validity was established through examinations of available evidence, expert reviews, and pilot studies.
Construct	• The studies above provided evidence for the 1st edition of the Sensory Profile School Companion. These studies verify that the School Companion provides relevant data about sensory processing for children who have various conditions.

(continued)

Table 12-16 (continued)

School Companion Sensory Profile 2 (SCSP2)	
Validity	
Construct	• When comparing the SCSP2 to the original Sensory Profile School Companion, the author reports significant correlation coefficients of .42 to .74; touch was not related.
Criterion	• For the 2nd edition, the author reports on comparisons between the SCSP2 and several other measures: ¤ Behavior Assessment System for Children, 2nd edition [school] ¤ Social Skills Improvement System [school] ¤ Vineland II Adaptive Behavior Scale [school] ¤ School Function Assessment ¤ Sensory Profile School Companion [first edition]
Standardization	• The SCSP2 was standardized across the United States with 679 students (teachers completed the forms). Ten percent of the standardization sample represented children with various disabilities; the overall sample was stratified based on the population distribution.
Utility	
Research Programs	• The SCSP2 is brief enough to be either a central or an ancillary measure for research protocols. It provides data on the student's sensory processing patterns during school, and so provides an additional perspective about what might be supporting or interfering with participation as a student.
Practice Settings	• Specifically designed for the practice setting of school, so it is very relevant to school-based practice. Having the teacher's perspective about how a student interacts based on sensory patterns is quite useful as the team designs interventions in the school contexts.
Strengths	• The SCSP2 is easy to administer and score. It is based on Dunn's Sensory Processing Framework[16] and so has a theoretical foundation based on research from the 1st editions of the Sensory Profile tests. Validity and reliability are strong for the second edition. • The SCSP2 contains items specifically for teachers and school settings, making this assessment relevant to this context and these activities. Scores for sensory systems, behaviors, and sensory patterns are consistent with the caregiver version, making it easy to compare across settings.
Complexities	• Online report generation requires that you collect additional information about the student's interests, the teacher's priorities, and goals so that these outcomes can be linked to sensory processing patterns identified during the assessment. • The SCSP2 is based on strengths perspectives; professionals may have to recalibrate their ways of characterizing findings. The SCSP2 is not designed to find things that are wrong or need to be fixed, but rather focuses on differences and similarities to the standardization sample. The impact of sensory patterns can only be determined in the context of the particular teacher's expectations of that student at school.

Table 12-17

Vineland Adaptive Behavior Scales, Second Edition (Vineland-II)

- Tier 2 and 3
- Three Versions: 1) Survey Forms: Survey Interview Form and Parent/Caregiver Rating Form; 2) The Expanded Interview Form, 3) The Teacher Rating Form

*We will be discussing the Teacher Rating Form – For the other versions of the form, please see the manual

Source	http://www.pearsonclinical.com/psychology/products/100000668/vineland-adaptive-behavior-scales-second-edition-vineland-ii-vinelandii.html
Key References	Sparrow et al[78]
Purpose	• The Vineland-II is a battery of assessments that provide adaptive behavior composites for people 0 to 90. Because this chapter focuses on assessment in the school setting, this box provides information on the Vineland-II, Teacher Rating Form Manual. For information on other Vineland assessments (ie, Survey Interview Form and Parent/Caregiver Rating Form; The Expanded Interview Form), please refer to the manual. The assessment is designed to measure adaptive behavior in the following domains: Communication, Daily Living Skills, Socialization, Motor Skills, and Maladaptive Behaviors.
Type of Client	• Individuals/students with adaptive behavior concerns.
Test Format	• Teacher Rating Forms—Record Booklet
Procedures	• Teacher completes booklet/questionnaire on the following domains: Communication (subdomains: receptive, expressive, and written), Daily Living Skills (personal, academic, and school/community), Socialization (interpersonal relationships, play and leisure time, coping skills), Motor Skills (gross and fine), and Adaptive Behavior Composite.
Time Required	• Teacher Rating Form: 20 minutes to complete, with 15 to 30 minutes for professionals to score and interpret. • ASSIST Software available for scoring
Reliability	
Test-Retest	• Test-retest: Domains average in the mid .80s; adaptive behavior composite is .91.
Internal Consistency	• Internal Consistency: 135 students tested; Domain average "very high" within the mid 90s, except for motor skills, which ranged from .86 to .92.
Inter-Rater	• Interrater Reliability: 180 students; domains range from mid .40s to high .60s. *For subdomain reports, see manual
Validity *Content* *Construct* *Criterion*	• Vineland-II compared to Vineland ABS Classroom Edition, the Weschler Intelligence Scale for Children 3rd and 4th Edition (WISC), the Adaptive Behavior Assessment System (ABAS) and the Behavior Assessment System for Children, 2nd Edition (BASC-2). • The Vineland-II TRF correlates high with the BASC-2 TRF and demonstrates an almost equal adaptive behavior score to that of the WISC IQ score. It also has a high correlation with the ABAS. • The Vineland-II was tested with the following clinical samples: ADHD, autism (verbal/non-verbal), emotional/behavioral disturbance, hearing impairment, learning disability, mental retardation (mild, moderate, severe/profound), visual impairment. • Results indicate the Vineland-II is able to distinguish among different clinical populations.

(continued)

Table 12-17 (continued)

Vineland Adaptive Behavior Scales, Second Edition (Vineland-II)

Standardization	• For the TRF, 277 students from 142 sites, with 6.5% received special education services. • Clinical samples: ADHD, autism (verbal/nonverbal), emotional/behavioral disturbance, hearing impairment, learning disability, mental retardation (mild, moderate, severe/profound), visual impairment.
Utility	
Research Programs	• Used widely in research
Practice Settings	• Schools, residential treatment programs, community-based programs
Strengths	• Used widely across disciplines • Can be used as pre-/posttest measure • Interviews can be used to gain multiple facets of participation • A variety of forms (survey, questionnaire, teacher, parent) can be used to gather information
Complexities	• Requires time to score and interpret.

References

1. Missiuna C, Pollock N, Levac D, et al. Partnering for Change: an innovative school-based occupational therapy service delivery model for children with developmental coordination disorder. *Can J Occup Therapy.* 2012;79(1):41-50.
2. Mossman Steiner A. A strength-based approach to parent education for children with autism. *J Positive Behavior Interventions.* 2011;13(3):178-190.
3. Seligman MEP. Positive psychology: fundamental assumptions. *The Psychologist.* 2003;16:126-127.
4. Saleeby D. *The Strengths Perspective in Social Work Practice.* 2nd ed. New York: Longman Publishers; 1996.
5. Dunn W, Koenig K, Cox J, et al. Harnessing strengths: daring to celebrate everyone's unique contributions. Part 1. *Developmental Disabilities Special Interest Section Quarterly.* 2013;36(1):1-3.
6. Dunn W, Koenig K, Cox J, et al. Harnessing strengths: daring to celebrate everyone's unique contributions. Part 2. *Developmental Disabilities Special Interest Section Quarterly.* 2013;36(2):1-3.
7. Hansen N, Philo C. The normality of doing things differently: bodies, spaces and disability geography. *Tijdschrift voor Economische en Sociale Geography.* 2007;98(4):493-506.
8. Fox L, Carta J, Strain PS, Dunlap G, Hemmeter ML. Response to intervention and the pyramid model. *Infants Young Children.* 2010;23(1):3-13.
9. Connell B, Jones M, Mace R, et al. *The Principles of Universal Design.* Raleigh, NC: North Carolina State University, The Center for Universal Design; 1997.
10. Basyk S, Demirijan L, Horvath F. Creating a Comfortable Cafeteria Program. 2014. Available at: https://www.drugfreeactionalliance.org/files/opec/OPEC_Comfy_Cafeteria.pdf. Accessed June 19, 2016.
11. Missiuna CA, Pollock NA, Levac DE, et al. Partnering for change: an innovative school-based occupational therapy service delivery model for children with developmental coordination disorder. *Can J Occup Ther.* 2012;79(1):41-50.
12. Schrank FA, Mather N, McGrew KS. *Woodcock-Johnson IV Tests of Achievement.* Rolling Meadows, IL: Riverside; 2014.
13. Coster W, Deeney TA, Haley S, Haltiwanger J. *School Function Assessment.* San Antonio, TX: The Psychological Corporation; 1998.
14. Dunn W. *The Sensory Profile.* San Antonio, TX: Pearson; 1999.
15. Alotaibi MN, Reed K, Nadar SM. Assessments used in occupational therapy practice: an exploratory study. *Occup Ther Health Care.* 2009;23(4):302-318.
16. Dunn W. *The Sensory Profile 2: Strengths Based Approach to Assessment and Planning.* San Antonio, TX: Pearson; 2014.
17. McLaren C, Rodger S. Goal attainment scaling: clinical implications for paediatric occupational therapy practice. *Austr Occup Ther J.* 2003;50(4):216-224.
18. Cusick A, McIntyre S, Novak I, Lannin N, Lowe K. A comparison of goal attainment scaling and the Canadian Occupational Performance Measure for pediatric rehabilitation research. *Pediatr Rehabil.* 2006;9(2):149-157.
19. Dunn W. *Best Practice Occupational Therapy for Children and Families in Community Settings.* Thorofare, NJ: SLACK Incorporated; 2011.
20. Wei Y, Oakland T, Algina J, MacLean WE. Multigroup, confirmatory factor analysis for the adaptive behavior assessment system-II. *Am J Retard.* 2008;113(3):178-186.
21. Rust JO, Wallace MA. Book review: Adaptive Behavior Assessment System. *J Psychoeduc Assess.* 2004;22(4):367-373.
22. American Psychiatric Association. *Diagnostic Criteria From DSM-IV-TR.* Arlington, VA: American Psychiatric Association Publishing; 2000.

23. Luckasson R, Coulter DL, Polloway EA, et al. *Mental Retardation: Definition, Classification, and Systems of Supports.* 9th ed. Washington DC: American Association on Mental Retardation; 1992.
24. Luckasson R, Borthwick-Duffy S, Buntinx WH, et al. *Mental Retardation: Definition, Classification, and Systems of Supports.* 10th ed. Washington DC: American Association on Mental Retardation; 2002.
25. Reynolds C, Kamphaus R. *Behavior Assessment for Children* (BASC-2). 2nd ed. Minneapolis, MN: Pearson, Inc; 2004.
26. Volker M. BASC-2 PRS profiles for students with high functioning autism spectrum disorders. *J Autism Dev Disord.* 2010;40(2):188-199.
27. Mahan S. Children and adolescents with autism spectrum disorders compared to typically developing controls on the BASC-2. *Res Autism Spectrum Disord.* 2011;5(1):119-125.
28. Titus J. Behavioral profiles of children with epilepsy: parent and teacher reports of emotional, behavioral, and educational concerns on the BASC-2. *Psychol Schools.* 2008;45(9):893-904.
29. Zeitlin S, Williamson G, Szczepanski, M. *Early Coping Inventory: A Measure of Adaptive Behavior.* Bensenville, IL: Scholastic Testing Service; 1988.
30. Simmons CD, Griswold LA, Berg B. Evaluation of social interaction during occupational engagement. *Am J Occup Ther.* 2010;64(1):10-17.
31. Søndergaard M, Fisher AG. Sensitivity of the evaluation of social interaction measures among people with and without neurologic or psychiatric disorders. *Am J Occup Ther.* 2012;66(3):356-362.
32. Dunn-Buron K, Wolfberg P. *Learners on the Autism Spectrum: Preparing Highly Qualified Educators.* Shawnee Mission, KS: Autism Asperger Publishing; 2008.
33. DuPaul GJ, Kern L, Volpe R, et al. Comparison of parent education and functional assessment-based intervention across 24 months for young children with attention deficit hyperactivity disorder. *School Psychol Rev.* 2013;42(1):56-75.
34. Kamps D, Wendland M, Culpepper M. Active teacher participation in functional behavior assessment for students with emotional and behavioral disorders risks in general education classrooms. *Behav Disord.* 2006;31(2):128-146.
35. Dumas HM, Fragala-Pinkham MA. Concurrent validity and reliability of the pediatric evaluation of disability inventory-computer adaptive test mobility domain. *Pediatr Phys Ther.* 2012;24(2):171-176.
36. Dumas H, Fragala-Pinkham M, Haley S, et al. Item bank development for a revised Pediatric Evaluation of Disability Inventory (PEDI). *Phys Occup Ther Pediatr.* 2010;30(3):168-184.
37. Haley SM, Coster WJ, Dumas HM, et al. Accuracy and precision of the Pediatric Evaluation of Disability Inventory computer-adaptive tests (PEDI-CAT). *Dev Med Child Neurol.* 2011;53(12):1100-1106.
38. Haley SM, Coster WJ, Dumas HM, Fragala-Pinkham MA, Moed R. *PEDI-CAT: Development, Standardization and Administration Manual.* Boston, MA: CRECare LLC; 2010.
39. Kao YC, Kramer JM, Liljenquist K, Tian F, Coster WJ. Comparing the functional performance of children and youth with autism, developmental disabilities, and without disabilities using the revised Pediatric Evaluation of Disability Inventory (PEDI) Item Banks. *Am J Occup Ther.* 2012;66(5):607.
40. Munkholm M, Löfgren B, Fisher AG. Reliability of the School AMPS measures. *Scand J Occup Ther.* 2012;19:2-8.
41. Fingerhut P, Madill H, Darrah J, Hodge M, Warren, S. Brief report—classroom-based assessment: validation for the School AMPS. *Am J Occup Ther.* 2002;56:210-213.
42. Atchison BT, Fisher AG, Bryze K. Rater reliability and internal scale and person response validity of the School Assessment of Motor and Process Skills. *Am J Occup Ther.* 1998;52:843-850.
43. Fisher AG, Bryze K, Hume V, Griswold LA. *School AMPS: School Version of the Assessment of Motor and Process Skills.* 2nd ed. Fort Collins, CO: Three Star Press; 2005.
44. Bowyer PL, Ross M, Schwartz O, Kielhofner G, Kramer J. *The Short Child Occupational Profile (SCOPE): Version 2.1.* Chicago, IL: Model of Human Occupation Clearinghouse; 2005.
45. Kielhofner G. *Model of Human Occupation: Theory and Application.* 4th ed. Philadelphia, PA: Lippincott, Williams and Wilkins; 2008.
46. Sakzewski L, Boyd R, Ziviani J. Clinimetric properties of participation measures for 5- to 13-year-old children with cerebral palsy: a systematic review. *Dev Med Child Neurol.* 2007;49(3):232-240.
47. American Occupational Therapy Association. *Occupational Therapy Services for Children and Youth Under the Individuals with Disabilities Education Act.* Bethesda, MD: AOTA; 1997.
48. Coster W. Occupation centered assessment of children. *Am J Occup Ther.* 1998;52:337-344.
49. Donohue MV. Social profile: assessment of validity and reliability with preschool children. *Can J Occup Ther.* 2005;72(3):164-175.
50. Donohue MV. Interrater reliability of the Social Profile: assessment of community and psychiatric group participation. *Aust Occup Ther J.* 54(1):49-58.
51. Mosey AC. The proper focus of scientific inquiry in occupational therapy: frames of reference. *OTJR.* 1989;9(4):195-201.
52. Parten MB. Social participation among pre-school children. *J Abnorm Soc Psychol.* 1932;27(3):243.
53. Shrout PE, Fleiss JL. Intraclass correlations: uses in assessing rater reliability. *Psychologic Bulletin.* 1979;86(2):420.
54. Gresham FM, Elliot SN. *Social Skills Improvement System.* Minneapolis, MN: Pearson, Inc; 2008.
55. Engel-Yeger B, Hus S, Rosenblum S. Age effects on sensory-processing abilities and their impact on handwriting. *Can J Occup Ther.* 2012;79(5):264-274.
56. Naish KR, Harris G. Food intake is influenced by sensory sensitivity. *PloS One.* 2012;7(8):e43622.
57. Ohl A, Butler C, Carney C. Test-retest reliability of the Sensory Profile Caregiver Questionnaire. *Am J Occup Ther.* 2012;66(4): 483-488.
58. Perez Robles R, Jane Ballabriga MC, Doval Dieguez E, da Silva PC. Validating regulatory sensory processing disorders using the Sensory Profile and Child Behavior Checklist (CBCL 11/2-5). *J Child Fam Stud.* 2012;21(6):906-916.
59. Reynolds S, Lane SJ, Thacker L. Sensory processing, physiological stress, and sleep behaviors in children with and without autism spectrum disorders. *OTJR.* 2012;32(1):246-257.
60. Shea C, Wu R. Finding the key: sensory profiles of youths involved in the justice system. *OT Practice.* October 7, 2013;9-13.

61. Abele-Webster LA, Magill-Evans JE, Pei JR. Sensory processing and ADHD in children with fetal alcohol spectrum disorder. *Can J Occup Ther.* 2012;79(1):60-63.
62. Davis AM, Bruce AS, Khasawneh R, Schulz T, Fox C, Dunn W. Validating regulatory sensory processing disorders using the Sensory Profile and Child Behavior Checklist (CBCL 11/2-5). *J Child Fam Stud.* 2012;56(2):156-160.
63. Fox C, Snow PC, Holland K. The relationship between sensory processing difficulties and behaviour in children aged 5 to 9 who are at risk of developing conduct disorder. *Emot Behav Diffic.* 2014;19(1):71-88.
64. Hildenbrand HL, Smith ACM. Analysis of the Sensory Profile in children with Smith-Magenis syndrome. *Phys Occup Ther Pediatr.* 2012;32(1):48-65.
65. Jewers R, Staley D, Shady G. Sensory processing differences in children diagnosed with Tourette's disorder. *Occup Ther Ment Health.* 2013;29(4):385-394.
66. Riby DM, Janes E, Rodgers J. Brief report: exploring the relationship between sensory processing and repetitive behaviours in Williams Syndrome. *J Autism Dev Disord.* 2013;43(2):478-482.
67. Shahar E, Zlotnik S, Ravid S, Engel-Yeger B. Sensory processing disabilities in childhood-onset generalized epilepsy. *J Pediatr Neurol.* 2013;11(2):83-88.
68. Van der Linde J, Franzsen D, Barnard-Ashton P. The sensory profile: comparative analysis of children with specific language impairment, ADHD and autism. *South African J Occup Ther.* 2013;43(3):34-40.
69. Taal MN, Rietman AB, Meulen SV, Schipper M, Dejonckere PH. Children with specific language impairment show difficulties in sensory modulation. *Logoped Phoniatr Vocol.* 2013;38(2):70-78.
70. Dar R, Kahn DT, Carmeli R. The relationship between sensory processing, childhood rituals and obsessive-compulsive symptoms. *J Behav Ther Exp Psychiatry.* 2012;43(1):679-684.
71. Gouze KR, Lavigne JV, Hopkins J, Bryant FB, Lebailly SA. The relationship between temperamental negative affect, effortful control, and sensory regulation: a new look. *Infant Ment Health J.* 2012;33(6):620-632.
72. Lidstone J, Uljarevic M, Sullivan J. Relations among restricted and repetitive behaviors, anxiety and sensory features in children with autism spectrum disorders. *Res Autism Spectrum Disord.* 2014;8(2):82-92.
73. O'Donnell S, Deitz J, Kartin D, Nalty T, Dawson G. Sensory processing, problem behavior, adaptive behavior, and cognition in preschool children with autism spectrum disorders. *Am J Occup Ther.* 2012;66(5):586-594.
74. Brown NB, Dunn W. Relationship between context and sensory processing in children with autism. *Am J Occup Ther.* 2010;64(3):474-483.
75. Buitendag K, Aronstam MC. The relationship between developmental dyspraxia and sensory responsivity in children aged 4 years through 8 years: part I. *South African J Occup Ther.* 2010;40(3):16-20.
76. Buitendag K, Aronstam MC. The relationship between developmental dyspraxia and sensory responsivity in children aged 4 to 8 years: part II. *South African J Occup Ther.* 2012;42(2):2-7.
77. Dunn W. Harnessing teacher's wisdom for evidence based practice: standardization data from the Sensory Profile School Companion. *J Occup Ther Schools Early Int.* 2008;1(3-4):206-214.
78. Sparrow SS, Cicchetti DC, Balla DA. *Vineland Adaptive Behavior Scales.* 2nd ed. Minneapolis, MN: Pearson Inc; 2006.

Legislative Resources

The following are legislative resources that mandate occupational therapy services, and provide regulations about how services are provided:

U.S. Department of Education for information about the laws: www.ed.gov .

http://sitemaker.umich.edu/356.zipkin/home University of Michigan resources about Special Education Legislation.

Section 504 of the Rehabilitation Act of 1973. http://www.hhs.gov/ocr/civilrights/resources/factsheets/504.pdf

Education for All Handicapped Children Act of 1975 (EHA) (PL 94-142) http://files.eric.ed.gov/fulltext/ED452659.pdf.

EHA Amendments, the Preschool Law of 1986 (PL 99-457) http://eric.ed.gov/?id=ED277172.

Individuals with Disabilities Education Act of 1990 (IDEA) (PL 101-476). (for the reauthorization of IDEA, 2004 see www.idea.ed.gov).

No Child Left Behind Act of 2002 (NCLB) (www.NoChildLeftBehind.gov LINK BROKEN).

Schoolwide Integrated Framework for Transformation (SWIFT) http://www.swiftschools.org/

Mine the Gold

Rehabilitation professionals from many disciplines have acknowledged the importance of activities of daily living (ADL) as foundational for all types of activities, participation, and occupations.

Become Systematic

Measures of ADL can be used to describe current abilities for clients of all ages. Many ADL measures can be used effectively to measure change over time and are useful across broad populations, making comparison over time and across practice areas possible.

Use Evidence in Practice

With standardized ADL measures, it is possible to measure change over time, and through that to potentially capture the effectiveness of rehabilitation interventions. Further, the combination of self-report and observational measures can provide data that can be combined in setting goals and intervention plans.

Make Occupational Therapy Contributions Explicit

ADL are frequently assessed and addressed in occupational therapy practice, across ages, conditions, and settings. Using standardized ADL measures can provide occupational therapists with concrete information to demonstrate the importance and value of attention to ADL.

Engage in Occupation-Based, Client-Centered Practice

Self-report measures can provide clients' perspectives on their performance, capacity, and satisfaction in their ADL. Used along with observation, an occupational therapist can design interventions to help clients address their basic self-care needs so that they can proceed to other areas of occupation.

CHAPTER 13

Measuring Occupational Performance in Basic Activities of Daily Living

Lori Letts, PhD, OT Reg. (Ont.) and Jackie Bosch, PhD, OT Reg. (Ont.)

What Are Activities of Daily Living?

Activities of daily living (ADL) are ubiquitous to the practice of occupational therapy. Almost to our detriment, they have become so much a part of our practice and our vernacular that we seldom pause to consider the true definition. Practice frameworks such as the AOTA framework[1] provide evidence of the fundamental nature of the concept by providing definitions that include words such as "taking care of one's body; fundamental to living; enable basic survival and well-being."[1(p S19)] While it seems that it should be easy to define the *basic activities of life*, these activities are dependent on a person's preferences, culture, environment, and stage of life.

The variance in definition is evident in the measures of ADL themselves because there are many measures available, yet none identical in content. For clinicians to evaluate ADL, they need to consider the factors that are important and choose a measure that best evaluates those components of ADL that are important to the client.

ADL are often divided into 2 broad categories. The first category, and the focus of this chapter, includes the most intimate self-care and personal care items, as defined previously. These activities can be called *basic* or *personal ADL* in some measures. Examples include toileting, bathing, dressing, and eating. The second is most commonly known as instrumental ADL (IADL). IADL are generally considered to be those "activities to support daily life within the home and community that often require more complex interactions than those used in ADLs."[1(p S19)] Examples of IADL include meal preparation, shopping, banking, driving, or using transportation. Assessment of IADL is often conducted through different measures than basic ADL measures, and in this text, IADL measures are reviewed in more detail in Chapter 14.

The Importance of Measuring Activities of Daily Living

Generally, occupational therapists want to measure basic ADLs to describe the client's current status, to set goals (eg, an intervention plan or determine a discharge setting), or because we think the status will change and change should be quantified. Therapists use ADL measures to do this because they either help them understand the client's ability or the burden of care. ADL measures are used not only to quantify ability, but for those measures that include direct observation, additional insights can be gained into the causes of the deficits. Ultimately, therapists use these measures to improve their ability to address ADL concerns of the client.

What Are the Usual Elements Included in Activities of Daily Living Measures?

Almost all measures of ADL include bathing, dressing, grooming, eating, and toileting. Functional mobility, communication, and bowel and bladder continence sometimes are included. The method for assessing each of these varies greatly between measures: observation vs self-report; simple (1 item per activity) to complex observations of activities broken into many components. Although the content areas seem similar, the methods by which they are assessed are really what makes variation between the measures.

Law M, Baum C, Dunn W, eds. *Measuring Occupational Performance: Supporting Best Practice in Occupational Therapy, Third Edition (pp 269-303).*

Strategies for Selecting Activities of Daily Living Measures

In considering which ADL measures to use, therapists have a number of possible sources for outcome measures. For example, a search of "activities of daily living" as the area of assessment on the Rehabilitation Measures Database (available at www.rehabmeasures.org) results in a list of over 80 measures. Thus, therapists have access to a large number of measures; some are for specific diagnostic groups, some embed ADL items within a measure of quality of life or symptoms. As such, therapists need to apply criteria to select the most appropriate measure.

In this chapter, ADL measures have been selected based on criteria that also might be important to clinicians (eg, a measure that has a summary score for ADL items, even if other areas are measured, some evidence of reliability testing having been completed, and so on). Our intent is to provide information on high-quality measures that are commonly used in research and/or practice.

Clinicians should decide on the most appropriate measure by considering the following:

- Content of the measure and items that are measured (for diagnosis, based on age)
- Method of measurement (eg, self-report or based on observations)
- Requirements of the setting
- Issues identified by the client
- Clinicians' abilities and time availability
- Use for clinical or research purposes

The instruments included in this chapter are clearly not the only ADL measures that should be used, but instead present a short list of the higher quality measures that should usually meet the basic criteria of ADL measurement.

Strategies for Communicating Assessment Results

Communicating results from standardized ADL assessments can be a challenge. Each of the ADL measures reviewed in this chapter characterize ADL abilities, capacities, or observations as a number. Although numbers are important in measurement and, with multiple administrations, they can provide indications of change, numbers can only be helpful if the meaning is understood by everyone who needs to use it. Clinicians using ADL scores need to ensure that people understand the meaning of the number. This might require educating team members, clients, and families on assessment results. This task is easier when norms exist; unfortunately, they are not available for many ADL measures. Commonly used instruments are often well known by team members, making communication of results within a team much easier.

Usefulness of the assessment results beyond specific clinical needs as a clinician is another consideration when selecting a measure. For example, there are some settings that require administration of specific measures like the Functional Independent Measure (FIM) as a method of outcome evaluation of the rehabilitation program.

In addition to scores, documentation of specific observations can be very helpful to illustrate the strengths and deficits experienced by the client during observations. These can also be helpful in communicating with teams, family members, and of course, clients. A combination of scores and examples or observational recordings may optimize understanding of a client's ADL function at any time.

Future Directions for Practice and Research

As previously mentioned, ADL have been measured by occupational therapists since the profession's early days, and there are many commonalities in terms of content across measures. It is not likely that there are major content gaps in ADL measurement; however, it has been challenging to ensure that the concept is measured precisely. One may question whether precision is necessary, but at times, it may mean an inability to detect actual and important change. Future directions for development of ADL measures should focus on the intent to improve precision while keeping efficiency and incorporating client preference.

In rehabilitation, the International Classification of Functioning, Disability and Health (ICF)[2] has become more prominent in guiding considerations and understandings of the factors that affect participation. As measures evolve, it may be important for consideration to be given to the nature of the items in new or revised ADL measures. At this point, measures may be inconsistent at times in their focus on activities, participation, body functions, and environmental factors. The Functional Autonomy Measurement System (SMAF) was originally developed using the International Classification of Impairments, Disabilities and Handicaps[3] as a framework; more recently, some research has explored how it fits with the newer ICF. In order to optimally understand ADL as either activity or participation, measures might be developed or revised to ensure that items are all focusing on activities and/or participation, for example. In this way, measures might be adopted more readily in research and program evaluation efforts.

That said, with an abundance of measures of ADL, we would argue that there is little need to develop new ADL measures. Rather, the focus of future research and practice should be adoption of the best of any number of well-researched existing measures. For example, both the FIM[4] and the Barthel[5] are well-researched ADL measures that can be used in evaluation and research, with evidence of reliability, validity, the ability to detect clinically important change, and efficiency of administration. A well-validated measure of both ADL and IADL, the Performance Assessment of Self-Care Skills (PASS),[6] is another example

Table 13-1

Activities Scale for Kids (ASK)

Source	http://www.activitiesscaleforkids.com/
Key References	Young[9]; Young et al[10,11]
Purpose	• A child self-report measure of physical disability that can be used as an outcome measure.

(continued)

of a well-researched measure that can be used by occupational therapists.

There continues to be a need for research that looks at the relationships amongst and between various ADL activities, leaving clinicians with limited information about ADL performance in general if there is not time to observe all activities. New developments in computer adaptive testing, such as with the Pediatric Evaluation of Disability Inventory (PEDI-CAT),[7] show promise in adding efficiency to instrument completion with fewer items to provide a sense of overall ADL performance. However, they must be used cautiously with children with cognitive impairment where a child may have an awareness problem or does not understand the question.[8]

Environmental considerations continue to be limited in most of the ADL measures reviewed in this chapter. In practice, clinicians would identify that dressing or bathing performance in a hospital setting is potentially quite different from the same activities conducted in familiar home environments, although most of the measures do not take environmental factors into consideration. Other approaches to consider environmental influences on performance may be needed when making determinations about clients' independence, or possible discharge environments, for example.

Overview of Measures of Activities of Daily Living Selection Criteria Review

A broad search of research literature and websites was conducted to identify possible measures of ADL for inclusion in this chapter. Because there were many available, a number of criteria were applied to limit the selections to those that had broad potential use in research and/or clinical practice. Measures were included in the review if there was the following:

- Some evidence for use in clinical practice or research
- An ADL score or subscore (ie, it could be part of a larger measure, but can be used as a stand-alone measure or with a subscore that is ADL-specific)
- At least one peer-reviewed study on reliability and validity
- Direct assessment of ADL activity (eg, opposed to assessing cognition and making an inference about ADL ability)

The measures of ADL reviewed in this chapter include the following:

- Activity Scales for Kids (ASK) (Table 13-1)
- Arnadottir OT–ADL Neurobehavioral Evaluation A-1 (Table 13-2)
- Arthritis Impact Measurement Scales (AIMS-2/SF) (Table 13-3)
- Barthel Index (Table 13-4)
- Functional Autonomy Measurement System (SMAF) (Table 13-5)
- Functional Independence Measure (FIM/Wee-FIM) (Table 13-6)
- Health Assessment Questionnaire (HAQ)/Children's Health Assessment Questionnaire (CHAQ) (Table 13-7)
- Juvenile Arthritis Functional Assessment Report (JAFAR)/Juvenile Arthritis Functional Assessment Scale (JAFAS) (Table 13-8)
- Juvenile Arthritis Self-Report Index (JASI)(Table 13-9)
- Katz Index of Activities of Daily Living (Table 13-10)
- Melville Nelson Self-Care Assessment (Table 13-11)
- Pediatric Evaluation of Disability Inventory (PEDI) (Table 13-12)
- Physical Self Maintenance Scale (PSMS) (Table 13-13)

Each measure offers opportunities for a therapist to consider how a client is able to manage basic ADLs. In comparing the measures, key features include whether a specific population or age group is the focus of the measure. In addition, some measures are more appropriate to use if evaluation of change is the focus of measurement. Administration approaches vary from observational to client/family self-report. In all, the included measures represent a range of measures of ADL that can readily be a starting point to select the most appropriate instrument to measure basic ADL.

Table 13-1 (continued)

Activities Scale for Kids (ASK)

Type of Client	• Children aged 5 to 15 years with musculoskeletal disorders without significant cognitive impairment.
Test Format	• Includes 30 items: personal care (3 items), dressing (4), eating and drinking (1), miscellaneous (2), locomotion (7), stairs (1), play (2), transfers (5), and standing skills (5). • There are 2 versions that can be used: the ASKp (performance measure) asks what the child "did do" in the last week; the ASKc (capability measure) asks what the child "could do" during the last week. • Each item is rated on a 5-point ordinal scale. An aggregate score is achieved by summing the item ratings.
Procedures	• Performance and capability versions may be administered together or separately to a single child or a group of children. • Children under 9 years of age may need a parent to read the questions for them. A clinician should not assist the child.
Time Required	• The manual states that it takes approximately 30 minutes to complete the ASK the first time, and as little as 10 minutes on subsequent administrations. • A study by Pencharz et al[12] noted a mean time of 9 minutes (range of 5 to 12 minutes).
Reliability	• Sample was drawn from rheumatology, orthopedic, and physical therapy clinics at children's rehabilitation hospitals in Ontario, Canada. Children with significant cognitive impairment were excluded.
Test-Retest	• N = 18 (mailed questionnaire sent to 40; 28 returned the first and 18 the second). An ICC of 0.97 was observed for the ASKp and 0.98 the ASKc[11]
Internal Consistency	• Correlation between items was 0.99 (Cronbach's alpha)[9]
Inter-Rater	• Children's and parents' scores were used to calculate intrarater reliability (n = 28); intraclass correlation coefficients (ICC) for child raters are reported to be 0.97 (ASKp) and 0.98 (ASKc), and for parent raters, they are 0.94 (ASKp) and 0.95 (ASKc).[9]
Validity	
Content	• Content validity was established through the instrument development process, which involved children, their parents, and expert review. Rasch analysis was also conducted to examine item characteristics.
Construct	• The ASK was compared to the Childhood Health Assessment Questionnaire (CHAQ) (the CHAQ is not the accepted standard method for measurement of function in this population; therefore, this was not considered criterion testing). The ASKp demonstrated a Pearson correlation of 0.81 with the CHAQ, and the ASKc demonstrated a Pearson correlation of 0.82.[10] • Demonstrated high ($r \geq 0.78$) and moderate ($r \geq 0.49$) correlations to the Pediatric Outcomes Data Collection Instrument (PODCI) and the Child Health Questionnaire Parent form (CHQ-PF-28), respectively[12] • The ASK was also compared to similar and dissimilar constructs of the HUI3 and demonstrated a Spearman's correlation of 0.43 and -0.03 respectively.[10] • It has also been shown that for children with no disability, scores on the ASK differ significantly from children with mild disability ($p = 0.005$).[13] Furthermore, scores for children with severe or moderate disability differ significantly from the ASK scores of those with mild disability ($p < 0.001$ for both).[13]

(continued)

Table 13-1 (continued)

Activities Scale for Kids (ASK)

Validity	
Criterion	• 24 children (n = 24) from rehabilitation clinics were asked to attend a clinic visit in which they completed half the questionnaire. Then, they demonstrated the activities from the questionnaire for clinicians who rated their performance (only ASKc was used). The result was a Pearson's correlation of 0.92 and an intraclass correlation of 0.89.[10]
Responsiveness to Change	• The ASK performance score demonstrated similar change scores to the CHAQ; however, the ASK-capability produced smaller change scores abilities.[10]
Standardization	• The manual is readily available from the author and provides information about the instrument development, reliability, validity, and administration.
Strengths	• The ASK is innovative in that it is based on child self-report and allows the user to decide if the focus is on performance, capability, or both. • The development process was rigorous and the psychometrics have been studied extensively. The correlations between other functional status measures and health status measures is promising.
Considerations	• Development and testing have been focused on children with musculoskeletal disorders; further exploration of its use with children with other impairments would be beneficial. • 18/30 performance questions can be marked "not applicable" and this would most likely apply to younger age ranges. It is unclear how this may affect change scores because ASKp is the more sensitive measure to change.
Final Word	• Since the first edition, the ASK seems to be used more in research settings, probably because of the ease of administration, its strong psychometric properties, as well as its ability to provide a method for examining both a child's capabilities and performance of functional tasks. To date, the clinical community has not followed suit.

Table 13-2

Arnadottir OT-ADL Neurobehavioral Evaluation (A-ONE)

Source	Arnadottir[14]
Key References	Arnadottir[15]; Gardarsdottir and Kaplan[16]; Rubio and Van Deusen[17]
Purpose	• Designed to detect neurobehavioral dysfunctions as well as functional levels (via ADL assessment).
Type of Client	• Designed for people over age 16 years who have central nervous system dysfunctions of cortical origin. It may be particularly useful with people with perceptual impairments.[17]
Test Format	• The A-ONE is divided into 2 parts. Part I includes the functional independence scale (FIS) and the neurobehavioral impairment scale (NIS). The functional independence scale includes dressing, grooming and hygiene, transfers and mobility, feeding, and communication. There are 22 items in this area, and each is rated on a 0 to 4 scale. The NIS has 2 subscales: the Neurobehavioral Specific Impairment Subscale (NSIS) and the Neurobehavioral Pervasive Impairment Subscale (NPIS). The NSIS includes ratings on 10 neurobehavioral items after each ADL task (eg, ideational apraxia, perseveration, abnormal tone). The NPIS determines the presence or absence of other neurobehavioral impairments observed throughout the assessment.

(continued)

Table 13-2 (continued)

Arnadottir OT-ADL Neurobehavioral Evaluation (A-ONE)

Type of Client	
Test Format	• Part II of the A-ONE attempts to localize possible lesion sites by comparing neurobehavioral observations to a chart on lesion sites.
Procedures	• Part I should be completed after 2 or 3 observations of clients engaging in ADL tasks in their natural environment. Part II is completed after Part I and requires no further administration with the client.
Time Required	• The manual states that Part I can be completed in approximately 25 minutes, although it may take longer to observe the person completing ADL tasks on 3 different occasions.
Reliability	
Test-Retest	• Part I values of 0.85 or higher (Spearmans' rank order correlation) when clients were tested 1 week apart[14]
Internal Consistency	• Not reported in the studies reviewed
Inter-Rater	• Part I average of 0.84 (Kappa scores)[14]
Validity	
Content	• Content validity was established in its development, which included comprehensive literature review and review by experts.[14]
Construct	• Examined the differences in ADL performance and neurobehavioral impairment between persons with left and right hemisphere damage; only scores on 3 (comprehension, speech, and shave/makeup) of the 18 ADL items on the FIS discriminated between the 2 groups (as was expected). On the NSIS, 13 of 39 items discriminated between the 2 groups.[15]
Criterion	• Part I of the A-ONE was found to discriminate between people with and without central nervous system dysfunction.
Responsiveness to Change	• Not reported in the studies reviewed
Standardization	• There are no standardized administration instructions, allowing clinicians to adapt the testing environment to meet clients' typical environments and use their own equipment. General guidelines are provided, and detailed information about scoring is included. • A small normative sample of 79 people from Iceland is reported in the manual, which included hospital staff volunteers and patients with acute, non-neurological problems.
Strengths	• Grounded in occupational therapy theory because neurological deficits are considered in the context of occupational performance. • Allows simultaneous assessment of ADLs and neurobehavioral functions.
Considerations	• Requires training (40 hours) to purchase forms and use, which may limit its accessibility to clinicians. • Part I would be strengthened by further validity testing and more study on its responsiveness to change.
Final Word	• Part I of the A-ONE would be useful to most clinicians working with clients with central nervous system impairments • Questions about scoring and responsiveness to change remain, making it difficult to determine the clinical utility of the measure

Table 13-3

Arthritis Impact Measurement Scales (AIMS) 2/Short Form (SF)

Source	http://www.proqolid.org/content/download/2883/14336/version/1/file/aims2.pdf Permission to be used must be obtained from Robert F. Meenan, MD, MPH, MBA, Dean of School of Public Health, Boston University. The AIMS2-SF is an appendix to the Guillemin[18] publication.
Key References	Guillemin[18]; da Mota Falcao et al[19]; Mason et al[20]; Meenan et al[21]; Meenan[22]
Purpose	• Original AIMS: Designed to measure health status in individuals with rheumatic diseases. • Revised version (AIMS2): Developed to improve the psychometric properties of the measure as well as incorporate client perception of performance into the assessment. • The AIMS2-SF is a shorter version of the AIMS2. • The CHAIMS was developed for use with children but did not demonstrate strong psychometric properties[23] and therefore will not be presented here.
Type of Client	• Adults with any type of rheumatic disease. It has also been used with clients with hemophilia.[24,25]
Test Format	• AIMS2: 12 subscales (57 items): mobility, walking and bending, hand and finger function, arm function, self-care tasks, household tasks, social activity, support from family and friends, arthritis pain, work, level of tension, and mood. There are 4 additional components: symptom, affect, social interaction, and role. In addition, satisfaction with health, impact of arthritis on health, areas of health most requiring improvement, and general questions on current health and expectations for the future are asked. Each section consists of 4 to 5 questions to total 78 questions (there are approximately 10 questions at the end that refer to demographic issues). • The majority of questions ask the respondents to rank their performance, ability, or feeling on a 5-point scale (the anchors of the scale vary with the questions being asked).[22] • The AIMS2-SF uses 26 of the original 78 items from the AIMS.[26]
Procedures	• Both the AIMS2 and the AIMS2-SF are designed to be self-administered.
Time Required	• AIMS2: Approximately 23 minutes[27] • AIMS2-SF: Approximately 5 minutes[18]
Reliability	
Test-Retest	• AIMS2: results ranged from 0.78 to 0.94 (intraclass correlation coefficient).[21] N = 127, patients with rheumatoid arthritis starting methotrexate treatment: results ranged from 0.73 to 0.90 (intraclass correlation coefficient).[26] Similar results were found for the Chinese, Persian, and Turkish verisons.[28-30] AIMS2-SF: Results ranged from 0.76 to 0.81 (intraclass correlation coefficient).[26] Similar results were found for the Dutch and German versions, the ICC exceeded 0.85 except for the affect scale (0.72).[31,32]
Internal Consistency	• AIMS2: for the 12 subscales results ranged from 0.72 to 0.91 (Cronbach's coefficient alpha) for subjects with rheumatoid arthritis and 0.74 to 0.96 for those with osteoarthritis.[21] The Chinese, Persian and Turkish versions demonstrated similar results.[28-30] • AIMS2-SF: The social interaction component demonstrated a Cronbach's alpha of 0.32. The other 4 components ranged from 0.74 to 0.87.[26] Ren et al[33] (n = 147 patients with osteoarthritis) also noted low internal consistency with social interaction (0.46, Cronbach's alpha) and scores ranging from 0.80 to 0.86 for affect, symptom, and physical components. Similar results were found for the Dutch and German versions.[31,32]
Inter-Rater	• Not applicable
Intra-Rater	• Not applicable

(continued)

Table 13-3 (continued)

Arthritis Impact Measurement Scales (AIMS) 2/Short Form (SF)

Validity	
Content	• AIMS2: 96% of the test subjects (n = 24) felt that the test was comprehensive.[21] • Similar scores between AIMS2-SF and AIMS2. Physical, symptomatic, and affect components demonstrated strongest correlations (0.24 to 0.59 AIMS2-SF; 0.14 to 0.60 AIMS2).[26]
Construct	• Significant differences in performance subscale scores between those subjects who reported the performance areas as a health status problem were found ($p < 0.001$) in all groups. In addition, subjects' responses were also dichotomized based on identification of the performance area as a priority. • AIMS2-SF: Klooster et al[34] conducted a factor analysis on data from 279 patients with rheumatoid arthritis and found distinct upper and lower extremity scores factors within the measure.
Criterion	• AIMS2: The AIMS2 physical function measures were moderately correlated with the Rapid Assessment of Disease Activity in Rheumatology (RADAR) measure (r = 0.11 to 0.52), while the AIMS2 arthritis pain scale was strongly correlated with the RADAR total joint score (r = 0.72 to 0.76).[20] This indicates that the AIMS2 physical functioning scale may be measuring constructs not present in the RADAR. AIMS2-SF: n = 1030 patients with rheumatoid arthritis: the AIMS2 and AIMS2-SF were both administered: intraclass correlations were lowest for Role (0.62), but = 0.85 for all remaining components.[35] The scale also showed moderate correlations with other general health status measures such as the Nottingham Health Profile, the Short Form-36, and the Sickness Impact Profile.[36]
Responsiveness to Change	• AIMS2: N = 31, attending an arthritis hydrotherapy program (primarily osteoarthritis and rheumatoid arthritis): values obtained at baseline, 10 weeks and 3 months, and compared to other measures (SF-36, WOMAC, VAS), no change detected.[37] Another study[38] found that the Italian version of the AIMS2 was more responsive to change than the SF-36, as well as 2 other utility measures. • AIMS2-SF: The studies by Haavardsholm et al[35] and Guillemin et al[26] both demonstrated similar results for the AIMS2-SF and AIMS2 in terms of responsiveness to change, indicating that the AIMS2-SF is at least as sensitive as the AIMS2. They also indicated that the physical and symptom components of both scales are most sensitive to change. • A study evaluating the sensitivity to change of the Dutch version of both measures noted that the physical, symptom, and affect components are sensitive to changes in perceived health.[31]
Standardization	• The manual notes that subjects should be given the questionnaire and asked to complete it, with no further instruction. • The AIMS2 has been translated in to the following languages: Chinese (non-dialect specific), Dutch, French, German, Greek, Hebrew, Italian, Japanese, Norwegian, Portuguese Russian, Spanish (Mexican), and Swedish. • The AIMS2-SF has been translated in to Turkish.

(continued)

Table 13-3 (continued)

Arthritis Impact Measurement Scales (AIMS) 2/Short Form (SF)

Strengths	• AIMS2 ¤ Considered an accepted standard method for measurement of health status for clients with rheumatoid arthritis ¤ Well-established reliability and validity. Although responsiveness was not demonstrated in 1 study, others studies have indicated that the measure is sensitive to change. ¤ Veenhof et al[27] reported that the questionnaire is understandable for all patients. ¤ Incorporates client satisfaction and client priorities for improvement. ¤ Assesses how many of the difficulties being experienced are attributable to arthritis. ¤ It is highly culturally adaptable and has been translated into many languages. A list of the available languages and psychometric properties can be found at the AIMS2 website. • AIMS2-SF ¤ All of the above, and easier to administer.
Considerations	• AIMS2 and AIMS2-SF ¤ The physical component includes both ADL and IADL. ¤ May have limited utility in both clinical and research settings because of the length of time required to administer the measure[39] ¤ The instrument is meant to be a general information source, so specific assessment would be required to determine the reason for the deficit. ¤ AIMS2 must be purchased.
Final Word	• The AIMS2 provides information on a client's level of occupational performance when occupational performance is being affected most by the disease progression of arthritis. As a specific ADL tool, further information would be required to clearly understand the problems identified. The AIMS2-SF has shown similar psychometric properties overall and for the physical component when compared to the AIMS2, yet it takes about one-fourth of the time to administer. • There are many well-conducted studies that validate the translated versions of both the AIMS-2 and AIMS2-SF in different languages, which lends support to the perceived clinical utility of the measure.

Table 13-4

Barthel Index (BI)

Source	Mahoney and Barthel[5] http://www.strokecenter.org/wp-content/uploads/2011/08/barthel.pdf
Key References	Collin et al[40]; Fricke and Unsworth[41]
Purpose	• To measure changes in functional status for clients undergoing inpatient rehabilitation.
Type of Client	• Adults with many diagnoses and physical disabilities (eg, stroke). Used in rehabilitation, acute, and community settings.
Test Format	• The original Barthel consists of 10 items (feeding, bathing, grooming, dressing, bowel control, bladder control, toilet transfers, chair/bed transfers, ambulation, and stair climbing).

(continued)

Table 13-4 (continued)

Barthel Index (BI)

Type of Client	
Test Format	• Scoring uses a 2- or 3-point ordinal scale. Scores for activities have been weighted (continence and mobility are the most heavily weighted), so final item scores range from 0 to 15. Total score on the assessment ranges from 0 to 100 in increments of 5. Many sources use a scoring system based on a total score of 20. • Modified by Shah et al[42] with a 5-point ordinal scale to be more sensitive to change. • A 5-item version[43] including transfers, bathing, toilet use, stairs, and mobility was developed as an outcome measure that appears to be psychometrically equivalent to the 10-item measure.
Procedures	• Raters should be rehabilitation professionals. Rating is completed using information from records or following direct observation of functional performance. • Telephone interview and self-report have both been explored.[44,45]
Time Required	• Scoring takes 2 to 5 minutes, but observation can require about 1 hour.
Reliability	• Excellent
Internal Consistency	• Original BI: Cronbach's coefficient alpha ranged from 0.87 to 0.92 at discharge for stroke and neurorehabilitation patients at admission and discharge.[42,43,46,47] • Modified BI: 0.90[42] • 5-item BI: Cronbach's coefficient alpha ranged from 0.71 to 0.88.[43,46] • First stroke survivors referred for inpatient rehabilitation (n=258); original BI: 0.87 at admission and 0.92 at discharge (Cronbach's coefficient alpha) Modified BI: 0.90 at admission and 0.93 at discharge.[42] Neurorehabilitation in patients (n=418); 0.89 for original BI and 0.88 for 5-item version (Cronbach's coefficient alpha).[43] Stroke rehabilitation inpatients (n=118) in Taiwan; original BI: 0.84 on admission and 0.85 on discharge; 5-item BI: 0.71 on admission and 0.73 on discharge (Chronbach's alpha).[46] Stroke rehabilitation inpatients (n=31); 0.87-0.95 (Cronbach's alpha).[47] • A study evaluating a Turkish version demonstrated internal consistency was 0.93 for stroke and 0.88 for spinal cord injury.[48]
Inter-Rater	• Individual items ranged from 0.71 to 1.00, with most above 0.85 (Spearman's rho correlation coefficients), and total scores were 0.99 or 1.00 (Pearson correlations coefficients).[49] • Inpatients referred to occupational therapy (n=25): ranges from 0.57 to 0.85 for individual items (kappa) and an overall statistics of 0.975 (intraclass correlation coefficient).[41] • A study by Heuschmann et al[50] evaluating the reliability of a German version of the BI found excellent inter-rater reliability (mean kappa=0.93). • A meta-analysis by Duffy et al[51] reported that the inter-observer reliability, primarily for clients with stroke, was good (weighted kappa=0.93).
Intra-Rater	• Hospitalized patients with stroke (n=7): ranges from .84 to .97 for 5 different therapists (kappa).[52]
Validity	
Content	• No specific method to ensure the content validity was reported. Laake et al,[53] using factor analysis, found a unidimensional score for stroke, but a 2-factor structure for geriatric and hip fracture patients. • In contrast, Valach et al[54] found a 3-factor structure for 147 post-stroke inpatients.

(continued)

Table 13-4 (continued)

BARTHEL INDEX (BI)

Validity	
Construct	• Individuals receiving scores of below 60 on the Barthel were dependent in self-care, and after stroke, people with scores greater than 45 were more likely to go home.[55] Initial scores predicted length of stay and rehabilitation outcome.[56] Granger et al[55] found initial scores post-stroke of over 40 were related to discharge home and over 60 to shorter stays.
Criterion	• Fortinsky et al[57] found the score was strongly related to the number of tasks in which a person was independent. Kwon et al[58] examined the relationship between original BI scores and an indicator of level of disability (n = 459 people on a stroke registry), and found that the BI differentiated all levels of disability except the 2 highest levels of function (demonstrating a potential ceiling effect). • Rehabilitation in patients (n = 127): 7 items of the BI predicted total scores on the Chedoke-McMaster Stroke assessment; total BI scores were predicted by 3 items of the same assessment.[54] • The Barthel has been compared to the Katz, the Kenny, the PULSES, and the FIM, all commonly accepted measures of ADL, and the correlations are generally good. Granger et al[55] report correlations with the PULSES to range from -.74 to -.90. • Fricke and Unsworth[41] report the BI correlated highly with the brief FIM (includes self-care, sphincter control, mobility, and locomotion sections only), with ranges between 0.86 and 0.90 with different raters. Gosman-Hedstron and Svensson[59] used 204 assessments post-CVA to establish high concordance between the FIM and BI. • Post et al[47] noted moderate to high correlations (r = 0.34 to 0.94) when BI scores compared to the Northwick Park Dependency Score and a global dependency rating (n = 31 stroke rehabilitation in patients).
Responsiveness to Change	• Numerous studies have examined responsiveness to change using a variety of statistics including effect size and standardized response mean. Overall, the data on responsiveness to change is promising for the FIM, although somewhat difficult to interpret because varying statistical methods have been used. • Effect sizes range from 0.37 (MS patients) to 0.95 (stroke patients).[43,60-62] • Standardized response mean: Stroke rehabilitation inpatients (n = 118) in Taiwan: original BI and 5-item BI: 1.2[46]; first time stroke inpatients (n = 50): 0.99.[63] Frail older adults (n = 265): 1.13 (standardized response mean); 0.46 (Norman's responsiveness statistic), indicating lower responsiveness than goal attainment scaling, but higher than other measures of function.[64] • Using 5 different approaches to examine responsiveness to change, the Modified BI was only slightly better than the original BI on most of the indicators.[65] When compared to the FIM on 4 statistical analyses of responsiveness, the BI was comparable for the entire sample and the FIM was slightly more sensitive for subjects who improved at least one level on the Rankin Index.[66] • People on a stroke registry who either improved or remained constant in function from 1 to 3 months post-stroke (n = 372): a minimal clinically important change of 1 unit on the Modified Rankin index was 16 units on the BI, effect size = 1.29.[66]
Standardization	• No published manual available; scoring instructions included in original article. Guidelines used in different reliability and validity studies are not always provided. • Other languages available: Chinese, Danish, French, German, Italian, Japanese, Korean, Persian, Spanish, and Turkish • One study[67] demonstrated that telephone administration is reliable in comparison to an in-person assessment (weighted Kappa of 0.90)

(continued)

Table 13-4 (continued)

Barthel Index (BI)

Standardization	• Heuschmann et al[50] reported a mean kappa of 0.79 for the German postal version and 0.80 for the German telephone version. • Shinar et al[49] and Korner-Bitensky and Wood-Dauphinee[44] found strong relationships between BI on self-report by telephone interview compared with observations on performance. Collin et al[40] found no systematic biases when comparing self-report, nurse report, and observation. • Richards et al[68] demonstrated similar scoring for those with nonclinical background compared to clinical staff
Strengths	• Widely used and familiar to many. • Covers the areas of ADLs comprehensively. • Used extensively in research. • Recent research suggests that the original and modified BI are responsive to change, especially for post-stroke inpatients. • Can be applied by both clinical and nonclinical staff with reasonable reliability[68]
Considerations	• Individual intervention plans may not be clear from examining the scores (not enough detail). • Adaptations have been made to items and scoring in the literature while still calling it the Barthel Index, so the literature must be read carefully. • Its ordinal scale has not been validated or shown to produce interval level measurements. • Potential ceiling and floor effects, especially for community-dwelling persons and diagnoses other than stroke; some question about construct validity in non-stroke population[69]
Final Word	• The original Barthel is a reliable measure that can describe self-care status and has some predictive validity. It is useful for group evaluation, program evaluation, and in research.

Table 13-5

Functional Autonomy Measurement System (SMAF)

Source	Centre d'expertise, Institut universitaire de gériatrie de Sherbrooke, 375, rue Argyll, Sherbrooke, QC Canada J1J 3H5
Key References	Desrosiers et al[70]; Hebert et al[71,72]
Purpose	• Designed to evaluate people's needs by measuring levels of disability and handicap. It considers not only the person's abilities and disabilities, but also the resources available to overcome the disabilities, and the stability of those resources.
Type of Client	• Designed for use with older adults in rehabilitation. Most studies have focused on people over age 65 years, although one had a subsample under age 65 years.
Test Format	• Organized into 5 sections: ADLs (7 items), mobility (6 items), communication (3 items), mental functions (5 items) and instrumental ADLs (IADLs) (8 items). Some mobility items (eg, transfers) also might be considered ADLs. Each item has a 4-point scale used to rate the level of independence. In the ADL, mobility, and IADL items, a 0.5 option was added in the revised version to indicate that a task can be done independently, but with some difficulty.[70]

(continued)

Table 13-5 (continued)

FUNCTIONAL AUTONOMY MEASUREMENT SYSTEM (SMAF)

Type of Client	
Test Format	• A shorter version without the IADL and outside mobility items is used for people living in institutional settings. The SMAF is available in English, French, Dutch, and Spanish. Some work has been undertaken to develop a social functioning component to the SMAF.[73] • An electronic version (eSMAF) is available in both French and English and is free when a restricted registered academic license is obtained.[74]
Procedures	• Completed based on interview and, in some cases, observation of the client completing the activities (this is determined based on the need judged by the rater). Research has been done with nurses, social workers, and occupational therapists completing it. • Once disability is rated, questions are considered related to whether the person has resources available to overcome the disability. Resources can be in the form of formal or informal help from people or assistive devices if these compensate for the disability. If the resources are available, the handicap score is 0. • The stability in future weeks of the resources is then considered. Scores are obtained by summing the items and can range from 0 (complete independence) to -87.
Time Required	• In the studies completed, the instrument requires about 40 minutes to complete.
Reliability	
Test-Retest	• People over age 65 years living in a range of residential settings for elderly people in Quebec (n=45): mean Kappa of 0.73 (ranging from 0.59 to -0.74), and ICCs of 0.95 (ranging from 0.78 to 0.96). ADL items were 0.74 (Kappa) and .96 (ICC).[70]
Internal Consistency	• Not reported in the studies reviewed
Inter-Rater	• People over age 65 years living in a range of residential settings for elderly people in Quebec (n=45): mean Cohen's weighted Kappa ranged from 0.61 to 0.81 with a mean of 0.68; ADL items were 0.81 (Kappa) and 0.95 (ICC).[70] Inpatients in acute/rehabilitation unit (n=94) with a slightly modified version of the SMAF: Kappas ranged from 0.74 to 0.86 between 3 raters.[75]
Validity	
Content	• Developed based on literature review of other measures and the judgement of the developers, and was linked to the WHO International Classification of Impairment, Disability and Handicap.[3] • It is not yet clear how the SMAF concepts of disability and handicap will conceptually link to the new WHO's International Classification of Function, Disability and Health (ICF).[2]
Construct	• Inpatients post CVA on an intensive functional rehabilitation program (n=132): FIM and SMAF total scores were highly correlated (0.93-0.95 at 4 points in time).[76] • Day hospital patients (n=27) and acute medical inpatients (n=29): modified SMAF total scores correlated with a new handicap scale 0.77 for inpatients and 0.64 for day hospital patients.[77] • Older adults visiting emergency departments (n=221): OARS ADL and SMAF ADL: 0.63 (Spearman correlations).[78]
Criterion	• Residents of a long-term care facility (n=99): SMAF ADL scores correlated with the required amount of nursing care, r=0.89.[71] • Inpatients on an acute rehabilitation unit (n=94): significant changes in SMAF scores were noted between admission and discharge.[75] • Inpatients (mostly older adults) admitted for treatment-rehabilitation with anxiety, depression or cognitive disorders (n=1385): gains of 5 points on the SMAF ADL score reduced the mean length of stay by a factor of 0.87 (independent effect).[79]

(continued)

Table 13-5 (continued)

Functional Autonomy Measurement System (SMAF)

Responsiveness to Change	• The ASK performance score demonstrated similar change scores to the CHAQ; however, the ASK-capability produced smaller change scores abilities.[10]
Standardization	• The manual is readily available from the author and provides information about the instrument development, reliability, validity, and administration.
Strengths	• Incorporates considerations of environmental resources and their stability, which is very useful for discharge planning or identifying service needs in community settings. • Can be administered by a multidisciplinary team. • It is one of the few instruments in which developers have worked to identify a significant change in score.
Considerations	• Further evidence of its use across different rehabilitation populations (particularly younger groups) is needed.
Final Word	• Provides very useful information, especially for discharge planning or identifying service needs in community settings in work with older adults.

Table 13-6

Functional Independence Measure (FIM) and WeeFIM

Source	Uniform Data System for Medical Rehabilitation, 232 Parker Hall, 3435 Main Street, Buffalo, NY 14214-3007; http://www.udsmr.org/ Note: The FIM and WeeFIM have been extensively researched. Not all research could be included in this review. A complete bibliography on each is available through this website.
Key References	The UDSMR website provides a comprehensive review of the instruments (FIM and WeeFIM): http://www.udsmr.org/Documents/The_FIM_Instrument_Background_Structure_and_Usefulness.pdf Details on validity and reliability of the measure: http://www.udsmr.org/Documents/UDSMR_Validity_Reliability_Of_The_FIM_Instrument.pdf There is also a comprehensive bibliography: http://www.udsmr.org/Documents/UDSMR_Bibliography_Of_The_FIM_Instrument.pdf
Purpose	• The FIM and WeeFIM are part of the Uniform Data System for Medical Rehabilitation (UDSMR).The FIM was designed to measure the degree of disability being experienced, changes over time, and the effectiveness of rehabilitation. • The WeeFIM was designed with similar purposes for children receiving rehabilitation services. • Both measure severity of disability defined in terms of the need for assistance.
Type of Client	• FIM: Can be used with any rehabilitation client age 7 years and older. • WeeFIM: Designed for children from age 6 months to 7 years.
Test Format	• The FIM and WeeFIM measures 18 items in 6 areas: self-care, sphincter control, mobility, locomotion, communication, and social cognition. • Each item is rated on a 7-point scale, from total assist to complete independence. Total scores range from 18 to 126. • FIM data can be described in terms of motor and cognitive subscales.

(continued)

Table 13-6 (continued)

Functional Independence Measure (FIM) and WeeFIM

Type of Client	
Procedures	• Both the FIM and the WeeFIM can be completed based on observations made by a clinician of any discipline, based on the client's usual rather than best performance. If observations are not possible, data can be collected through interview or medical record review. • A self-report FIM is reported in the literature; however, the FIM authors caution against the use of self-report or completion of the measure by untrained raters[80] • An AlphaFIM is available that measures 6 items (4 motor and 2 cognitive) and is designed for use in the acute care to facilitate appropriate transfer to rehabilitation settings.
Time Required	• The instruments can be completed in 15 to 20 minutes, but observation of tasks may require more time.
Reliability	• Reliability of the FIM and WeeFIM are both excellent, with studies conducted to evaluate internal consistency, inter-rater and intrarater or test-retest reliability, and results consistently high.
Test-Retest	• FIM: not reported in studies reviewed • WeeFIM: ICC for total score = 0.98 (items ranged from 0.91 to 0.99)[81,82] • WeeFIM: Pearson r values ranged from 0.83 to 0.99[83]
Internal Consistency	• FIM: neurorehabilitation inpatients (n = 149): alph = 0.95 for total FIM, 0.94 for motor component and 0.89 for cognitive component[44] • FIM: stroke inpatients (n = 118): Cronbach's alpha = 0.88 at admission and 0.91 at discharge for the motor subscale[46] • WeeFIM: children who had been preterm infants (n = 149): 0.90 (Cronbach's alpha)[83]
Inter-Rater	• FIM: ICC = 0.96 for total scores and ranged from 0.89 to 0.94 for items. Reliability was higher in a subset of 24 facilities with more training[84,85] • FIM: Mean Kappa for items ranged from over 0.40 to 0.56 (social interaction items were lowest), and ICC was 0.92 for the summary motor items[86] • WeeFIM: Pearson r ranged from 0.74 to 0.96.[83] Also tested between raters with short and long delay; ICC for short was 0.97 (items ranged from 0.82 to 0.94), and for long delay was 0.94 (items ranged from 0.73 to 0.90)[82] • WeeFIM: Children receiving inpatient and outpatient rehabilitation (n = 20): 0.93 (ICC) for self-care, and ranged from 0.82 to 0.94 on the other subscales[87]
Intra-Rater	• FIM: patients of an MS research clinic (n = 35): self-care items kappas ranged from 0.55 to 0.78, with ICC for total FIM of 0.94[88]
Validity	• Across numerous explorations of validity of the FIM and WeeFIM, both instruments consistently have results suggesting good validity.
Content	• Both were developed based on judgmental and statistical methods. • FIM: Rasch analysis on 27,699 rehabilitation patient FIM scores demonstrated 2 main constructs: motor (13 items) and cognitive (5 items)[89] • FIM: Ravaud et al[90] criticize the use of a summary score for the FIM because it is not based on a unidimensional construct • WeeFIM: well children (n = 170), Rasch analysis confirmed the same 2 scales as the FIM—motor and cognitive[83]

(continued)

Table 13-6 (continued)

Functional Independence Measure (FIM) and WeeFIM

Validity	
Convergent	• FIM: compared to the Barthel, FIM (motor) scores; Kappa = 0.92 at admission and 0.88 at discharge[91] • Total FIM and total PULSES correlations were -0.82 at admission and -0.88 at discharge[92] • WeeFIM: compared to PEDI subscales, WeeFIM self-care score Spearman correlation coefficients were 0.94 for self-care functional scale and 0.96 for self-care caregiver assistance[87] • WeeFIM total scores correlation was 0.92 (Spearman) with the total on the Battelle Developmental Inventory and 0.89 with the Vineland Adaptive Behavior Scales[93]
Predictive	• FIM: Admission motor FIM scores were the most significant predictors of motor status at discharge; admission functional status was consistently related to discharge functional status and length of stay, although the strength of the associations varied across impairment groups[89] • The strongest predictor of discharge location was admission FIM scores[94]; scores of over 80 were associated with likely discharge to home rather than a skilled nursing facility[95] • Timbeck and Spaulding[96] conducted a review and concluded that FIM admission scores can predict discharge FIM scores, outcome disability, and discharge location. • WeeFIM: scores were significantly related to the amount of effort required to provide assistance to the child (0.69 to 0.96) and the time given to assist (0.40 to 0.88)[97]
Construct	• FIM: scores were found to be linked to time required for help in ADL each day in patients with MS,[4] stroke,[98] and post-traumatic brain injury.[99] • Orthopedic inpatients: FIM self-care and total scores were significantly correlated with physical therapy and occupational therapy visits and units as well as length of stay.[100] Kwon et al[59] found that the motor-FIM differentiated between 3 levels of disability (demonstrating a potential ceiling effect). • WeeFIM: strong correlations were found between item scores and age[101]; FIM scores were able to distinguish children with major impairments and no impairments and were related to parents' perceptions of the children's health status.[83] • Compared to a parent-report measure of the amount of assistance required, WeeFIM total scores had correlation of 0.91 and self-care correlation of 0.83. WeeFIM total scores were the major predictor of amount of assistance provided when included in a multiple regression analysis.[102]
Responsiveness to Change	• Research has been published focusing on the ability of the FIM to detect clinically important change, and to detect change in populations that are expected to change. The results indicate that the FIM and WeeFIM can be useful as an outcome measure, particularly with a post-stroke population. • A minimal clinically important change of 1 unit on the Modified Rankin index was 11 units on the FIM, effect size = 1.29.[66] • When compared to the Barthel Index on 4 statistical analyses of responsiveness, the FIM was comparable for the entire sample and slightly more sensitive for subjects who improved at least 1 level on the Rankin Index.[66] Similarly, Houlden et al[62] reported that the Barthel Index and the total and physical FIM scores showed similar responsiveness and that the cognitive FIM score was least responsive.

(continued)

Table 13-6 (continued)

FUNCTIONAL INDEPENDENCE MEASURE (FIM) AND WEEFIM

Responsiveness to Change	• Other studies that have examined the responsiveness of the FIM found effect sizes of 0.30 for patients with MS, 0.82 for patients with stroke (n=283),[61] and 1.62 for self-care in orthopedic inpatients (n=28).[100] • Standardized response mean for the FIM self-care and sphincter control categories was 0.77 and 0.97 for the total score (both slightly smaller than the SMAF).[76] • WeeFIM: using 5 statistical analyses to examine responsiveness, the authors report that the WeeFIM was responsive to change (eg, effect size was 0.62, standardized response mean=.31).[103]
Standardization	• The manual (guide for the Uniform Data Set for Medical Rehabilitation) is available from the publisher. • Training for both the FIM and WeeFIM are required, with self-study of the manual, viewing videotapes, attendance at workshops, and a certification process with model case studies. Sites using the FIM must be licensed. Users subscribe annually to the UDSMR and specific details on cost can be obtained through the website. • Translations for the FIM are available for the following languages: Afrikaans, Finnish, French, German, Italian, Spanish, Swedish, and Turkish. • Translations for the WeeFIM are available in Dutch and Turkish • A study evaluating the cultural adaptability of the WeeFIM demonstrates that the measure can be a useful and reliable instrument for assessing functional independence in Thai children.[104] • In Turkey, a similar study evaluating the cultural adaptability of the FIM also demonstrated that the measure can be successfully adapted cross-culturally.[105] • Although there are no norms for the FIM, there are performance profiles[98] and articles on function-related and resource-utilization groups.[106,107] • Norms for the WeeFIM were compiled based on 417 children with no developmental delay.[108] In 2002, Wong et al[109] also examined the utility of the WeeFIM in Chinese children and created a normative WeeFIM profile suitable for healthy Chinese children (n=445).
Strengths	• Excellent reliability and validity for the FIM • Widely used in North America, particularly in inpatient stroke setting • Can be used in a variety of rehabilitation settings with all types of patients, and can be rated by many team members.
Considerations	• Comparison across patient groups should be done cautiously as one study[110] suggests that adjustments for differential item functioning may be required when comparing different patient populations. • Cost and training required for use of the FIM and the WeeFIM may be a barrier to accessing the instruments in some settings.
Final Word	• The FIM is a well-studied measurement tool that has an extensive infrastructure to support use and interpretation.

Table 13-7

HEALTH ASSESSMENT QUESTIONNAIRE (HAQ)/ CHILDREN'S HEALTH ASSESSMENT QUESTIONNAIRE (CHAQ)

Source	HAQ: The questionnaire and manual (HAQ-PAK) can be found at http://patienteducation.stanford.edu/research/haq20.html CHAQ: The questionnaire can be found as a figure (Figure 1) in Singh et al.[111] The additional questions and revised scoring for the CHAQ can be found in Norgaard et al.[112]
Key References	HAQ: Bruce and Fries[113]; CHAQ: Singh et al[111]
Purpose	• HAQ: The HAQ was originally designed to be a comprehensive outcome measure for people with rheumatic disease, but has more recently been described as a generic functional outcome measure.[114] The HAQ described in this section will be the Improved HAQ, which consists of 20 questions on ADL rated using a 5-point scale, 4 questions on use of assistive devices and 1 question each on pain, general health, and assistance with activities. • CHAQ: To measure functional status in children with juvenile rheumatoid arthritis, ages 1 to 19 years.[111]
Type of Client	• Improved HAQ: Originally designed for adults with rheumatic diseases, but expanded to include all adults with reason for disability[115] • CHAQ: Used with clients having wide range of rheumatic diagnoses as well as dermatomyositis and spina bifida[113]
Test Format	• Note: Further development of the HAQ has resulted in slight changes to the wording of questions and a larger range of scoring options (5 instead of 4). Newer versions continue to include the use of assistive devices or help from another as part of the measure, but incorporating the scoring for these items slightly differently than the original version.[114] Therefore, if comparing HAQ scores across time points or trying to compare results of different studies, it is important to ensure the same version of the measure was used. • Improved HAQ: As described previously, which consists of 20 questions on ADL rated using a 5-point scale, 4 questions on use of assistive devices and 1 question each on pain, general health, and assistance with activities. • Improved HAQ: Although the original HAQ has been translated into over 60 languages,[113] it is unclear if the Improved HAQ has been translated. • CHAQ: Similar to the HAQ in the 8 categories but the authors have modified the questions within the categories slightly to ensure there are relevant questions for all age groups.[111] It also includes visual analog scales for pain and overall functioning. The CHAQ has been translated into over 12 different languages.[113]
Procedures	• Improved HAQ: Usually self-administered but can be given face-to-face or by telephone interview. Scoring is described in detail in the manual and although it is not simple, clear instructions are provided.[114] • CHAQ: Parent proxy or self-administered
Time Required	• Improved HAQ: 5 minutes[114] • CHAQ: Less than 10 minutes to complete[111]
Reliability	
Test-Retest	• Improved HAQ: Bruce and Fries[113] in their 2003 review, provide a comprehensive list of the over 350 studies that have been completed reviewing the issues of reliability, validity, and responsiveness to change for the HAQ. The measures have been studied with a variety of populations. Test-retest reliability ranges between 0.87 and 0.99, and inter-rater reliability (interviewer administered versus self-administered) ranges from 0.85 to 0.95. Reliability of the Improved HAQ compared to the original HAQ demonstrated slightly better reliability of the Improved HAQ.[115]

(continued)

Table 13-7 (continued)

Health Assessment Questionnaire (HAQ)/ Children's Health Assessment Questionnaire (CHAQ)

Reliability	
Test-Retest	• CHAQ: n = 13 children with JRA. Spearman's correlation coefficient of 0.79 ($p < 0.002$).[111] Feldman et al[116] demonstrated an intraclass correlation of 0.87 in 37 children with juvenile dermatomyositis.
Internal Consistency	• HAQ: Not discussed in articles reviewed. • CHAQ: n = 72 children who had juvenile rheumatoid arthritis (JRA). Cronbach's alpha (overall) was 0.941[111]
Validity	
Content	• Improved HAQ: The content areas covered in the new measure are very similar to the previous measures and, therefore, the process of validating the content of the original can be applicable to the Improved HAQ. The original measure developed in 1978 was reviewed by expert panels, then tested in studies of both subjective and objective assessment. There is expert consensus that the test possesses both face and content validity.[113,117,118] • CHAQ: Initially determined by 7 rheumatologists and 8 health care professionals including occupational and physical therapists.[111]
Construct; Convergent	• Improved HAQ: Specific studies have not been conducted using the Improved HAQ; however, the original version demonstrated good construct and convergent validity[113,118,119] and given the similarity in content, similar values would be expected for the Improved HAQ. • CHAQ: n = 72 children who had juvenile rheumatoid arthritis (JRA), compared to Steinbrocker functional class, physical symptoms (joint count stiffness) and physician's assessment, values ranged from (Kendall's tau b) 0.54 to 0.77, all significant at the $p < 0.0001$ level. N = 37 children with JDM, compared to disease severity Spearman's correlation was 0.71 ($p < 0.002$), compared with proximal muscle strength rs = -0.57 ($p < 0.002$), shoulder abduction rs = 0.051 ($p < 0.01$), knee extension rs = -0.40 ($p = 0.05$), and grip strength rs = -0.079 ($p < 0.20$).
Criterion	• Improved HAQ: Has been widely studied and significantly correlated (0.71 to 0.95) with a wide variety of measures, including disease specific, generic health status, biochemical markers and measures of self-report. • CHAQ: No criterion measure is available to compare.
Responsiveness to Change	• Improved HAQ: Again, the majority of research has been done using the original version. The responsiveness to change has been well documented and the studies indicate that the measure is responsive to change.[113,117,118,120] As well, evidence exists for the minimal clinically important difference ranging from 0.10 to 0.22.[113] The more recent study by Fries et al[121] found that the Improved HAQ has similar responsiveness to the original HAQ and may have fewer floor effects. • CHAQ: Brown and Wallen[122] studies are inconclusive as a study by Ruperto et al[123] in children with juvenile chronic arthritis did not demonstrated responsiveness when compared with physician and parent global assessments, articular variables, and laboratory indicators. Conversely, both Singh et al[111] and Feldman et al[121] did demonstrate responsiveness.
Standardization	• Improved HAQ: Although population norms have been established for the original HAQ,[120] these are not available for the improved HAQ. • CHAQ: Not discussed in articles reviewed.

(continued)

Table 13-7 (continued)

Health Assessment Questionnaire (HAQ)/ Children's Health Assessment Questionnaire (CHAQ)

Strengths	• Improved HAQ: ¤ Better version of the HAQ, which is widely used in research as well as clinical practice ¤ Extensive development process and excellent psychometric properties ¤ Validated translations available in 60 languages. • CHAQ: ¤ Thorough development and strong psychometric properties across a few different diagnostic groups. ¤ Thorough validation of translations with more than 25 languages available
Considerations	• Improved HAQ: There are many versions and while the version discussed may be the best, its uptake into both clinical practice and research is not yet known. • CHAQ: Responsiveness to change has not been established.
Final Word	• HAQ: A very good functional status measure that is applicable to those with rheumatic conditions as well as those without. It is a well-developed self-report measure that provides information on the clients' perception of ability, which could be complimentary to observational measures. • CHAQ: This tool is simple to use and does provide reliable and valid results. Its use as an outcome measure is questionable because of the varying results in testing in terms of responsiveness to change.

Table 13-8

Juvenile Arthritis Functional Assessment Report (JAFAR)/ Juvenile Arthritis Functional Assessment Scale (JAFAS)

Source	JAFAR: Howe et al[124]; JAFAS: Lovell et al[125]
Key References	See above
Purpose	• The purpose of both is to measure disability due to juvenile rheumatoid arthritis (JRA).
Type of Client	• JAFAR & JAFAS: Children with JRA age 7 to 16 years.
Test Format	• JAFAR: There is a child report (JAFAR-C) and parent report version (JAFAR-P), both of which contain the same 23 questions in which either the child or parent reports on a 3-point scale as to whether the child is always, sometimes, or almost never able to complete the functional task. • JAFAS: 10 functional tasks that the child is asked to perform in front of an observer. Time to task completion is considered in the scoring.
Procedures	• JAFAR-C: Administered by a health professional using simple instructions. JAFAR P: Self-administered. • JAFAS: Therapist administered with specific standardized procedures as well as equipment.
Time Required	• JAFAR-C or -P: 5 minutes to complete and 3 minutes to score. JAFAS: 10 minutes to complete.

(continued)

Table 13-8 (continued)

Juvenile Arthritis Functional Assessment Report (JAFAR)/ Juvenile Arthritis Functional Assessment Scale (JAFAS)

Reliability	
Test-Retest	• JAFAR-C & -P: Not reported in articles reviewed • JAFAS: Not reported in articles reviewed
Internal Consistency	• JAFAR-C: Cronbach's alpha ranged from 0.83 to 0.85.[124,126] • JAFAR-P: Cronbach's alpha ranged from 0.81 to 0.96.[124-126] • JAFAS: Cronbach's alpha of 0.91.[127]
Inter-Rater	• JAFAR-C & -P: Not applicable • JAFAS: Inter-rater: n=21 children, aged 5 to 16 years with JRA, Kappa values for each question ranged from 0.07 to 1.00.[126]
Validity	
Content	• JAFAR-C & -P: Developed by the same panel of experts who developed the JAFAS. Item selection was done based on work done on JAFAS. • JAFAS: Content was initially taken from the Arthritis Impact Measurement Scale (AIMS), Health Assessment Questionnaire (HAQ), and the McMaster Health Index.[125] An expert panel chose items and pilot tested prior to development of final test.
Construct	• JAFAR-C & -P: n=72 children, n=70 parents compared to JAFAS scores; JAFAR-C, 0.69 (PCC); JAFAR-P, 0.69.[124] • JAFAS: n=52, children 5 to 16 years of age with JRA, compared to the Physician's Global Assessment of Disease activity, JAFAR- C, 0.36, JAFAR-P, 0.34 and compared with joint count JAFAR-C, 0.29, JAFAR-P, 0.30.[126]
Convergent	• JAFAR-C & -P: n=72 (children) and n=70 (parents), correlations with a visual analog pain scale were 0.57 (Pearson's correlation coefficient) and 0.61, respectively[124]; several other studies in comparable populations demonstrated similar results with JAFAR-C & P when compared to joint counts and biochemical markers.[128-130] • JAFAS: n=71 children with JRA, compared to number of involved joints, correlation of 0.40, compared to Steinbrocker functional class 0.59, compared to disease activity status, -0.32. The authors note the direction of these correlations were as expected.[125]
Responsiveness to Change	• In a study comparing the JAFAR-C, JAFAR-P, and JAFAS to the Children's Health Assessment Questionnaire (CHAQ), British authors noted that the CHAQ demonstrated an effect size of almost twice that of the other measures.[126] • Robinson et al[131] noted similar change scores between the CHAQ and the JAFAR in a sample of 21 children with JRA.
Standardization	• JAFAR: Not discussed in the articles reviewed. • JAFAS: Specific procedures for administration available. No norms discussed in articles reviewed.
Strengths	• The JAFAR-C & -P as well as the JAFAS have undergone rigorous psychometric testing and demonstrate good reliability and validity. • All 3 are easy to administer; however, the JAFAR C & P do take less and time and do not require special equipment. • The JAFAR-C & -P are being used in research.

(continued)

Table 13-8 (continued)

Juvenile Arthritis Functional Assessment Report (JAFAR)/ Juvenile Arthritis Functional Assessment Scale (JAFAS)

Considerations	• The authors note that the JAFAS should be considered as a separate measure to either of JAFARs; however, they used the JAFAS as the comparator for construct validity, indicating that they are measuring similar constructs. • Special equipment is required to administer the JAFAS.
Final Word	• Although similar in construct because it is easier to administer, takes less time to complete, and provides the same information, the JAFAR C or P would seem to be the measure of choice. We continue to watch for future research regarding responsiveness as there is some doubt about this.

Table 13-9

Juvenile Arthritis Self-Report Index (JASI)

Source	Wright V, Law M, Crombie V, Goldsmith C, Dent P, Shore A. The JASI. Available from vwright@hollandbloorview.ca
Key References	Wright et al[132,133]
Purpose	• The JASI is designed as a self-report measure of daily living and mobility activities of school-aged children with juvenile rheumatoid arthritis (JRA).
Type of Client	• The instrument was tested with children from 8 years of age and up.[132] It is designed for school-aged children and adolescents with JRA.
Test Format	• The JASI is divided into 2 parts. In Part 1, children are asked to rate their performance on 100 items in 5 categories: self-care, domestic, mobility, school, and extracurricular. Each item is rated on a 7-point ordinal scale. In Part 2, the children identify and rate their performance on activities of most importance to them.
Procedures	• The instructions are reviewed with the child, and sample items are administered. If the child can understand the ratings and read the questions, he or she can complete it independently. If there are difficulties with reading, the administrator reads the items to the child.
Time Required	• Administration time ranges from 30 to 45 minutes.
Reliability	
Test-Retest	• Part 1: ICC = 0.99 at 2 to 3 weeks and 0.98 for a subgroup of 11 subjects at 3 months. • Part 2: short-term reliability was 0.57 (weighted Kappa) after 2 to 3 weeks.[132]
Internal Consistency	• Not reported in studies reviewed
Inter-Rater	• Not reported in studies reviewed
Validity	
Content	• Content validity was established through the instrument development process, which incorporated the use of experts including clinicians, children, parents, and teachers.[133]

(continued)

Table 13-9 (continued)

Juvenile Arthritis Self-Report Index (JASI)

Validity	
Construct	• JASI scores were correlated with a number of measures used in pediatrics with a sample of 36 children with JRA: joint pain (r=-0.15), arthritis status (r=0.24); active joint count (r=-0.51); morning stiffness (r=-0.62); Bruininks subtest 8 (r+0.55 with n=30); grip strength (r=0.60); presence of hip synovitis (r=-0.62); hip flexion contracture (r=-0.65); timed walk (r=-0.66); Keitel upper extremity score (r=-0.72); ACR functional rating (r=-0.75); timed run (r=-0.79); total Keitel index (r=-0.89); Keitel lower extremity score (r=-0.91). Only the relationship to pain was less than expected.[132] • Comparisons were also made between self-report by children and observational scores completed by clinicians (n=30) for 60 of the items on the JASI that could be observed. Mean weighted Kappa score was 0.66 (indicating fair to good agreement); and further analysis indicated that there was not a strong bias for children to rate their performance higher than the clinicians.
Convergent	• Not reported in studies reviewed.
Responsiveness to Change	• The JASI demonstrated similar responsiveness to change as the JAFAR and the CHAG.[134]
Standardization	• There is no manual that accompanies the instrument.
Strengths	• The JASI is innovative in its use of self-report. • Useful for treatment planning with priorities identified by the child in Part 2.
Considerations	• No information on validity for those under 8 years of age.
Final Word	• The JASI is useful as an initial assessment to assist in treatment planning. It can contribute to client-centered practice because the children report their abilities in a variety of daily activities, but it does take longer to administer than the JAFAR and the CHAQ.

Table 13-10

Katz Index of Activities of Daily Living

Source	Katz et al[135]
Key References	Brorsson and Asberg[136]; Asberg and Sonn[137]
Purpose	• Designed to describe levels of function, to predict future function and level of care, and to evaluate programs.
Type of Client	• Developed from observations of older adults after hip fractures, but has been used with adults with musculoskeletal and neurological impairments, and with community-dwelling older adults.
Test Format	• The original form includes 6 items that cover feeding, continence, transfer, toileting, dressing, and bathing. • Each item is rated on a 3-point scale (independence, receives assistance, dependent), which is converted to an independent/dependent rating (with the "receives assistance" falling under independent for some items and dependent for others).

(continued)

Table 13-10 (continued)

Katz Index of Activities of Daily Living

Type of Client	
Test Format	• A summary letter score on a Guttman scale, based on a hierarchy of the order in which ADL skills are lost and regained, is then used to indicate the types of ADL skills with which the person has difficulty. • With community-dwelling older adults, efforts have been made to add IADL items to the Katz, so that it is more sensitive to the types of difficulties that people have in daily living.[137-139]
Procedures	• The instrument was originally developed so that scoring was based on the 2-week period prior to the evaluation and can be administered based on interview and/or observation of some components. • A 5-item version (omitting continence) has been tested as a telephone interview.[140]
Time Required	• Because the instrument administration is not standardized, it is difficult to estimate how long it would require. A 2-week observation is recommended prior to completion.
Reliability	
Test-Retest	• Not reported in the studies reviewed.
Internal Consistency	• Random sample of South Carolina residents (n=6472): using a 5-item telephone instrument, a Kuder-Richardson 20 statistic of 0.87.[140] • Frail elderly persons (n=83): urinary continence item deleted: Cronbach's alpha: 0.56.[141]
Inter-Rater	• Examined based on the number of differences between raters, and, in all cases, the inter-observer variability was low.[136]
Validity	
Content	• Content covers the main areas of ADLs most commonly cited, although the authors do not justify item selection. • The Guttman scaling was originally based on developmental and anthropological hierarchies. A very high percentage (~96%) of subjects could be classified by the index.[135] • Brorsson and Asberg[136] report coefficients of scalability ranging from 0.74 to 0.88.
Construct	• Compared to the amount of assistance required from a non-family attendant, there was a significant difference between those rated more independent than those less independent.[142] • Hypotheses have also been tested related to the order of recovery and these generally followed the scaling. • Katz ratings were also found to predict length of stay in hospital, type of discharge, actual residence 1-year post-assessment, and mortality in clients in acute care.[136] Scores were also predictive of discharge location, length of stay in rehabilitation, and mortality in a sample of clients post-stroke,[143] and in a sample of patients post-amputation.[144]
Responsiveness to Change	• Not reported in the studies reviewed.
Standardization	• There are no formal instructions to administer and no manual. Information is included about the ratings in a number of the original journal articles.
Strengths	• Quick to complete and easy to score. • Considering its brevity, reliability, and validity are good. • Adaptations to add IADLs may make the instrument more useful in community settings.
Considerations	• 2-week observations before scoring are unrealistic in many settings. • May be less useful for planning individual intervention plans because its brevity makes it difficult to identify specific areas for intervention.[145]
Final Word	• A brief measure that may be susceptible to a ceiling effect and limited evidence of responsiveness to change.

Table 13-11

Melville Nelson Self-Care Assessment (SCA)

Source	http://www.utoledo.edu/healthsciences/depts/rehab_sciences/ot/melville.html; Occupational therapists are free to download the self-care assessment as long as copyright is acknowledged.
Key References	Nelson et al[146]
Purpose	• Provides an objective measure of self-care performance and support.
Type of Client	• Designed for use with patients in subacute and skilled nursing facilities.
Test Format	• Observational measure that is part of the Melville-Nelson Occupational Therapy Evaluation System for Skilled Nursing Facilities (SNF) and Subacute rehabilitation, which also included demographics and history information and the Self-Identified Goal Assessment.[147] • Each of the 7 sections (bed mobility, transfers, dressing, eating, toilet use, personal hygiene, and bathing) is rated on self-performance and the support needed. For self-performance, each occupation is broken into sub-occupations (eg, eating is broken into finger food, utensil, and drink). For each sub-occupation, a number of tasks are considered within (eg, finger food is broken into grasp, to mouth, open mouth, and in mouth). • Higher scores on self-performance indicate that more assistance is needed. A total score can also be calculated (maximum total is 140). • For each of the 7 self-care tasks, a single support score is also rated depending on the type of support needed (eg, from no setup or physical help to 2-person physical help required). A total support score is not calculated.
Procedures	• Observation of each of the self-care occupations is required to rate the SCA. • Any items that are not applicable to the client are not scored, so scores reflect only applicable items (although it is not clear how this not-applicable status is indicated on the form).
Time Required	• Administration time not described in the research reviewed. Observation of all components is required, which could take anywhere from 1 to 3 hours, depending on the client.
Reliability	
Test-Retest	• Not reported in the studies reviewed.
Internal Consistency	• Not reported in the studies reviewed.
Inter-Rater	• Patients receiving subacute rehabilitation (n=68), 8 raters in 4 teams (1 certified occupational therapist and 1 occupational therapy graduate student in each): ICC for total self-performance was 0.94, and for specific individual areas ranged from 0.77 to 0.98. For support, the ICCs ranged from 0.57 to 0.89.[146]
Intra-Rater	• Not reported in the studies reviewed.
Validity	
Content	• The content of the SCA intentionally follows the Minimum Data Set (MDS), an assessment required at long-term care facilities in the US, to ease administration for occupational therapists already completing the MDS for reimbursement purposes.
Construct	• In a sample of 40 patients receiving subacute rehabilitation, discharge total self-performance SCA was correlated with caregiving time in home, FIM scores, and Klein Bell scores.[146]
Convergent	• Patients receiving subacute rehabilitation (n=68): Total SCA self-performance scores were correlated with the FIM (Spearman rank order correlation [rho] with total FIM was -0.85) and Klein Bell (rho=-.085). • Correlations for the 7 subscales of the SCA were also correlated with the relevant items from the FIM and Klein-Bell and all were statistically significant correlations. Correlations between SCA support scores and FIM and Klein Bell components were similar.[146]

(continued)

Table 13-11 (continued)

Melville Nelson Self-Care Assessment

Responsiveness to Change	• Responsiveness to change was determined by examining effect sizes (2 different statistics) for a sample of 68 patients receiving subacute rehabilitation evaluated at admission and discharge. Eleven of 15 variables on the SCA showed significant change from admission to discharge. Effect sizes varied depending on how they were calculated, but were generally high for transfers, dressing, and toileting and lower for eating, personal hygiene, and bathing.[146]
Standardization	• The manual/protocol can be downloaded from the source website.
Strengths	• Consistency with the MDS items makes completion of the SCA straightforward for clinicians in settings requiring the MDS and should facilitate team communication. • Observation of details within each sub-occupation provides clinicians with rich information for intervention planning.
Considerations	• Although the SCA is part of the Melville Nelson Occupational Therapy System for Skilled Nursing Facilities and Subacute Rehabilitation, it is not clear how the SCA relates to those other components, or how the 3 components should be used together. • A ceiling effect was noted for discharge scores on the SCA, which is hypothesized to be related to the inclusion of the MDS items only, which tend to focus on basic rather than more complex ADL activities.
Final Word	• The SCA appears to offer occupational therapists working in long-term care facilities and subacute rehabilitation an observation-based ADL assessment with enough detail to generate intervention plans. Further research is required on its psychometric properties. Information on its responsiveness suggests that it will be most useful for patients who are expected to have long stays with many self-care issues.

Table 13-12

Pediatric Evaluation of Disability Inventory (PEDI)

Source	http://www.pearsonclinical.com/psychology/products/100000505/pediatric-evaluation-of-disability-inventory-pedi.html The PEDI-CAT can be purchased from www.pedicat.com at an annual fee of $89.00 USD.
Key References	Feldman et al[148]; Haley et al[149]; Iyer et al[150]
Purpose	• Designed for 3 purposes: 1) to describe a child's functional status; 2) for program evaluation of inpatient, outpatient, and school-based programs; and 3) to monitor change in individuals or groups of children with functional disabilities.
Type of Client	• Designed for children between 6 months and 7.5 years (or older if their functional development is significantly delayed). It can be used with many diagnostic groups.
Test Format	• Organized into 3 measurement dimensions: functional skills, caregiver assistance, and modifications. Each of these is organized into self-care, mobility, and social function. • The functional skills measure is organized hierarchically based on the order in which skills are typically achieved by children. Each item is scored on a capable/not capable dichotomous scale. • The caregiver assistance scale explores the amount of assistance the child requires in task areas that are more general than the specific items in the functional skills area. Each item is rated on a 6-item scale from total assistance to independence. • The modifications scale considers the frequency that modifications (either typical modifications used by children or specific modifications used by children with disabilities) are used.

(continued)

Table 13-12 (continued)

Pediatric Evaluation of Disability Inventory (PEDI)

Type of Client	
Test Format	• Recently, 10- and 15-item computer adaptive testing (CAT) versions have been studied and demonstrated added efficiency, while retaining the psychometric properties of the measure.[7]
Procedures	• Either parents or professionals (health or educational) can complete the instrument. Parents can typically complete the functional skills component independently, as long as someone familiar with the PEDI reviews it with them afterward. • The caregiver assistance and modifications scales are more demanding to understand and may be completed best with structured interview with parents. • There is a computer program available to assist with scoring or it can be scored manually. Raw scores, normative standard scores, or scaled scores can be used. • It is possible to use only specific components of the instrument if appropriate for the child. Research indicates the self-care classification system seemed to reflect clinically important changes in skills between admission and discharge from an inpatient rehabilitation setting[151]
Time Required	• It can take 45 to 60 minutes to complete the instrument by interviewing parents; 20 to 30 minutes if a professional is completing it based on observations of the child.
Reliability	• Overall, the reliability of the PEDI is excellent. A number of studies have been undertaken by the developers as well as others, although the sample sizes tend to be small.
Test-Retest	• Children with varying severities of cerebral palsy aged 3 to 7 years (n = 21); 4 respondents (primary caregiver, classroom teacher, occupational therapist, and physical therapist) rated the child on 2 occasions 3 weeks apart; intraclass correlation coefficients all over 0.95 for total scores and above 0.80 for the 3 domains.[152] • Chen et al[153] and Erkin et al[154] also demonstrated excellent test-retest reliability (ICC: 0.96 to 0.998).
Internal Consistency	• Using the normative sample (n = 412), Cronbach's alpha ranged from 0.95 to 0.99.[149] • A study evaluating the reliability and validity of a Chinese version of the PEDI reported a high internal consistency (Cronbach's alpha = 0.90 to 0.99).[153] Similarly, a study evaluating a Turkish version of the PEDI also demonstrated a high internal consistency (Cronbach's alpha: 0.98).[154]
Inter-Rater	• Intraclass correlation coefficients ranged from 0.96 to 0.99.[149] • Children with disabilities (n = 12); intraclass correlation coefficients ranged from 0.84 to 1.00.[155] • Comparison of responses from parent and rehabilitation team members; intraclass correlation coefficients ranged from 0.74 to 0.96, except the social function modifications scale (0.30).[149] • Children receiving inpatient or outpatient rehabilitation (n = 41): 0.83 (ICC) for self-care, and 0.89 for self-care caregiver assistance.[87] • Children receiving occupational or physical therapy in the midwest United States (n = 17); comparing parent and therapist ratings; intra-class correlation coefficients ranged from 0.2 to 0.93 for functional skill scales; 0.15 to 0.95 on the caregiver assistance scales (in both cases most were over 0.6).[156]
Intra-Rater	• Children receiving occupational or physical therapy in the Midwest United States (n = 23); 2 interviews conducted by the same interviewer 1 week apart; intraclass correlation coefficients ranged from 0.67 to 1.00 on the functional skill scales, and 0.68 to 0.90 for the caregiver assistance scale.[156]
Validity	• The validity of the PEDI overall is quite strong, with a mix of studies conducted by the developers and others.
Content	• When the instrument was developed, the content was evaluated by expert ratings of 31 people who reviewed its content. As well, Rasch modeling has been used to validate the content in terms of the developmental sequence of the tasks involved.[149]

(continued)

Table 13-12 (continued)

Pediatric Evaluation of Disability Inventory (PEDI)

Validity	
Construct	• The developers examined the relationship between age and PEDI scores and found support for the hypothesis that scores increased with age. These data were also used to support hypotheses about the ability of the PEDI to differentiate between functional skills and caregiver assistance as separate constructs.[149] • Children with spina bifida (n=63): PEDI scaled scores on ADL correlated with parent ratings of ADL independence.[157] • Children with CP seen at a paediatric therapy center (n=18): PEDI scores were correlated with the Melbourne Assessment of Unilateral Upper Limb Function with r=.939 for the PEDI self-care component.[158]
Convergent	• PEDI scores have been compared to a number of other developmental instruments with positive results, including the Battelle Developmental Inventory Screening Test (results ranged from 0.62 to 0.97)[148]; the WeeFIM (results ranged from 0.80 to 0.97)[155]; and from .76 to .94 (Spearman correlations) when PEDI self-care scores were compared to WeeFIM subscales,[87] the Gross Motor Function Measure (0.75 to 0.85),[152] and the Peabody Developmental Motor Scales (0.24 to 0.95).[156] • Chen et al[153] demonstrated that a Chinese version of the measure had a high correlation with the WeeFIM (Spearman's p: 0.92 to 0.99).
Responsiveness to Change	• PEDI scores were compared across time in 2 clinical samples. The scores changed in the expected direction in the 2 clinical groups, providing an indication of the PEDI's responsiveness.[149] • Children with spastic diplegia undergoing selective dorsal rhizotomy (n=18): scaled scores on the functional and caregiver assessment scales changed significantly between preoperative and 6 and 12 months postoperative assessments (normative scores did not change significantly).[159] • Children discharged from inpatient rehabilitation (n=53): in a sample of 53 children discharged from inpatient rehabilitation, a change of 11 points in the scaled score was estimated to be the minimal clinically important difference.[150] • A study evaluating the responsiveness of the PEDI in children with cerebral palsy found that the measure had effect size and standardized response means greater than 0.8.[160]
Standardization	• The manual for the PEDI[149] is comprehensive. Norms are included based on a sample of 412 children from the northeastern United States. Clinical interpretation of scores is discussed by Haley et al.[161] • Dutch, Norwegian, Spanish, and Swedish versions are described in the literature with some psychometric testing done on most of the translations.[159,162-165]
Strengths	• Well-developed and standardized instrument. • Appears to comprehensively evaluate function in young children. • Could be used to develop individual program plans, as well as program evaluation. • Computer adaptive testing of the self-care and social functions scales demonstrated good reliability and validity meaning that these 2 scales can be reliably used in time-constrained settings.[166,167]
Considerations	• A ceiling effect may occur in some instances in ADL function for children with minimal impairment.[151] • Several studies evaluating the cross-cultural validation of the measure have recommended that adapting and norming the measure to a specific culture is necessary before using the instrument in clinical practice.[168-170]

(continued)

Table 13-12 (continued)

Pediatric Evaluation of Disability Inventory (PEDI)

Final Word	• Overall, the PEDI appears to be an excellent tool to evaluate ADLs as one component of function—and taps into both the capacity to complete tasks, as well as the amount of assistance and types of modifications used to enable function. Information about the minimal clinically important difference provides useful information for clinical and evaluative purposes. The PEDI-CAT could be a useful tool if funding allows.

Table 13-13

Physical Self-Maintenance Scale (PSMS)

Source	Lawton and Brody[171]
Key References	Edwards[172]; Rubenstein et al[173]
Purpose	• Designed to measure basic self-care skills.
Type of Client	• It was designed for use with older clients (over 60 years).
Test Format	• Consists of 6 items: toileting, feeding, dressing, grooming, physical ambulation, and bathing. In its original format, there are 4 levels of independence noted, but the person is scored 1 for independence and 0 if he or she requires other assistance. However, many users have adopted a 4-point rating scale. • Japanese version available[174]
Procedures	• The instrument can be administered based on observation or self-report. However, Settle and Holm[151] note that without observation, the clinical usefulness of the PSMS is diminished for individual program planning.
Time Required	• 20 to 30 minutes.
Reliability	• Overall, the reliability of the PSMS is excellent. A number of studies have been undertaken by the developers as well as others, although the sample sizes tend to be small.
Test-Retest	• Patients (impaired and nonimpaired) (n=44); correlation of 0.91 (Pearson r).[171] • Patients on a geriatric assessment or reactivation unit over 65 (n=30), 1 week between ratings: 0.56 (ICCs). Edwards[172] notes that changes in status may have changed in some subjects in 1 week.
Internal Consistency	• Adults over 60 years old from a variety of institutional and community service provider agencies (n=265): reproducibility coefficient of 0.96 reported.[171]
Inter-Rater	• Patients over 60 with various self-care deficits (n=36); correlation of 0.87 (Pearson r).[171] • Patients on a geriatric assessment or reactivation unit over 65 (n=30); 0.96 (ICCs).[172] • Community-dwelling and institutionalized older adults (n=76): 92% agreement.[175]
Validity	
Content	• The items included in the PSMS were derived from literature review and primarily the Langley-Porter Neuropsychiatric Institute ADL Scale. It covers the main areas of personal ADLs.
Criterion	• Not reported in the studies reviewed.
Construct	• Edwards[172] found that the PSMS distinguished between seniors discharged home vs those discharged to institutional settings. • In 2 studies,[172,173] significantly different scores were noted for self-report vs direct observation, indicating that the 2 methods of data collection cannot be used interchangeably.

(continued)

Table 13-13 (continued)

PHYSICAL SELF-MAINTENANCE SCALE (PSMS)

Validity	
Convergent	• The PSMS has been examined in terms of its relationship to a number of other instruments. Geriatric inpatients (n = 180): Lawton & Brody IADL Scale (r = 0.61); physicians' ratings of physical capacity (r = 0.62); mental status questionnaire (r = 0.38), and a behavior and adjustment rating scale (r = 0.38).[171] • Patients on a geriatric assessment or reactivation unit over 65 (n = 30): the mini-mental status exam (r = 0.19), the FIM (r = 0.70), the geriatric depression scale (r = 0.25).[172] • Community-dwelling and institutionalized older adults (n = 76): OSOT perceptual assessment r = 0.435 and MMSE r = 0.246 (Spearman correlation), demonstrating a relationship between perceptual and (to a lesser extent) cognitive status and ADL performance.[175]
Responsiveness to Change	• Frail older adults (n = 265): responsiveness of the PSMS discussed compared to goal attainment scaling, the Barthel, and IADL measure and a quality of life index. Statistics on the responsiveness of the total PSMS are not provided; the PSMS is more responsive than the Barthel on 3 of 4 indicators of responsiveness.[65]
Standardization	• There are no formal instructions and no manual. • Although not norms, Lawton[176] cites mean scores on the PSMS as 20.61 for a sample of 253 community residents, 20.77 for a sample of 173 older adults living in public housing, 19.26 for 99 people receiving in-home services and 18.51 for 65 people on institutional waiting lists. These data are based on 7 items (transferring and getting outside were added and grooming removed) rated on a 3-point scale for each item.
Strengths	• Brief and flexible use, covers major areas of ADLs. • Adequate reliability and validity. • For individual program planning, it would be best to use it with observation of task performance (there are not enough items or detail within the items to give a therapist direction for intervention).
Considerations	• There is not enough information about its responsiveness to change, which limits its usefulness in evaluation.
Final Word	• The PSMS is a useful instrument that covers basic self-care skills in older adults and can be used at individual or group levels for description and evaluation.

REFERENCES

1. American Occupational Therapy Association. Occupational therapy practice framework: domain and process. 3rd ed. *Am J Occup Ther.* 2014;68(Suppl 1):S1-S48.
2. World Health Organization. *International Classification of Functioning, Disability and Health.* Geneva: WHO; 2001.
3. World Health Organization. *International Classification of Impairments, Disabilities and Handicaps.* Geneva: WHO; 1980.
4. Granger CV, Cotter AC, Hamilton BB, Fiedler RC, Hens MM. Functional assessment scales: a study of persons with multiple sclerosis. *Arch Phys Med Rehabil.* 1990;71:870-875.
5. Mahoney SI, Barthel DW. Functional evaluation: the Barthel index. *Md State Med J.* 1965;14:61-65.
6. Rogers JC, Holm MB. Daily living skills and habits of older women with depression. *Occup Ther J Res.* 2000;20S:68S-85S.
7. Haley S, Coster W, Dumas H, et al. Accuracy and precision of the Pediatric Evaluation of Disability Inventory computer-adaptive tests (PEDI-CAT). *Dev Med Child Neurol.* 2011;53:1100-1106.
8. Kramer JM, Coster WJ, Kao YC, Snow A, Orsmond GI. A new approach to the measurement of adaptive behavior: development of the PEDI-CAT for children and youth with autism spectrum disorders. *Phys Occup Ther Pediatr.* 2012;32(1):34-47.
9. Young NL. *The Activities Scale for Kids (ASK) Manual.* Toronto, ON: The Hospital for Sick Children; 2009.
10. Young NL, Williams JI, Yoshida KK, Wright JG. Measurement properties of the Activities Scale for Kids. *J Clin Epidemiol.* 2000;53:125-137.
11. Young NL, Yoshida KK, Williams JI, Bombardier C, Wright JG. The role of children in reporting their physical disability. *Arch Phys Med Rehabil.* 1995;76:913-918.

12. Pencharz J, Young NL, Owen JL, Wright JG. Comparison of three outcomes instruments in children. *J Pediatr Orthop.* 2001;21:425-432.
13. Plint AC, Gaboury I, Owen J, Young NL. Activities Scale for Kids: an analysis of normals. *J Pediatr Orthop.* 2003;23:788-790.
14. Arnadottir G. *The Brain and Behavior: Assessing Cortical Dysfunction Through Activities of Daily Living (ADL).* St. Louis, MO: C. V. Mosby; 1990.
15. Arnadottir G. *Measuring the impact of body functions on occupational performance: Validation of the ADL-focused Occupation-based Neurobehavioral Evaluation (A-ONE).* Unpublished doctoral Dissertation, Department of Communication Medicine and Rehabilitation, Occupational Therapy, Umea University; 2010.
16. Gardarsdottir S, Kaplan S. Validity of the Arnadottir OT-ADL neurobehavioral evaluation (A-ONE): performance in activities of daily living and neurobehavioral impairments of persons with left and right hemisphere damage. *Am J Occup Ther.* 2002;56:499-508.
17. Rubio KB, Van Deusen J. Relation of perceptual and body image dysfunction to activities of daily living of persons after stroke. *Am J Occup Ther.* 1995;49:551-559.
18. Guillemin F. Functional disability and quality-of-life assessment in clinical practice. *Rheumatology.* 2000;39(Suppl):14-23.
19. da Mota Falcao D, Ciconelli RM, Ferraz MB. Translation and cultural adaptation of quality of life questionnaires: an evaluation of methodology. *J Rheumatol.* 2003;30:379-385.
20. Mason JH, Meenan RF, Anderson JJ. Do self-reported arthritis symptom (RADAR) and health status (AIMS2) data provide duplicative or complementary information? *Arthritis Care Res.* 1992;5:163-172.
21. Meenan RF, Mason JH, Anderson JJ, Guccione AA, Kazis LE. The content and properties of a revised and expanded Arthritis Impact Measurement Scales Health Status Questionnaire. *Arthritis Rheum.* 1992;35(1):1-10.
22. Meenan RF. *AIMS2 User's Guide and the AIMS2.* Boston, MA: Boston University; 1990.
23. Coulton CJ, Zborowsky E, Lipton J, Newman AJ. Assessment of the reliability and validity of the arthritis impact measurement scales for children with juvenile arthritis. *Arthritis Rheumatol.* 1987;30:819-824.
24. Szende A, Schramm W, Flood E, et al. Health-related quality of life assessment in adult haemophilia patients: a systematic review and evaluation of instruments. *Haemophilia.* 2003;9:678-687.
25. van Meeteren NLU, Strato IHM, van Veldhoven NHMJ, et al. The utility of the Dutch Arthritis Impact Measurement Scales 2 for assessing health status in individuals with haemophilia: a pilot study. *Haemophilia.* 2000;6:664-671.
26. Guillemin F, Coste J, Pouchot J, et al. The French Quality of Life in Rheumatology Group. The AIMS2-SF: a short form of the Arthritis Impact Measurement Scales 2. *Arthritis Rheumatol.* 1997;40:1267-1274.
27. Veenhof C, Bijlsma J, Van den Ende C, Van Dijk G, Pisters M, Dekker J. Psychometric evaluation of osteoarthritis questionnaires: a systematic review of the literature. *Arthritis Rheumatol.* 2006;55:480-492.
28. Chu E, Chiu K, Wong R, Tang W, Lau C. Translation and validation of Arthritis Impact Measurement Scales 2 into Chinese: CAIMS2. *Arthritis Rheumatol.* 2004:51(1);20-27.
29. Mousavi SJ, Parnianpour M, Askary-Ashtiani AR, Hadian MR, Rostamian A, Montazeri A. Translation and validation study of the Persian version of the Arthritis Impact Measurement Scales 2 (AIMS2) in patients with osteoarthritis of the knee. *BMC Musculoskelet Disord.* 2009;10:95
30. Atamaz F, Hepguler S, Oncu J. Translation and validation of the Turkish version of the arthritis impact measurement scales 2 in patients with knee osteoarthritis. *J Rheumatol.* 2005;32(7):1331-1336.
31. Taal E, Rasker J, Riemsma R. Psychometric properties of a Dutch short form of the Arthritis Impact Measurement Scales 2 (Dutch-AIMS2-SF). *Rheumatol.* 2003;42(3):427-434.
32. Rosemann T, Korner T, Wensing M, Schneider A, Szecsenyi J. Evaluation and cultural adaptation of a German version of the AIMS2-SF questionnaire (German AIMS2-SF). *Rheumatol.* 2005;44(9):1190-1195.
33. Ren XS, Kazis L, Meenan RF. Short-form Arthritis Impact Measurement Scales 2: tests of reliability and validity among patients with osteoarthritis. *Arthritis Care Res.* 1999;12:163-171.
34. Klooster P, Veehof M, Taal E, Van Riel P, Van de Laar M. Confirmatory factor analysis of the Arthritis Impact Measurement Scales 2 short form in patients with rheumatoid arthritis. *Arthritis Rheum.* 2008;59(5):692-698
35. Haavardsholm EA, Kvien TK, Uhlig T, Smedstad LM, Guillemin F. A comparison of agreement and sensitivity to change between AIMS2 and a short form of AIMS2 (AIMS2-SF) in more than 1000 rheumatoid arthritis patients. *J Rheum.* 2000;27:2810-2816.
36. Carr A. Adult measures of quality of life. *Arthritis Rheum.* 2003;49(5S):S113-S133.
37. Lineker SC, Badley EM, Hawker G, Wilkins A. Determining sensitivity to change in outcome measures used to evaluate hydrotherapy exercise programs for people with rheumatic diseases. *Arthritis Care Res.* 2000;13:62-65.
38. Salaffi F, Stancati A, Carotti M. Responsiveness of health status measures and utility-based methods in patients with rheumatoid arthritis. *Clin Rheum.* 2002;21:478-487.
39. Gignac M, Cao X, McAlpine J, Badley E. Measures of disability. *Arthritis Rheum.* 2011;63(S11):S308-S324.
40. Collin C, Wade DT, Davies S, Horne V. The Barthel ADL index: a reliability study. *Int Disabil Stud.* 1988;10:61-63.
41. Fricke J, Unsworth CA. Interrater reliability of the original and modified Barthel Index and a comparison with the Functional Independence Measure. *Aust Occup Ther J.* 1996;43:22-29.
42. Shah S, Vanclay F, Cooper B. Improving the sensitivity of the Barthel Index for stroke rehabilitation. *J Clin Epidemiol.* 1989;42:703-709.
43. Hobart JC, Thompson AJ. The five item Barthel index. *J Neurol Neurosurg Psychiatry.* 2001;71:225-230.
44. Korner-Bitensky N, Wood-Dauphinee S. Barthel index information elicited over the telephone: is it reliable? *Am J Phys Med Rehabil.* 1995;74:9-18.
45. Sinoff G, Ore L. The Barthel activities of daily living index: Self reporting versus actual performance in the old-old (>75 years). *J Am Geriatr Soc.* 1997;45:832-836.

46. Hsueh IP, Lin JH, Jeng JS, Hsieh CL. Comparison of the psychometric characteristics of the functional independence measure, 5 item Barthel index, and 10 item Barthel index in patients with stroke. *J Neurol Neurosurg Psychiatry.* 2002;73:188-190.
47. Post MW, Visser-Meily JM, Gispen LS. Measuring nursing needs of stroke patients in clinical rehabilitation: a comparison of validity and sensitivity to change between the Northwick Park Dependency Score and the Barthel Index. *Clin Rehabil.* 2002;16:182-189.
48. Kucukdeveci AA, Yavuzer G, Tennant A, et al. Adaptation of the modified Barthel Index for use in physical medicine and rehabilitation in Turkey. *Scand J Rehabil Med.* 2000;32(2):87-92.
49. Shinar D, Gross GR, Bronstein KS, et al. Reliability of the ADL Scale and its use in telephone interview. *Arch Phys Med Rehabil.* 1987;68:723-728.
50. Heuschmann P, Kolominisky-Rabas P, Nolte C, et al. The reliability of the German version of the Barthel-index and the development of a postal and telephone version for the application on stroke patients. *Fortschritte Der Neurologie Psychiatrie.* 2005;73(2):74-82.
51. Duffy L, Gajree S, Langhorne P, Stott D, Quinn T. Reliability (inter-rater agreement) of the Barthel Index for assessment of stroke survivors: systematic review and meta-analysis. *Stroke.* 2013;44:462-468.
52. Loewen SC, Anderson BA. Reliability of the modified motor assessment scale and the Barthel index. *Phys Ther.* 1988;68:1077-1081.
53. Laake K, Laake P, Hylen Ranhoff A, Sveen U, Wyller TB, Bautz-Holter E. The Barthel activities of daily living index: factor structure depends upon the category of patient. *Age Ageing.* 1995;24:393-397.
54. Valach L, Signer S, Hartmeier A, Hofer K, Steck GC. Chedoke-McMaster stroke assessment and modified Barthel Index self-assessment in patients with vascular brain damage. *Int J Rehabil Res.* 2003;26:93-99.
55. Granger CV, Dewis LS, Peters NC, Sherwood CC, Barett JE. Stroke rehabilitation: analysis of repeated Barthel index measures. *Arch Phys Med Rehabil.* 1979;60:14-17.
56. Shah S, Cooper B. Commentary on "A critical evaluation of the Barthel index". *Br J Occup Ther.* 1993;56:70-72.
57. Fortinsky RH, Granger CV, Selzer GB. The use of functional assessment in understanding home care needs. *Med Care.* 1981;19:489-497.
58. Kwon S, Hartzema AG, Duncan PW, Min-Lai S. Disability measures in stroke: relationship among the Barthel Index, the Functional Independence Measure, and the Modified Rankin Scale. *Stroke.* 2004;35:918-923.
59. Gosman-Hedstrom G, Svesson E. Parallel reliability of the functional independence Measure and the Barthel ADL index. *Disabil Rehabil.* 2000;22:702-715.
60. Wright J, Cross J, Lamb S. Physiotherapy outcome measures for rehabilitation of elderly people: responsiveness to change of the Rivermead Mobility Index and Barthel Index. *Physiotherapy.* 1998;84:216-221.
61. van der Putten JJ, Hobart JC, Freeman JA, Thompson AJ. Measuring change in disability after inpatient rehabilitation: comparison of the responsiveness of the Barthel index and the Functional Independence Measure. *J Neurol Neurosurg Psychiatry.* 1999;66:480-484.
62. Houlden H, Edwards M, McNeil J, Greenwood R. Use of the Barthel Index and the Functional Independence Measure during early inpatient rehabilitation after single incident brain injury. *Clin Rehabil.* 2006;20(2):153-159.
63. Salbach NM, Mayo NE, Higgins J, Ahmed S, Finch LE, Richards CL. Responsiveness and predictability of gait speed and other disability measures in acute stroke. *Arch Phys Med Rehabil.* 2001;82:1204-1212.
64. Rockwood K, Howlett S, Stadnyk K, Carver D, Powell C, Stolee P. Responsiveness of goal attainment scaling in a randomized controlled trial of comprehensive geriatric assessment. *J Clin Epidemiol.* 2003;56:736-743.
65. Hocking C, Williams M, Broad J, Baskett J. Sensitivity of Shah, Vanclay and Cooper's modified Barthel Index. *Clin Rehabil.* 1999;13:141-147.
66. Wallace D, Duncan PW, Lai SM. Comparison of the responsiveness of the Barthel Index and the motor component of the Functional Independence Measure in stroke: the impact of using different methods for measuring responsiveness. *J Clin Epidemiol.* 2002;55:922-928.
67. Della Pietra G, Savio K, Oddone E, Reggiani M, Monaco F, Leone M. Validity and reliability of the Barthel index administered by telephone. *Stroke.* 2011;42:2077-2079.
68. Richards S, Peters T, Coast J, Gunnell D, Darlow M, Pounsford J. Inter-rater reliability of the Barthel ADL index: how does a researcher compare to a nurse? *Clin Rehabil.* 2000;14(1):72-78.
69. De Morton N, Keating J, Davidson M. Rasch analysis of the Barthel index in the assessment of hospitalized older patients after admission for an acute medical condition. *Arch Phys Med Rehabil.* 2008;89:641-647.
70. Desrosiers J, Bravo G, Hebert R, Dubuc, N. Reliability of the revised functional autonomy measurement system (SMAF) for epidemiological research. *Age Ageing.* 1995;24:402-406.
71. Hebert R, Carrier R, Bilodeau, A. The functional autonomy measurement system (SMAF): description and validation of an instrument for the measurement of handicaps. *Age Ageing.* 1988;17:293-302.
72. Hebert R, Spiegelhalter DJ, Brayne, C. Setting the minimal metrically detectable change on disability rating scales. *Arch Phys Med Rehabil.* 1997;78:1305-1308.
73. Pinsonnault E, Desrosiers J, Dubuc N, Kalfat H, Colvez A, Delli-Colli N. Functional autonomy measurement system: development of a social subscale. *Arch Gerontol Geriatr.* 2003;37:223-233.
74. Boissy P, Brière S, Tousignant M, Rousseau E. The eSMAF: a software for the assessment and follow-up of functional autonomy in geriatrics. *BMC Geriatrics.* 2007;7:2.
75. Rai GS, Gluck T, Wientjes HJFM, & Rai SGS. The functional autonomy measurement system (SMAF): a measure of functional change with rehabilitation. *Arch Gerontol Geriatr.* 1996;22:81-85.
76. Desrosiers J, Rochette A, Noreau L, Bravo G, Hebert R, Boutin C. Comparison of two functional independence scales with a participation measure in post-stroke rehabilitation. *Arch Gerontol Geriatr.* 2003;37:157-172.
77. Rai GS, Kiniorns M, Burns W. New handicap scale for elderly in hospital. *Arch Gerontol Geriatr.* 1999;28:99-104.
78. McCusker J, Bellavance F, Cardin S, Belzile E. Validity of an activities of daily living questionnaire among older patients in an emergency department. *J Clin Epidemiol.* 1999;52:1023-1030.

79. Berod AC, Klay M, Santos-Eggimann B, Paccaud F. Anxiety, depressive or cognitive disorders in rehabilitation patients: effect on length of stay. *Am J Phys Med Rehabil.* 2000;79:266-277.
80. Granger C, Harper C, Duffey E. The FIM-SR (self-report) is not the FIM instrument. *Arch Phys Med Rehabil.* 2007;88:266-267.
81. Ottenbacher KJ, Taylor ET, Msall ME, et al. The stability and equivalence reliability of the functional independence measure for children (WeeFIM). *Dev Med Child Neurol.* 1996;38:907-916.
82. Ottenbacher KJ, Msall ME, Lyon NR, Duffy LC, Granger CV, Braun S. Interrater agreement and stability of the functional independence measure for children (WeeFIM): use in children with developmental disabilities. *Arch Phys Med Rehabil.* 1997;78:1309-1315.
83. Msall ME, DiGaudio KM, Duffy LC. Use of functional assessment in children with developmental disabilities. *Phys Med Rehabil Clin N Am.* 1993;4:517-527.
84. Granger CV, Hamilton BB. UDS Report: the uniform data system for medical rehabilitation report of first admissions for 1990. *Am J Phys Med Rehabil.* 1992;71:108-113.
85. Hamilton BB, Laughlin JA, Fiedler RC, Granger CV. Interrater reliability of the 7-level functional independence measure (FIM). *Scand J Rehabil Med.* 1994;26:115-119.
86. Daving Y, Andren E, Nordholm L, Grimby G. Reliability of an interview approach to the Functional Independence Measure. *Clin Rehabil.* 2001;15:301-310.
87. Ziviani J, Ottenbacher KJ, Shephard K, Foreman S, Astbury W, Ireland P. Concurrent validity of the Functional Independence Measure for Children (WeeFIM) and the Pediatric Evaluation of Disabilities Inventory in children with developmental disabilities and acquired brain injuries. *Phys Occup Ther Pediatr.* 2001;21:91-101.
88. Sharrack B, Hughes RAC, Soudain S, Dunn G. The psychometric properties of clinical rating scales used in multiple sclerosis. *Brain.* 1999;122(2):141-159.
89. Heinemann AW, Linacre JM, Wright BD, Hamilton BB, Granger CV. Relationships between impairment and physical disability as measured by the functional independence measure. *Arch Phys Med Rehabil.* 1993;74:566-573.
90. Ravaud J-F, Delcey M, Yelnik A. Construct validity of the Functional Inde-pendence Measure (FIM): questioning the unidimensionality of the scale and the "value" of FIM scores. *Scand J Rehabil Med.* 1999;31:31-41.
91. Kidd D, Stewart G, Baldry J, et al. The functional independence measure: a comparative validity and reliability study. *Disabil Rehabil.* 1995;17:10-14.
92. Marshall SC, Heisel B, Grinnell D. Validity of the PULSES profile compared with the Functional Independence Measure for measuring disability in a stroke rehabilitation setting. *Arch Phys Med Rehabil.* 1999;80:760-765.
93. Ottenbacher KJ, Msall ME, Lyon N, et al. Measuring developmental and functional status in children with disabilities. *Dev Med Child Neurol.* 1999;41:186-194.
94. Oczkowski WJ, Barreca S. The functional independence measure: Its use to identify rehabilitation needs in stroke survivors. *Arch Phys Med Rehabil.* 1993;74:1291-1294.
95. Black TM, Soltis T, Bartlett C. Using the functional independence measure instrument to predict stroke rehabilitation outcomes. *Rehabil Nursing.* 1999;24:109-114.
96. Timbeck RJ, Spaulding SJ. Ability of the Functional Independence Measure to predict rehabilitation outcomes after stroke: a review of the literature. *Phys Occup Ther Geriatr.* 2003;22(1):63-76.
97. Msall ME, DiGaudio K, Rogers BT, et al. The functional independence measure for children (WeeFIM): conceptual basis and pilot use in children with developmental disabilities. *Clin Pediatr.* 1994;33:421-430
98. Granger CV, Cotter AC, Hamilton BB, Feidler RC. Functional assessment scales: a study of persons after stroke. *Arch Phys Med Rehabil.* 1993;74:133-138.
99. Granger CV, Divan N, Fiedler RC. Functional assessment scales: a study of persons after traumatic brain injury. *Am J Phys Med Rehabil.* 1995;74:107-113.
100. Aitken DM, Bohannon RW. Functional independence measure versus short form-36: relative responsiveness and validity. *Int J Rehabil Res.* 2001;24(1):65-68.
101. Braun SL, Granger CV. A practical approach to functional assessment in paediatrics. *Occup Ther Practice.* 1991;2(2):46-51.
102. Ottenbacher KJ, Msall ME, Lyon N, et al. Functional assessment and care of children with neurodevelopmental disabilities. *Am J Phys Med Rehabil.* 2000;79:114-123.
103. Ottenbacher KJ, Msall ME, Lyon N, et al. The WeeFIM instrument: its utility in detecting change in children with development disabilities. *Arch Phys Med Rehabil.* 2000;81:1317-1326.
104. Jongit J, Komsopapong L, Saikaew T, et al. Reliability of the functional independence measure for children in normal Thai children. *Pediatr Int.* 2006;48:132-137.
105. Kucukdeveci AA, Yavuzer G, Elhan AH, Sonel B, Tennant A. Adaptation of the Functional Independence Measure for use in Turkey. *Clin Rehabil.* 2001;15:311-319.
106. Eilertsen TB, Kramer AM, Schlenker RE, Hrincevich CA. Application of Functional Independence Measure-function related groups and resource utilization groups-version III systems across post-acute settings. *Med Care.* 1998;36:695-705.
107. Sandstrom R, Mokler PJ, Hoppe KM. Discharge destination and motor function outcome in severe stroke as measured by the functional independence measure/function-related group classification system. *Arch Phys Med Rehabil.* 1998;79:762-765.
108. Msall ME, DiGaudio K, Duffy LC, LaForest S, Braun S, Granger CV. WeeFIM: normative sample on an instrument for tracking functional independence in children. *Clin Pediatr.* 1994;33:431-438.
109. Wong V, Wong S, Chan K, Wong W. Functional Independence Measure (WeeF-IM) for Chinese children: Hong Kong Cohort. *Pediatrics.* 2002;109(2):E36-E36.
110. Dallmeijer A, Dekker J, Roorda L, et al. Differential item functioning of the Functional Independence Measure in higher performing neurological patients. *J Rehabil Med.* 2005;37:346-352.
111. Singh G, Athreya BH, Fries JF, Goldsmith DP. Measurement of health status in children with juvenile rheumatoid arthritis. *Arthritis Rheum.* 1994;37:1761-1769.
112. Norgaard M, Thastum M, Herlin T. The relevance of using the Childhood Health Assessment Questionnaire (CHAQ) in revised versions for the assessment of juvenile idiopathic arthritis. *Scand J Rheumatol.* 2013;42(6):457-464.

113. Bruce B, Fries JF. The Stanford Health Assessment Questionnaire: a review of its history, issues, progress and documentation. *J Rheumatol.* 2003;30:167-178.
114. Stanford University School of Medicine, Division of Immunology & Rhematology. *The Health Assessment Questionnaire (HAQ)© and the Improved HAQ.* 2009. http://aramis.stanford.edu/downloads/HAQ%20Instructions%20%28ARAMIS%29%206-30-09.pdf
115. Maska L, Anderson J, Michaud K. Measures of functional status and quality of life in rheumatoid arthritis. *Arthritis Care Res.* 2011;63(S11):S4-S13.
116. Feldman BM, Ayling-Campos A, Luy L, Stevens D, Silverman ED, Laxer RM. Measuring disability in juvenile dermatomyositis: validity of the childhood health assessment questionnaire. *J Rheumatol.* 1995;22:326-331.
117. Ramey DR, Raynauld J-P, Fries JF. The Health Assessment Questionnaire 1992: status and review. *Arthritis Care Res.* 1992;5:119-129.
118. Ramey D, Fries J, Singh G. The Health Assessment Questionnaire 1995—status and review. In Spilker B, ed. *Quality of Life and Pharmacoeconomics in Clinical Trials.* 2nd ed. Philadelphia, PA: Lippincott-Raven; 1996:227-237.
119. Citera G, Arriola M, Maldonado-Cocco J, et al. Validation and crosscultural adaptation of an argentine Spanish version of the health assessment questionnaire disability index. *J Clin Rheumatol.* 2004;10:110-115.
120. Krishnan E, Sokka T, Hakkinen A, Hubert H, Hannonen P. Normative values for the Health Assessment Questionnaire Disability Index. *Arthritis Rheum.* 2004;50:953-960.
121. Fries JF, Cella D, Rose M, Krishnan E, Bruce B. Progress in assessing physical function in arthritis: PROMIS short forms and computerized adaptive testing. *J Rheumatol.* 2009;36:2061-2066.
122. Brown GT, Wallen M. Functional assessment tools for paediatric clients with juvenile chronic arthritis: an update and review for occupational therapists. *Scand J Occup Ther.* 2002;9:23-34.
123. Ruperto N, Ravelli A, Migliavacca D, et al. Responsiveness of clinical measures in children with oligoarticular juvenile arthritis. *J Rheumatol.* 1999;26:1827-1830.
124. Howe S, Levinson J, Shear E, et al. Development of a disability measurement tool for juvenile rheumatoid arthritis: the Juvenile Arthritis Functional Assessment Report for Children and Their Parents. *Arthritis Rheum.* 1991;34:873-880.
125. Lovell DJ, Howe S, Shear E, et al. Development of a disability measurement tool for juvenile rheumatoid arthritis: the Juvenile Arthritis Functional Assessment Scale. *Arthritis Rheum.* 1989;32:1390-1395.
126. Tennant A, Kearns S, Turner F, Wyatt S, Haigh R, Chamberlain MA. Measuring the function of children with juvenile arthritis. *Rheumatology.* 2001;40:1274-1278.
127. Bekkering W, Ten Cate R, Van Rossum M, Vliet Vlieland T. A comparison of the measurement properties of the Juvenile Arthritis Functional Assessment Scale with the childhood health assessment questionnaire in daily practice. *Clin Rheumatol.* 2007;26:1903-1907.
128. Baildam EM, Holt PJ, Conway SC, Morton MJ. The association between physical function and psychological problems in children with juvenile chronic arthritis. *Br J Rheumatol.* 1995;34:470-477.
129. Spadaro A, Riccieri V, Sili Scavalli A, et al. Interleukin-6 and soluble interleukin-2 receptor in juvenile chronic arthritis: correlations with clinical and laboratory parameters. *Revue du Rhumatisme.* 1996;63:153-158.
130. van der Net J, Prakken AB, Helders PJ, et al. Correlates of disablement in polyarticular juvenile chronic arthritis: a cross sectional study. *Br J Rheumatol.* 1996;35:91-100.
131. Robinson RF, Nahata MC, Hayes JR, Rennebohm R, Higgins G. Quality-of-life measurements in juvenile rheumatoid arthritis patients treated with entracept. *Clin Drug Investig.* 2003;23:511-518.
132. Wright FV, Kimber JL, Law M, Goldsmith C, Crombie V, Dent P. The Juvenile Arthritis Functional Status Index (JASI): a validation study. *J Rheumatol.* 1996;23:1066-1079.
133. Wright FV, Law M, Crombie V, Goldsmith CH, Dent P. Development of a self-report functional status index for juvenile rheumatoid arthritis. *J Rheumatol.* 1994;21:536-544.
134. Brown GT, Wright FV, Lang BA, et al. Clinical responsiveness of self-report functional assessment measures for children with juvenile idiopathic arthritis undergoing intraarticular corticosteroid injections. *Arthritis Care Res.* 2005;53:897-904.
135. Katz S, Ford AB, Moskowitz RW, Jackson BA, Jaffe MW. Studies of illness in the aged: the index of ADL: a standardized measure of biological and psychosocial function. *JAMA.* 1963;185(12):94-99.
136. Brorsson B, Asberg KH. Katz index of independence in ADL: reliability and validity in short-term care. *Scand J Rehabil Med.* 1984;16:125-132.
137. Asberg KH, Sonn U. The cumulative structure of personal and instrumental ADL: a study of elderly people in a health service district. *Scand J Rehabil Med.* 1988;21:171-177.
138. Iwarsson S, Isacsson A. On scaling methodology and environmental influences in disability assessments: the cumulative structure of personal and instrumental ADL among older adults in a Swedish rural district. *Can J Occup Ther.* 1997;64:240-251.
139. Spector WK, Katz S, Murphy JB, Fulton JP. The hierarchical relationship between activities of daily living and instrumental activities of daily living. *J Chronic Dis.* 1987;40:481-489.
140. Ciesla JR, Shi L, Stoskopf CH, Samuels ME. Reliability of Katz's activities of daily living scale when used in telephone interviews. *Eval Health Prof.* 1993;16:190-204.
141. Reuben DB, Valle LA, Hays RD, Siu AL. Measuring physical function in community-dwelling older persons: a comparison of self-administered, interviewer-administered, and performance-based measures. *J Am Geriatr Soc.* 1995;43:17-23.
142. Katz SK, Downs TD, Cash HR, Grotz RC. Progress in development of the index of ADL. *Gerontologist.* 1970;10:20-30.
143. Hulter-Asberg KH, Nydevick I. Early prognosis of stroke outcome by means of Katz index of activities of daily living. *Scand J Rehabil Med.* 1991;23:187-191.

144. Hermodsson Y, Ekdahl C. Early planning of care and rehabilitation after amputation for vascular disease by means of Katz Index of Activities of Daily Living. *Scand J Caring Sci.* 1999;13:234-239.
145. Settle C, Holm MB. Program planning: the clinical utility of three activities of daily living assessment tools. *Am J Occup Ther.* 1993;47:911-918.
146. Nelson DL, Melville LL, Wilkerson JD, Magness RA, Grech JL, Rosenberg JA. Interrater reliability, concurrent validity, responsiveness and predictive validity of the Melville-Nelson Self-Care Assessment. *Am J Occup Ther.* 2002;56:51-59.
147. Melville LL, Baltic TA, Bettcher TW, Nelson DL. Patients' perspectives on the Self-Identified Goals Assessment. *Am J Occup Ther.* 2002;56:650-659.
148. Feldman AB, Haley SM, Coryell J. Concurrent and construct validity of the Pediatric Evaluation of Disability Inventory. *Phys Ther.* 1990;70:602-610.
149. Haley SM, Coster WJ, Ludlow LH, Haltiwanger JT, Andrellos, PJ. *Pediatric Evaluation of Disability Inventory (PEDI) Version 1.0: Development, Standardization and Administration Manual.* Boston, MA: Trustees of Boston University, Center for Rehabilitation Effectiveness; 1992.
150. Iyer LV, Haley SM, Watkins MP, Dumas HM. Establishing minimal clinically important differences for scores on the Pediatric Evaluation of Disability Inventory for inpatient rehabilitation. *Phys Ther.* 2003;83:888-898.
151. Dumas HM, Haley SM, Fragala MA, Steva BJ. Self-care recovery of children with brain injury: descriptive analysis using the Pediatric Evaluation of Disability Inventory (PEDI) functional classification levels. *Phys Occup Ther Pediatr.* 2001;21:7-27.
152. Wright FV, Boschen KA. The Pediatric Evaluation of Disability Inventory: validation of a new functional assessment outcome instrument. *Can J Rehabil.* 1993;7:41-42.
153. Chen K, Hsieh C, Sheu C, Hu F, Tseng M. Reliability and validity of a Chinese version of the Pediatric Evaluation of Disability Inventory in children with cerebral palsy. *J Rehabil Med.* 2009;41:273-278.
154. Erkin G, Elhan A, Aybay C, Sirzai H, Ozel S. Validity and reliability of the Turkish translation of the Pediatric Evaluation of Disability Inventory (PEDI). *Disabil Rehabil.* 2007;29:1271-1279.
155. Reid DT, Boschen K, Wright V. Critique of the Pediatric Evaluation of Disability Inventory. *Phys Occup Ther Pediatr.* 1993;13(4):57-93.
156. Nichols DS, Case-Smith J. Reliability and validity of the Pediatric Evaluation of Disability Inventory. *Pediatr Phys Ther.* 1996;8:15-24.
157. Tsai PY, Yang TF, Chan RC, Huang PH, Wong TT. Functional investigation in children with spina bifida—measured by the Pediatric Evaluation of Disability Inventory (PEDI). *Childs Nerv Syst.* 2002;18:48-53.
158. Bourke-Taylor H. Melbourne Assessment of Unilateral Upper Limb Function: construct validity and correlation with the Pediatric Evaluation of Disability Inventory. *Dev Med Child Neurol.* 2003;45:92-96.
159. Nordmark E, Jarnlo G, Hagglund G. Comparison of the Gross Motor Function Measure and Pediatric Evaluation of Disability Inventory in assessing motor function in children undergoing selective dorsal rhizotomy. *Dev Med Child Neurol.* 2000;42:245-252.
160. Vos-Vromans D, Ketelaar M, Gorter J. Responsiveness of evaluative measures for children with cerebral palsy: the Gross Motor Function Measure and the Pediatric Evaluation of Disability Inventory. *Disabil Rehabil.* 2005;27:1245-1252.
161. Haley SM, Ludlow LH, Coster WJ. Pediatric Evaluation of Disability Inventory: clinical interpretation of summary scores using Rasch rating scale methodology. *Phys Med Rehabil Clin N Am.* 1993;4:529-540.
162. Berg M, Jahnsen R, Froslie KF, Hussain A. Reliability of the pediatric evaluation of disability inventory (PEDI). *Phys Occup Ther Pediatr.* 2004;24(3):61-77.
163. Custers JW, Van der Net J, Hoijtink H, et al. Discriminative validity of the Dutch Pediatric Evaluation of Disability Inventory. *Arch Phys Med Rehabil.* 2002;83:1437-1441.
164. Gannotti ME, Cruz C. Content and construct validity of a Spanish translation of the Pediatric Evaluation of Disability Inventory for children living in Puerto Rico. *Phys Occup Ther Pediatr.* 2001;20:7-24.
165. Wassenberg-Severijnen JE, Custers JW, Hox JJ, Vermeer A, Helders PJ. Reliability of the Dutch Pediatric Evaluation of Disability Inventory (PEDI). *Clin Rehabil.* 2003;17:457-462.
166. Coster WJ, Haley SM, Ni P, Dumas HM, Fragala-Pinkham MA. Assessing self-care and social function using a computer adaptive testing version of the pediatric evaluation of disability inventory. *Arch Phys Med Rehabil.* 2008;89:622-629.
167. Haley S, Coster W, Kao Y, et al. Lessons from use of the Pediatric Evaluation of Disability Inventory: where do we go from here? *Pediatr Phys Ther.* 2010;22:69-75.
168. Chen KL, Tseng MH, Hu FC, Koh CL. Pediatric evaluation of disability inventory: a cross-cultural comparison of daily function between Taiwanese and American children. *Res Dev Disabil.* 2010;31:1590-1600.
169. Berg M, Aamodt G, Stanghelle J, Krumlinde-Sundholm L, Hussain A. Cross-cultural validation of the Pediatric Evaluation of Disability Inventory (PEDI) norms in a randomized Norwegian population. *Scand J Occup Ther.* 2008;15:143-152.
170. Srsen KG, Vidmar G, Zupan A. Applicability of the Pediatric Evaluation of Disability Inventory in Solvenia. *J Child Neurol.* 2005;20:411-416.
171. Lawton MP, Brody EM. Assessment of older people: self-maintaining and instrumental activities of daily living. *Gerontologist.* 1969;9:179-186.
172. Edwards MM. The reliability and validity of self-report activities of daily living scales. *Can J Occup Ther.* 1990;57:273-278.
173. Rubenstein LZ, Schairer C, Wieland GD, Kane, R. Systematic biases in functional status assessment of elderly adults: effects of different data sources. *J Gerontol.* 1984;39(6):686-691.
174. Hokoishi K, Ikeda M, Maki N, et al. Interrater reliability of the Physical Self-Maintenance Scale and the Instrumental Activities of Daily Living Scale in a variety of health professional representatives. *Aging Mental Health.* 2001;5:38-40.
175. Boyd A, Dawson DR. The relationship between perceptual impairment and self-care status in a sample of elderly persons. *Phys Occup Ther Geriatr.* 2000;17(4):1-16.
176. Lawton MP. Scales to measure competence in everyday activities. *Psychopharmacol Bull.* 1988;24(4):609-614.

Mine the Gold

Instrumental activities of daily living (IADL) are the stepping stones between basic ADL and participation, or advanced ADL. Successful and safe performance of IADL are also critical determinants of a client's ability to remain in the community and age in place.

Become Systematic

Systematically screening for IADL disability is important because a large proportion of a client's day is spent performing IADL. Therefore, systematically screening all clients for IADL disability is just good practice.

Use Evidence in Practice

One method of using evidence in practice is to start an "IADL evidence" notebook in which articles are filed and categorized by IADL domains. These articles can then be used for a weekly staff journal club.

Make Occupational Therapy Contributions Explicit

When working with clients, reporting at team meetings, or documenting in the medical record, make your profession known. When screening clients about their IADL, let them know that you are interested in how they perform "skills for the job of living."

Engage in Occupation-Based, Client-Centered Practice

IADL are innately occupation-based activities. By ascertaining which IADL are most important to each client—which ones they want to do, need to do, or are expected to do—your practice becomes client centered.

CHAPTER 14

Measuring Performance in Instrumental Activities of Daily Living

Margo B. Holm, PhD, OTR/L, FAOTA, ABDA and Joan C. Rogers, PhD, OTR/L, FAOTA

"People may doubt what you say, but they will always believe what you do." –Anonymous

Occupational performance measurement is hierarchical, with each progressive level indicative of higher levels of occupational functioning. The body-oriented basic activities of daily living (BADL; eg, eating, grooming, dressing, continence, transfers) are at the lowest level of the hierarchy. The middle level focuses on instrumental ADL (IADL; eg, meal preparation, medication management, laundry, shopping, money management, home maintenance, transportation), or those activities needed to maintain one's home and function in the community. The top level of the hierarchy focuses on advanced ADL (AADL; eg, running a mile, traveling, socializing) or those activities that typically place substantive physical, cognitive, or psychosocial demands on people.[1] With the advent of the Functional Independence Measure (FIM)[2] and its companion tool, the Inpatient Rehabilitation Facility—Patient Assessment Instrument (IRF-PAI),[3] often linked to third party insurance payments, the focus of occupational performance measurement became the BADL. The BADL became paramount because they are the essential daily living tasks needed for discharge to the home. However, for clients to function in their homes and participate in their communities, the focus of occupational performance measurement needs to be broadened to the IADL and AADL. AADL activities are not necessary for survival. They contribute to the quality of one's life. Clinically, discharge disposition does not depend on the AADL, but it does depend on the IADL—can the client perform needed IADL independently, safely, and adequately to return home and remain in the community? If not, how will those IADL be accomplished? Research on IADL can help identify which activities, and at what level, best predict the functional performance needed for a successful return to the community, as well as provide guidance about interventions that will improve performance of IADL.

Overview of Instrumental Activities of Daily Living

Lawton and Brody[4] coined the term *IADL* in the late 1960s and identified 8 IADL that could be assessed by asking the client or a knowledgeable family member about the ability to use the telephone, shop, prepare food, maintain the house, do laundry, use transportation, manage medications, and handle finances. Since that time, numerous measures of IADL performance have been developed and IADL tasks have expanded beyond the original 8 IADL (Table 14-1). Lawton and Brody's IADL were generic categories of activities (eg, laundry), with more specific criteria listed under each category that yielded a score (eg, does personal laundry completely = 1; launders small items, rinses socks, stockings, etc = 1; all laundry must be done by others = 0). With advances in IADL measurement, items have become more specific, methods of data collection have expanded, and determination of psychometric properties has become more robust. In addition, research studies have used IADL assessment results to measure change in functional status, categorize levels of disability, and predict future levels of client functioning.

Law M, Baum C, Dunn W, eds. *Measuring Occupational Performance: Supporting Best Practice in Occupational Therapy, Third Edition* (pp 305-331).

Instrumental Activities of Daily Living Categories and Items

IADL beyond the original 8 activities have expanded to include categories such as health, leisure, small repairs, managing appliances, errands, caring for others, and volunteering (see Table 14-1). IADL assessment items have also become more specific, such as playing a game of skill, repotting a plant, vacuuming 2 rooms, preparing a letter, obtaining critical information from a newspaper, prioritizing tasks by importance, and filling out forms (see Table 14-1). Over time, more items have focused on community and social involvement, such as inviting people to his or her home, going out to public places, explaining how to do a mulitstep task to others, and using a calendar to keep track of appointments (see Table 14-1).

The Fundamentals of Instrumental Activities of Daily Living Data: Skills, Habits, and Satisfaction

Most IADL assessments measure skills, not habits. Skills and habits are different, although intrinsically linked. Few assessments measure satisfaction. Daily living routines are made up of skilled behaviors. When a discrepancy in IADL exists between clients' current performance and what is desired, required, or expected of the clients, it is important to ascertain whether the discrepancy is due to a skill deficit or a habit deficit. It is also helpful to ascertain how satisfied the clients are with their current performance because if they are satisfied with their discrepant performance, they may not be motivated to improve it.

Skills

Skills are task-specific abilities to perform the requirements of a task proficiently.[5] Proficiency standards may be determined by the client (eg, "I can't do it the way I used to"), or by family members, assisted living centers, employers, communities, or society. Because skills are task-specific, lack of proficiency in one task, or one step of a task does not mean that a client is not proficient in other tasks or others steps of the task. When asking a client about IADL skills, an assessment item usually begins with, "Can you..." With performance-based assessments, clients are usually asked, "Can you show me how you..." or, "Can you demonstrate how you..." Skills usually can be measured using an interview or a performance-based assessment in a single clinical session. When a client's IADL skill performance in the clinic differs from what is wanted, needed, or expected, it is important to find out why by considering the following:

- Did the client ever learn to perform the task, has the client not performed the task recently, or was another method used (eg, client uses money orders, not checks)?
- Are the task tools familiar to the client (eg, electric vs gas stovetop)?
- Is the environment consistent with the client's environment (eg, faucets to the left as client enters the tub)?
- Does the presence of the practitioner make the client nervous or paranoid because of being observed?
- Does the client have a new health condition or impairment that may be negatively influencing IADL skill?

Habits

Repetition of several skills in a sequence constitutes a *routine*, and repetition of a routine over time constitutes a *habit*.[6] Habits are patterns, developed over time, which can increase efficiency in the performance of everyday tasks. Habits are unique to each person. When interviewing a client about IADL habits, an assessment item usually begins with, "Do you..." or "How frequently do you..." However, because habits are unique to each person and they occur over time, they are more difficult to measure in a single clinical performance-based assessment session. When a client's IADL habits do not match what is wanted, needed, or expected, it is important to find out why by considering the following:

- Does the environment preclude the client from enacting usual routines because the task objects, family members, and the usual environment are not present to trigger the daily routines?
- Does the client even have effective routines and habits?
- Does the client have obligatory routines and habits (eg, handwashing ritual) that prevent the client from carrying out IADL tasks proficiently?
- Does the client have a new health condition or impairments that may be negatively influencing IADL performance?
- Does the client want or need to routinely do the task?

Satisfaction

Patient-reported outcomes, such as "satisfaction," have received increasing attention in health care, as have client-centered outcomes in occupational therapy. Satisfaction with current IADL performance for those tasks clients want to do, need to do, or are expected to do needs to be assessed. Likewise, changes in performance during and following occupational therapy interventions need to be assessed to confirm that our interventions are not just technically on target, but also on target based on the perspective of the client. When satisfaction with current performance is less than desirable, it is important to find out why by considering the following:

- What aspect of task performance causes dissatisfaction (eg, increased length of time needed to complete the task; Too much effort is now needed to perform the task; Task quality is not the same as it used to be)?
- Is dissatisfaction associated with a new health condition or impairment, or has the client been dissatisfied for a longer period of time?

- Has the client's or family member's level of dissatisfaction with task performance caused the client to stop performing the task?

Methods of Collecting Instrumental Activities of Daily Living Data

Self-Report

Clients know the most about their IADL performance because they enact it daily or weekly. However, recency of task performance can influence accuracy of responses, especially if a task has not been performed recently. Clients may also overestimate their performance if they fear they may have to move from their homes if they are deemed "disabled." In contrast, clients may also underestimate their performance if they are seeking services that will be granted if they have a specific level of "disability." If clients are unwilling or unable to self-report, proxies are often asked to provide IADL data.

Proxy Report

The usefulness of the IADL information gathered from proxies is dependent on how familiar they are with the client's IADL skills and habits. Those who live with the client would be most familiar, as would family, friends, or whomever spends the most time with the client when the client is engaged in IADL activities. One surrogate measure of familiarity with the client's performance, and to validate the proxy's responses, is to ask, "How many hours per day do you spend with the client?" However, a proxy can spend 4 to 6 hours per day with a client and never see the client prepare a meal, manage medications, or cope with finances. Again, the recency of observing the client perform the IADL tasks in question must be clarified. Bias may influence proxy responses. Family proxies are known to see the client as more disabled than professionals working with the client, and spouses tend to see the client as more disabled than other family members. Because spouses and family members are often caregivers, their perspectives often reflect their own exhaustion.[7]

Observation of Clinic Performance

Although interviewing the client or the client's proxy about IADL performance is an excellent method of screening for IADL performance ability and disability, observation of the client's performance provides details necessary for intervention planning that an interview cannot provide. For example, although the client or proxy may report that the only problem with meal preparation is standing tolerance, observation of the client's performance may indicate that the client mixes up which burners are on and neglects to turn them off before sitting down to eat. Because of costs, most IADL performance-based assessments are administered in the clinic setting. However, the clinic is not the "lived-in" environment, and clinic IADL performance is not always equivalent with home performance. Among clients with arthritis, percent agreement indicated that performance in the clinic equaled performance in the home only 55.4% of the time for cognitively-oriented IADL (eg, managing medications), and only 52.0% for the more physically-oriented IADL (eg, taking out the garbage). When performance was not equal, the clinic performance underestimated home performance.[8] Among wheelchair users, percent agreement among observers indicated that performance in the clinic equaled performance in the home 42.1% to 89.5%, depending on the tasks. When performance was not equal, clinic performance overestimated home performance, most likely because of the prosthetic clinic environment (wide hallways, smooth floors, lower countertops).[9] Telerehabilitation, with the use of high-quality video equipment, has extended the clinic environment to distant clinical sites, and thus extended the expertise of practitioners with specific IADL assessment skills.[10,11] To achieve ecological validity when performance testing in the clinic, it is important to clarify the client's familiarity with the task objects being used in the assessment as well as how well the physical arrangement of the assessment setting mirrors the "lived-in" environment.

Observation of Home Performance

Because home is the "lived-in" environment, it is more ecologically valid than a clinic for performance-based assessments of IADL. The "lived in" environment allows the practitioner to observe how clients interact with their own task objects and in the environment where the tasks usually take place. In their homes, clients will also slip into their task routines, and the practitioner can observe whether the routine promotes or hinders task efficiency and safety. It also allows the practitioner to observe the point of task breakdown or risk, which can lead to an appropriate intervention. However, observation of home performance is not always possible because of cost, distance, and the fact that many clients do not want to be assessed in their homes. Cost and distance issues can be ameliorated successfully with telerehabilitation. For example, following a telerehabilitation home intervention for stroke survivors, client self-reports indicated significant improvements.[12] Hoenig et al[13] also used telerehabilitation to provide occupational therapy and physical therapy. They found that, of the interventions recommended, 89% of the adaptive strategy, 53% of the assistive technology, and 46% of the environmental modifications were implemented by the clients.

Psychometric Properties to Look for in Instrumental Activities of Daily Living Measures

Validity

Validity of an assessment establishes the degree to which it measures what it claims to measure, the trustworthiness of the score meaning and interpretation, and the assessment's concordance with a gold standard. The most common types of validity reported for clinical assessments are content, construct, and criterion validity.[14,15]

- *Content validity*: The content validity of an IADL assessment must take into consideration the universe being sampled (ie, IADL), the relevance of the content to an IADL assessment, and whether the universe is sufficiently sampled. Thus, some IADL assessments focus only on meal preparation, while others have multiple domains (eg, housecleaning, outdoor home maintenance). Often, item selection is based on a literature review, a review of other assessments, or empirical methods such as factor analysis and item response theory (IRT). It is the practitioner's responsibility to make sure that there is a match between a specific IADL assessment and the IADL performance needs, wants, and expectations of the client.[15]
- *Construct validity*: Construct validity is the ability of an assessment to measure a concept or construct, such as IADL. However, IADL assessment tools can measure different constructs, such as difficulty, assistance needed, independence, satisfaction, and self-efficacy. When assessing the construct validity of an IADL assessment, construct validation can take numerous forms, including the known group method (eg, does the assessment differentiate between those with mild and severe arthritis based on the construct of difficulty?). Convergent validity, discriminant validity, factor analysis, and IRT are 4 other empirical methods of determining construct validity. Convergent validity is conducted to ascertain whether the assessment outcomes correlate strongly with another tool known to measure the same underlying construct (eg, satisfaction). Divergent validity is conducted to ascertain whether there are low correlations between the assessment and another tool known to measure a different concept (eg, self-efficacy vs musicality). With IRT, infit and outfit statistics are also reported and indicate the variance between the observed responses and the model-predicted responses. Each of these methods of measuring construct validity contribute to the trustworthiness that the score of the IADL assessment represents the construct being measured.[16,17]
- *Criterion validity*: For criterion validity, an IADL assessment may be compared with a "criterion" assessment—one that measures the construct in question. However, assessments are often developed because no other assessment measures the exact construct; therefore, multiple "criterion" assessments may be correlated with the new assessment to yield the data needed to confirm the construct validity. For example, if there were no assessments that measured satisfaction with IADL performance, once the new assessment was developed, the scores could be correlated with "criterion" assessments that measure related constructs of independence, self-efficacy, and difficulty. If the level of satisfaction with IADL performance correlates well with high levels of independence and self-efficacy and low levels of difficulty, then the new tool would be said to have "criterion" validity.

Reliability

According to psychometric experts, clinical assessments that are used to guide intervention should have, at minimum, moderate reliability coefficients > 0.51 to 0.75.[17] Typical reliability coefficients that are reported for assessments are test-retest reliability, internal consistency, and inter-rater reliability.[14,15]

- *Internal consistency*: Internal consistency values indicate the homogeneity of the assessment items, in total or in part. IADL assessments often consist of content areas that are not conceptually consistent (eg, financial management vs small repairs); therefore, subtest or domain scores may be reported and more valid than total score internal consistency. Internal consistency is usually reported as a Cronbach's alpha, and a desirable range is between 0.70 and 0.90, indicating good internal consistency of items without redundancy.[17]
- *Test-retest reliability*: Test-retest reliability data indicate the stability of assessment scores over time. The time between test and retest is dependent on what is being measured and the duration of time that the content is not expected to change (eg, 3 days, 1 week). Test-retest reliability is usually reported as percent agreement, Pearson's r correlation, Spearman rank order correlation, or an intraclass correlation coefficient (ICC). If the assessment tool is not stable, then practitioners can misinterpret the data it yields and end up reporting that a client's disability status has declined when, in fact, it is the assessment that does not allow for consistent measurement.
- *Inter-rater reliability*: Inter-rater reliability, or interobserver reliability, indicates the consistency with which 2 or more practitioners observing the same client's performance, at the same time, generate the same scores. Inter-rater reliability is usually reported as percent agreement, Pearson's r correlation, the kappa statistic, or an ICC. Nonagreement among practitioners (low correlations) may be due to one or more of the raters, and reasons for the differences need to be examined. For example, one practitioner may not be adhering to the scoring criteria, or one practitioner may be too lenient or too rigorous a scorer. However, it is important for all practitioners working together to have excellent inter-rater reliability, so that when work schedules require that one practitioner administers the admission assessment and another the discharge assessment, the practitioners' abilities as raters are interchangeable.[17]

Item Response Theory Item Reliability and Person Reliability

The item reliability index indicates the expected replicability of the IADL item ordering if these items were administered to another sample of the same size, with the same traits (eg, stroke survivors). The person reliability index indicates the expected replicability of the ordering of the clients if the clients were administered another assessment measuring the same IADL construct (eg, independence).

Responsiveness

An assessment must not only be valid and reliable, but for its clinical utility, it must also be responsive to a meaningful minimal change in IADL performance over time (ie, pre- to post-intervention). Responsiveness can be measured statistically using the minimal detectable difference (MDD) and the minimal clinically important difference (MCID). Responsiveness criteria for a specific assessment can vary based on the MCID for specific populations and settings as well as the design of the study (eg, type and duration of the intervention, sample, etc).

Several Factors That May Affect Instrumental Activities of Daily Living Performance Assessment

Research has documented multiple factors that impact IADL performance, with studies using self-report, proxy report, or performance-based assessments for collecting IADL data. Table 14-2 includes examples of demographic, health, assistance, environmental, methodological, and cultural factors that may affect IADL performance.

Importance of Measurement for Instrumental Activities of Daily Living

For hospitalized clients who wish to return to the community, and clients receiving care in outpatient clinics or through home health services, there is an ethical obligation to screen for IADL disability using self-report or proxy report. For those domains or tasks where reported performance is discrepant from the level of performance the client needs to, wants to, or is expected to demonstrate, performance-based assessment needs to follow. Because IADL are within occupational therapy's scope of practice, if clients are discharged to the community or in the community without an IADL assessment and subsequently harm themselves, the occupational therapy practitioners could be held accountable.

Most adults also do not spend the majority of their days on BADL, but rather on IADL, work, and leisure activities. Therefore, just based on the proportion of time spent on IADL and leisure, if reported IADL performance is discrepant or at risk, it is important and ethical for practitioners to assess IADL.

If there is a caregiver for the client, it is also important to assess whether the caregiver can safely and adequately assist the client with IADL tasks that remain discrepant, without putting both the client and the caregiver at risk. Even though the caregiver claims to have the ability to assist the client, if an IADL task will require both the client and the caregiver to perform the task, then the caregiver needs to be assessed, educated, and trained.

Factors to Remember

The sequence of IADL assessment should be client-centered and logically start with a self-report of meaningful IADL that the client wants to do, needs to do, or is expected to do. Then, the practitioner needs to query about habits for the identified IADL—"How frequently are they performed and when was the last time you performed them [recency]?" The next query should be the perceived level of skill when performing IADL. The practitioner can query clients by asking them, "Even though you haven't performed this IADL recently, could you perform it in an emergency?" or, "Given your current health status, could you perform this IADL independently, safely, and adequately?" Finally, the practitioner needs to query about clients' satisfaction with their current performance, and whether they have stopped performing valued IADL because they (or family members) were not satisfied with how independently, safely, or adequately they were performed.

Strategies for Selecting Measures for Instrumental Activities of Daily Living

Screen First, Then Choose

Once the practitioner has screened for habits, skills, and satisfaction with a client's meaningful IADL, the choice of one or more appropriate standardized, valid, and reliable IADL assessments—matched to the client's needs, wants, and expectations—should become clear.

Choose Measures That Are Relevant

If a client is going to be discharged to an assisted living facility, it is important to know the facility's admission criteria (eg, are all residents expected to manage their own medications?) and assess whether the client can perform those tasks safely and adequately. Because "assistance" at an assisted living facility comes with a price tag, other IADL such as using the small stovetop and the mini-microwave should be assessed to confirm that the client is not at risk. Likewise, if a client is being discharged to a long-term care facility (LTCF), there is no need at this time to assess meal preparation, medication management, or household maintenance tasks if the client is expected to reside there.

Strategies for Reporting About Instrumental Activities of Daily Living

- Develop reporting forms that provide summary data, with room for explanations (Table 14-3). Team members do not have the time to read long and rambling documentation, but they want to know critical information. Development of reporting forms often has to be approved by the medical records department, so the process can take time.
- Identify tasks that need no assistance, and level of assistance for at-risk tasks. It is important to identify those IADL tasks that clients can perform independently, as well as those for which the client needed assistance. For tasks requiring assistance, the type (eg, verbal vs physical) of assistance required is important for the client and family members to understand. Terms such as minimal, moderate, and maximal are too vague to be understood by clients and families, and a misunderstanding may put the client at risk.
- Identify tasks that pose a safety risk to the client and/or the caregiver. For clients and their caregivers to be vigilant about safety risks, it is necessary to identify which tasks pose safety risks as well as the type of safety risk (eg, left the stovetop burner on).
- Highlight the overall level of supervision needed. If clients have numerous safety risks and/or cognitive impairments, it is important to make clear to the clients and their families that 24/7 supervision is needed. If 24/7 supervision is not needed, then it is important to identify which tasks will require supervision to ensure that the client and/or others and the environment will not be harmed when the client performs them.
- Document caregiver training and level of skill. When it is determined that a client will need assistance, then the practitioner has the responsibility for assessing whether the caregiver has the skills needed to assist the client safely. If it is determined that the caregiver is unsafe when assisting the client, this needs to be documented and explained to the caregiver, and another caregiver needs to be recruited.

Future Directions for Practice and Research in Instrumental Activities of Daily Living

- Because IADL independence, safety, and adequacy are important for community living and "aging in place," occupational therapy practitioners need to advocate to include IADL in their overall assessment and interventions plans. Just because they are not included in the FIM or the IRF-PAI does not mean that IADL are not relevant to clients, especially after their discharge and return to the community.
- IADL are also the stepping stone to community and social participation. Several IADL assessments include items related to socialization (eg, invite people to your home) and community participation (eg, volunteer job). With an increased emphasis on participation as an outcome of rehabilitation, IADL can be significant enablers of participation.
- One of the common legal criteria for competency in conservatorship or guardianship hearings is people's ability to care for themselves, or BADL and IADL abilities. Occupational therapy practitioners should be the professionals of choice to conduct those evaluations. Inpatient settings providing services to mental health clients and those with cognitive impairments usually have access to magistrates who conduct competency hearings, and occupational therapy practitioners can be called on to testify regarding BADL and IADL deficits. In one instance, the practitioner reported that the client said she could manage all of her BADL and IADL, and the magistrate's response was, "I don't care what the client says she can do, I want to know what you have observed her doing."
- In a 2007 editorial in the *American Journal of Geriatric Psychiatry*, Reynolds wrote that research:

  > has now taught us that decisional capacity in the elderly, as evidenced by consent to treatment or behavioral evidence of independent, safe, and adequate IADL performance, is correlated with executive impairments and, in the case of IADL, by speed of information processing. Additional work of this kind is likely to move us forward to reliable, valid, and useful tools for assessment of decisional capacity for everyday functional challenges and could also assist in developing empiric models to enhance rehabilitation and recovery from the mental and neuropsychiatric disorders of old age. This is what really matters, to our patients and to us.[18(p 90)]

- Research also can lead to better predictive validity of occupational therapy IADL assessments. IADL assessment data and outcome data are at opposite ends of the same continuum, with interventions in the middle. The ability of an assessment to predict whose IADL status will change the most for a given intervention would move our measurement science forward considerably.
- IRT can also move our IADL measurement science forward by identifying those IADL assessment items that are easier or more difficult for specific populations of clients. IRT can also decrease client assessment burden by identifying the item difficulty hierarchy for an IADL assessment. The practitioner can then start the assessment at the midpoint of the items that are meaningful to the client, with the assumption that items below the midpoint are easier (which may not always be the case), and adjust the assessment items

Table 14-1

ORIGINAL AND NEWER IADL MEASURES WITH ADDED CATEGORIES AND TASKS, OVER TIME

IADL Sources	*Sample New IADL Categories/Tasks Added Over Time*	*Assessment Method*
Lawton and Brody[4] Instrumental Activities of Daily Living Scale (IADLS)	• Ability to use the telephone • Shopping • Food preparation • Housekeeping • Laundry • Mode of transportation • Responsibility for own medications • Ability to handle finances	• Self-report • Proxy report
McGourty (Thomson)[19] Kohlman Evaluation of Living Skills (KELS)	• Safety and health • Leisure	• Performance
Pfeffer et al[20] Functional Activities Questionnaire (FAQ)	• Assembling tax records, business affairs, papers • Playing a game of skill, working on a hobby • Preparing a balanced meal • Keeping track of current events • Paying attention to/understanding a book, TV • Remembering appointments, holidays • Traveling out of the neighborhood; drive; bus	• Proxy report
Fisher[21] Assessment of Motor and Process Skills (AMPS)	• Making a tossed salad • Ironing a shirt, garments, and setting up/taking down • Repotting a plant, plant care • Handwashing dishes • Making snacks, sandwiches, eggs, salads, soup, pasta dishes, and fried food • Vacuuming 2 rooms/vacuuming inside of a car, mopping • Raking leaves, weeding	• Clinic performance • Home performance

(continued)

up or down the hierarchy accordingly based on the client's responses.

- Finally, research on IADL measurement can help to clarify when self-report or proxy report can be substituted reliably for performance-based assessment. Practitioners need to know for which IADL items will self-report be accurate, and for whom. Practitioners also need more evidence to document the discrepancy between self-report of IADL and performance-based assessment of IADL to convince third-party insurance payers that, for specific IADL, the potential risk to the client outweighs the cost of performance-based assessment.

Overview of Measures of Instrumental Activities of Daily Living

Measures of IADL reviewed in this chapter were designed to assess IADL, have adequate psychometric properties, and have scales relevant to IADL disability (eg, independence, level of assistance, safety, adequacy) (Tables 14-4 through 14-13). Most are performance-based assessments, although some are self-report or proxy report. Most have been developed by occupational therapists or teams that included an occupational therapist. Measures were excluded if only a small part of the assessment focused on IADL, or the primary focus of the assessment was impairment or participation.

Table 14-1 (continued)

Original and Newer IADL Measures With Added Categories and Tasks, Over Time

IADL Sources	*Sample New IADL Categories/Tasks Added Over Time*	*Assessment Method*
Lowenstein et al[22] Direct Assessment of Functional Status (DAFS)	• Telling time • Preparing a letter • Transportation signage • Counting currency • Shopping recall	• Clinic performance
Rogers and Holm[23] Performance Assessment of Self-Care Skills (PASS)	• Taking out the garbage; locking/unlocking door • Changing bed linens • Obtaining critical information (audio/radio/TV) • Obtaining critical information (visual/newspaper) • Small repairs • Manage oven, stovetop, sharp utensils • Playing bingo	• Clinic performance • Home performance
Law et al[24] Canadian Occupational Performance Measure (COPM)	• Client generates tasks	• Self-report
Willis[25] Everyday Problems Test	• Interpreting bills • Interpreting Medicare forms • Interpreting tax forms • Interpreting health information	• Clinic performance
Spector and Fleishman[26] Research article	• Get on/off a bus • Get in/out of a car • Use a step stool	• Self-report
McHorney and Cohen[27] Research article	• Scrub floors • Carry groceries • Iron clothes • Go to the bank	• Self-report
Sheehan et al[28] Research article	• Shop/run errands	• Self-report
Jette et al[29]; Haley et al[30] Late Life Function and Disability Instrument (LLFDI)	• Invite people to home • Care for others • Visit friends and family • Go out to public places • Keep contact with others • Take care of errands • Take care of health • Volunteer job	• Self-report
Farias et al[31] Research article	• Recalling conversations a few days later • Ability to develop a strategy in a game of skill • Prioritizing tasks by importance	• Proxy report

(continued)

Table 14-1 (continued)

Original and Newer IADL Measures With Added Categories and Tasks, Over Time

IADL Sources	*Sample New IADL Categories/Tasks Added Over Time*	*Assessment Method*
Jette et al[32] Activity Measure for Post-Acute Care (AM-PAC)	• Explaining how to do a several-step task • Following a 10- to 15-minute lecture • Reading a book with over 100 pages • Reading/ following instructions for new appliance • Filling out forms (eg, insurance) • Using a calendar to keep track of appointments • Putting together a shopping list of 10 to 15 items	• Self-report • Proxy report
Classen et al[33] Fitness to Drive Screening Measure	• Driving history profile • Driving skills	• Proxy report

Table 14-2

Several Factors That May Affect IADL Performance Assessment

Factors	*Examples of Evidence*
Age	• After controlling for multiple demographic variables, those aged 75 to 84 years were 3 times more likely to have an IADL deficit, and those aged 85 years and older were 8 times more likely to have an IADL deficit than those aged 65 to 74 years.[34] • For middle-aged adults (ages 55 to 69 years), from 2001 to 2009, hobbies and leisure and sports and exercise increased and yardwork and repairs decreased. Also, as disability increased, time spent on "sleep/naps, walking, paid work, household, repairs/yard, shopping, entertainment, sports/ exercise" helping others, and hobbies/leisure decreased. As disability increased, less time was spent on IADL and more time was spent on ADL.[35(p 194)]
Race/ethnicity/ culture	• Among US Medicare beneficiaries, 18.9% of White/non-Hispanics reported needing assistance from another, compared to 27.2% of Black/non-Hispanics, 32.5% of Hispanics, and 19.0% of Other (mostly Asians).[36] • Culture can also have an impact on preferences for reducing IADL disability. In a US national survey of community-dwelling adults age 55 years and older, when comparing White non-Hispanic to the Other race/ethnic category, respondents in the Other race/ethnic category were more likely to prefer personal assistance (with or without equipment assistance), which may reflect cultural differences in the availability and willingness of family to help.[37]
Income	• When income levels were examined among US Medicare beneficiaries, 30.1% of those with the lowest income (< 15,000) reported needing assistance from another, as did 21.6% of the second lowest quartile ($15,000 to $30,000), 12.8% of the third lowest quartile ($30,000 to $60,000), and 8.8% of the highest income quartile (> $60,000).[36]
Education	• Older adults with a high school diploma have lower disability rates than those who did not complete high school. Those over the age of 50 with a high school diploma had lower odds of having an IADL deficit than those with a GED diploma.[34]

(continued)

Table 14-2 (continued)

Several Factors That May Affect IADL Performance Assessment

Factors	*Examples of Evidence*
Health status	• The number of chronic health conditions has been linked to IADL performance. US Medicare population estimates indicate that those with 4 or more chronic conditions identified needing assistance from others, whereas those with < 2 chronic conditions reported that they were fully able.[36] • In stroke survivors, age (< 70 years), gender (male), upper limb strength (Motricity Index > 75), and a Barthel Index > 9 at 10 days post-stroke predicted a 100% functional recovery of IADL at 6 months.[38] • Performance-based, cognitively-oriented IADL were able to distinguish levels of independence task adequacy between participants with Parkinson's disease (PD) without dementia and participants without PD. IADL that were most discriminating were medication management, shopping, and sharp utensil use.[39]
Cognitive/mood status	• A study comparing cognitively normal older adults with those with dementia and mild cognitive impairment (MCI) found that those with dementia had significantly greater IADL disability than the cognitively normal older adults, as did those with MCI compared to the cognitively normal older adults. Tasks that relied heavily on memory were affected the most.[31] • The Everyday Problems Test (performance-based) and the Scales of Independent Behavior-Revised (self- and proxy-reported) tools differentiated between those with no cognitive impairment and those with MCI.[40] • Using Functional Activities Questionnaire (FAQ) proxy reports, those with amnesic MCI had greater IADL disability on 6/10 FAQ items, and those with non-amnesic MCI had greater disability on 8/10 FAQ items.[41] • Two performance-based IADL (shopping and checkbook balancing) on the Performance Assessment of Self-Care Skills were able to discriminate between older adults with normal cognitive function and those with MCI.[42] • Established habits and commitments kept older adults with late life depression engaged in some IADL activities during their depressive episodes.[43]
Physical status	• Tiring during IADL performance, taking too much time to perform IADL, and pain during IADL performance all contribute to IADL disability. In a US national survey of adults age 55 years and older, 43.6% identified extended task time as their greatest symptom of IADL disability; 41.5% identified tiring during task performance, and 27.1% identified pain.[37] • Respondents to a US national survey of adults age 55 years and older[37] ranked 8 IADL tasks that yielded the most disability symptoms: heavy housework (37.9%); shopping (23.5%); light housework (15.4%); preparing meals (14.4%); getting to places outside of a walking distance (14.3%); managing medication (8.5%); money management (8.2%); and using the telephone (6.5%).
Sensory status	• Patients with airway obstruction and dyspnea are most likely to have fewer "IADL disability-free years of life left" than those with normal lung function.[44] • IADL disability affected 18.3% of normal vision controls compared to 25% of those with bilateral visual field loss from glaucoma and 44.7% of those with bilateral visual acuity or severe unilateral acuity loss from age-related macular degeneration.[45]

(continued)

Table 14-2 (continued)

Several Factors That May Affect IADL Performance Assessment

Factors	*Examples of Evidence*
Medications	• Medications and medication dosages can affect IADL performance. For example, higher dosages (13.3 mg/24h vs 9.5 mg/24 h) of the rivastigmine patch (Exelon) for those with dementia resulted in less IADL decline over 48 weeks.[46]
Assistance (personal/devices)	• The use of assistance (personal and devices) has been found to decrease IADL disability • Severity of disability (eg, unable vs some difficulty vs a lot of difficulty) was the most important factor affecting IADL improvement with assistance (ie, personal assistance, equipment assistance, both) in US community-dwelling adults age 55 years and older.[37] • Among a US national sample of community-dwelling adults with disabilities, age 55 years and older, 43.4% reported a reduction in task difficulty with IADL assistance and 19.8% reported that task difficulty was resolved with IADL assistance.[37] • Verbrugge and Sevak[37] also found a hierarchy of assistance: both personal and equipment assistance > equipment assistance > personal assistance for reducing the severity of task disability.
Environment	• Among clients with arthritis, percent agreement indicated that performance in the clinic equaled performance in the home only 55.4% of the time for cognitively-oriented IADL, and only 52.0% for the more physically-oriented IADL.[8] • Among 20 older adults living in the community who were assessed with the Assessment of Motor and Process Skills, motor skills remained stable between the 2 environments, but 10 of the 20 participants performed process skills better in their homes.[47]
Method of assessment	• Among community-dwelling older women being treated for depression, their perceived IADL habits, perceived IADL skills, and demonstrated IADL skills were not congruent. In general, perceived skills were greater than perceived habits, which in turn were greater than demonstrated habits.[48] • Older non-depressed controls were compared with participants with depression and MCI and participants with depression and no cognitive impairments to ascertain if self-reported habits and skills were concordant with performance-based observation of IADL in their homes. No differences were found for mobility and BADL tasks, but concordance for the more complex IADL tasks was close to chance.[49] • When comparing responses of older drivers, family member proxies and certified driver rehabilitation specialists, family member proxy reports were most concordant with the certified driver rehabilitation specialists.[50] • *Also see Environment*

Table 14-3

Performance-Based Observational Assessment of Functional Status

Mrs. A was assessed in her home on June 5, 2016. The following tasks that were meaningful to the client were assessed, and the maximum level of assistance needed to initiate, continue, or complete each functional task were checked for that task, as well as each domain. Number of tasks for which performance was unsafe or inadequate were reported for each domain.

Independent: No assists from another person **Safe**: Task was performed in a manner that placed neither persons nor the environment at risk **Adequate**: Task was performed efficiently and the task process and end product matched the quality criteria	No Assists (Independent)	Verbal Assists	Physical Assists	Total Assist (unable)	Performance UNSAFE	Performance Inadequate	Not Assessed
Bed mobility							X
Stair mobility							X
Tub/shower mobility							X
Toilet mobility							X
Indoor walking							X
Functional Mobility Domain					N/A	N/A	X
Oral hygiene							X
Dressing							X
Trimming toenails							X
BADL Domain					N/A	N/A	X
Carrying out the garbage			X		X	X	
Sweeping the floor							X
Changing bed linens							X
Cleanup after meal preparation							X
IADL Domain—Physical Emphasis			X		1	1	
Shopping—cash exchange			X			X	
Bill paying by check		X					
Checkbook balancing		X					
Preparing bills to be mailed		X					
Telephone use	X						
Medication management				X		X	
Obtain critical information—Radio							X
Obtain critical information—Newspaper							X
Small repairs (flashlight)							X
Home safety awareness		X			X	X	
Bingo							X
Stovetop use		X			X		
Oven use		X					
Use of sharp utensils	X						
IADL Domain—Cognitive emphasis				X	2	3	

Performance Assessment of Self-Care Skills (PASS) Reporting Form

* = Refused to attempt the task; therefore coded as Unable; N/A = Not applicable, tasks not assessed

(continued)

Table 14-3 (continued)

Performance-Based Observational Assessment of Functional Status

Assessment

Functional Mobility: Not assessed

BADL: Not assessed

Physical IADL: Performance carrying out the garbage required physical assist (tripped); task performance unsafe and inadequate

Cognitive IADL: No assistance was required for telephone use and use of sharp utensils. Verbal cues needed with several tasks. Performance unsafe for home safety awareness (caught foot on rug) and stovetop use (left burner on). Performance inadequate for cash exchange, medication management, and home safety awareness.

Of the 11 IADL tasks assessed, assistance was required for 9, 3 were not performed safely, and 4 did not meet adequacy criteria.

Plan

Intervention will focus on cognitive and physical IADL. A family meeting will be scheduled following reassessment to discuss potential supervision needs.

Table 14-4

Activity Measure—Post-Acute Care (AM-PAC)

Source	http://www.bu.edu/bostonroc/instruments/am-pac/ http://pac-metrix.com/am-pac-resources/am-pac-ecat/ http://pac-metrix.com/am-pac_short-form/
Key References	Haley et al[51]; Haley et al[52]; Haley et al[53]; Jette et al[54]; Cheville et al[55]
Purpose	• The purpose of the AM-PAC is to measure changes in basic mobility, daily activity, and applied cognition throughout the continuum of care.
Type of Client	• The AM-PAC is designed for adult clients, or a proxy if necessary.
Test Format	• The AM-PAC has 2 formats: Computerized Adaptive Testing (CAT), and a paper and pencil Short Form. The format for the items begins with, "How much difficulty do you [does the client] currently have..." Responses are 1 = Unable, 2 = A lot, 3 = A little, and 4 = None.
Procedures	• CAT: Clients sign on to a computer and respond to the questions on the screen. The CAT program adjusts which items will be administered next based on the response to each question. The CAT pool of items has 131 mobility items, 88 daily activity items, and 50 applied cognition items. • Short Form: There are 3 versions of the Short Form depending on which scales and populations are relevant to the client.
Time Required	• CAT: Each scale takes from 2 to 3 minutes to respond, and the proprietary software program scores the AM-PAC and generates a profile of difficulty for all tasks. This process yields a "severity modifier" that can be linked to Medicare G-code modifiers. The CAT version also yields a client profile based on 5 stages of difficulty. • Short Form: It takes approximately 10 minutes to respond to the 10 items. Practitioners need to convert the raw scores to T-scale scores using the proprietary forms. This process yields a "severity modifier" that can be linked to Medicare G-codes modifiers.

(continued)

Table 14-4 (continued)

Activity Measure—Post-Acute Care (AM-PAC)

Standardization	• Both formats of the AM-PAC use standardized procedures and materials.
Reliability	
Test-Retest	• Not applicable—self-report. For responsiveness, the AM-PAC was also compared to the Physical Function Test, the Short Physical Performance Battery, the 6-minute walk test, and a timed gait speed test over a 12-week period with clients recovering from a unilateral surgical hip repair. The AM-PAC exceeded all measures in responsiveness over the 12-week period.
Internal Consistency	• Rasch person reliabilities ranged from 0.83 to 0.97, and item reliabilities ranged from 0.91 to 0.99. Confidence intervals (95%) around the total item pool were small, indicating the precision of the scores.
Inter-Rater	• Not applicable; once clients on the CAT select the first response, the computer generates the next questions. Not reported for the Short Form.
Validity	
Content	• The content validity of the AM-PAC is based on the International Classification of Functioning, Disability and Health (ICF[56]), as well as patient and practitioner feedback. Item response theory was used to test the items, scoring, and stages of the AM-PAC. The Basic Mobility items focus on ambulation, transfers, bending, carrying and lifting, and locomotion with a device. The Daily Activities items focus on feeding, meal preparation, and grooming/dressing. The Applied Cognition items focus on communication, print information, and complex instructions.
Construct	• Both the CAT and Short Form versions were able to correctly classify clients into functional stages throughout their recovery process.
Criterion	• The AM-PAC was compared to the Functional Independence Measure (FIM) and, in each case, equaled or exceeded the ability of the FIM to correctly stage clients in the recovery process.
Utility	
Research Programs	• The AM-PAC has been used as an outcome measure in multiple studies. As a measure that is valid across settings and recovery times, it has great utility for outcomes research.
Practice Settings	• The AM-PAC has been used in hospitals, outpatient clinics, rehabilitation centers, nursing homes, and clients' homes. Because it is applicable across settings, it has great clinical utility.
Strengths	• The AM-PAC is unique in that its administration time is usually less than 10 minutes, it is valid and reliable, and it can generate profiles that can be converted to match Medicare G-code modifiers. The 2 methods of administration increase its availability for settings that do not have computers for client assessment.

Table 14-5

Assessment of Motor and Process Skills (AMPS)

Source	http://www.innovativeotsolutions.com/content; http://www.ampsintl.com/AMPS/related/AONE.php
Key References	Fisher[57]; Park et al[47]; Doble[58]; Bray et al[59]; Merritt[60]
Purpose	• The purpose of the AMPS is to assess motor and process skills of clients by having them engage in several BADL or IADL tasks.

(continued)

Table 14-5 (continued)

Assessment of Motor and Process Skills (AMPS)

Type of Client	• The AMPS is appropriate for adolescent and adult populations, and more recently, children.
Test Format	• The AMPS is a performance-based assessment that can be administered in the clinic or home.
Procedures	• Practitioners wishing to use the AMPS must first enroll in a 5-day training program. They are then provided with the proprietary software needed to score client performance, and compare client motor and process skills to reference groups. To administer the AMPS, practitioners ask clients to select several ADL or IADL tasks from a menu of 50+ tasks for the evaluation. In the clinic, a standardized setup is used. As clients perform the chosen tasks, they are rated on 16 motor skills and 20 process skills. As they observe the client's performance, practitioners consider a client's unsafe performance, need for assistance, and task breakdown. Motor and process skills are scored with a 1 for deficient performance and/or task breakdown, a 2 for ineffective performance, a 3 for questionable performance, and a 4 for competent performance.
Time Required	• The AMPS uses many-faceted Rasch (MFR) modeling to analyze client motor and process skill performance using the AMPS proprietary software and anchor database. No information could be found for scoring and reporting time.
Standardization	• The AMPS requires raters to be trained, and the software adjusts for differences in rater severity. The AMPS has standardized procedures for each task. The AMPS has been standardized on over 110,000 international clients.
Reliability	
Test-Retest	• AMPS test-retest reliability was reported as r=0.88 for motor skills and r=0.86 for process skills.
Internal Consistency	• Adequate internal consistency is supported by MFR analyses.
Inter-Rater	• Of all AMPS-calibrated raters, 97% demonstrated acceptable goodness-of-fit to the MFR AMPS model, indicating high rater reliability.
Validity	
Content	• Content validity is based on the everyday ADL and IADL tasks that community-based adults perform in their homes. Furthermore, because clients can select which tasks they wish to perform, the content is specifically valid for them.
Construct	• The Rasch model indicates that each of the skills (motor, process) are unidimensional. Multiple validity studies have found that the AMPS can differentiate between age groups, genders, diagnostic subgroups, and across environments. Research has shown the AMPS to be valid across cultures.
Criterion	• The AMPS has also demonstrated criterion validity in several studies, including discriminating those clients who were safe/not safe at home and in the clinic based on the SAFER tool. A separate study used a matched sample to evaluate whether the AMPS could determine the need for assistance to live in the community, which it predicted with fair to good Receiver Operating Curve values.
Utility	
Research Programs	• Multiple research programs in the United States, Europe, New Zealand, Australia, and Asia have used and continue to use the AMPS as an assessment and intervention outcome measure, as well as to distinguish between diagnostic group characteristics.
Practice Settings	• Several thousand practitioners have been trained in the AMPS, and the data from the AMPS serves to inform and support their clinical judgments.
Strengths	• The AMPS provides impairment-oriented outcome data gathered from observations of clients performing everyday tasks. The AMPS has a history of well-designed item response theory research studies, using MFR analysis. This allows trained practitioners to have access to databases of reference groups for client comparisons. The AMPS also controls for differences among rater severity.

Table 14-6

Canadian Occupational Performance Measure (COPM)

Source	http://www.thecopm.ca/
Key References	Carswell et al[61]; Eyssen et al[62]; Colquhoun et al[63]
Purpose	• The purpose of the COPM is designed to identify problems in ADL/IADL performance and document change following interventions.
Type of Client	• The COPM is designed for use by adolescents and adults, but has also been used with children.
Test Format	• The COPM uses a semi-structured interview format.
Procedures	• Practitioners interview clients to help them identify meaningful problematic activities. For each problematic activity, clients are asked to rate (1) importance of the activity [I], (2) ability to perform the activity [P], and (3) satisfaction with the way the activity is performed [S]. Each scale ranges from 1 to 10, with 1 = not important at all [I], not able to do it [P], not satisfied at all [S], and with 10 = extremely important [I], able to do it extremely well [P], extremely satisfied [S]. P and S scores are then multiplied by the I score prior to making any intervention decisions with the client.
Time Required	• Administration time for the COPM depends on the number of problems identified by the client as well as the ability of the client to reflect on each scale (I, P, S).
Standardization	• The COPM uses a standardized semi-structured interview format with standardized materials.
Reliability	
Test-Retest	• Test-retest reliability has been reported as r = 0.89 for P and 0.88 for S, and ICCs of 0.81 for P and 0.76 for S. The responsiveness of the COPM has also been reported for performance and satisfaction scales, using Receiver Operating Curves. The area under the curve was reported as 0.85 for both.
Internal Consistency	• Not applicable because each client identifies unique problems
Inter-Rater	• Not applicable because each client identifies unique problems
Validity	
Content	• Content validity was based on a review of 136 instruments, of which 39 were used as models.
Construct	• Multiple studies comparing the COPM with measures of gross and fine motor ability and function have indicated construct validity. The constructs of performance and satisfaction have also been validated in multiple studies.
Criterion	• The COPM has been positively associated with multiple valid assessments, including the Oswestry Disability Scale, the Health Assessment Questionnaire, and the DASH-DLV.
Utility	
Research Programs	• The COPM has been used in multiple studies as a primary and secondary assessment and as a primary and secondary outcome measure. It has also been used as the gold standard against which other assessments are compared. Over 100 research papers have been published that focus on the COPM, or include the COPM in the design of the study. Because of its client-centered approach, it is an excellent tool for clinical research.
Practice Settings	• Practice settings: The COPM has been used in hospitals, clinics, outpatient and community programs, and schools, as well as with traditional and emerging practice areas.
Strengths	• The COPM is unique in its client-centeredness. It is also unique in its 3 scales (I, P, S). As such, it engages clients immediately and research has established its validity and reliability with multiple populations being assessed in multiple settings.

Table 14-7

Direct Assessment of Functional Status—Revised (DAFS-R)

Source	Graham J. McDougall, PhD, RN, FAAN, The University of Texas at Austin, School of Nursing, 1700 Red River St, Austin, TX 78701. E-mail: gmcdougall@mail.nur.utexas.edu
Key References	Lowenstein, et al[22]; McDougall et al[64]; Pereira et al[65]
Purpose	• The DAFS-R is designed to be a measure of high-level cognitive IADLs and is designed to be administered to older adults in a clinic.
Type of Client	• The DAFS-R is designed for use with older adults.
Test Format	• The DAFS-R is a performance-based measure
Procedures	• Practitioners present clients with 9 IADL subscales (phone, letter, money handling, balancing a checkbook, shopping recall, shopping recognition, identifying medication, pillbox, and refill) and items in each scale receive 1 point for a correct response. The best score on the DAFS-R is the maximum score of 55 points.
Time Required	• Administration time for the DAFS-R has been reported as 25 to 40 minutes depending on the client's ability. Scoring and reporting time were not reported.
Standardization	• The administration and materials used with the DAFS-R are standardized.
Reliability	
Test-Retest	• Depending on the scale, test-retest reliability ranged from 0.50 to 0.92 (kappas) for cognitively impaired subjects and 0.78 to 1.00 for nonimpaired subjects.
Internal Consistency	• Cronbach's α for each of the subscales ranged from 0.67 to 0.68.
Inter-Rater	• Inter-rater reliabilities ranged from 0.91 to 1.00 (kappas) for cognitively impaired subjects and stable at 1.00 for nonimpaired subjects.
Validity	
Content	• The content validity is based on the original DAFS. However, because of ceiling effects on the original DAFS, the DAFS-R deleted easy items and added 3 medication management tasks. The choice of medication tasks was based on a literature review of medication management problems experienced by older adults.
Construct	• The DAFS-R was able to differentiate between older adults with no cognitive impairment, those with mild cognitive impairment, and those with mild dementia. Convergent validity was established with the Blessed Dementia Rating Scale (BDRS), and the mini-BDRS, which is a proxy report.
Criterion	• The ability of the DAFS-R to differentiate cognitive levels was based on comparison with Rivermead scores and correlations with MMSE scores.
Utility	
Research Programs	• The DAFS-R has been translated and adapted with culturally relevant examples to yield the DAFS-BR (Brazilian Revised). The DAFS-BR was also shown to distinguish between clients with different levels of cognitive impairment.
Practice Settings	• The DAFS has been consistently used in geriatric clinics.
Strengths	• The DAFS-R assesses the more complex and cognitively challenging IADL for older adults, with tasks that are realistic.

Table 14-8

Everyday Problems Test (EPT)

Source	https://sharepoint.washington.edu/uwsom/sls/researchers/Pages/EptTests.aspx
Key References	Jobe et al[66]; Gross et al[67]; Rebok et al[68]
Purpose	• The purpose of the EPT is to assess memory and reasoning skills associated with daily living tasks in 7 categories: health (medications), meal preparation/nutrition, phone usage, consumer (shopping), financial management, household management, and transportation.
Type of Client	• The EPT is designed for use with adults.
Test Format	• The EPT comes in 2 forms: multiple choice and open-ended, which requires 2- to 3-word responses. The EPT has 2 test versions: 84-item and 42-item for flexibility in the comprehensiveness of the assessment. The EPT can be administered on an individual basis or in small- to moderate-sized groups with a proctor.
Procedures	• The practitioner presents the client with stimuli (eg, a recipe, a nutrition information chart, directions for use of cough syrup, Medicare benefits payment schedule) and the client is asked questions that require interpretation of the stimuli information. Each correct item receives 1 point, and higher scores indicate better performance.
Time Required	• The EPT is untimed. Scoring is done by hand, and inter-rater reliability should be established for the open-ended format. Scoring is done by summing the correct answers within each category/scale. Reporting consists of comparing the EPT results to the norms, which are categorized by age, gender, and education. T-scores are computed for comparison purposes.
Standardization	• The EPT administration procedures and scoring are standardized.
Reliability	
Test-Retest	• Test-retest coefficients for the open-ended formats were $r=0.95$ for the 84-item format and $r=0.93$ for the 42-item format. For the multiple choice format, coefficients were $r=0.91$ for the 84-item format and $r=0.83$ for the 42-item format.
Internal Consistency	• Internal consistency: Cronbach's α for the 84-item open-ended format were 0.94; 0.89 for the 42-item open-ended format; 0.93 for the 84-item multiple choice format; and 0.89 for the 42-item multiple choice format
Inter-Rater	• Not reported
Validity	
Content	• Content validity was based on expanding 7/8 categories of the Lawton and Brody[4] IADL scale (laundry not included).
Construct	• Convergent validity was established by comparing responses of subjects with fewer IADL limitations and those with more IADL limitations based on Lawton and Brody's scale. Those with fewer limitations had significantly higher EPT scores [$F(1,371)=5.37$, $p<.05$], and those with more IADL limitations had significantly lower EPT scores.
Criterion	• Older adults were observed performing 21 everyday tasks in their homes that were represented on the EPT. Correlation between the EPT total and the total score for the in-home assessment was 0.67, indicating that the EPT was assessing the same constructs.
Utility	
Research Programs	• The EPT has been used as a primary and secondary outcome measure in multiple cognitive training research studies (eg, ACTIVE Cognitive Intervention Trial). It is a functional memory and reasoning measure that reflects everyday items that need interpretation, and can be added to occupational therapy research studies examining interventions focused on cognition.

(continued)

Table 14-8 (continued)

Everyday Problems Test (EPT)

Utility	
Practice Settings	• The EPT is a relevant clinical tool because its stimuli reflect everyday materials that require interpretation, and it can provide data about how a client compares with age, gender, and education cohorts.
Strengths	• The EPT is an engaging memory and reasoning assessment that will resonate with clients because it uses stimuli that they encounter every day.

Table 14-9

Executive Function Performance Test (EFPT)

Source	Baum et al[69]
Key References	Hahn et al[70]
Purpose	• The purpose of the EFPT is to document the level of support needed by clients with cognitive impairments to complete a task (originally a cooking task).
Type of Client	• The EFPT is designed for use with clients with cognitive impairments.
Test Format	• Performance-based assessment for the clinic
Procedures	• The EFPT requires clients to complete 4 everyday tasks: cooking (making oatmeal), using the telephone, managing medications, and paying a bill. The practitioner observes task performance, provides support as necessary, and rates the client on the following categories: initiation, organization, performance of all steps, sequencing, judgment and safety, and completion. Scoring reflects the level of support provided by the practitioner for each category and ranges from 0 (independently competent) to 3 (totally incapable). The lower the score, the better the performance. An alternate version of the EFPT (aEFPT) added alternate cooking, telephone use, medication management, and money management items.
Time Required	• Time for administration was 35 minutes for the EFPT with post-stroke clients and 47 minutes for the aEFPT.
Standardization	• The EFPT and the aEFPT use standardized setups and scoring.
Reliability	
Test-Retest	• ICC = 0.94 for the total score of the EFPT.
Internal Consistency	• Cronbach's α among stroke survivors for the EFPT was α = 0.94. Alphas for the subtests were cooking = 0.86, paying bills = 0.78, managing medications = 0.88, and using the telephone = 0.77.
Inter-Rater	• Inter-rater reliability (ICCs) ranged from 0.79 to 0.94 for the EFPT.
Validity	
Content	• The content validity is based on everyday tasks that require initiation, organization, inclusion of all steps, sequencing, judgment, and safety.
Construct	• Construct validity of the EFPT was established by comparing 3 groups (controls, mild stroke, moderate stroke). The EFPT successfully discriminated among the groups in the hierarchy expected: controls performed significantly better than those with mild stroke, who performed better than those with moderate stroke. The same occurred for the rating categories, except for initiation.

(continued)

Table 14-9 (continued)

Executive Function Performance Test (EFPT)

Validity	
Criterion	• Concurrent criterion validity of the EFPT was examined by correlating the EFPT scores of the stroke survivors with several cognitive measures, with correlations ranging from r=0.39 to −0.59. Similarly, for the aEFPT, correlations ranged from rs=0.53 to 0.69.
Utility	
Research Programs	• The EFPT has been used in research studies involving clients with stroke, multiple sclerosis, and schizophrenia.
Practice Settings	• The EFPT was designed for use in a clinic setting.
Strengths	• The EFPT and aEFPT provide impairment-oriented outcome data gathered from observations of clients performing everyday tasks. As such, practitioners can use the category scores (eg, initiation, sequencing) to generalize potential limitations in other cognitively oriented tasks that may also require support, and include them in the assessment plan.

Table 14-10

Fitness to Drive Screening Measure (FTDS; AKA, the Safe Driving Behavior Measure)

Source	http://www.fitnesstodrivescreening.com/
Key References	Classen et al[33]; Winter et al[71]; Classen et al[72]; Classen et al[73]; Classen et al[50]; Classen et al[74]; Classen et al[75]
Purpose	• The FTDS is a screening assessment to be completed by family members and/or caregivers to assist in the identification of potentially at-risk older drivers.
Type of Client	• The FTDS is a proxy-report assessment (family members or caregivers)
Test Format	• The FTDS is an online screening assessment.
Procedures	• Once the proxy is online, the FTDS requires completion of 3 sections: 1) demographics of the proxy rater and demographics of the driver; 2) driving history profile (eg, driving frequency); and 3) rating of driving skills. A video explains the content of the FTDS and what the results will include. There is also a short "training" video to clarify terms that will be used in the driving skills portion of the assessment. Driving skills are rated using an ordinal scale consisting of Very Difficult, Somewhat Difficult, A Little Difficult, and Not Difficult. Item response theory is used to generate the scores and categorized the driver into 1 of 3 categories: 1) accomplished driver, 2) routine driver, or 3) at-risk driver. A keyform with the driver's score and skill levels for each item is then presented, with recommendations for the driver to consider.
Time Required	• The FTDS takes approximately 25 minutes to complete.
Standardization	• The FTDS uses standardized procedures.

(continued)

Table 14-10 (continued)

FITNESS TO DRIVE SCREENING MEASURE (FTDS; AKA, THE SAFE DRIVING BEHAVIOR MEASURE)	
Reliability	
Test-Retest	• Not reported
Internal Consistency	• Rasch person reliability (>0.92) and item reliability (>0.93) was found for caregivers, occupational therapists, and certified driver rehabilitation specialists (CDRS). A Cronbach's α of >0.96 was achieved.
Inter-Rater	• Drivers, family members, and CDRS practitioners achieved weak but significant ICCs (0.253, $p < .001$). However, the ICCs between the family members and the older drivers was only 0.141 ($p = .023$), and between family members and CDRS evaluators was stronger and significant (0.394, $p < .001$), which is most likely why the current version of the FTDS uses proxy reports only. MFR analyses indicated that the CDRS practitioners were the most rigorous evaluators, followed by family members.
Validity	
Content	• Content validity was established for the original measure using the literature, 3 theoretical models of driving safety, and a review of existing measures. The refined version of the measure was based on input from caregivers, occupational therapists, and CDRS.
Construct	• The FTDS showed good person separation (>3.49) and item separation (>3.60), indicating that the assessment distinguishes between drivers of different skill levels (person separation), and items of differing difficulty levels.
Criterion	• Concurrent criterion-related validity was established by comparing FTDS levels against an on-road assessment (pass/fail). Using receiver operating curve analyses, the area under the curve (AUC) for drivers was 0.62, but for family members, the AUC was 0.73, again confirming that proxy reports of older driver skills are more valid.
Utility	
Research Programs	• Research programs: The FTDS has been examined and included in multiple research studies and is supported by the American Automobile Association and the American Association of Retired Persons. Driving is an important IADL that needs to be included in comprehensive IADL assessments.
Practice Settings	• Practice settings: the FTDS can be used in any setting that has access to a computer, the Internet, and a printer. Because of the 2 videos included in the assessment, it may be important to have a headset available or a private room in which to complete the FTDS.
Strengths	• The FTDS is a valid and reliable measure of potential at-risk driving behaviors. It is a free online program that engages the users immediately with the introductory video. Moreover, upon completion of the FTDS, the software program generates a key form of the items, areas of risk, and recommendations that can be printed out immediately.

Table 14-11

Kohlman Evaluation of Living Skills (KELS)

Source	American Occupational Therapy Association www.aota.org
Key References	Thomson[76]; Burnett et al[77]
Purpose	• The purpose of the KELS is to assess IADL skills required for community living.
Type of Client	• The KELS is designed for use with adults.
Test Format	• Combination of interview and performance-based assessment.
Procedures	• The client is presented with questions and tasks about self-care, safety, health, money management, community mobility, telephone use, employment, and leisure participation, and the newest version (under construction) includes an electronic banking item. Scoring for each item is a 0 for independent and a 1 for needs assistance.
Time Required	• Administration takes approximately 30 to 45 minutes, depending on the client's ability.
Standardization	• The KELS procedures and materials are standardized.
Reliability	
Test-Retest	• Not reported
Internal Consistency	• Not reported
Inter-Rater	• Percent agreement among raters ranged from 74% to 94%.
Validity	
Content	• Content validity is based on the literature and ADL/IADL necessary for community living.
Construct	• Studies have shown that the KELS was able to distinguish between older adults with and without self-neglect who were living in the community, as well as those who lived independently in the community vs in sheltered living environments.
Criterion	• Scores on the KELS were positively correlated with scores on the Bay Area Functional Performance Evaluation (r=0.84), and with the Global Assessment Scale (r=0.78 to 0.89).
Utility	
Research Programs	• The KELS is currently being revised, and research is being conducted at 40 clinical sites to update its psychometric properties.
Practice Settings	• The KELS is currently being used in hospitals, nursing homes, outpatient programs, and community-based settings.
Strengths	• The KELS provides practitioners with practical information about a client's IADL skills that are necessary for community living.

Table 14-12

Performance Assessment of Self-Care Skills (PASS)

Source	PASS@shrs.pitt.edu to request copies
Key References	Rogers et al[8,49]; Chisholm[78]; Holm and Rogers[79]; Reynolds et al[80]; Foster[39]; Rodakowski et al[42]
Purpose	• The purpose of the PASS is to measure current status in any of 5 functional mobility (FM), 3 BADL, and 18 IADL (14 with a cognitive orientation, 4 with a physical orientation). The responsiveness of the PASS enables it to be used to assess short- and long-term changes in functional status. There is also an item development template that practitioners can use to develop and test new items.

(continued)

Table 14-12 (continued)

Performance Assessment of Self-Care Skills (PASS)

Type of Client	• The PASS is designed to be used with adolescents and adults.
Test Format	• The PASS has 2 versions: performance-based in the clinic, and performance-based in the home.
Procedures	• For the clinic and home versions, practitioners ask clients to demonstrate how they perform from 1 to 26 of the core items (each item stands alone), and rate the client on each task and subtask for independence, safety, and adequacy of performance. Ratings for each construct range from 0 (unable, unsafe, inadequate) to 3 (independent, safe, adequate). Independence is the mean of all subtasks for an item, and safety and adequacy are scored for the total item. The higher the score, the greater the independence, safety, and adequacy for a task.
Time Required	• Depending on the number of items administered for the performance-based versions, administration, scoring, and reporting can take from 20 minutes (3 to 4 items) to 2 hours (26 items).
Standardization	• Administration is standardized. For both performance-based versions, the assessment conditions, practitioner directions, and hierarchy of assists are standardized, as well as the scoring protocol.
Reliability	
Test-Retest	• PASS Clinic test-retest reliability was r=0.92 for Independence; 0.89 percent agreement for Safety, and r=0.82 for Adequacy. PASS Home test-retest reliability was r=0.96 for Independence; 0.90 percent agreement for Safety, and r=0.97 for Adequacy. The responsiveness of the PASS has been demonstrated for both short-term changes in stroke survivors ($p<.01$) for independence and adequacy, and for long-term changes in older adults ($p<001$) for independence and adequacy. Safety remained the same (high) for both times.
Internal Consistency	• Cronbach's α was 0.82 for the PASS Clinic and 0. 85 for the PASS Home.
Inter-Rater	• PASS Clinic inter-rater reliability percent agreement was 0.92 for Independence, 0.93 for Safety, and 0.90 for Adequacy. PASS Home inter-rater reliability percent agreement was 0.96 for Independence, 0.97 for Safety, and 0.88 for Adequacy
Validity	
Content	• Items from the OARS Multidimensional Functional Assessment, the Instrumental Self-Maintenance Scale, the Comprehensive Assessment and Referral Evaluation, and the Functional Assessment Questionnaire were operationalized for the performance-based PASS versions. The self-report and proxy report questionnaires are based on the performance-based PASS versions.
Construct	• Factor analysis confirmed the 3 measurement constructs: independence, safety, and adequacy. Methodological studies have also established the degree to which performance in the home (gold standard) matched self-reports, proxy reports, clinical judgments, and performance in the clinic, and the direction of bias (overestimation, underestimation). The PASS successfully distinguished between healthy subjects and diagnostic samples as well as between diagnostic samples.
Criterion	• Task analysis was used to identify critical tasks, subtasks, and usual sequence of performance.

(continued)

Table 14-12 (continued)

Performance Assessment of Self-Care Skills (PASS)

Utility	
Research Programs	• Research with the PASS has focused on methodological studies of differences in IADL performance based on method of data collection (eg, self-report vs performance), as well as a primary or secondary pre-/post-measure following medical, surgical, rehabilitation, and psychiatric interventions. The self-report and proxy report questionnaires have been used clinically and in a number of methodological studies.
Practice Settings	• The PASS performance-based measures have been used in a variety of settings, including the intensive care unit, hospitals, rehabilitation centers, outpatient clinics, homes, and long-term care facilities. The PASS focuses on FM, BADL, and IADL performance and is appropriate for healthy and diagnostic populations. One item or all 26 items can be administered depending on the needs, wants, and expectations of the client and the team.
Strengths	• Each PASS item stands alone, and practitioners can administer any number of items. There is also an item development template so practitioners can develop and text new items. Separate ratings of safety and adequacy in addition to independence are unique.

Table 14-13

Test of Grocery Shopping Skills (TOGSS)

Source	ehamera@kumc.edu
Key References	Hamera and Brown[81]; Rempfer et al[82]; Brown et al[83]
Purpose	• The purpose of the TOGSS is to assess grocery shopping skills in a community-based context.
Type of Client	• The TOGSS was initially designed for use with clients with schizophrenia.
Test Format	• The TOGSS is a performance-based assessment with 2 forms—1 for pretest and 1 for post-test.
Procedures	• The client is given a shopping list with 10 items of different sizes, brands, and costs, the locations of which are distributed throughout the store. The list is attached to a clipboard, and a pen is provided. The accuracy scores were based on: a) the total number of correct items, b) at the correct size, and c) the number of items at the lowest price. One point is given for each scale item that is correct, with a maximum score of 30. The TOGSS yields 3 scores: 1) accuracy, 2) efficiency (tracking of repeat trips down previously visited aisles and wrong aisles), and 3) time (measured from entering the store to completing checkout).
Time Required	• Once at the grocery store, time for administration ranged from 40 minutes to 105 minutes in the validity/reliability sample.
Standardization	• The TOGSS procedures and materials are standardized.
Reliability	
Test-Retest	• Alternate forms reliability between Form 1 and Form 2 for correct item was r=0.69, for correct size was r=0.83, and for lowest price was r=0.60. Overall test-retest reliability with Forms 1 and 2 was r=0.69.
Internal Consistency	• Not reported
Inter-Rater	• Inter-rater reliability was reported as r=0.99.

(continued)

Table 14-13 (continued)

Test of Grocery Shopping Skills (TOGSS)

Validity	
Content	• Content validity was established by interviewing consumers with schizophrenia about: a) where they usually shopped, b) what issues were important when deciding what to purchase, c) what foods they usually purchased, and d) the problems they encountered when grocery shopping.
Construct	• When the TOGSS was correlated with the Test of Drug Store Shopping, total accuracy scores for the 2 assessments were strongly correlated (r=0.91, Form 1; r=0.86, Form 2), suggesting that the TOGSS is an assessment of generalized shopping skills. Multiple cognitive assessments, knowledge of grocery shopping, and performance of grocery shopping (TOGSS) were examined. Results indicated that providing knowledge of grocery shopping skills can serve as a bridge between cognitive skills and performance of grocery shopping skills.
Criterion	• Six cognitive measures (Rey Auditory Verbal Learning Test, Letter Cancellation, Stroop Color-Word Task, Controlled Oral Word Association Test, the Wisconsin Card Sorting Task, Allen Cognitive Levels Test) were correlated with TOGSS. Several of the cognitive measures were significantly correlated with the TOGSS accuracy scores and efficiency scores, indicating that cognition is important for successful shopping.
Utility	
Research Programs	• The TOGSS is a unique assessment in that it is context-based in a community grocery store. The findings that knowledge was a mediator of cognition and performance has merit for planning interventions related to shopping and other IADL.
Practice Settings	• This is a community-based assessment in a grocery store.
Strengths	• The TOGSS was designed based on patient input and is an ecologically valid tool. However, not all settings will take the risk of having practitioners assess clients in the community, which may limit the utility of the TOGSS.

References

1. Rosen SL, Reuben DB. Geriatric assessment tools. *Mt Sinai J Med.* 2011;78:489-497.
2. Uniform Data System for Medical Rehabilitation (UDSMR). *Functional Independence Measure Training Manual.* Buffalo, NY: UDSMR; 1997.
3. Uniform Data System for Medical Rehabilitation (UDSMR). *Inpatient Rehabilitation Facility Patient Assessment Instrument (IRF-PAI) Training Manual.* Buffalo, NY: UDSMR; 2001.
4. Lawton MP, Brody EM. Assessment of older people: self-maintaining and instrumental activities of daily living. *Gerontologist.* 1969;9(3):179-186.
5. Fleishman EA. Human abilities and the acquisition of skill. In: Bilodeau EA, ed. *Acquisition of Skill.* New York: Academic Press; 1966:147-167.
6. Kielhofner G, Burke JP. Components and determinants of human occupation. In: Kielhofner G, ed. *A Model of Human Occupation.* Baltimore: Williams & Wilkins; 1984:12-36.
7. Rubenstein LZ, Schairer C, Wieland GD, Kane R. Systematic biases in functional status assessment of elderly adults: effects of different data sources. *J Gerontol.* 1984;39:686-691.
8. Rogers JC, Holm MB, Beach S, et al. Concordance of four methods of disability assessment using performance in the home as the criterion method. *Arthritis Rheum.* 2003;49:640-647.
9. Sarsak H. *Functional Assessment of Wheeled Mobility and Seating Interventions: Relationship of Self-Report and Performance-Based Assessments.* [dissertation]. Pittsburgh: University of Pittsburgh; 2014.
10. Schein R, Schmeler M, Holm MB, Saptano A, Brienza, D. Telerehabilitation wheeled mobility and seating assessments compared with in person. *Arch Phys Med Rehabil.* 2010;91:874-878.
11. Schein R, Schmeler M, Holm MB, Saptano A, Brienza D. Telerehabilitation assessment using the Functioning Everyday with a Wheelchair-Capacity instrument. *J Rehabil Res Dev.* 2011;48(2):115–124.
12. Chumbler NR, Quigley P, Li X, et al. Effects of telerehabilitation on physical function and disability for stroke patients: a randomized, controlled trial. *Stroke.* 2012;43:2168-2174.
13. Hoenig H, Sanford JA, Butterfield T, Griffiths PC, Richardson P, Hargraves, K. Development of a teletechnology protocol for in-home rehabilitation. *J Rehabil Res Dev.* 2006;43:287-298.

14. Fieo RA, Austin EJ, Starr JM, Deary IJ. Calibrating ADL-IADL scales to improve measurement accuracy and to extend the disability construct into the preclinical range: a systematic review. *BMC Geriatrics.* 2011;11:42.
15. Moore DJ, Palmer BW, Patterson TL, Jeste DV. A review of performance-based measures of functional living skills. *J Psych Research.* 2007;41:97-118.
16. Bond TG, Fox CM. *Applying the Rasch Model: Fundamental Measurement in the Human Sciences.* 2nd ed. Mahwah, NJ: Lawrence Erlbaum; 2007.
17. Portney LB, Watkins MP. *Foundations of Clinical Research: Applications to Practice.* 3rd ed. Upper Saddle River, NJ: Pearson Prentice Hall; 2009.
18. Reynolds CF III. Assessing the capacity to make everyday decisions about functional problems: where does the field go from here? *Am J Geriatric Psych.* 2007;15(2):89-91.
19. McGourty LK. *The Kohlman Evaluation of Living Skills.* Bethesda, MD: AOTA; 1979.
20. Pfeffer RI, Kurosaki TT, Harrah CH Jr, Chance JM, Filos S. Measurement of functional activities in older adults in the community. *J Gerontol.* 1982;37:323-329.
21. Fisher AG. *Assessment of Motor and Process Skills, Volume 1: Development, Standardization and Administration Manual; Volume 2: User Manual.* Fort Collins, CO: Three Star Press; 1989.
22. Lowenstein DA, Amigo E, Duara R, et al. A new scale for the assessment of functional status in Alzheimer's disease and related disorders. *J Gerontol Psychol Sci.* 1989;44(4):114-121.
23. Rogers JC, Holm MB. *Performance Assessment of Self-Care Skills.* Pittsburgh, PA: University of Pittsburgh; 1989.
24. Law M, Baptiste S, Carswell-Opzoomer A, McColl MA, Polatajko H, Pollock N. *Canadian Occupational Performance Measure.* Toronto: CAOT Publications ACE; 1991.
25. Willis SL. Manual for the Everyday Problems Test. Seattle, WA: University of Washington; 1993. https://sharepoint.washington.edu/uwsom/sls/researchers/Pages/EptTests.aspx. Accessed October 3, 2016.
26. Spector WD, Fleishman JA. Combining activities of daily living with instrumental activities of daily living to measure functional disability. *J Gerontol B Psychol Sci Soc Sci.* 1998;53:46-57.
27. McHorney CA, Cohen AS. Equating health status measures with item response theory: illustrations with functional status items. *Med Care.* 2000;38:43-59.
28. Sheehan TJ, DeChello LM, Garcia R, Fifield J, Rothfield N, Reisine S. Measuring disability: application of the Rasch model to activities of daily living (ADL/IADL). *J Outcome Meas.* 2002;5:839-863.
29. Jette AM, Haley SM, Coster WJ, et al. Late life function and disability instrument: I. Development and evaluation of the disability component. *J Gerontol A Biol Sci Med Sci.* 2002;57:209-216.
30. Haley SM, Jette AM, Coster WJ, et al. Late life function and disability instrument: II. Development and evaluation of the function component. *J Gerontol A Biol Sci Med Sci.* 2002;57:217-222.
31. Farias, S. T., Mungas, D., Reed, B. B., Harvey, D., Cahn-Weiner, D., & DeCarli, C. (2006). MCI is associated with deficits in everyday functioning. *Alzheimer Dis Assoc Disord.* 2006;20:217-223.
32. Jette AM, Haley SM, Coster WJ, Ni P. Activity Measure for Post-Acute Care (AM-PAC). Boston, MA: Boston Rehabilitation Outcomes Measurement; 2007. http://www.bu.edu/bostonroc/instruments/am-pac/. Accessed October 3, 2016.
33. Classen S, Winter SM, Velozo C, et al. Item development and validity testing for a Safe Driving Behavior Measure. *Am J Occup Ther.* 2010;64:296-305.
34. Liu SY, Chavan NR, Glymour MM. Type of high-school credentials and older age ADL and IADL limitations: is the GED credential equivalent to a diploma? *Gerontologist.* 2012;53:326-333.
35. Verbrugge LM, Liu X. Midlife trends in activities and disability. *J Aging Health.* 2014;26:178-206.
36. Freedman VA, Kasper JD, Spillman BC, Agree EM, Mor V, Wallace RB. Behavioral adaptation and late-life disability: a new spectrum for assessing public health impacts. *Am J Public Health.* 2014;104:e88-e94.
37. Verbrugge LM, Sevak P. Disability symptoms and the price of self-sufficiency. *J Aging Health.* 2004;16:688-722.
38. Cioncoloni D, Martini G, Piu P, et al. Predictors of long-term recovery in complex activities of daily living before discharge from the stroke unit. *NeuroRehabil.* 2013;33:217-223.
39. Foster ER. Instrumental activities of daily living performance among people with Parkinson's disease without dementia. *Am J Occup Ther.* 2014;68:353-362.
40. Burton CL, Strauss E, Bunce D, Hunter MA, Hultsch DF. Functional abilities in older adults with mild cognitive impairment. *Gerontology.* 2009;55:570-581.
41. Teng E, Becker BW, Woo E, Cummings JL, Lu PH. Subtle deficits in instrumental activities of daily living in subtypes of mild cognitive impairment. *Dement Geriatr Cogn Dis.* 2010;30:189-197.
42. Rodakowski J, Skidmore ER, Reynolds CF III, et al. Can performance on daily activities discriminate between older adults with normal cognitive function and those with mild cognitive impairment? *J Am Geriatr Soc.* 2014;62:1347-1352.
43. Leibold ML, Holm MB, Raina KD, Reynolds CF, Rogers JC. Activities and adaptation in late life depression: a qualitative study. *Am J Occup Ther.* 2014;68:570-577.
44. Locke E, Thielke S, Diehr P, et al. Effects of respiratory and non-respiratory factors on disability among older adults with airway obstruction: the cardiovascular health study. *COPD.* 2013;10:588-596.
45. Hochberg C, Maul E, Chan ES, et al. Association of vision loss in glaucoma and age-related macular degeneration with IADL disability. *Invest Ophthalmol Vis Sci.* 2012;53:3201-3206.
46. Grossberg G, Cummings J, Frölich LI, et al. Efficacy of higher dose 13.3 mg/24 h Rivastigmine patch on instrumental activities of daily living in patients with mild-to-moderate Alzheimer's disease. *Am J Alzheimers Dis Other Demen.* 2013;28:583-591.
47. Park S, Fisher AG, Velozo CA. Using the Assessment of Motor and Process Skills to compare occupational performance between clinic and home settings. *Am J Occup Ther.* 1993;48:697-709.
48. Rogers JC, Holm MB. Daily-living skills and habits of older women with depression. *Occup Ther J Res.* 2000;20:68S-85S.

49. Rogers JC, Holm MB, Raina KD, et al. Disability in late-life major depression: Patterns of self-reported task abilities, task habits, and observed task performance. *Psychiatry Res.* 2010;178:475-479.
50. Classen S, Wang Y, Winter SM, Velozo CA, Lanford DN, Bédard M. Concurrent criterion validity of the Safe Driving Behavior Measure: a predictor of on-road driving outcomes. *Am J Occup Ther.* 2013;67:108-116.
51. Haley SM, Coster WJ, Andres PL, Kosinski M, Ni P. Score comparability of short forms and computerized adaptive testing: simulation study with the Activite Measure for Post-Acute Care. *Arch Phys Med Rehabil.* 2004;85:661-666.
52. Haley SM, Andres PL, Coster WJ, Kosinski M, Ni P, Jette AM. Short-form Activity Measure for Post-Acute Care. *Arch Phys Med Rehabil.* 2004;85:649-660.
53. Haley SM, Siebens HI Coster WJ, et al. Computerized adaptive testing for follow-up after discharge from inpatient rehabilitation: I. Activity outcomes. *Arch Phys Med Rehabil.* 2006;87:1033-1042.
54. Jette AM, Ni P, Rasch EK, et al. Evaluation of patient and proxy responses on the Activity Measure for Postacute Care. *Stroke.* 2011;43:824-829.
55. Cheville AL, Yost KJ, Larson DR, et al. Performance of an item response theory-based computer adaptive test in identifying functional decline. *Arch Phys Med Rehabil.* 2012;93:1153-1160.
56. World Health Organization. *International Classification of Functioning, Disability and Health (ICF).* Geneva, Switzerland: Author; 2001.
57. Fisher AG. The assessment of IADL motor skills: An application of many-faceted Rasch analysis. *Am J Occup Ther.* 1993;47:319-329.
58. Doble SE. Test-retest reliability of the Assessment of Motor and Process Skills in elderly adults. *Occup Ther J Res.* 1999;3:203-215.
59. Bray K, Fisher AG, Duran L. The validity of adding new tasks to the Assessment of Motor and Process Skills. *Am J Occup Ther.* 2001;55:409-415.
60. Merritt BK. Validity of using the Assessment of Motor and Process Skills to determine the need for assistance. *Am J Occup Ther.* 2011;65:643-650.
61. Carswell A, McColl MA, Baptiste S, Law M, Polatajko H, Pollock N. The Canadian Occupational Performance Measure: a research and clinical literature review. *Can J Occup Ther.* 2004;71:210-222.
62. Eyssen I, Steultjens M, Oud T, Bolt E, Maasdam A, Dekker J. Responsiveness of the Canadian Occupational Performance Measure. *J Rehabil Res Devel.* 2011;48:517-528.
63. Colquhoun HL, Lette LJ, Law MC, MacDermid JC, Missuna CA. Administration of the Canadian Occupational Performance Measure: effect on practice. *Can J Occup Ther.* 2012;79:120-128.
64. McDougall GJ, Becker H, Vaughan PW, Acee TW, Delville CL. The revised Direct Assessment of Functional Status for independent older adults. *Gerontologist.* 2010;50:363-370.
65. Pereira FS, Oliveira AM, Diniz BS, Forlenza OV, Yassuda MS. Cross-cultural adaption, reliability and validity of the DAFS-R in a sample of Brazilian older adults. *Arch Clin Neuropsychol.* 2010;25:335-343.
66. Jobe JB, Smith DM, Ball K, et al. ACTIVE: a cognitive intervention trial to promote independence in older adults. *Controlled Clin Trials.* 2001;22:453-479.
67. Gross AL, Rebok GW, Unverzagt FW, Willis SL, Brandt J. Cognitive predictors of everyday functioning in older adults: results from the ACTIVE cognitive intervention trial. *J Gerontol B Psychol Sci Soc Sci.* 2011;66:557-566.
68. Rebok GW, Ball K, Guey LT, et al. Ten-year effects of the advanced cognitive training for independent and vital elderly cognitive training trial on cognition and everyday functioning in older adults. *J Am Geriatr Soc.* 2014;62:16-24.
69. Baum C, Tabor Connor L, et al. Reliability, validity, and clinical utility of the Executive Function Performance Test: a measure of executive function in a sample of people with stroke. *Am J Occup Ther.* 2008;62:446-455
70. Hahn B, Baum C, Moore J, et al. Development of additional tasks for the Executive Function Performance Test. *Am J Occup Ther.* 2014;68:e242-e246.
71. Winter SM, Classen S, Bédard M, et al. Focus group findings for a self-report Safe Driving Behavior Measure. *Can J Occup Ther.* 2011;78:72-79.
72. Classen S, Wen P, Velozo C, et al. Psychometrics of the Self-Report Safe Driving Behavior Measure for older adults. *Am J Occup Ther.* 2012;66:233-241.
73. Classen S, Wen P, Velozo C, et al. Rater reliability and rater effects of the Safe Driving Behavior Measure. *Am J Occup Ther.* 2012;16:69-77.
74. Classen S, Winter SM, Velozo CA, Hannold L. Stakeholder recommendations to refine the Fitness-to-Drive Screening Measure. *Open J Occup Ther.* 2013;1(4):Article 3. http://scholarworks.wmich.edu/ojot/vol1/iss4/3. Accessed October 3, 2016.
75. Classen S, Velozo C, Winter SM, Wang Y, Bedard M. Psychometrics of the Fitness-to-Drive Screening Measure. *Occup Ther J Res.* 2015;35(1):42-52.
76. Thomson LK. *The Kohlman Evaluation of Living Skills.* 3rd ed. Bethesda, MD: AOTA; 1979/1993.
77. Burnett J, Dyer CB, Naik AD. Convergent validation of the Kohlman Evaluation of Living Skills as a screening tool of older adults' ability to live safely and independently in the community. *Arch Phys Med Rehabil.* 2009;90:1948-1952.
78. Chisholm D. *Disability in Older Adults with Depression.* [dissertation]. Pittsburgh, PA: University of Pittsburgh; 2005.
79. Holm MB, Rogers JC. Performance assessment of self-care skills. In Hemphill- Pearson BJ, ed. *Assessments in Occupational Therapy Mental Health: An Integrative Approach.* 2nd ed. Thorofare, NJ: SLACK Incorporated; 2008:101-110.
80. Reynolds CF III, Butters MA, Lopez O, et al. Maintenance treatment of depression in old age: a randomized, double-blind, placebo-controlled evaluation of the efficacy and safety of Donepezil combined with antidepressant pharmacotherapy. *Arch Gen Psychiatr.* 2011;68:51-60.
81. Hamera E, Brown CE. Developing a context-based performance measure for persons with schizophrenia: the Test of Grocery Shopping Skills. *Am J Occup Ther.* 2000;54:20-25.
82. Rempfer MV, Hamera ED, Brown CE, Cromwell RL. The relations between cognition and the independent living skill of shopping in people with schizophrenia. *Psychiatr Res.* 2003;117:103-112.
83. Brown CE, Rempfer MV, Hamera E, Bothwell R. Knowledge of grocery shopping skills as a mediator of cognition and performance. *Psychiatr Serv.* 2006;57:573-575.

Mine the Gold

A long-standing assumption in occupational therapy literature is that occupational balance, or an appropriate mix of occupations, promotes health. What that mix looks like is subjectively defined and shaped by the individual's values, goals, personal perspective on time, and sociocultural environment.[1,2] There is a temporal aspect to occupational balance, but time use alone is an overly simplistic approach that fails to capture these subjective elements. A lack of congruence between occupations and the individual's perspective on balance is referred to as *occupational imbalance*, and includes both overabundance and too little occupation.[3] Literature in psychology, social ecology, education, occupational science, and occupational therapy suggest that a state of occupational balance is beneficial to health and well-being, and correspondingly, that occupational imbalance leads to distress and illness.[2,4-7]

Become Systematic

Sometimes clients may feel unable to effectively manage their occupational roles or occupations associated with those roles, as if their lives are "out of control." By creating a structure for analyzing time use, we provide the opportunity to reframe this thinking and take action to regain a sense of efficacy over daily routines and performance of occupations. Exploring individual perceptions regarding the meaning attributed to roles and occupations helps clients make informed choices to achieve or maintain a more satisfying sense of balance. Increasingly, tools developed for and by occupational therapists are available to measure occupational balance. A systematic approach to measuring occupational balance is one that is theoretically informed and empirically based, yet flexible, because time use as a concept is subjectively determined by each person.

Use Evidence in Practice

Evidence is equivocal regarding occupational balance as a single bidirectional construct (a continuum with balance and imbalance as polar opposites) vs 2 distinct dimensions that occur independently and should be measured separately (level of balance and imbalance on separate scales).[8,9] The latter approach asks individuals to consider 2 aspects: the extent to which they experience balance (a positive, harmonious state where occupations are congruent with values or compatible/facilitatory) and their experience of imbalance (a negative state where occupations are incongruent with values or compete/interfere with one another). Another approach to measurement is the discrepancy approach, which examines the difference between actual time use and desired time use.[10] As measurement approaches are tested, theories about occupational balance are refined.

Make Occupational Therapy Contributions Explicit

In this *Third Edition*, we emphasize occupational balance measures designed or under development by occupational therapists because they focus on goal-directed activities in the context of people's daily lives. This occupation focus helps make the occupational therapy contribution to health explicit. Additional tools exist in other disciplines to capture elements of time use and occupational balance or occupational patterns (eg, role conflict/overload, role theory in the psychological literature), but the unique focus or philosophy of occupational therapy may be lacking. Most of the measures selected attend to construct and criterion validity against the assumption that a satisfying balance or variety of occupations is predictive of well-being. As the measures are used more widely, this assumption can be empirically tested.

Engage in Occupation-Based, Client-Centered Practice

As a construct, occupational balance is wholly client-centered and dependent on the activities, occupations, roles, goals, and aspirations of the individual. However, these self-report measures often require a level of cognition, health literacy, and introspection that may not be present in all clients, and in general, occupational balance has been defined in ways relevant to wealthy, Western cultures. Little is known about occupational balance across cultures or in populations fighting for survival (eg, as a result of poverty or political conflict). Although these tools may not be practical with some client groups, a strong understanding of occupational balance may inform skilled observation and interviews with clients to "get at" occupational performance issues related to balance and time use. This focus may empower clients to make changes that support their recovery, rehabilitation, or life goals.

CHAPTER 15

Measuring Time Use and Occupational Balance

Catherine Backman, PhD, OT(C), FCAOT and Mary Forhan, PhD, OT(C)

Overview

Key Concepts

Measuring occupational balance is an interesting and thought-provoking endeavor. Scholars in fields such as social ecology, sociology, education, vocational counseling, and psychology have examined time use and the meaning attributed to many aspects of everyday activity.[4,11-14] People strive toward a satisfactory balance of everyday activities, but it is difficult to articulate precisely what a reasonable balance of occupations looks like. Thus, while it is possible to calculate "norms" for time use in a given population, the traditional standardized test with normative data is unlikely to be developed for the concept of occupational balance.

Underlying measurement approaches is the assumption that occupational balance is indicated by feelings of satisfaction, contentment, or pleasure (leading to health and happiness), while imbalance is characterized by feelings of distress or boredom as a result of being over- or underoccupied (leading to illness and unhappiness). Beyond noting that occupational balance is subjective, there is a lack of consensus on definitions, yet all relate it to well-being. Sheldon[10] observes the circuitousness of this theoretical discussion and proposes the possibility that occupational balance and well-being are the same construct.

A primary focus of occupational therapy interventions has been on enabling participation in meaningful occupations from the perspective of the roles individuals carry out in their day-to-day lives.[15] These roles help describe how, why, and where individuals spend their time. Descriptions of, or instructions for, measurement tools cited in this chapter may refer to roles when inviting clients to report on what they do or reflect on the pattern of activities in which they engage over time. Literature in psychology has addressed role balance, role conflict, and role overload, concepts akin to occupational balance and imbalance.

In an essay on balance in occupation, Christiansen[16] offers 3 perspectives to thinking about balance, each of which suggests different approaches to measurement. The first relates to time use or how we structure our days and weeks. Diaries are a measurement approach compatible with this perspective. The comment that "I have no time" to do obligatory or desired activities seems to be a symptom of "I lack balance" in my life. Thus, time use approaches may provide data that more precisely identify the problem and potential solutions. Recent advances on the time use perspective include discrepancy approaches: comparing the diary of actual time use with the desired allocation of time and calculating the discrepancy between the two.[10] Christiansen's second perspective considers chronobiology, or the naturally occurring rhythms of day and night, and their associated physiological responses. Although this perspective poses a theoretically interesting approach to understanding balance, no promising measurement tools were found to illustrate this perspective. The third perspective is a social ecology approach, which considers the environmental, social, and personal facilitators and restraints to engagement in various occupations and their impact on one another. Self-report questionnaires and introspective/self-reflection systems are measurement approaches that tap into this perspective, asking individuals to describe in some detail what they do, how well, and with whom, and to judge the fit with their values or preferences and the interaction of occupations or overall occupational pattern. In this chapter, we focus our reviews on measures that collect information about the spending of time, the way in which people structure their day, and also measures that are guided by a social ecological approach.

Law M, Baum C, Dunn W, eds. *Measuring Occupational Performance: Supporting Best Practice in Occupational Therapy, Third Edition (pp 333-349).*

Importance of Measurement in Time Use and Occupational Balance

Achieving or working toward a balance among work, play, rest, and other activities deemed satisfying or salient is a familiar goal for many people, regardless of ability. Individuals subjectively define occupational balance in terms of how they choose to spend time on valued, obligatory, and discretionary activities.[17] Therefore, measurement of such a construct is naturally client-centered and takes into account individual variation regarding what constitutes a "balanced" life. There are an infinite number of satisfying lifestyles, and the purpose of measuring occupational balance is to help people discover a balance that is right for them.

Philosophically, time use and occupational balance are important to measure because they reflect a fundamental value underlying the profession: occupation is a determinant of health. To support clients' occupational engagement in health-promoting ways requires understanding their pattern of occupation and perceived satisfaction with their mix of occupations, measuring what matters most to the client, whether individual or group/community. This is achieved by measuring time use and occupational balance. Occupational balance will not be important to all stages in the occupational therapy process or all settings where occupational therapists work, but given the relationship with well-being,[2] it appears that risks to overall health may, in part, stem from certain patterns of occupational engagement. The tools offered here are useful during the assessment phase of the occupational therapy process to clarify occupational performance issues requiring intervention. For example, if symptoms seem to interfere with a client's ability to satisfactorily perform needed or desired activities, the Occupational Questionnaire[18] or NIH Activity Record[19] may help to clarify the extent of the problem and suggest possible modifications to time use, such as planning ahead. Alternatively, if a client indicates dissatisfaction with his or her perceived imbalance of work and play, completing a Personal Projects Analysis[20] might yield useful information about current goal-directed activities that support the occupational therapist in coaching the client toward a more satisfying balance of activities. Subsequent administration of these measures helps document changes as a result of intervention or other factors. As research tools, all of the instruments appear to provide information regarding how individuals engage in occupation and, therefore, are likely to enhance our understanding about activity patterns associated with health and illness.

Factors to Remember

Measuring occupational balance is not as straightforward as the measurement of impairment (such as joint motion or muscle strength), nor is it observable like the discrete aspects of occupational performance (such as capacity to prepare a meal). It is not possible to place someone's daily occupations on a scale and observe whether balance has been achieved. However, it is possible to use various data collection procedures to obtain information about engagement in occupation and use this as a basis for problem identification and resolution with clients. Measurement of time use and occupational balance is compatible with a coaching approach—the assessment is integrally involved in the intervention and may not be applicable as an outcome measure in some instances. The tools reviewed in this chapter may be helpful to clients in examining how they spend time and the characteristics of the activities in which they engage, and guide changes to time use, activity choices, or activity patterns in order to achieve greater satisfaction.

Little is known about the influences of culture, economics, and literacy on occupational balance. Most of the tools presented have been developed with relatively affluent populations and influenced by Western ideologies about work and leisure. This does not mean that these measures of occupational balance will not apply to other client groups, but as with all measurement approaches, the user needs to judge the relevance of the tool selected and interpret accordingly.

Strategies for Selecting Measures of Time Use and Occupational Balance

We recommend screening to identify occupational balance as a potential issue prior to selecting a tool. This may be done in the context of an interview where the client's description suggests issues that match the purpose of a specific tool or class of tools. For example, a time use diary helps to better understand activity patterns and links between activities and illness symptoms or issues with pacing and prioritizing occupations. Another approach is to ask specific questions. Forhan and Backman[21] report on the use of 3 stand-alone items proposed by clients and scored on a 1 to 10 response scale:

1. How satisfied are you in your ability to perform your main work activity?
2. How satisfied are you with the balance of time you spend on work, self-care, leisure, and rest?
3. At the end of the day, how satisfied are you that you have accomplished what you set out to do? (1 = not at all; 10 = completely satisfied)

Although not tested as screening tools, these items have demonstrated both test-retest reliability and construct validity. Low ratings on these questions suggest the need for more descriptive tools on occupational balance.

Selecting a tool requires a match between client needs and priorities (or research purpose) and the characteristics of the tool. Some tools are more comprehensive than others; for example, the Life Balance Index[22] has items crossing more domains than the Occupational Balance Questionnaire,[23] but both take less than 20 minutes.

Others, such as Personal Projects Analysis[20] and the Intergoal Relations Questionnaire,[24] require individuals to identify and analyze their current activities and consequently take longer to administer and score. Indeed, Little refers to analysis of personal projects as representative of balancing acts.[6] These are practical considerations that need to be weighed against the quality and depth of data the occupational therapist believes necessary to support intervention planning and implementation.

Strategies for Reporting About Time Use and Occupational Balance

When reporting on time use and occupational balance of clients, it is important to document the following: the name of the tool used, the score(s) obtained (if applicable), and a brief summary interpreting the results. The interpretation should be connected to the specific occupational performance issue(s) previously documented for the client. For example, if the occupational performance issue relates to difficulties planning time for specific activities and fulfilling obligations, the Occupational Questionnaire may be applicable. State the reason for using the Occupational Questionnaire, summarize the findings on time spent on the categories of occupation, sense of competency, and occupational interests, and provide a short interpretation in support of the intervention plan.

Future Directions for Practice and Research on Time Use and Occupational Balance

The goal of supporting clients to achieve balance among work, play, self-care, and rest is as old as the profession.[25] However, it may no longer capture the way we think about occupational balance today. Contemporary approaches to balance consider patterns of occupation and interactions across occupations, but not only in the "big 4" categories of work, play, self-care, and rest. Instead, occupations are classified in ways compatible with personal philosophies, and the congruence between occupations and values or interests influence choices, decisions, and perceived satisfaction. As we move through life stages, our perception of what is important, meaningful, and deserving of our time and energy changes. The measurement of occupational balance is inexact, and the interpretation of the data generated by the methods discussed in this chapter requires careful consultation with the client in order to be useful in documenting current status and change over time. Because culture, motivation, and life stage are all likely to influence one's perception of balance, the roles of society, personality, and age may all be interesting lines of inquiry in future studies of occupational balance. It has also been suggested that the issue of balance is of concern to a privileged segment of society[12] because occupational choice and allocation of time is a luxury that is not affordable to individuals living in poverty. For example, in this latter instance, Whiteford[26] proposes that occupational balance is irrelevant to survival. However, a small portion of survival—physiologic need—has been identified as a domain in Matuska's[22] approach to balance, and this is indicative of evolution in research.

Csikszentmihalyi's[27] concepts of "flow" and "optimal experience" advance the social ecological approach to balance because of the consideration of context or environmental influences under which people act. Experience Sampling Method (ESM)[28,29] is a measurement approach that contributes to theoretical understanding of optimal experience. Building on this foundation, Jonsson and Persson[30] proposed an alternative perspective on flow theory analysis that they refer to as an *experiential model of occupational balance*. Their model has 3 dimensions shown to be useful in analyzing the dynamic cycle of balanced experiences in everyday life that promote health and well-being. Further research along this line of inquiry may yield new measures for practice. The lifestyle balance model initially proposed by Matuska and Christiansen[7] has been revised and is now referred to as the *life balance model*.[31] This model is gaining momentum in the occupational therapy and science literature and demonstrates preliminary validity.[31] Dür et al,[9] Eakman,[32,33] Stamm et al,[34] and Wagman and Håkansson[23,35] are examples of scholars pushing the research agenda for improved theoretical understanding of occupational balance and better measurement tools.

There are challenges to measuring a concept that is subjective (and, some argue, lacks a definition with clear consensus). Backman and Anaby[8] outlined a research agenda that included questions related to the dimensionality of balance: are balance and imbalance opposing anchors on a single continuum, or do they coexist as independent dimensions? That is, is it possible to experience balance and imbalance at the same time? Narratives of balance suggest that a person may believe his or her daily pattern of occupation reflects his or her values and interests but may not meet external demands, an example of balance and imbalance coexisting. To what degree does this affect health outcomes? Future measurement development in this area may develop or refine tools so they are compatible with theoretical definitions, operationalized, discriminative, and applicable to various populations.[8]

The continued use and development of measures such as those described here, especially with diverse populations, will provide a greater understanding of how occupational balance contributes to health and well-being. It also would be of interest to explore the concept of balance outside of industrialized nations. If occupation is a determinant of health, then a greater understanding of how people configure occupation in their daily lives would assist occupational therapists to enhance health for individual clients, communities, and populations.

Overview of Measures of Time Use and Occupational Balance

Selection Criteria

Measures presented here relate to either time use or occupational balance and have either been developed by occupational therapists or used (as reported in literature) by occupational therapists. This decision helped reduce the number of measures and ensure they had an occupation-based focus. Measures were excluded if they did not report at least preliminary validity data indicative of measuring the stated construct. Not all of the selected measures were ready for clinical use at the time of publication, but they were included if the authors indicated developmental work was ongoing and the tool was available on request to other researchers. Measures were excluded if the effort required was deemed impractical for practice. Experience Sampling Method (ESM)[28] was excluded because it involves random paging of individuals who then record what they are doing and respond to specific questions about the activity, although it was recognized to have research utility for in-depth studies of time use and the occupational experiences.

List of Measures Reviewed

The following tools are reviewed in Tables 15-1 through 15-8.

Time Use

- Occupational Questionnaire (OQ) (Table 15-1)
- National Institutes of Health (NIH) Activity Record (ACTRE) (Table 15-1)
- Structured Observation and Report Technique (SORT) (Table 15-2)

Occupational Balance

- Life Balance Inventory (LBI) (Table 15-3)
- Occupational Balance Questionnaire (OBQ) (Table 15-4)
- Occupational Balance-Questionnaire (OB-Quest) (Table 15-5)
- Meaningful Activity Wants and Needs Assessment (MAWNA) (Table 15-6)
- Intergoal Relations Questionnaire (IRQ) (Table 15-7)
- Personal Projects Analysis (PPA) (Table 15-8)

A typical way to assess time use is with diaries or daily logs, such as the Occupational Questionnaire (OQ)[18] and the National Institutes of Health Activity Record (ACTRE).[19] For both the OQ and the ACTRE, the client completes a diary by indicating the primary activity pursued in each half-hour increment of the day. The diary is kept for 2 days. Attributes of the activities and, in the case of the ACTRE, symptoms associated with each activity, are assessed with specific questions following each entry on the diary sheet. Both of these tools provide an inventory of the types of activities the client pursues and may provide additional insight regarding how much time is spent on discretionary vs obligatory activities, possible sources of client dissatisfaction with time allocated to various activities, and ways to modify time use. The OQ has been updated with descriptors in place of the original numerical ratings for commenting on occupations (eg, responses for the item rating importance are coded extremely important, important, take it or leave it, rather not do it, or total waste of time).[15]

Harvey and Pentland[36] summarize data from time use studies to describe what people do, for how long, and with whom. Most diaries are designed in half-hour increments and kept for periods of 2 to 7 days, and structured diaries are generally considered reliable. Diaries can be flexible, allowing for additional questions about the nature of the activities recorded, such as whether other people were involved in the activity. There is a great deal of data from population studies about time use, and many nations collect these data through regular national health and social surveys. Comparisons regarding time use and categories of occupations can then be made across subpopulations, such as age groups, genders, or regional communities. It is important to note that time use studies tend to focus on the primary activity in which the person was engaged at a particular moment in time, although some diary formats also ask about secondary activities. The nature of occupation is such that multiple tasks may be occurring simultaneously, even tasks related to different occupations. For example, a mother may be simultaneously assisting her children with homework while preparing dinner and sorting through bills to pay. Studies of mothers in particular have noted how occupations may be embedded in one another.[37] Similar approaches include a "yesterday diary" where the client is interviewed about the day prior, from the time he or she arose until the end of the day. It differs from other diaries in that time is not recorded in uniform increments, but the person is asked what he or she did, how long it took, what he or she did next, and so on. Claessens and colleagues[38] provide a review of time management approaches to measurement and their effect on performance.

Another time use measure is the Structured Observation and Report Technique (SORT),[39] a subscale of the Longitudinal Functional Assessment System, which measures health status and functional performance of people with disabilities. The SORT is a cued recall record of the activities engaged in during a day and can be administered using either an interview or a diary format. Information about what the individual did, where, with whom, and for how long is recorded using the tool. Children's time use can be measured by interviewing the parents and validating the activities with the child. The SORT provides rich and specific data about activity patterns in individuals.

Newer tools designed by occupational therapists include questionnaires directly asking about perceived occupational balance. The LBI is longer and more comprehensive than the OBQ and OB-Quest, but first asks whether the item is relevant to the respondent; if not, the item is skipped and not included in the scoring. The LBI subscales are health, relationships, identity, and challenge, but empirical work to date suggests that the meaning of activities (eg, cooking) within the LBI may relate to more than 1 subscale.[22] Thus, both the life balance model upon which it is based and the tool itself are expected to evolve with continued research. In contrast, the OBQ is a short, 13-item questionnaire directed to the client's satisfaction with amount and variation of occupation, without specifying which occupations.[23] It is a new tool that shows promise for clinical utility but has not yet been used in clinical settings. Similarly, the OB-Quest[9] is a brief 10-item questionnaire that is generic (not specific to occupation or population). It differs from the previous 2 measures in that items were generated from a large number of narratives of people living with chronic illness and the general population in an effort to ensure the theoretical construct being measured (occupational balance) was grounded in the patient perspective. However, the 10-item version is the result of testing an earlier version of the tool, and while this is a natural progression for building validity, it has not yet been used clinically.

The MAWNA[33] was informed by the discrepancy approach to balance advanced by Sheldon.[10] It focuses on "wants" and "needs" and the discrepancy between occupations in which the individual is currently engaged and his or her perceived desirable state. It requires the simultaneous measurement of meaningful occupation, in this case, the Engagement in Meaningful Activities Survey (EMAS).[32] A main limitation to the interpretation of data from the MAWNA is that it has been tested primarily with university students, although the companion tool, EMAS, has been used with older adults.

The social ecological perspective to studying occupation includes methods that examine engagement in goal-directed tasks, including environmental, social, and personal resources and restraints that influence occupation. In this way, the nature of occupation is described and the relationship among daily occupations can be studied. The IRQ[24] requires that the respondent identify 4 goal-directed activities and then analyze the impact of each activity on the other 3. This helps explore balance in terms of a cluster of occupations of immediate relevance to the individual. The IRQ is compatible with a conceptualization that considers balance and imbalance as 2 distinct characteristics, and in a study of working age adults using this approach, it was noted that imbalance, but not balance, was inversely associated with well-being.[40]

PPA[20] (Table 15-8) is a widely-used social ecological approach. It is not designed to account for the time people spend on activities, but instead focuses on the characteristics and inter-relationships of the projects (occupations) in which the person is engaged. Briefly, PPA consists of 3 steps: project elicitation, rating the projects on various dimensions, and a cross-impact matrix. The project elicitation step asks the client to identify all goal-directed activities he or she is currently pursuing or about to begin working on. Projects may be in any area of life and range in scope from finding a job to getting a manicure. In step 2, the client selects the 10 most relevant projects and rates them on a number of dimensions, such as the importance, enjoyment, and difficulty associated with each project. The approach is flexible enough to allow the addition or deletion of project characteristics in this step so that the characteristics of greatest interest to client and therapist are rated. Step 3, the cross-impact matrix, asks the client to consider the relative impact of each project on each of the other projects. A project can have a positive, negative, or neutral effect on the client's pursuit of other projects.

Both IRQ and PPA require a fair amount of introspection and have the potential to identify problematic occupations, desirable occupations, and conflict within an individual's system of occupations. Therefore, they may provide useful information for working with clients toward achieving a more satisfactory balance in daily occupations.

As outlined in Tables 15-1 through 15-8, a variety of tools exist to evaluate time use and occupational balance, and reflect differing levels of effort on the client's part to complete and the therapist's part to apply to practice. Although time use can be observed by others, interpretations of satisfactory allocation of time and perceptions of occupational balance are inherently subjective. Little is known about their usefulness in guiding therapeutic approaches with a variety of populations. Several new measures of occupational balance have been introduced in recent research but have not yet infiltrated practice settings. Future research might examine the utility of these tools in different practice settings, with more varied populations (sociocultural and diagnostic), and how well they capture change or indicate important intervention outcomes. Theoretically, additional questions might be explored, such as the following:

- Are occupational balance and imbalance 2 opposing points on a 2-dimensional scale, or are they 2 separate unidimensional scales?
- To what extent is occupational balance a discrete construct, or is it the same as happiness or well-being constructed through an occupation-based lens?

Exploration of these and other research directions will advance the measurement of occupational balance and time use and their application to occupational therapy.

Table 15-1

Occupational Questionnaire (OQ) and NIH Activity Record (ACTRE)

Source	Human Occupation Clearinghouse: http://www.moho.uic.edu Under "Products," choose "Free Resources" then "Occupational Questionnaire" or "NIH Activity Record." OQ is downloaded from this site; ACTRE can be requested from NIH using the link on this site.
Key References	Gerber and Furst[19]; Kielhofner[15]; Smith et al[18]
Purpose	• Descriptive and evaluative. • Both are daily logs for documenting occupations/time use by half-hour intervals. The OQ describes clients' perceptions of type of occupation (eg, work, play, rest) and sense of competence, value, and enjoyment attributed to each occupation. The ACTRE expands the OQ with items rating the impact of pain and fatigue on the listed occupations.
Type of Client	• Adolescents and adults.
Test Format	• Self-report, paper-based questionnaire. A structured diary with 30-minute increments for listing occupations, then columns with questions to categorize the occupation and rate characteristics. In English.
Procedures	• Instructions printed on form. Verbal instructions and practice with a sample form are recommended prior to client taking it home for completion over 2 days. • OQ: list the primary occupation for each 30-minute time slot then answer 4 additional questions on a 4- or 5-point nominal or ordinal scale (depending on the question). Scored by calculating the proportion of time spent on each of 4 occupational categories and means for each occupational characteristic. • ACTRE: in addition, pain and fatigue are rated for their impact on each occupation and means calculated.
Time Required	• Approximately 20 to 25 minutes for client to complete one 24-hour diary. Recommend use for 5 to 10 minutes at mealtimes and bedtime to record activities up to that point of the day; 10 minutes to score.
Standardization	• Instructions provided. No published norms.
Reliability	
Test-Retest	• Percent agreement for OQ in sample of 20 American older adults: 87% for occupational category; 77% for personal causation/sense of competence; 81% for value/importance; and 77% for interest/enjoyment[18]
Internal Consistency	• Not reported
Inter-Rater	• Not applicable
Validity	
Content	• Theoretically informed by concepts in the Model of Human Occupation. Client chooses the occupations to report, suggesting content is relevant to the individual assessed
Construct	• Preliminary concurrent validity of OQ established in a pilot study of 18 college students who also completed the Household Work Study Diary. Percent agreement for personal causation 92%, values 86%, interests 84%[18]
Criterion	• Hypothesized association with life satisfaction was supported in a study of 60 adults aged 65 to 99 years with small but statistically significant correlations[18]

(continued)

Table 15-1 (continued)

Occupational Questionnaire (OQ) and NIH Activity Record (ACTRE)

Validity	
Criterion	• In a pilot study of 21 American adults with rheumatoid arthritis, the ACTRE was administered with 3 different "gold standard" measures to validate personal causation/competence, enjoyment, pain, and fatigue ratings. Spearman correlation coefficients were calculated, but only significance levels were reported. All expected correlations were statistically significant except for fatigue during specific times of day.
Utility	
Research Programs	• Time consuming but potentially useful for gathering detailed time use data with an occupation focus. Preliminary reliability and validity based on very small samples; pilot testing recommended.
Practice Settings	• Has potential for systematic approach to understanding and managing time use/achieving occupational balance, inclusive of common symptoms of chronic illness, possibly informing self-management strategies. Test-retest reliability should be established before use as an outcome measure.
Strengths	• Structured diary on time use may reveal patterns of activity that serve to guide identification of occupational performance issues and intervention plans in ways that cannot be captured by less detailed description of daily routines.
Complexities	• Takes commitment to record information every half hour or to recall in 4- to 5-hour chunks. May affect data integrity.

Table 15-2

Structured Observation and Report Techniques (SORT)

Source	Rintala et al[39]
Key References	Spencer et al[41]; Quittner and Opopari[42]
Purpose	• Descriptive. • SORT describes the unique constellation of an individual's daily activities, including what they did, where, with whom, and how.
Type of Client	• Children, adolescents, and adults of all ages.
Test Format	• Self-report questionnaire administered using an interview.
Procedures	• Respondents are asked to report on the activities they have completed over a specific period of time, usually the past 24 hours, and asked about other people present and the location of the activity.
Time Required	• The interview takes 15 to 45 minutes. Time to code and score is not reported.
Standardization	• Instructions for administration are in the source article. No published norms.
Reliability	
Test-Retest	• Not reported.
Internal Consistency	• Reported as impractical to assess.
Inter-Rater	• Percent agreement between coders of activities ranged from 77% to 86%[39]

(continued)

Table 15-2 (continued)

Structured Observation and Report Techniques (SORT)

Validity	
Content	• By virtue of data collection method, content validity should be present.
Construct	• Self-report of activity agreed with independent observers from 77% to 83% of the time. • The SORT discriminates between different life experiences such as living at home or being in the hospital.
Criterion	• The SORT has predicted activity levels post-discharge from a rehabilitation hospital, with a high correlation between in-hospital measures of independent activity and post-discharge measures. • When used with mothers, the SORT differentiates the time spent by mothers with a child with a chronic illness in comparison to healthy siblings.[42]
Utility	
Research Programs	• As a research tool, has potential to describe how individuals spend their time.
Practice Settings	• Used with individual clients, SORT can assist with describing patterns of time use and balance of occupations across ADL or self-care; work or productive activities, including household management tasks; and play and leisure activities.
Strengths	• Although originally designed for use with children and adolescents, SORT is a tool that can be used with clients across the lifespan. • In situations where a client has difficulties with reporting, a parent or other family member can be asked to clarify information. • SORT was one of the first systematic approaches to describing activity patterns in children.
Complexities	• Requires further published information to assist with administration and interpretation, particularly for use with adults and older adults.

Table 15-3

Life Balance Inventory (LBI)

Source	Matuska[22] LBI can be accessed online at http://minerva.stkate.edu/LBI.nsf
Key References	Matuska and Christiansen[7]; Matuska[31]; Matuska et al[43]
Purpose	• To measure the congruence between one's actual activity configuration and desired activity configuration, consistent with a specific theoretical model and definition of life balance. Life balance is defined as "a satisfying pattern of daily activity that is healthful, meaningful, and sustainable...within the context of [one's] current life circumstances."[7(p 11)]
Type of Client	• Adults
Test Format	• Self-report. Free online tool. Available in English.
Procedures	• There are 53 items, but only those activities one currently does or wishes to do are completed using a 5-point scale. Online tool includes and scores a short stress scale. • The author of the LBI owns the raw data which are retained in a secure database when individuals complete the online tool.
Time Required	• 10 to 15 minutes

(continued)

Table 15-3 (continued)

Life Balance Inventory (LBI)

Standardization	• Instructions embedded in online format and scored automatically from 1.00 (very unbalanced, lack of congruence) to 3.00 (very balanced, congruence between actual and desired activities). Online tool reports overall life balance score and 4 subscales, along with a legend for interpretation: physiological health, relationship, identity, and challenge subscales, corresponding to the needs-based dimensions of the life balance model.
Reliability	
Test-Retest	• Not reported
Internal Consistency	• Cronbach's alpha = 0.89 in first pilot test (n = 282)[22] • Cronbach's alpha = 0.97 in second pilot test (n = 458)[22]
Inter-Rater	• Not applicable
Validity	
Content	• Item generation based on life balance model and broadly phrased activities encompassing occupational performance areas; reviewed by 6 occupational therapy scholars and 52 friends, family, and students to eliminate redundancy and add missing activity categories. Pilot tested with n = 282 American adults (90% female, 98% white, mean age 43 years) and Rasch analysis applied. Mean square values for all items between 1.82 and .82 indicating each item contributed to the overall score[22] • Rasch analysis indicated all items fit model expectations, mean square values between 1.82 and .82. Sample n = 458 American adults (55% female, 25% non-White, age range 18 to 90 years, mean age 41 years)[22]
Construct	• Confirmatory factor analysis with n = 458 inconclusive: did not support the 4 subcategories (comparative fit index, CFI = .70; CFI of .90 or better indicates a good fit); and several items had weak factor loadings onto the expected subscales. Subcategories were retained for further testing because they were informed by the theoretical model of life balance.[22] • Structural equation models examined relationships among the total LBI, stress, well-being, and basic psychological need satisfaction, demonstrating expected associations between a congruence definition of life balance and the other variables.[22]
Criterion	• In a sample of 1048 American adults, LBI total scores were associated with life stress, Spearman's r = -0.52; subscale scores had slightly lower correlations. In multiple regression analysis, the combination of subscale scores explained 30% of the variance in life stress, while the LBI total score explained 25% of the variance; when controlling for age, gender, and race, the combination of subscale scores explained 31% of variance. Caution urged because demographic characteristics were available for less than half the sample.[43]
Utility	
Research Programs	• Use of online tool may not be appropriate given data are stored in an American database; author might be contacted for permission to use and scoring instructions. Comprehensiveness (53 items) needs to be weighed against respondent burden. No test-retest reliability data yet reported and, therefore, may not be suitable for intervention or repeated measures studies. Suitable for one-time assessment when congruence definition of balance matches research objectives.
Practice Settings	• Easy to access online tool, scored immediately. May be useful as an intervention tool (rather than measurement tool) to address satisfying pattern of activities in Western cultures. Lack of test-retest reliability suggests caution for monitoring progress over time.

(continued)

Table 15-3 (continued)

LIFE BALANCE INVENTORY (LBI)

Strengths	• Theoretically driven. Exploration of congruence or match between actual and desired activities is compatible with many views of occupational balance.
Complexities	• The notion of a bipolar scale (1 = very imbalanced, 3 = very balanced) vs 2 separate scales for imbalance and balance has been challenged elsewhere. Applicability to diverse personal characteristics not yet established (males, varied socioeconomic and cultural groups).

Table 15-4

OCCUPATIONAL BALANCE QUESTIONNAIRE (OBQ)

Source	Wagman and Håkansson[23] Tool available in Swedish from the authors for research purposes.
Key References	Wagman and Håkansson[35]
Purpose	• To measure perceived satisfaction with the amount and variety of occupations
Type of Client	• Adults
Test Format	• Self-report, paper-based questionnaire • 13 items rated on 6-point Likert scale (0 to 5)
Procedures	• Client completes the questionnaire • Items are summed for a total score, but may also be used individually
Time Required	• Not stated. Likely less than 10 minutes.
Standardization	• Not stated
Reliability	• In well-educated convenience samples of Swedish adults, n = 67, 70% women (sample A) and n = 153, 61% women (sample B)
Test-Retest	• Individual items, kappa coefficients of 0.61 to 0.83 (sample B) • Total score, Spearman's rho = 0.93 (sample B) • Average of 1 week between test and retest
Internal Consistency	• Cronbach's alpha = 0.94 (sample A), 0.92 (sample B)
Inter-Rater	• Not applicable
Validity	
Content	• Items development informed by a conceptual framework that defined occupational balance as comprising 4 aspects: variety across occupations, amount of occupation, congruence with personal resources, and meaning of occupations. All aspects influence one's perception of a satisfactory balance or pattern of occupation. The relevance of the 13 items was assessed by 21 occupational therapists using a content validity index; the proportion of occupational therapists giving the highest and lowest ratings of relevance is compared to arrive at a number between 0 and 1. Ratings for items ranged from 0.71 to 1.0 with an average rating of 0.90 indicating strong validity in terms of relevance to occupational balance.

(continued)

Table 15-4 (continued)

Occupational Balance Questionnaire (OBQ)

Validity	
Construct	• It was hypothesized that OBQ scores would be moderately associated with self-reported Health (single ordinal item) and Life Satisfaction (single ordinal item), suggesting that occupational balance is health-related (overlapping) but distinct from these constructs, using sample B (n = 153, see above). • Spearman rho = 0.58 (p = .01) for Health • Spearman rho = 0.52 (p = .01) for Life Satisfaction
Criterion	• Not reported
Utility	
Research Programs	• A quick, easy self-report tool to include when occupational balance is a variable of interest, with promising preliminary psychometric properties.
Practice Settings	• A quick, easy self-report tool that is easily scored, can be completed in a waiting room or in advance of a visit, and can be used to stimulate discussion and monitoring of occupational performance issues related to balance.
Strengths	• Conceptually based, short self-report tool. No/low cost
Complexities	• Health literacy may be an issue for some client groups

Table 15-5

Occupational Balance Questionnaire (OB-Quest)

Source	Dür et al[9]; The tool with response choices is reproduced in Tables 4 (English) and 5 (German) of the above citation. Developed in German and translated to English by native speakers using forward and backward translation procedures.
Key References	See above
Purpose	• Outcome measure to assess presence/absence of indicators of occupational balance from the person
Type of Client	• Adults
Test Format	• Self-report, paper-based
Procedures	• 10 items with 3-point response scale. Response phrasing is specific to each item, but is interpreted loosely as 1 = positive, 2 = little bit negative, 3 = very negative. Items individually scored (no summed, average, or total score)
Time Required	• Not stated. Appears to be less than 10 minutes
Standardization	• Not stated
Reliability	
Test-Retest	• Not stated
Internal Consistency	• Cronbach's alpha = 0.57 on earlier version with n = 251 Austrian adults with and without a health condition
Inter-Rater	• Not applicable

(continued)

Table 15-5 (continued)

Occupational Balance Questionnaire (OB-Quest)

Validity	
Content	• Thorough analysis of qualitative interviews with 90 Austrian adults (15 each of 5 chronic conditions and 15 with no illness) to identify 8 key components of occupational balance from the patient or person perspective. Wording of 8 initial items vetted by n = 20 potential clients in pilot test, and 1 item deleted.
Construct	• Rasch reliability (fit) statistics were satisfactory for 5 items; 2 were deleted and Cronbach's alpha improved to the 0.57 reported above. The 2 misfit items were considered compound items and split into 2 new items each, as was 1 other item, to result in final 10-item questionnaire in both German and English. • It is important to note that reliability and validity have not yet been reported on this final version.
Criterion	• Not reported
Utility	
Research Programs	• Short tool easily integrated into self-report approaches. Uncertainty about dimensionality and scoring may make it premature for hypothesis testing.
Practice Settings	• Ten questions that may lead to identification of lifestyle/balance issues across activities, rest, sleep, and capacity to adapt activity in response to environmental circumstances.
Strengths	• Concepts based on client perspectives.
Complexities	• Rigorous psychometric properties not yet established on final version of the tool but shows promise.

Table 15-6

Meaningful Activity Wants and Needs Assessment (MAWNA)

Source	Eakman[33]
Key References	Eakman[32]
Purpose	• Assess perceived need for meaningful experiences in occupation; intended to be used with a measure of meaningful occupation as a discrepancy approach to life balance. On its own, gives indication of goal achievement, enjoyment, and social connections.
Type of Client	• Adults, nonspecific. Initially tested with 250 undergraduate and graduate student respondents to an invitation sent to a random sample at an American university, largely White, female, mean age 31 years.
Test Format	• Self-report. Online survey. Instructions sufficient to create a paper version.
Procedures	• Individuals respond to 21 items using a 4-point scale (0 = I do not want or need more of this in my life; 1 = I would like more of this in my life; 2 = I really want more of this in my life; 3 = I truly need more of this in my life).
Time Required	• Not stated. Likely less than 15 minutes to complete and score.
Standardization	• Not stated

(continued)

Table 15-6 (continued)

Meaningful Activity Wants and Needs Assessment (MAWNA)

Reliability	• n=49 college students, subset of n=250 American college students, 91% White, 65% female, mean age 31 years.
Test-Retest	• ICC=0.89, $p<0.001$; 95% CI=0.85, 0.92 (2 weeks)
Internal Consistency	• Cronbach's alpha=0.95
Inter-Rater	• Not applicable
Validity	
Content	• Initial items and scoring pilot-tested, revised, and response formats confirmed by Rasch analysis (n=29 graduate students). Items developed to measure 3 theoretically-derived aspects of meaning, confirmed by factor analysis. Hypothesized that items would load on 3 subscales: competence and goal achievement, pleasure and enjoyment, social connectedness.
Construct	• See Content.
Criterion	• Low but statistically significant correlations with life satisfaction, r=-0.29; depression, r=0.33; psychological needs for autonomy, r=-0.33; competence, r=-0.32; and relatedness, r=-0.28; all in expected directions. n=250 American college students described previously.
Utility	
Research Programs	• Relatively short to administer, easy to score. Useful if content matches research purpose. Caveat: has only been tested with college students.
Practice Settings	• Relatively short to administer, easy to score. High literacy required. May generate discussion to identify occupational performance issues related to desire/need for meaningful occupation and how time is spent or priorities set.
Strengths	• Conceptually strong.
Complexities	• Used with companion measure, Engagement in Meaningful Activities Survey (EMAS) to identify discrepancy between desired occupations and current engagement in occupations in order to estimate life balance from an occupation perspective.

Table 15-7

Intergoal Relations Questionnaire (IRQ)

Source	Riediger et al[24] The IRQ is reproduced in the article appendix.
Key References	Anaby et al[40]; Riediger and Freund[44]
Purpose	• Measures 2 constructs related to pursuit and achievement of client-identified goals based on the impact of a goal on other goals: (a) interference among goals in terms of time, energy, and financial constraints, and incompatible goal attainment strategies; and (b) facilitation among goals in terms of goal relations and overlap of goal attainment strategies.
Type of Client	• Adults
Test Format	• Self-report, paper-based

(continued)

Table 15-7 (continued)

Intergoal Relations Questionnaire (IRQ)

Type of Client	
Procedures	• Given examples of goals and life domains, client lists 4 goals, pairs each goal with each of the other 3 (12 pairs), and then rates interference (4 items) and facilitation (2 items) for each pair. Sample interference items: "how often can it happen that, because of the pursuit of Goal A, you do not invest as much time/energy/money into Goal B as you would like?" Sample facilitation items: "how often can it happen that you do something in the pursuit of Goal A that is simultaneously beneficial for Goal B?" Scored using 5-point scale, from 1 (never/very rarely) to 5 (very often). There is a total of 72 items (6 items for 12 goal pairs). Means are calculated to arrive at interference and facilitation subscale scores.
Time Required	• Not stated
Standardization	• Minimal instructions in journal articles
Reliability	
Test-Retest	• Not reported
Internal Consistency	• Cronbach's alpha = .94 interference; .90 facilitation, in a sample of n = 111 German adults (n = 53 adults 20 to 30 years, mean age 24; n = 58 adults 60 to 78 years, mean age 65; 60% female)[44]
Inter-Rater	• Not applicable
Validity	
Content	• Informed by goal pursuit literature but actual item generation not reported.
Construct	• Tested hypothesis that intergoal facilitation and interference are distinct characteristics; this was supported by a 2-factor solution with IRQ scores from sample of 111 German adults[44] • Intergoal facilitation differs between younger and older adults (older adults report greater facilitation across goals)[24]
Criterion	• Intergoal facilitation and interference are differentially associated with subjective well-being and pursuit of goals: • IRQ facilitation subscale was associated with goal pursuit but not well-being; IRQ interference subscale was not associated with goal pursuit but was consistently negatively associated with well-being, R^2 values between .23 and .42.[44] • In a group of 24 Israeli adults, IRQ interference was negatively associated with life satisfaction (r = -.5) but IRQ facilitation was not.[40]
Utility	
Research Programs	• Two dimensions (variables) related to balance are captured in a single tool, potentially reducing respondent burden. Although a self-report tool, may require a high level of literacy to complete.
Practice Settings	• Potentially useful to establish baseline issues related to goal attainment, and to assess outcome of interventions aimed at reducing interference and enhancing facilitation. However, lack of test-retest reliability tempers use as an outcome measure.
Strengths	• Client-centered: focused on 4 goals (occupations) selected by the client as currently relevant. Considers impact of goals on one another, potentially getting at the root of perceived balance from a goal-oriented perspective.
Complexities	• May be a sophisticated concept for some users and require verbal guidance to complete the self-report tool.

Table 15-8

Personal Projects Analysis (PPA)

Source	Little[20]
Key References	Christiansen et al[45,46]; Little[13,47]; Little and Gee[48]; Little et al[49]; Palys and Little[50]
Purpose	• Descriptive. PPA was developed for studying the stages of project inception, planning, action, and termination, as well as interproject impact and linkages with values and actions.
Type of Client	• Adolescents and adults of all ages.
Test Format	• Self-report; paper and pencil questionnaire administered with verbal or written instructions.
Procedures	• Respondent completes a 3-part questionnaire. Part 1 is a list of all goal-directed projects in which the client is currently engaged or about to begin. In Part 2, the 10 most pertinent projects are rated on a 0 to 10 scale for various dimensions such as importance, enjoyment, and time adequacy. (There is some flexibility here about how many dimensions are rated; a core set of 17 has been reported). Part 3 is a cross-impact matrix in which each project is assessed regarding its impact on every other project. • Scoring consists of categorizing the listed projects from Part 1, calculating means for each project dimension in Part 2, and summing the cross-impact matrix ratings from Part 3. • The cross-impact score indicates relative concordance or conflict within a project system, and is therefore a possible indicator of "occupational balance."
Time Required	• 30 to 40 minutes for clients • 10 to 15 minutes for scoring
Standardization	• A PPA workbook is available online from the author's website (www.brianrlittle.com/wp-content/uploads/2011/10/ppa-workbook.doc) for research and testing purposes only. Formats for Parts 1 and 2 are reprinted in Little[20]; the format for the cross-impact matrix is in Christiansen et al.[46] The author, Brian Little, maintains a bank of comparative data.
Reliability	
Test-Retest	• Adequate
Internal Consistency	• Adequate for project dimensions, averaging 0.70 (coefficient alpha), ranging from 0.53 for project stress to 0.77 for value congruency[51]
Inter-Rater	• Not applicable, given nature of the method of assessment.
Validity	
Content	• Clients are able to report any and all projects; therefore, it is highly client-centered. • 17 core dimensions appear to cover a broad range of characteristics of goal-directed activities. • The method is sufficiently flexible that other dimensions may be added. • Factor analysis suggests that project dimensions load on 5 factors: meaning, structure, community, efficacy, and stress, each of which appear to be relevant content. Efficacy and (absence of) stress were the most predictable factors of well-being and depression.
Construct	• PPA factor structure correlates moderately with the NEO Personality Inventory and the Sense of Coherence Scale. Specific correlations are too numerous to list; see Little references for details.
Criterion	• It has been hypothesized that PPA scores would be associated with life satisfaction and depression. This has been established in several studies; see Christiansen et al[46] and Little et al[49] for summaries. • Project efficacy and project (absence of) stress were the most predictable factors of well-being and depression.[48]

(continued)

Table 15-8 (continued)

PERSONAL PROJECTS ANALYSIS (PPA)

Utility	
Research Programs	• Researchers have used PPA as a method to explore problems in the areas of environmental planning, developmental transitions, adaptation to chronic illness and pain and to predict adherence to treatments. It is flexible and allows for additional occupational characteristics to be added (match variables to research purpose).
Practice Settings	• PPA can be used to assess the content, appraisal, prioritization, and impact of personal projects with individual clients. It takes time but offers detailed descriptive information.
Strengths	• Easy to obtain and administer (to those with adequate reading and comprehension ability). • Comprehensive descriptions of occupations relevant to the individual client. An increasing number of studies in the literature, from a range of investigators, are adding to the rigor of this method of assessment.
Complexities	• Requires good literacy and cognitive skills on the part of the client; not suitable for those with cognitive impairment. • Time to complete may be burdensome in some situations, depending on client priorities.

REFERENCES

1. Backman CL. Occupational balance: exploring the relationships among daily occupations and their influence on well-being. *Can J Occup Ther.* 2004;71:202-209.
2. Backman CL. Occupational balance and well-being. In: Christiansen CH, Townsend EA, eds. *Introduction to Occupation: The Art and Science of Living.* 2nd ed. Upper Saddle River, NJ: Prentice Hall; 2010:231-249.
3. Stadnyk RL, Townsend EA, Wilcock AA. Occupational justice. In: Christiansen CH, Townsend EA, eds. *Introduction to Occupation: The Art and Science of Living.* 2nd ed. Upper Saddle River, NJ: Prentice Hall; 2010:329-358.
4. Amundson NE. Three-dimensional living. *J Employment Counseling.* 2001;38:114-127.
5. Håkansson C, Matuska K. How life balance is perceived by Swedish women recovering from a stress-related disorder: a validation of the Life Balance Model. *J Occup Science.* 2010;17:112-119.
6. Little BR. Foreword. In: Christiansen C, Matuska K, eds. *Life Balance: Multidisciplinary Theories and Research.* Thorofare NJ: SLACK Incorporated; 2009:xv-xix.
7. Matuska KM, Christiansen CH. A proposed model of lifestyle balance. *J Occup Science.* 2008;15:9-10.
8. Backman CL, Anaby D. Research directions for advancing the study of life balance and health. In: Christiansen C, Matuska K, eds. *Life Balance: Multidisciplinary Theories and Research.* Thorofare NJ: SLACK Incorporated; 2009.
9. Dür M, Steiner G, Fialka-Moser V, et al. Development of a new occupational balance-questionnaire: incorporating the perspectives of patients and healthy people in the design of a self-reported occupational therapy balance outcome instrument. *Health Qual Life Outcomes.* 2014;12:45.
10. Sheldon KM. Defining and validating measures of life balance: suggestions, a new measure, and some preliminary results. In: Christiansen C, Matuska K, eds. *Life Balance: Multidisciplinary Theories and Research.* Thorofare NJ: SLACK Incorporated; 2009.
11. Caproni P. Work/life balance: you can't get there from here. *J Applied Behavioral Science.* 1997;33:46-56.
12. Kerka S. The balancing act of adult life. ERIC Digest No. 229, Article EDO-CE-01-229. http://www.ericdigests.org/2002-3/act.htm. Accessed June 19, 2016.
13. Little BR. Persons, contexts and personal projects. In: Wapner S, Demick J, Yamamoto T, Minami H, eds. *Theoretical Perspectives in Environment-Behavior Research.* New York: Kluwer Academic; 2000.
14. Perrons D. The new economy and the work-life balance: conceptual explorations and a case study of new media. *Gender, Work Organization.* 2003;10:65-93.
15. Kielhofner G. *A Model of Human Occupation: Theory and Application.* 4th ed. Philadelphia: Lippincott Williams & Wilkins; 2008.
16. Christiansen CH. Three perspectives on balance in occupation. In: Zemke R, Clark F, eds. *Occupational Science: The Evolving Discipline.* Philadelphia: F. A. Davis; 1996:431-451.
17. Backman C. Occupational balance: measuring time use and satisfaction across occupational performance areas. In Law M, Baum C, Dunn W, eds. *Measuring Occupational Performance: Supporting Best Practice in Occupational Therapy.* Thorofare, NJ: SLACK Incorporated; 2001:203-213.
18. Smith NR, Kielhofner G, Watts JH. The relationship between volition, activity pattern, and life satisfaction in the elderly. *Am J Occup Ther.* 1986;40:278-283.
19. Gerber LH, Furst GP. Validation of the NIH Activity Record: a quantitative measure of life activities. *Arthritis Care Res.* 1992;5:81-86.

20. Little BR. Personal projects: a rationale and method for investigation. *Environ Behavior.* 1983;15:273-309.
21. Forhan M, Backman C. Exploring occupational balance in adults with rheumatoid arthritis. *OTJR.* 2010;30:133-141.
22. Matuska K. Description and development of the Life Balance Inventory. *OTJR.* 2012;32:220-228.
23. Wagman P, Håkansson C. Introducing the occupational balance questionnaire (OBQ). *Scand J Occup Ther.* 2014;21:227-231.
24. Riediger M, Freund AM, Baltes PB. Managing life through personal goals: intergoal facilitation and intensity of goal pursuit in younger and older adulthood. *J Gerontol B Psychol Sci Soc Sci.* 2005;60(2):P84-P91.
25. Bryden P, McColl MA. The concept of occupation: 1900 to 1974. In: McColl MA, ed. *Theoretical Basis of Occupational Therapy.* Thorofare, NJ: SLACK Incorporated; 2003.
26. Whiteford G. Occupational deprivation: understanding limited participation. In Christiansen CH, Townsend EA, eds. *Introduction to Occupation: The Art and Science of Living.* Upper Saddle River, NJ: Prentice Hall; 2010:303-328.
27. Csikszentmihalyi M. *Finding Flow.* New York: Basic Books; 1997.
28. Larson R, Csikszentmihalyi M. The experience sampling method. In: Reis HT, ed. *Naturalistic Approaches to Studying Social Interaction.* San Francisco: Jossey-Bass; 1983.
29. Csikszentmihalyi M, Larson R. Validity and reliability of the Experience-Sampling Method. *J Nerv Ment Dis.* 1987;175(9):526-536.
30. Jonsson H, Persson D. Towards an experiential model of occupational balance: an alternative perspective on flow theory analysis. *J Occup Science.* 2006;13:162-173.
31. Matuska KM. Validity evidence for a model and measure of life balance. *OTJR.* 2012;32:229-237.
32. Eakman AM. Measurement characteristics of the Engagement in Meaningful Activities Survey in an age-diverse sample. *Am J Occup Ther.* 2012;66(2):e20-e29.
33. Eakman AM. The meaningful activity wants and needs assessment: a perspective on life balance. *J Occup Science.* 2015;22(2):210-227.
34. Stamm TA, Lovelock L, Stew G, et al. I have a disease, but I am not ill: a narrative study of occupational balance in people with rheumatoid arthritis. *OTJR.* 2009;29(1):32-39.
35. Wagman P, Håkansson C. Exploring occupational balance in adults in Sweden. *Scand J Occup Ther.* 2014;21(6):415-420.
36. Harvey AS, Pentland W. What do people do? In: Christiansen CH, Townsend EA, eds. *Introduction to Occupation: The Art and Science of Living.* Upper Saddle River, NJ: Prentice Hall; 2004:63-90.
37. Larson EA. The orchestration of occupation: the dance of mothers. *Am J Occup Ther.* 2000;54:269-280.
38. Claessens BJC, van Eerde W, Rutte CG, Roe RA. A review of the time management literature. *Personnel Rev.* 2007;36:255-276.
39. Rintala DH, Uttermohlen DM, Buck EL, et al. Self-observation and report technique (SORT): description and clinical applications. In Halpern AS, Fuhrer MJ, eds. *Functional Assessment in Rehabilitation.* Baltimore, MD: Paul H. Brookes; 1984:205-221.
40. Anaby DR, Backman CL, Jarus T. Measuring occupational balance: a theoretical exploration of two approaches. *Can J Occup Ther.* 2010:77:280-288.
41. Spencer J, Hersch G, Shelton M, et al. Functional outcomes and daily life activities of African American elders after hospitalization. *Am J Occup Ther.* 2002;56(2):149-159.
42. Quittner AL, Opopari LC. Differential treatment of siblings: interview and diary analyses comparing two family contexts. *Child Dev.* 1994;65:800-814.
43. Matuska K, Bass J, Schmitt JS. Life balance and perceived stress: predictors and demographic profile. *OTJR.* 2013;33:146-158.
44. Riediger M, Freund AM. Interference and facilitation among personal goals: differential associations with subjective well-being and persistent goal pursuit. *Pers Soc Psychol Bull.* 2004;30:1511-1523.
45. Christiansen C, Backman C, Little BR, Nguyen A. Occupational and well-being: a study of personal projects. *Am J Occup Ther.* 1999;53:91-100.
46. Christiansen CH, Little BR, Backman C. Personal projects: a useful approach to the study of occupation. *Am J Occup Ther.* 1998;52:439-446.
47. Little BR. Personality science and self-regulation: personal projects as integrative units. *Applied Psychology.* 2006;55:419-427.
48. Little BR, Gee TL. Personal projects analysis. In: Salkind N, ed. *Encyclopedia of Measurement and Statistics.* Thousand Oaks, CA: Sage Publications; 2007.
49. Little BR, Salmela-Aro K, Phillips SD. *Personal Project Pursuit: Goals, Action, and Human Flourishing.* Mahwah, NJ: Lawrence Erlbaum Associates; 2007.
50. Palys TS, Little BR. Perceived life satisfaction and the organization of personal project systems. *J Pers Soc Psychol.* 1983;44:1221-1230.
51. Little BR, Lecci L, Watkinson B. Personality and personal projects: linking big five and PAC units of analysis. *J Personal.* 1992;60:501-525.

Mine the Gold

Colleagues within and outside the profession of occupational therapy have long acknowledged the influences of attitudinal, cultural, institutional, physical, and social environmental factors on human behavior, on participation in occupation, and on health and well-being. Since the publication of the International Classification of Function, Disability and Health (ICF) in 2001,[1] there has been greater attention toward developing and using assessments of environmental factors in occupational therapy and rehabilitation practice.

Become Systematic

These measures enable occupational therapists to gather specific information about the environmental factors that support or limit occupational performance and engagement.

Use Evidence in Practice

Use of environmental assessments aids therapists in understanding the complex relationships between persons, their occupations, and the environmental context.

Make Occupational Therapy Contributions Explicit

Occupational therapists focus on environmental factors that support performance and engagement, and make changes in the environment to improve performance and engagement.

Engage in Occupation-Based, Client-Centered Practice

The successful performance of day-to-day occupations is often dependent on a supportive environment and environmental resources. Assessment and consideration of environmental factors allows clients to achieve their goals for occupational performance and engagement.

CHAPTER 16

Measuring Environmental Factors

Patricia Rigby, PhD, OT Reg. (Ont.); Oana Craciunoiu, MScOT, OT(C); Jill Stier, MA, OT Reg. (Ont.); and Lori Letts, PhD, OT Reg. (Ont.)

Occupational therapists often see their clients within the environmental context where daily occupations occur, including their clients' home, school, community, and workplace.[2] The environment provides a context for occupational performance and engagement, and environmental factors influence human behavior. Thus, environment is integral to occupational therapy practice models and frameworks[3-8] and the ICF.[1]

In occupational therapy, *environment* is broadly defined to include physical, social, cultural, attitudinal, economic, and organizational elements. The environment is also considered at various levels, from the level of individuals; to their families, community, workplace, and school; and beyond to the macro level of social and institutional policies and structures.[5,9] Activities and occupations undertaken by people typically occur within multiple environments. They are influenced by, and in turn have an impact on, environmental factors. This reciprocal relationship of the person, his or her environment, and occupation is considered to be transactional.[5] The transactional relationship is so interwoven and interdependent that it cannot be teased apart. In occupational therapy, the outcome of a congruent person-environment-occupation (PEO) relationship, or good PEO fit, is optimal occupational performance and engagement.[3,5] Conversely, environmental barriers can reduce the PEO fit and negatively influence occupational performance. A major goal of occupational therapy interventions is to improve PEO fit, or the enabling factors that influence clients' experiences doing or engaging in an occupation. Environmental resources, in many instances, can be accessed easily and environmental barriers may be amenable to change or removal.[10]

The ICF classifies environmental factors as assistive products and technology; the natural and human-made environments; supports and relationships; attitudes; and services, systems, and policies.[1] These factors are included in the ICF to encourage the identification (through assessment) of environmental barriers and facilitators to the performance of daily occupations. The ICF also recognizes the importance of the environment in distinguishing between capacity and performance. Therapists want to know what their client is capable of doing within a supportive, "ideal" setting—their capacity to "do." This "ideal" barrier-free setting may be created within a clinic and may include resources that can support their client's functioning. In contrast, *performance* is what a person does in his or her current environment (eg, the person's home, community, or workplace). The gap between performance and capacity is examined to identify the aspects of the environment that facilitate or create barriers to performance. The ICF Checklist Version 2.1a includes an environmental factors section in which environmental facilitators and barriers can be identified.[11] Therapists can employ this approach by comparing occupational performance across environments (eg, comparing bath transfers in the hospital with bath transfers in a client's home) to identify the environmental resources or modifications that can be made to optimize performance (eg, the installation of grab bars and the help of a trained attendant to assist with the bath transfer).

It is critical that therapists be cognizant that occupational performance and engagement may differ from one environmental context to another. The therapist should not assume that a client would perform better in a controlled clinic setting. In fact, clients may demonstrate more optimal performance in environments in which they are comfortable and familiar, using familiar cues and supports to optimize performance. Therapists should consider potential differences in performance across various settings, and factor exploration of environmental variables into their assessment plans. These ideas will be explored further in this chapter.

Law M, Baum C, Dunn W, eds. *Measuring Occupational Performance: Supporting Best Practice in Occupational Therapy, Third Edition (pp 351-390).*

Environmental factors can be equally important to consider when the occupational therapist is dealing with groups or populations as the "client." In occupational therapy practice, for example, consultation or support can be given to more than one client (the client may be a group or type of person). For example, therapists can be involved in assessing public environments for accessibility for people with disabilities,[12] universal design,[13] or with a focus on age-friendly environments. In these situations, the general characteristics of the type of person intended to use the environment are considered, and environmental factors are assessed in relation to that general population. In this way, therapists may be in an excellent position to modify environments in order to meet the needs of many users, rather than a single client.

Overview of Measuring Environmental Factors

Key Concepts

The environment is multidimensional and complex and can be categorized in the many different ways described in the introduction to this chapter. This is a critically important concept to keep in mind because these categories can help organize a therapist's approach to assessment of environmental factors. The therapist can start by identifying the contextual focus for the assessment, whether it is the home, school, community setting, or workplace. At times, the contextual focus is across settings because the occupational issues and/or goals that the therapist is addressing with his or her client may involve more than one of these settings. This is illustrated in the case scenario in Box 16-1.

As noted earlier, the performance and engagement in daily occupations may differ from one setting to another, depending on a constellation of environmental factors. Thus, the therapist must take into consideration various environmental factors, whether attitudinal, cultural, physical, social, or institutional. As therapists know, environmental factors can support and enable, or contribute obstacles and constrain occupational performance and engagement. It is important that therapists use tools that allow them to identify barriers, supports, and resources in the environment. This is critical to intervention planning because the removal of barriers and access to environmental supports and resources can happen at the micro level of individuals, their immediate and extended family, their community, and beyond to the macro level of social and institutional policies and structures. In the case of Sue Lee, the environmental assessments focus on home, school, and community settings, with a focus on physical, social, attitudinal, and institutional aspects of the environment.

Another key concept is that occupational therapists view environment as part of the PEO transaction. However, this can pose challenges for measurement, and some tools will focus on discrete elements of the environment. Thus, it is critical that the therapist ensure that these discrete elements are examined in relation to that PEO transaction. In addition, the PEO relationship is dynamic and influenced by the passage of time and different settings.[3,5] The degree of PEO fit can change throughout the course of 1 day, 1 week, and over a lifetime. For example, Sue Lee may not experience optimal performance in daily self-care and school-related occupations during the first several weeks after she starts school as she becomes familiar with her new apartment and college environment. Occupational therapists would expect her occupational performance to improve as environmental resources are accessed, modifications are made, and she becomes more familiar with and skilled in navigating these new environments.

Importance of Measurement of Environmental Factors

It is commonly understood by occupational therapists that environmental factors can support or constrain the participation and inclusion of many people in the various occupations of daily life.[10,14-16] Physical access barriers, physical and social risks to personal safety, and social stigma and discrimination are still common and the most obvious environmental barriers. Social and organizational structures as well as lack of resources to make accommodations for people with occupational performance issues also pose barriers to programs and services within communities. There also are many institutional resources and services and social support systems that enable and support individuals in their homes and participation in their communities. As noted earlier, the environment and its influence on occupational performance and engagement is featured in prominent occupational therapy models and frameworks that guide practice. Thus, it is critically important that therapists include the assessment of environmental factors in their assessment protocol. By examining how features of the environment support or constrain occupational performance and engagement, the therapist acquires vital information to guide intervention planning with his or her client. This was illustrated in Tomas' efforts to understand how environmental factors such as physical accessibility and attitudes have the potential to constrain Sue's performance as a student at college. He then can use the findings to collaborate with Sue to implement plans to optimize her performance as she settles into school routines and gains greater autonomy.

There is a growing body of research that demonstrates that environmental interventions can have a very positive impact on occupational performance outcomes, and that the environment can be more amenable to change than a person.[10,15,17-19] For example, there is considerable evidence that environmental interventions to improve home safety help prevent falls in older adult populations.[15,20] In other studies, participation in social- and

Box 16-1

Case Study of Sue Lee

Sue is a 22-year-old woman who has a L5 level spinal cord injury with resultant paraplegia. Sue had been living at home with her parents in a bungalow following her discharge from the rehabilitation center. She uses a wheelchair for mobility. She had gained greater autonomy in her self-care and daily life in general, including meal preparation, shopping, and going out with friends. Sue felt that she was ready to go back to school and was accepted into a child life specialist program at a college in the city. She wanted to move closer to the college and live independently while attending school. Sue had been advised that the job demands of a child life specialist require a fair bit of mobility; however, she was determined to enter this program and to move into independent housing near the college. Sue's parents were supportive of her wishes, but anxious for her.

Sue and Tomas, her community-based occupational therapist, identified the following broad occupational goals that required occupational therapy attention:

- Move into student housing near campus and manage daily routines independently of her parents
- Be able to access transportation to and from the campus and on campus
- Attend classes on campus

Tomas needed to analyze the factors that would influence Sue's ability to attend college and live independently in a residential setting. He began by selecting 2 assessments of the environment to examine obstacles and facilitators that could affect Sue's occupational performance. He selected the Facilitators and Barriers Survey/Mobility (FABS/M)[21] because it identifies the attitudinal and physical obstacles and facilitators to participation in daily occupations in the home and community. Using the FABS/M with Sue at home, Tomas found that Sue's home and local community environments, in addition to the support from her parents, are facilitators to her daily life. In particular, there were many aspects of her current living arrangement that facilitate her daily occupations, including physical accessibility and access to community resources and services. Many barriers to her participation were also identified, including some negative previous experiences with paid personal attendants as well as Sue's own willingness to access help from friends and peers. The FABS/M results provided Tomas, Sue, and her parents with a helpful starting point for a discussion about various accessibility issues and resources Sue would need for her move to attend the college and participate in the program.

Sue and her parents used the FABS/M as a resource to guide their appraisal of the environment during a few visits they made to the college campus and student housing. Tomas met with them after those visits and reviewed issues identified on the FABS/M. Examples of obstacles identified included poor accessibility in some of the school buildings and specific access issues in student housing; transportation on campus and to and from campus; and accessibility within the community close to campus. Facilitators included the availability of home care and attendant care services; access to student loans and scholarships; and accessible community resources such as libraries, a popular coffee shop, and some entertainment facilities close to campus.

Tomas also used the Housing Enabler[22] during a visit to the apartments available through the college's student housing service. This tool provides a comprehensive assessment of the housing environment while considering the client's functional limitations and dependence on mobility aids. In this way, an environmental assessment can be structured and planned around aspects that may act as the greatest barriers to occupational performance. Because Sue uses a wheelchair for mobility and has resultant limited reaching ability, the tool identified several potential obstacles to her independent living that were not issues in her family home. These obstacles included entrances to the apartment building and to her suite; maneuvering space within the apartment; height of kitchen and bathroom cabinets; and availability of grab bars and a place to sit in the shower/bath.

These findings enabled Sue and her parents, together with Tomas, to identify and prioritize plans to prepare for Sue's move, and to access resources to support Sue. Their efforts enabled Sue to transition to college and campus life. After Sue had been at college for 1 month, Tomas met with her to follow up and examine the next steps to further support her occupational performance at school.

community-based occupation improves after the removal of environmental barriers.[23,24] Furthermore, O'Brien et al[16] argue that the environment (eg, barriers and negative social attitudes) may create disability as much, if not more than, the individual's impairments. This is illustrated in the case study of Sue Lee, who could manage most of her self-care without assistance at her parents' home, but physical accessibility obstacles posed barriers to her independence in the student apartment. Several modifications were required to enable her to regain autonomy in self-care. In addition, Sue experienced negative social attitudes from classmates and teachers at college in relation to her career goals. Many environmental resources can be accessed easily, and environmental barriers quite often respond more readily to change than using interventions that focus on fixing a client's impairments. While it is still important to optimize a client's abilities through remediation and adapt and modify occupations to achieve a good PEO fit, the environment should also be a major focus for occupational therapy interventions.

Factors to Remember When Measuring the Environment

It is difficult for any single instrument to measure something as multifaceted and complex as the environment and its dynamic influence on human behavior. Observational assessments provide a snap-shot of an environmental setting at a single point in time. Depending on the tool used, the therapist may be gathering discrete details about the environment in isolation of a client, or observations of the client performing an occupation within the environment. The validity of the findings can be strengthened by comparing similar information gathered at multiple points in time and establishing patterns of relationships, by ensuring that all of the important contributing factors are included in the evaluation, and by using tools that include an interview format in which clients or their proxy rate typical experiences with environmental factors across a time frame. It also is valuable to consider tools that incorporate a semi-structured interview or discussion with a client and his or her caregivers to further explore how the environment is influencing occupational performance and engagement. Most importantly, therapists can improve on their ability to assess the influence of the environment on occupational performance by having the environment rather than the person with disabilities be the focus or unit of measurement, and by concentrating their examination on what is occurring at the person-environment and occupation-environment interfaces.

It is also important to learn about a client's lived experience and become aware of what it means to a client to engage in and perform specific occupations within particular contexts. The concepts of place identity and place attachment can influence human behavior in various contexts, and are worth considering when assessing, interpreting assessment results, and planning environmental interventions. These concepts are rather complex, but in a nutshell, they arise from an individual's cognitions about daily experiences in the physical world in which he or she lives.[25,26] This physical world has attitudinal, cultural, physical, and organizational features. These cognitions influence one's attitudes, feelings, ideas, memories, and personal values about a place. Experiences in a place are stored in memory, and influence one's perceptions of place, whether good or bad. Time and experience in a place are important for deepening the meanings and emotional ties to a place.[27] These memories, in turn, influence feelings, attitudes, and beliefs about that place, and other places that share similar features.[25] Place attachment is built through one's personal experiences and connections to a place.[28] Place identity is a reflection of one's personal connection to a place, which shapes one's overall identity and one's sense of belonging and purpose.[27]

Both place identity and place attachment become important for occupational therapists to take into consideration, in particular if there is resistance to making environmental modifications. If a person has lived in a specific home for a long time, items that the therapist may perceive as clutter may in fact represent important family memories. Furniture that appears to be a barrier to optimal occupational performance may have sentimental value that needs to be respected. By asking key questions to get at the meaning of place for a client in specific situations, the therapist can come to appreciate why a client may be reluctant to make modifications to the environment or access certain types of environmental resources. This open discussion may enable conversations about adaptations and resources that are acceptable to the client.

Strategies for Selecting Environmental Measures

In selecting any assessment, the first step is to focus on the purpose of the assessment. See Chapter 4 for a discussion of this issue in detail. For environmental assessments, the purpose of the assessment may be determined by the focus of either the setting or the type of environmental factor that the therapist and client believe should be explored. For example, as in the scenario with Sue Lee, as Sue and Tomas begin to explore her housing options at college, an assessment of the physical accessibility of housing environments may be appropriate. However, in exploring transportation, an assessment of transit with a focus on physical and attitudinal environmental factors may be most appropriate. If a therapist wants to assess a client's ability to manage safely at home after discharge from the hospital, an assessment of physical and social supports with a focus on safety and the PEO transaction may be most appropriate.

The purpose also may be influenced by the societal and practice contexts in which the occupational therapist and client are situated.[6] The nature of the societal context includes the cultural, institutional, physical, and social environment. For example, in the case of Sue Lee, an environmental assessment that considers family and peer support and physical accessibility around campus is necessary as she enters the college setting. Additionally, the purpose may be influenced by the occupational therapist's practice context. For example, a therapist providing direct service to individuals or small groups of clients may use different accessibility instruments than a therapist involved in a consultative role to look at accessibility of a public building.

In most situations, an assessment must be located that fits with the client-centered approach to practice, and have good clinical utility. For example, the tool must be reasonably priced and culturally relevant, have adequate instructions, have clear scoring criteria, and be completed in a reasonable time frame dependent on the purpose of the assessment. Assessments also should have acceptable measurement properties. Ideally, environmental assessments would have evidence to support their content and/or construct validity, as well as reliability.

There are no measures that are comprehensive and address all environmental factors. Thus, depending on the purpose, it is appropriate in many situations to use a combination of tools that complement each other, with little overlap.

The influence of time and the complexity of issues raised in this chapter mean that simple, short environmental assessments may not provide the depth and accuracy of information necessary for therapists to accurately evaluate environmental effects on occupational performance. Specific, well-designed instruments may not always be available and choices may need to be made from among less than optimal measures. Under these circumstances, it is particularly important to be informed about the strengths and limitations of the available instruments.

Strategies for Reporting About Environmental Factors Influencing Occupational Performance and Engagement

When considering and sharing the results of environmental assessments, it is important to summarize what was assessed and what was found as a result of the assessment. Because environmental assessment can be diverse and broad, findings to be shared must return to the focus of the assessment (eg, the setting or the environmental focus).

Focusing on summaries of major environmental supports and barriers can be a very helpful way to share and discuss findings with clients or teams. For example, in the scenario of Sue Lee, Tomas could engage with Sue and her parents in an overview of the strengths and limitations of the campus environment in supporting students with disabilities. This might include supports through the university itself and a notation about the accessibility of libraries, classrooms, and campus eating establishments.

Depending on the context, it is common for the occupational therapist to formulate recommendations (usually in collaboration with the client) for environmental modifications based on environmental assessment results.[29,30] These recommendations are an important component of documentation. In formulating recommendations, it is important that recommendations are justified based on the assessment findings or other evidence, such as accessibility or universal design principles. Further, they need to be clear, specific, and framed in a way that the client (whether an individual or group) perceives them to be implementable. Often, recommendations are prioritized based on clear and transparent criteria. For example, recommendations for environmental modifications are often prioritized to ensure the safety of clients in the environment as a primary criterion. Ease of implementation may be a secondary means of prioritizing. For example, it may be easier for signage to be installed to promote orientation in a congregate living setting, rather than immediately replacing all carpets or flooring. Recommendations might be set so that easier adaptations are framed for short-term implementation, while more major modifications are framed as long-term recommendations. Cost associated with recommendations is also a consideration; often therapists suggest alternatives representing a range of costs that might achieve similar results based on clients' expressed goals.

Overview of Measures of Environmental Factors

Selection Criteria for Review

This chapter includes a wide variety of assessments of the environment, many of which have been developed by and for occupational therapists or others in rehabilitation, and those that therapists commonly use in practice and/or research. Some tools may not be familiar to therapists, but they may find these tools very useful in research and some practice settings, particularly when providing consultation regarding the needs of groups with common occupational issues. Most of the measures focus on adult and older adult settings; however, there are some excellent tools that focus on settings specific to children. Because the definition of environment is so broad, tools were selected from each of the categories of home, community, workplace, and school; and to assess attitudinal, physical, social, and institutional environmental factors. Tools that can be used with various client populations such as those with cognitive, mental health, physical, and sensory impairments were also included. Another criterion was to include tools that address environmental factors influencing occupational performance, participation in life situations, and/or social inclusion.

The tools selected for this chapter are the best that are currently available; they possess adequate to excellent measurement properties and clinical utility. A few promising new measures that have the potential to measure the person-environment relationship in a clinically useful manner, but for which sufficient psychometric information is not yet available, were also included. Tools were excluded if they were not easy to access, lacked administration and scoring instructions, or did not have evidence of adequate measurement properties.

List of Measures of Environmental Factors

Twenty-seven measurement tools are included in this chapter and listed in setting categories in Table 16-1. This table also identifies the broad environmental factors assessed by each instrument. Fourteen tools underwent a full review and are presented in alphabetical order in Tables 16-2 to 16-15. Most of these are either commonly used in practice and/or research, or would be an excellent addition to the therapist's toolkit. The others are briefly described in the following 2 sections. We have included only a few pertinent measures of social support because this topic is more fully addressed in Chapter 17; some child-specific measures are described more fully in Chapters 9, 10, and 12.

Recently Developed Instruments

Several promising new assessments of the person and environment have recently been developed and are worth mentioning here. For example, the European Child Environment Questionnaire (ECEQ) was developed for a large European study to assess the attitudinal, institutional, physical, and social environmental factors influencing the participation and quality of life of children with cerebral palsy.[31] This is a promising new tool that has been used successfully in research and may, in the future, be useful in clinical practice.[32]

The Measure of Environmental Qualities of Activity Settings (MEQAS)[33] was designed to measure the place- and opportunity-related qualities of leisure activity settings for young people. It is a 32-item observer-rated measure and is unique because it focuses on the activity setting as the conceptual unit of analysis. In an activity setting, activity happens in the context of the setting in which it occurs; thus, activity and environment are intertwined. Environmental qualities of the activity setting afford opportunities for youth participation. The MEQAS authors also developed a companion measure, the Self-reported Experiences of Activity Settings (SEAS), which enables youth to report their experiences in an activity setting.[34] These measures can be used by occupational therapists to design and assess youth leisure programs, particularly for "at risk" youth and those with disabilities.

Measures Worthy of Consideration by Occupational Therapists

There are a number of measures available for occupational therapy practice with older adults who live in sheltered care or nursing home environments. For example, the Therapeutic Environment Screening Survey for Nursing Homes (TESS-NH)[35] has been used in several recent studies[36,37] and is described in Table 16-12. The Multiphasic Environmental Assessment Procedure (MEAP)[38] is a comprehensive measure of sheltered care settings that has instruments that focus on the physical and architectural features of the setting as well as the policy and programs offered, and includes 5 different instruments based on resident and staff reports, direct observations, and record reviews. The instrument is standardized, with norms from 262 community and 81 veteran facilities, and has excellent reliability and validity.

The Measure of Quality of the Environment (MQE) Version 2[39] is a valid and reliable tool that is based on a modified ICF format.[40] It uses an interview format to evaluate the environment's facilitators and obstacles that influence a client's accomplishment of daily activities and social participation at home, in the workplace, and in the community. This assessment was developed for persons with physical disabilities but could be used with individuals with a variety of challenges. The long version (84 items) takes between 30 to 60 minutes to complete, while the short version takes only 10 minutes. The assessment was developed in French, and is also available in English, German, and Turkish. This useful tool can assist therapists, together with their clients of all ages, to identify both facilitators and obstacles to the client's participation in daily activities.

Maintaining Senior's Independence: A Guide to Home Adaptations[41] is a very useful tool for occupational therapists. It was developed to identify barriers to participation as a result of the physical and social home environment of older adults, and to provide adaptation strategies to support the independent participation in routine activities of daily living. It is administered through a semi-structured interview and includes observations of the client within his or her home. It addresses self-care and IADL in relation to environmental barriers. It also provides possible solutions for each of the 73 items, which the client and occupational therapist can review and discuss during the assessment.

The Environment-Independence Interaction Scale (EIIS)[42] was developed to measure features of the rehabilitation environment that affect human performance. It is appropriate for adults receiving rehabilitation services in either home or institutional settings. The scale is organized into 4 domains: physical, temporal, social, and cultural environmental factors. There are 4 parallel versions of the EIIS: home-family, home-professional care provider, institutional-family, and institutional-professional care provider. Information on the EIIS can be obtained from the University of Kansas School of Nursing, 3901 Rainbow Blvd., Kansas City, KA 66160-7502.

There are several tools that address children's environmental settings. Bundy[43] developed The Test of Environmental Supportiveness (TOES), which should be used together with her Test of Playfulness[44] to provide occupational therapists with a comprehensive picture of the play experience of any child, whether or not the child has a disability. This tool examines both the human and nonhuman factors that help or hinder a child's play. This tool is described in detail in Chapter 10. The Participation and Environment Measure for Children and Youth (PEM-CY) is a parent-report measure that allows parents to identify and appraise environmental factors that support or hinder their child's participation in their home, community, and school.[45] This tool is described in detail in Chapter 9.

A group of environmental rating scales published by the Frank Porter Graham (FGP) Child Development Institute, University of North Carolina at Chapel Hill (http://ers.fpg.unc.edu) was designed for use in child-care programs to assist in program design and evaluation, as well as staff training and supervision. The 4 measures are as follows:

1. Infant-Toddler Environment Rating Scale, Revised Edition[46] for children from birth to 2.5 years
2. Early Childhood Environment Rating Scale, Revised Edition[47] for children ages 2.5 to 5 years
3. Family Child Care Rating Scale, Revised Edition[48]
4. School-Age Care Environment Rating Scale, Updated Edition[49] for ages 5 to 12 years

The subscales in each tool address such environmental factors as space, furnishings, program structure, care routines, and resources to support child activities. Similarly, the authors of the HOME have developed Child Care HOME Inventories to assess the quality of home-based child-care settings where children are looked after by care providers who are not their parents.[50] These 2 measures (Infant and Toddler version and Early Childhood version) are structured like the HOME inventories, and focus on environmental affordances, and the child's opportunities and experiences in that setting. Therapists working in child-care settings may find these tools useful, particularly for roles involving program consultation and evaluation.

There are measures of the environment that are used in different fields of practice in which occupational therapists may work. An occupational therapist may want to become familiar with the measure even when he or she may not be the person administering it. For example, the Readily Achievable Checklist: A Survey for Accessibility (http://www.ada.gov/checkweb.htm) was developed for owners and managers of public buildings and businesses to identify barriers in their facilities. This survey tool is based on the Americans with Disabilities Act Accessibility Guidelines (ADAAG) and provides easy- to-use measurement guides to identify accessibility barriers, and suggestions for "readily achievable" access solutions. The occupational therapist can assist businesses to use this tool and set priorities for achieving accessibility.

Future Directions for Development and Utilization of Assessments of Environmental Factors

From this review, several areas for development were identified for measurement of the environment for both occupational therapy practice and research. Although there are quite a few measures of the environment that have been developed and tested, there are some gaps in areas of environmental focus addressed through available assessments. For example, while there are numerous home-based assessments of the environment in use by occupational therapists, there are fewer well-developed environmental measures focused on the community or public sphere. This includes not only physical accessibility, but assessments that incorporate social, attitudinal, and institutional supports and barriers. In particular, Brownson et al[51] argue that sociopolitical variables are also important to consider in concert with assessments of the physical environment. They describe the need to include sociopolitical variables in addition to measures of the built environment, and advocate for systematic attention to measuring social and cultural environments, and measures of policies that govern built environments. The broader cultural environment and macro-level political environment also appear to be largely unaddressed in current assessments of environmental factors and may provide interesting insights into barriers and facilitators to occupational performance.

Furthermore, there is a need for many of the assessments to be tested further in terms of measurement properties. This includes more research to ensure applicability to different types of environments and adoption within different cultural contexts, or with varying populations. This would help ensure a broader application of each instrument, and offer occupational therapists stronger measures from which to choose the most appropriate for each client situation. In addition, many assessments have been developed and used in research but are not as widely used in clinical practice. A focus on clinical utility as instruments are developed, tested, and revised is warranted. This may be addressed in part through research on versions of assessments that are either shortened to the most important items, or with computerized adaptive testing that adapts items based on earlier responses, allowing an efficient assessment of the construct being measured.

As occupational therapy practice expands, there may be a need for development of environmental measures appropriate for use in those emerging practice contexts. In particular, as occupational therapists make inroads into areas of consultation such as post-secondary education institutions and workplaces, broad environmental measures may be valuable to establish needs and recommendations for environmental interventions. Further, environmental assessments will be important in measuring outcomes. Thus, efforts to develop measures for clinical purposes, and to encourage their adoption in clinical contexts, are warranted.

Table 16-1

Measures of Environment

Category	Name of Measurement Tool	Factors Assessed
Adult and Older Adult Settings		
Home	HOME-FAST	Physical
	Maintaining Seniors Independence	Physical, Social
	SAFER & SAFER-HOME	Physical, Social
	The Housing Enabler	Physical
	Westmead Home Safety Ax (WeHSA)	Physical
Residential Setting	Environment Audit Tool (EAT)	Institutional, Physical
	Multiphasic Environmental Assessment Procedure	Institutional, Physical
	Therapeutic Environment Screening Survey for Nursing Homes (TESS-NH)	Institutional, Physical, Social
Home and Community	Home & Community Environment Survey (HACE)	Attitudinal, Physical
	Measure of Quality of Environment (MQE)	Attitudinal, Physical
Community	Facilitators and Barriers Survey/Mobility (FABS/M)	Attitudinal, Physical
	Readily Achievable Checklist	Physical
Workplace	Work Environment Impact Scale (WEIS)	Physical, Social
	Work Environment Scale (WES)	Institutional, Social
Home, Community, Workplace	Life Stressors & Social Resources Inventory—Adult and Youth (LISRES-A, LISRES-Y)	Social
	Craig Hospital Inventory of Environmental Factors	Attitudinal, Institutional, Physical, Social
	Measure of Quality of the Environment	Attitudinal, Institutional, Physical, Social
	Multidimensional Scale of Perceived Social Support (MSPSS)	Social
Child Settings		
Home	Home Environment: Home Observation for Measurement of the Environment (HOME)	Attitudinal, Physical, Social
Home and Community	Test of Environmental Supportiveness (TOES)	Physical, Social
	Measure of Ludic Behaviour	Physical, Social
	Measure of Environmental Qualities of Activity Settings (MEQAS)	Attitudinal, Physical, Social
Home, Community, School	European Child Environment Questionnaire (ECEQ)	Attitudinal, Institutional, Physical, Social
	Participation and Environment Measure – Child & Youth version (PEM-CY)	Attitudinal, Institutional, Physical, Social
Community (child care settings)	Environment Rating Scales: Infant-Toddler version, Early Childhood version, Family Child Care version, School-age Care version.	Institutional, Physical, Social
	Child Care HOME Inventories	Attitudinal, Institutional, Physical, Social
School	School Setting Interview	Physical, Social

Despite the need for ongoing development and adoption of assessments of the environment in practice, there is evidence to suggest that this area of assessment continues to evolve in practice. Assessing the environment is used throughout the occupational therapy practice processes to identify supports and barriers to occupational performance, and to plan and evaluate the effectiveness of environmental modifications to support optimal performance in context.

Table 16-2

Craig Hospital Inventory of Environmental Factors (CHIEF and CHIEF Short Form)

Source	The Centre for Outcome Measurement in Brain Injury at Craig Hospital http://tbims.org/combi/chief; http://www.tbims.org/combi/chief/CHIEF.pdf
Key References	Whiteneck et al[52]; Dijkers et al[53]; Fougeyrollas[54]; Whiteneck et al[55]; Fleming et al[56]
Purpose	• To evaluate environmental characteristics that hinder accomplishment of daily activities and social roles; to measure how individuals with a disability characterize the severity of perceived environmental barriers to social participation.
Type of Client	• Individuals with physical and/or sensory impairments including individuals with a variety of neurological issues (eg, stroke, traumatic brain injuries, spinal cord injuries). Only standardized tool that assesses environmental barriers with traumatic brain injured clients.[56]
Test Format	• Self-administered or administered by interview, either in person or by phone; can be administered through a proxy with client participation, should not be administered to proxy alone. • CHIEF: 25 items across 5 subscales: attitude and support; services and assistance; physical and structural; policies; work and school. • CHIEF Short Form: 12 items across the 5 subscales.
Procedures	• No training required to administer. Clear, comprehensive instructions; easy to administer, score, and interpret. • Frequency measured on 5-point scale, ranging from 0 = never to 4 = daily problem. Magnitude measured on a 3-point scale ranging from 0 = no problem to 2 = big problem. Frequency and magnitude ratings are averaged to obtain a total score (0 to 8). The higher the score, the greater the impact by environmental barriers.
Time Required	• Self-administered: 10 minutes, interviewer administered is approximately 15 minutes. CHIEF Short Form when self-administered: 5 minutes, and interviewer administered: approximately 10 minutes.
Standardization	• Published manual, including psychometric properties. http://tbims.org/combi/chief
Reliability	
Test-Retest	• Moderate to high ratings: ICC of 0.93 for total score; individual item scores for frequency and magnitude scales range from .033 to 0.88[52] • Brazilian Version: Used with children and adolescents with cerebral palsy: 0.28 to 1.0 for frequency score and 0.30 to 0.98 for the magnitude score. ICC ≥ 0.92[57] • Chinese version: ICC = 0.85 with chronic stroke clients[58]
Internal Consistency	• Field test of 10-item CHIEF for Children-Parent Version: Time 1 administration: 0.76, time 2: 0.78, ICC = 0.73 for total score[59] • Cronbach's α values with the disability sample was .93 for the total score and ranged from 0.76 to 0.81 for the subscales.[52]
Inter-Rater	• Persian Version: Greater than 96% of items correlated strongly with its own subscale rather than other subscales (r > 0.40). ICC > 0.70 and the values of the SEM were ≤ 1 for the score of subscales and total score. Cronbach's α = 0.86.[60] • Brazilian Version: each question: 0.28 to 1.0 for frequency score, 0.30 to 0.98 for magnitude score. ICC ≥ 0.92. • Chinese Version: Chronbach's α = 0.92[58] • Participant-proxy agreement analysis indicated that proxies not be asked to complete CHIEF when participants are unavailable to do so; proxy-participant agreement ICC range = 0.41 to .070 (total score ICC of 0.62).

(continued)

Table 16-2 (continued)

Craig Hospital Inventory of Environmental Factors (CHIEF and CHIEF Short Form)	
Validity	
Content	• Based on literature review and expert consultation consisting of 4 advisory panels (total of 32 participants), each focusing on a different area of disability issue (mobility, self-care, communication, and learning). Excellent representation from experts included academics, researchers, representatives from advocacy and policy implementation groups, and consumers.
Construct	• Demonstrated differences in reported frequency and magnitude of environmental barriers between groups with a variety of impairments and activity limitations[52,61] • High correlation between CHIEF and other measures for physical barriers, attitudinal barriers significantly correlated with relationship changes.[56] Average scores of 0.86 were found when compared individuals with severe disabilities with and without injuries.[62] • Perceived environmental barriers of elderly Taiwanese individuals were associated with difficulties in BADL and IADL.[63]
Criterion	• The impact of a child's disability on family and the perceived environmental supports and barriers predicted physical health-related quality of life in children with physical disabilities aged 6 to 14 years, when the Child Health Questionnaire was administered. Environmental barriers were assessed using the Chief.[64]
Utility	
Research Programs	• Environmental barrier items could be further researched with the aging population as it relates to participation limitations[63] and in the development of policies for individuals with traumatic brain injury.[56] • The adapted 10-item CHIEF for Child-Parent version needs further research.
Practice Settings	• No cost, available online from the Craig Hospital website. • Translated into Chinese. Has been used in Taiwan and Korea. Swedish, Portuguese, and Persian versions were created. Easy to use, comprehensive measure that can be interpreted easily and used with a variety of different diagnoses and cultures. • Can be used at the individual level to assess environmental barriers for those who have difficulties with BADL and IADL. • The adapted 10-item CHIEF shows promise in the clinical setting.
Strengths	• Very useful to assess the frequency and magnitude of a broad range of environmental barriers. • Manual: Instructions are clear, comprehensive, and available; outlines specific procedures for administration, scoring, interpretation; evidence of reliability and validity. • Based on ICF and addresses participation • Can be used for assessment and research that is both population- and individual-based. • Excellent evidence of psychometric properties • Consistent with a client-centered perspective • Can be used with a variety of different cultures

(continued)

Table 16-2 (continued)

CRAIG HOSPITAL INVENTORY OF ENVIRONMENTAL FACTORS (CHIEF AND CHIEF SHORT FORM)	
Complexities	• Had originally intended to measure both environmental facilitators and barriers, but focuses only on the environmental factors as barriers. Further research is needed to compare measures such as the CHIEF, that focus on barriers, with those such as the MQE, that also consider the positive aspects of the environment when used in the stroke population.[58] • Further validation with children is recommended. • Scale for assessing magnitude of barriers has only 3 points (no, little, or big problem), which makes it difficult to statistically analyze relationships. • May not be sensitive to small changes (floor effect). • Further evaluation of psychometric properties needed including problems with attitudes/policy category.[56] • When used as an adapted form for use with parents of children with cerebral palsy aged 5 to 16 years in New Zealand, the questionnaire was easy to use but there were reported difficulties in the interpretation of some items,[65] and use of examples may help clarify items.[57]

Table 16-3

FACILITATORS AND BARRIERS SURVEY/MOBILITY (FABS/M)	
Source	Available with appendix of the journal publication: Gray et al[66] Cost: Free with access to journal publication.
Key References	See above
Purpose	• To identify facilitators and barriers to participation that persons with lower limb mobility impairments encounter in their lived environment by means of a self-report survey • May be used at an individual level to develop community participation intervention and as an outcome measure[66]
Type of Client	• Populations with lower limb mobility limitations, age from adolescent to older adult; able to complete self-report survey from cognitive perspective; validated with 5 diagnostic groups (SCI, CP, MS, stroke, polio)[66]
Test Format	• 133 instrument items describe 6 domains: 1) personal mobility device; 2) home built features; 3) community built and natural features; 4) community destinations access; 5) community facilities access; 6) attitudes. • Ordinal scale response format for majority of items.
Procedures	• Self-report survey for those with no cognitive impairments. • Can be administered by interview; formal training requirements are not reported[66] • Interview format supports discussion about findings; this can lead to identification of intervention strategies.
Time Required	• Approximately 60 minutes to complete; this may vary depending on population characteristics.
Standardization	• Normative data provided in Gray et al.[66] Manual is not published.

(continued)

Table 16-3 (continued)

FACILITATORS AND BARRIERS SURVEY/MOBILITY (FABS/M)

Reliability	
Test-Retest	• Moderate to high reliability across 6 domains (n=604)[66]
Internal Consistency	• Cronbach α low to high values across 6 domains (moderate for community built features, attitudes; low for natural features; high for community destination access, facilities)[66]
Inter-Rater	• Not established
Validity	
Content	• Instrument items formed from qualitative interview data based on the ICF framework; purposive sample included a) persons from 5 diagnostic populations (spinal cord injury [SCI], cerebral palsy [CP], multiple sclerosis [MS], stroke, polio); b) using a range of mobility devices; c) significant others and health care professionals providing care.[66]
Construct	• Pilot tested (n=40, 5 diagnostic groups); adjusted to improve scoring and comprehension clarity[66] • FABS/M scores distinguished between diagnostics groups (SCI, CP, MS, stroke, polio) and mobility device user groups[66]
Criterion	• Not established
Utility	
Research Programs	• Survey-based administration method may be feasible for large-scale rehabilitation studies and community advocacy projects. • Instrument items may be applicable to future studies exploring barriers and facilitators to participation during initial encounters with environmental demands.
Practice Settings	• Can be used at the individual level to develop community participation interventions and also an outcome measure of the effectiveness of those interventions. • English language and cognitive demands to complete survey may limit access to some populations.
Strengths	• Focused specifically for people with lower limb mobility impairments and limitations. • Scores can be aggregated across diagnostic groups and/or mobility device groups for broader view of environmental factors influencing participation.
Complexities	• Exclusively language-based method of survey (eg, no illustrative figures provided), language and cognitive barriers should be considered. • Cognitive demands should be considered with easily fatigued populations. • Psychometric properties established in one study with a purposive sample of 5 diagnostic groups; instrument has limited generalizability to other groups[66]; further measurement studies recommended. • Considerations should also be given to time since impairment occurred; instrument items were not developed from a sample of persons newly interacting with the environment; some barriers to participation may have occurred in the distant past and not have been identified.[66]

Table 16-4

Home and Community Environment (HACE) Instrument

Source	http://www.medicaljournals.se/jrm/content/?doi=10.1080/16501970410014830 Contact: Dr. Julie J. Keysor, Associate Professor, Department of Physical Therapy and Athletic Training, Boston University. E-mail: jkeysor@bu.edu Cost: Free.
Key References	Keysor et al[67]
Purpose	• To provide a self-report assessment of physical and social characteristics of an individual's home and community environment
Type of Client	• Initial psychometric evidence established with a sample of community-dwelling adults and older adults[67] • Future directions aim to expand to incorporate populations with more complex functional limitations (eg, wheelchair use).
Test Format	• 36 instrument items cover 6 conceptual domains: 1) home mobility; 2) community mobility; 3) basic mobility devices; 4) communication devices; 5) transportation factors; 6) attitudes. • Item response options vary within and between each of the 6 conceptual domains (eg, home mobility item response options consist of dichotomous [yes/no] items; attitudes items response options consist of ordinal scale items).
Procedures	• In research phase, trained assessors administer HACE items.[67] Can be completed as self-report in the community context.
Time Required	• Approximately 10 minutes for administration and scoring; total administration time may vary with environmental context.
Standardization	• Not a standardized assessment. No norms established. A manual has not been published.
Reliability	
Test-Retest	• Median percent agreement for 6 domains ranged from 75% to 100%; median Kappa values ranged from 0.47 to 1.0.[67]
Internal Consistency	• Not established
Inter-Rater	• Not established
Validity	
Content	• Instrument items compiled from literature review, expert consultation, and field-testing[67]
Construct	• Authors extracted attractive features from existing measures[67]
Criterion	• Not established
Utility	
Research Programs	• Promising instrument that may be used with future population-based rehabilitation outcome studies; short administration time (approximately 10 minutes) and limited scoring demands make it feasible for large-scale data collection where study costs and participant burden are critical considerations.[67]
Practice Settings	• Instrument primarily for population-based research. However, it may be used with individual clients to characterize aspects of the physical and social environment that restrict or facilitate participation in the home and community.

(continued)

Table 16-4 (continued)

Home and Community Environment (HACE) Instrument

Strengths	• Encouraging initial psychometric evidence supports the HACE as a promising self-report instrument. • Promising instrument for use with large-scale rehabilitation outcomes studies.
Complexities	• Measurement properties require further investigation in studies with varying geographical and cultural characteristics, and with larger, diverse samples. Plus, longitudinal data are needed to understand how the person-environment interaction limits or facilitates participation in activities of daily living. • Initial psychometric properties established in only one sample; thus generalizability of findings is limited. • Limited to those with English speaking abilities and intact or minimal level of cognitive impairment.

Table 16-5

Home Observation for Measurement of the Environment (HOME) (Revised Edition, 2003)

Source	Caldwell and Bradley[68]; http://fhdri.clas.asu.edu/home/index.html
Key References	Bradley et al[69-71]; Totsika and Sylva[72]
Purpose	• To describe and discriminate the quality and quantity of stimulation and support for cognitive, social, and emotional development available to a child in the home environment. • To profile the child's opportunities and experiences at home.
Type of Client	• Children and adolescents aged 0 to 15 years with all diagnoses. There are separate versions for 4 different age groupings. Respondents may include caregivers, service providers, and other professionals.
Test Format	• Semi-structured interview and naturalistic observation during home visit; noninvasive, but requires active participation of child and caregiver.
Procedures	• Easy to administer and score; more complex to interpret. Training tapes are available and recommended. There are different subscales for each version of the measure: ¤ Infant/toddler (0 to 3 years): responsivity; acceptance; organization; learning materials; involvement; variety ¤ Early childhood (3 to 6 years): learning materials; language stimulation; physical environment; responsivity; learning stimulation; modeling of social maturity; variety in experience; acceptance ¤ Middle childhood (6 to 10 years): responsivity; encouraging maturity; learning materials; active stimulation; emotional climate; physical environment; parental involvement; family participation ¤ Early adolescence (10 to 14 years): physical environment; learning materials; modeling; instructional activities; regulatory activities; variety of experience; acceptance; responsivity • Items are presented as statements to be scored as YES or NO. Items can be rated by observing the child and caregiver in the home and/or by asking the caregiver questions.

(continued)

Table 16-5 (continued)

HOME Observation for Measurement of the Environment (HOME) (Revised Edition, 2003)	
Procedures	• Scoring: Each subscale's score is simply the number of "yes" responses. Higher number of "yes" scores indicates a more enriched home environment in relation to the child's contextual and organismic features. Scores falling in the lower quarter of the scoring range indicates the environment may pose a risk to aspects of the child's development.
Time Required	• 45 to 90 minutes to administer and score.
Standardization	• Both an administrative manual and a summary of research are available. • Norms: 0 to 15 years. Norms available for typical children and for children with multiple handicaps[68]
Reliability	• Reviews of research on HOME can be found in numerous publications noted on HOME website (http://fhdri.clas.asu.edu/home/)[69,71,73]
Test-Retest	• Not examined due to nature of the test.[69] Long-term stability between 6 to 24 months on total score was moderate: r=0.64.
Internal Consistency	• Cronbach's α for Infant/toddler version=0.89 total score and 0.44 to 0.89 for subscores; early childhood version=0.93 total score and 0.53 to 0.88 for subscores; middle childhood version=0.90 total score and 0.53 to 0.90 for subscores; early adolescent version=above 0.90 for total score[68]
Inter-Rater	• Average of 90% agreement in 3 studies and 90% to 96% in another.[74] Bradley[75] reports agreement never fell below 80%. Many researchers in various countries have conducted examined interrater agreement within their studies and have found >80% agreement.[76]
Validity	
Content	• Factor analysis aided in the formation of empirically distinct, psychometrically sound, conceptual subscales. Items clustered to fit groupings supported by research and theory. Field testing was conducted with each version of the tool with large samples to address item clarity and relevance.
Construct	• More than 2 studies that demonstrated confirmation of theoretical formulations. HOME was able to discriminate children of different IQ levels. Correlations between HOME scores and IQ levels, poverty levels, and prematurity[73,77]
Criterion	• Small to moderate correlations were found between HOME and 7 socioeconomic status variables, including poverty levels.
Utility	
Research Programs	• Has been used in a wide variety of research and clinical settings throughout North and South America (including the Caribbean), in several European and Asian countries, in Australia, and in at least 2 African nations. It can and has been used for epidemiology studies and to evaluate the impact of intervention programs. Reviews of research on the HOME can be found in several studies.[69,71,73,77]
Practice Settings	• Very useful for examining the amount of stimulation available to a child in the home environment in relation to child development and opportunities for the child to learn. The specific findings from this tool are useful for guiding intervention planning. The interview component provides a good starting point from which to collaborate with a parent regarding how to modify the home setting.

(continued)

Table 16-5 (continued)

Home Observation for Measurement of the Environment (HOME) (Revised Edition, 2003)

Strengths	• Has been used successfully in practice and in research. Strong psychometric properties. • Easy to administer and score; nonthreatening to parent or child • Can complete and score at the same time. • Very useful for describing the main areas of the child's home environment; broader and more useful than other instruments. • Interviews provide time limits: focus on specific occurrences of specific day or week, which means that the occupational therapist can elicit more objective information on the actual occurrences in the child's life rather than on the parent's mental representations/feelings about the occurrences. However, there is still a time at the end of the interview for the parent to express his or her perspective. • Has been used to study at-risk populations and non-normative populations and can detect differences in a child's development due to poverty and prematurity.
Complexities	• Information obtained by only one parent on one occasion might not be representative of a child's full life conditions. • Binary measurement scale is easy for interviewer to score, but does not give occupational therapists enough information to make informed judgments.

Table 16-6

Home Falls and Accidents Screening Tool (HOME FAST)

Source	Mackenzie et al[78]; the Appendix includes HOME FAST items along with definitions. http://www.bhps.org.uk/falls/documents/HomeFast.pdf Cost: Free
Key References	Mackenzie et al[79-81]; Mehraban et al[82]
Purpose	• Screening instrument designed to identify community-dwelling older adults at risk of falls as a result of home hazards.
Type of Client	• Developed for use with a community-based population of older adults.
Test Format	• 25-item screening tool; nominal scoring; naturalistic observation.
Procedures	• Clinicians use judgment and observation to identify home hazards.[80]
Time Required	• Approximately 20 to 30 minutes to administer and score; total time will vary according to clinical setting and purpose. • 25 items are scored as "hazard," "not a hazard," or "not applicable." Definitions are provided for each item to assist with scoring.
Standardization	• No manual has been published. No norms exist.
Reliability	
Test-Retest	• Not established
Internal Consistency	• Cronbach's α for the overall scale was 0.95.[80]

(continued)

Table 16-6 (continued)

HOME FALLS AND ACCIDENTS SCREENING TOOL (HOME FAST)

Reliability	
Inter-Rater	• Fair to good level of agreement between raters in one study (n = 40, overall kappa = 0.62); noteworthy, raters ranged in degree of professional qualifications; one item "hazardous outside paths" demonstrates poor agreement (n = 40, kappa = 0.30); level of agreement is stable among raters regardless of number of hazards present in the home.[80]
Validity	
Content	• Instrument development consisted of compilation of large item pool from published home hazards checklists literature review, field testing (n = 83 older adults), reduction of items by expert panel consultation.[78] • Content was further examined through a cross-national validation (Australia, Canada, and United Kingdom) that asked occupational therapists, physiotherapists, and nurses to respond to a survey regarding the content and weighting of HOME FAST items.[79]
Construct	• Initial evidence suggests that some HOME FAST items (ie, 7 of 25) may be useful in identifying relative risk for falls associated with exposure to home hazards (CI = 99%, n = 19).[78]
Criterion	• Not established
Predictive	• One study evaluated predictive validity (n = 727, age > 70 years)[81]; logistic regression modeling revealed having a fall per unit increase in HOME FAST score (odds ratio 1.106, 95% CI, p = 0.006)
Responsiveness	• One study evaluated the responsiveness of the HOME FAST to change in the home environment (n = 727, age > 70 years)[81]; changes in prevalence of items show p ≤ 0.05 from baseline to follow-up.
Utility	
Research Programs	• Investigators are extending the utility of the HOME-FAST by introducing a self-report version (HOME-FAST SR) that will assist older adults to identify their own falls risk.[82] • Initial research findings suggest HOME-FAST SR shows promise to become a feasible tool to be used in community-based self-evaluation of home environment falls risk. HOME-FAST SR was designed using expert review, pretesting, piloting testing; psychometric investigation (n = 568, age > 67 years) shows moderate agreement among self-reported (HOME-FAST SR) and professional ratings (HOME-FAST).
Practice Settings	• Noninvasive, easily accessible screening instrument. • Can be used to identify older adults at risk of falls, and to facilitate referral for a more detailed assessment and/or recommendations for interventions.
Strengths	• Quick administration/scoring as a screening assessment. • Validated internationally (Australia, UK). • Promising psychometric properties as a screening tool.
Complexities	• Encouraging psychometric properties; however, it is important to consider that further research in this area is required with larger sample sizes and with longitudinal information rather than mostly cross-sectional data. • Initial evidence suggests that identification of hazards and subsequent home modification intervention can reduce the odds of falls by 1% to 2% for every point score. • It is noteworthy to critically reflect on falls risk as a multidimensional phenomenon with multiple contributing factors when interpreting findings.

Table 16-7

The Housing Enabler

Source	http://enabler.nu/ Cost: variable according to currency conversion (starting at $360 USD for multiple user license).
Key References	Carlsson et al[83]; Fänge and Iwarsson[84]; Iwarsson et al[15,85,86]
Purpose	• To describe, evaluate, and predict the congruence or fit between an individual with a mobility impairment and the home environment.
Type of Client	• Designed for but not limited to use with older adults, suitable for any diagnostic category. Additional populations include caregivers and other professionals (eg, architects and planners). Suitable for individual testing or assessment at a group/population level.
Test Format	• Semi-structured interview; noninvasive observation of performance in the home environment. • Phase 1 consists of 15 items concerning individual's functional limitations: functional abilities (13), dependence on mobility aids (2). • Phase 2 consists of 188 items divided into 4 environmental subscales: outdoor conditions (33); entrances (49); indoor conditions (100); and communication (6).
Procedures	• Training in administration/scoring procedures highly recommended; available from contact with the authors. Administration involves: ¤ Phase 1 (personal component of accessibility) assesses individual's functional limitations, including dependency on mobility devices, using interview and observation. ¤ Phase 2 (environment component of accessibility) identifies barriers in the environment (outdoor/indoor/communication). ¤ Phases 1 and 2 use dichotomous ratings (nominal); Phase 1 and 2 subscores can be used independently. ¤ Phase 3 various predefined assessment items compute to produce a total person-environment fit score predicting the degree of accessibility challenges (ordinal: 4-point Likert scale), score can be validated through additional performance testing.
Time Required	• Approximately 2 hours to administer, depending on functional limitations and the physical environment. Phase 1 and Phase 2 do not require a quantitative measure of the degree of accessibility challenges; the presentation of results constitutes a systematic checklist. Phase 3 constitutes calculation of a total score; use of Housing Enabler 1.0 scoring software highly advised.
Standardization	• Manual available in English through author at the University of Lund, Sweden and outlines: ¤ Administration procedures ¤ Scoring and interpretation ¤ Evidence of psychometric properties ¤ Available norms
Reliability	
Test-Retest	• ICC = 0.92 to 0.98[85]
Internal Consistency	• Not established

(continued)

Table 16-7 (continued)

THE HOUSING ENABLER

Reliability	
Inter-Rater	• Three studies reported the following[85]: 1. Pilot 1 (n=416 occupational therapists and 1 building) 100% agreement for 46% environmental items and 81% to 94% agreement for 27% items. 2. Pilot 2 (n=440 occupational therapists and 26 cases) overall mean Kappa=0.76 for person and 0.55 for environment. 3. Pilot 3 (n=430 occupational therapists and 30 cases) mean Kappa 0.82 for person, 0.68 for environment (188 items), and 0.87 for accessibility problems; ICC range=0.92 to 0.98. • Moderate to good percentage agreement and kappa results (n=64) from a multinational population (5 European countries, raters of various professional backgrounds) for personal component and environment parts.[86]
Validity	
Content	• Item selection based on literature review and expert opinion; adjusted after pilot studies. Epidemiological data required when used with populations.
Construct	• Theoretical agreement for person-environment relationship and for construct of housing accessibility[87,88]
Criterion	• Swedish accessible housing standards provide the gold standard against which the environmental assessments are measured. • Iwarsson et al[89] found the person-environment fit score is strong predictor of falls in older adults (odds ratio=1.02, p=0.03, n=834).
Responsiveness	• In 3 separate studies, person-environment fit scores captured significant differences between baseline and follow-up time frames.[84,90,91]
Utility	
Research Programs	• Useful for cross-national research exploring housing accessibility[86] • The Housing Enabler Screening Tool was recently developed and is much quicker to administer and score.[83] Initial pilot testing and psychometric properties show that it is a promising new instrument. Available in English at www.enabler.nu
Practice Settings	• Very useful for examining home accessibility. • Results can be used to guide interventions at an individual level, and advocacy efforts at a policy level to overcome environmental barriers to accessibility. • Instrument and manual adapted for use in 7 languages, including cross-national adaptation to norms and region specific guidelines for housing standards. More extensively used in European countries.
Strengths	• Meticulous development; established psychometric properties. • Ongoing use in both clinical and varied research settings. • Easily accessible from up-to-date website.
Complexities	• Phase 2 is time-consuming to administer and requires familiarity with assessing functional demands, physical barriers in the physical environment, and knowledge of accessibility standards. • Without the use of Housing Enabler 1.0 software, calculation of Phase 3 (person-environment fit score) predictive score is complex and susceptible to calculation error due to large amount of data processing.

Table 16-8

Life Stressors and Social Resources Inventory— Adult and Youth (LISRES-A; LISRES-Y)

Source	Psychological Assessment Resources Inc., PO Box 998, Odessa, FL 33556; 1-800-331-8378 www.parinc.com
Key References	Moos[92]; Moos et al[93,94]; Holanah et al[95]
Purpose	• To provide a profile of an individual's life context, including his or her life stressors and social resources. • Used to monitor stability and changes; can compare individuals and groups and evaluate the effect life events have on an individual's functioning and situation.
Type of Client	• LISRES-A: Adults 18 years and older. • Healthy adults; or those with mental health, substance abuse, or medical issues. • LISRES-Y: Youths 12 to 18 years. • Healthy teenagers; or those with conduct disorders, psychiatric or medical conditions.
Test Format	• LISRES-A: Self-report or interview of positive and negative life stressors and social resources in 8 domains: physical health, spouse/partner, finances, work, home/neighborhood, children, friends and social activities, and extended family. • LISRES-Y: 8 domains of life experiences: physical health, home and money, school, parents, siblings, extended family, boyfriend/girlfriend, friends, and social activities. • 200 items in 8-page item booklet using dichotomous and Likert-type scales, documented in 2-part answer/profile form. • Manual with 10 reusable item booklets and 50 answer/profile forms = $210 USD plus shipping. • Manual = $46 USD; Reuseable item booklets = $46 /10 pkg; Hand-scorable Answer/Profile Forms = $72/25 package plus tax and shipping. Adult and Youth versions are the same price.
Procedures	• Structured interview administered in groups or individually. Can be administered in groups or individually as a structured interview with individuals who have a minimum of sixth grade reading and comprehension • No formal training required. • LISRES A: 16 subscales: 9 life stressors (provides an index of negative life events) and 7 social resources (provides an index of positive life events). Subscales can be used independently. No summary score or total score.
Time Required	• 30 to 60 minutes to administer, 20 minutes to score. • Manual instructions are clear, comprehensive, available, outlines procedures for administration, scoring and interpretation.
Standardization	• Norms: LISRES-A: Based on a sample of 1884 adults (1181 men and 703 women). • LISRES-Y based on a sample of 400 youth.
Reliability	
Test-Retest	• At 4- and 7-year follow-ups: moderate to high for all scales except work, negative and positive events.
Internal Consistency	• LISRES A: Stressor scales—0.77 to 0.93; Social Resources scales -0.50 to 0.92. • LISRES Y: Stressor Scales—66 to 0.92; Social Resources scales-0.78 to 0.93. • Evaluation of subsets with a parallel set of items of quality of relationships in high-risk alcohol consumption in older adults with spouse—Chronbach's $\alpha = 0.90$; quality of relationships with extended family members—Chronbach's $\alpha = 0.80$; adequacy of finances—Chronbach's $\alpha = 0.84$[93]

(continued)

Table 16-8 (continued)

Life Stressors and Social Resources Inventory—Adult and Youth (LISRES-A; LISRES-Y)

Reliability	
Internal Consistency	• Family's adaptation to a traumatic brain injury in young children stressors—Chronbach's α = 0.71; and resources—Chronbach's α = 0.60.[96] The social environment correlates with perceived family stress after a traumatic brain injury.[96]
Inter-Rater	• N/A
Validity	
Content	• Based on review of the literature and research with 2 pilot studies (18 months apart) involving clients with the following: depression, alcoholism, arthritis, and healthy adults.
Construct	• Socio-demographic variables correlate with stressors and resources consistently across numerous studies. • Discriminative between diagnoses, treatment outcomes, and health in adults with substance abuse, depression, and cardiac and arthritic conditions • Theoretical constructs concerning inter-relationships amongst stress, resources, and coping are well supported in research. • Evaluation of AA self-help groups confirmed friendly networks and coping style mediates effects of group.[97] Increased peer support associated with less distress and police involvement for alcoholics.[98] Older moderate drinkers of alcohol who engaged in episodic heavy drinking had increased mortality.[95] The quality of the spousal relationship and financial resources increased the risk of alcohol consumption in older adults.[93]
Criterion	• A child's social environment had an effect on math achievement.[99] • Initial support of a cumulative risk index to predict family burden following childhood traumatic brain injury with use of LISRES-A.[100]
Responsiveness	• N/A
Utility	
Research Programs	• Used to evaluate stress, resources, and coping. Much research on individuals with alcohol-related issues. Some research on caregivers of children with traumatic brain injuries.
Practice Settings	• Occupational therapists are well poised to research the relationship between alcohol consumption, stressor/supports on occupational performance. • Can be used with individuals with a variety of physical health and mental health issues including depression, substance abuse, cardiac, arthritic conditions, or traumatic head injury. • Limited use in occupational therapy practice settings, but could be used in settings where stress, resources, and coping influence occupational performance issues. • The client's narrative regarding stressors and supports can be explored using this assessment. • Occupational therapists can take more of an active role in the assessment of individuals with substance abuse issues using this assessment. • An assessment of stressors and supports can become standard practice in the university setting to optimize students' occupational performance.

(continued)

Table 16-8 (continued)

Life Stressors and Social Resources Inventory—Adult and Youth (LISRES-A; LISRES-Y)

Strengths	• Examines both stressors and social supports of adults and youth • Well standardized. • Excellent evidence of psychometric properties. • Internally consistent, valid tool with different populations. • Relatively inexpensive to purchase • Fairly quick and easy to administer, score, and interpret. • Can be used for assessment and research that is both population- and individual-based.
Complexities	• No items on spirituality. • Very little research on populations of different cultures.

Table 16-9

The Multidimensional Scale of Perceived Social Support (MSPSS)

Source	Zimet et al[101]
Key References	Stanley et al[102]; Zimet et al[103]; Canty-Mitchell and Zimet[104]
Purpose	• To assess perceptions of social support adequacy from family, friends, and significant other.
Type of Client	• Adolescents, adults, and older adults. • Used with a variety of psychiatric conditions (eg, generalized anxiety, depression, schizophrenia), postsurgical treatment (eg, cardiac, cancer, end-stage renal disease), ABI caregivers, marginalized groups (eg, incarcerated women). • Measure used in a variety of countries including US, Turkey, Italy, China, Hong Kong, and South Asia.
Test Format	• List of 12 statements of relationships with family, friends, and significant other. A 7-point Likert-type scale ranging from "very strongly disagree" (1) to "very strongly agree" (7) are rated.
Procedures	• Responses are averaged to create total and subscale scores. Higher scores indicate higher perceived social support. • No training required.
Time Required	• 2 to 5 minutes.
Standardization	• No published manual • Published norms for the general adult Western population[105]; general adult Italian[106,107]; Chinese students[108]; psychiatry, surgical, and general population in Turkey[109]; adolescents in Hong Kong[110] and Europe[103]; US young and older adults with and without generalized anxiety[102]; young adults with and without significant psychopathology living in the community[111]; and US surgical patients with and without depression[112-114]

(continued)

Table 16-9 (continued)

THE MULTIDIMENSIONAL SCALE OF PERCEIVED SOCIAL SUPPORT (MSPSS)

Reliability	
Test-Retest	• After 2 to 3 months with 69 undergraduate psychology students: subscales (0.72, 0.85, 0.75), total score (0.85)[101] • Malaysian medical students 0.77,[115] Tamil version 0.71[115] • With 94 older adults with no diagnosable psychiatric disorder, subscales (friends 0.73, family 0.74) and total scale (0.70) were adequate, except significant other subscale was low (0.54),[102] adolescent youth's mental health in South Africa (0.50 to 0.70)[116]
Internal Consistency	• Cronbach's α in these studies ranged consistently from 0.81 to 0.91 • Cronbach's α in following studies: adult Asian population with schizophrenia, 0.90 to 0.91[117]; Malaysian medical students, 0.89[118]; Tamil version, 0.92[115]; Thai version used with medical students and psychiatric patients, 0.91 and 0.87, respectively; South Asian population, 0.92[119]
Inter-Rater	• N/A
Validity	
Content	• Principal component factor analysis confirmed subscale groupings with different groups and cultures[101-103,108,109,111,120]
Construct	• Demonstrated positive relationships with health; compared to generalized anxiety in older adults,[102] to significant psychopathology in young adults,[111] or to depression in surgical patients[112-114] • Positive relationships between marriage and significant other subscale with no differences on family or friend subscales for pediatric residents; positive relationships with family subscale and frequency among adolescents sharing concerns with mother[103] • Marginalized groups have lower perceived social support (psychiatry[109]; incarcerated women[121]). • Total scores correlate with self-esteem and life satisfaction[122,123]; spirituality and religiosity[124] • 3-factor structure demonstrated high validity and reliability in adult outpatients in Singapore[117]
Criterion	• Not applicable
Utility	
Research Programs	• Used extensively in research programs (eg, used in research to distinguish between groups), and clinically to identify needs • Can be used as an outcome measure to evaluate treatment interventions
Practice Settings	• Could be used for needs assessment and as outcome measurement in the clinical setting
Strengths	• Easy to administer and score in a short time • Evidence for use across a variety of cultures • Consistent with client-centered practice • One of the most widely used self-report social support measures
Complexities	• Need to be wary of socially desirable responses • Requires evaluation of sensitivity to change

Table 16-10

Safety Assessment of Function and the Environment for Rehabilitation Tool (SAFER) and Safety Assessment of Function and the Environment for Rehabilitation—Health Outcome Measurement and Evaluation (SAFER-HOME V3)

Source	VHA Rehab Solutions, Toronto, Canada. E-mail: info@vha.ca Website: http://www.vha.ca/resources/publications-for-sale Cost: $100.00 (manual and 10 forms)
Key References	Letts and Marshall[125]; Chui et al[126]; Letts et al[127]; Chui and Oliver[128]
Purpose	• The SAFER Tool was developed to identify safety concerns of individuals in the home environment and collect information to plan interventions and recommendations to improve safety. • The SAFER-HOME V3 is designed to measure change in safety over time (to evaluate the effectiveness of interventions to improve home safety). • The SAFER-HOME V3 has replaced the SAFER Tool.
Type of Client	• Originally developed for psychogeriatric population; later, it was expanded to meet the needs of adult clients with physical disabilities. Frequently used for clients with multiple comorbidities, diverse diagnosis, and complex needs.
Test Format	• Interview with client and/or caregivers, observation of task performance, naturalistic observation. • SAFER Tool consists of 97 items categorized into 14 domains: living situation, mobility, kitchen, fire hazards, eating, household, dressing, grooming, bathroom, medication, communication, wandering, memory aids and general.[125] • SAFER-HOME V3 consists of 74 items categorized into 12 domains: living situation; mobility; kitchen; environmental hazards; household; eating; bathroom and toilet; medication, addiction and abuse; leisure; communication and scheduling; personal care and wandering.[126]
Procedures	• Semi-structured interview and naturalistic observation carried out in home environment.
Time Required	• Approximately 45 to 90 minutes to administer depending on the home environment context; time allotted for interpretation of scores and intervention recommendations will vary according to complexity of the context. Paper/pencil reporting format. • SAFER Tool items are scored on 2-point scale as "problem" or "not a problem."[125] • SAFER-HOME V3 items are scored on a 4-point ordinal scale as: "no problem," "mild problem," "moderate problem," or "severe problem."[126]
Standardization	• The SAFER Tool and SAFER HOME are not standardized in administration format. A manual is available, describing background information, administration instructions, guidelines for considering each item, potential recommendations for each item if identified as a problem, and 4 example case studies. Norms are not available. Manual provides information about a reference group of occupational therapy clients (n = 563, mean age = 78 years).
Reliability	
Test-Retest	• SAFER Tool: Kappa or % agreement = acceptable to excellent for 90 items (n = 38, mean age = 77 years)[127] • SAFER HOME: No data available

(continued)

Table 16-10 (continued)

Safety Assessment of Function and the Environment for Rehabilitation Tool (SAFER) and Safety Assessment of Function and the Environment for Rehabilitation—Health Outcome Measurement and Evaluation (SAFER-HOME V3)

Reliability	
Internal Consistency	• SAFER Tool: Kuder-Richardson 20 estimate = 0.83[125] • SAFER-HOME V2: Cronbach's α for total scores = 0.86; subscales range from 0.54 to 0.79[128]
Inter-Rater	• SAFER Tool: Kappa statistic = acceptable (59 of 66 items)[127] • SAFER HOME: No data available
Validity	
Content	• For both the SAFER Tool and the SAFER-HOME V1-3, content validity established through review by experts and clinicians as well as statistical analysis of completed measures
Construct	• SAFER Tool: Total scores have been associated with cognitive status and independent living in houses, but not directly to ADL or IADL. • SAFER-HOME V2: Total scores were compared to functional status scores using the SMAF. The correlation was weak, which confirmed that the SAFER HOME V2 is measuring more than functional abilities.[128]
Criterion	• Not established
Responsiveness	• Not established. It is hypothesized that the SAFER-HOME V3 will be more sensitive to change as a result of a 4-point rating response format for each item.
Utility	
Research Programs	• Promising instrument to facilitate rehabilitation research as an outcome measure that uniquely considers the person-environment relationship
Practice Settings	• Instrument available for purchase in both English and French • Manual provides case study examples and administration/scoring guidance • Commonly used in occupational therapy practice in Canada; however, length of administration may be a barrier for use in some practice settings
Strengths	• Both instruments are unique in that they focus on all areas of function to provide a comprehensive analysis of home safety. • Both instruments emphasize the interaction between the person and the physical and social home environment to assist clinicians in optimizing intervention strategies. • Both the SAFER Tool and SAFER-HOME show promising psychometric properties.
Complexities	• Lengthy administration may be a problem for easily fatigued populations. • Unique focus on the person-environment interactions to evaluate skills/abilities of the person in the context of the home environment • Limited research on responsiveness to change, which may limit utility as an outcome measure

Table 16-11

School Setting Interview (SSI) Version 3.0 (2005)

Source	Available in English in the US and Canada from MOHO: http://www.cade.uic.edu/moho/productDetails.aspx?aid=10 Cost: $40 USD Available in Europe and other English speaking countries from the Swedish Association of Occupational Therapists.
Key References	Egilson and Hemmingsson[129]; Hemmingsson et al[30,130,131]
Purpose	• To examine the level of person-environment fit of students with disabilities to facilitate the planning of occupational therapy interventions in schools • The SSI focuses on physical and social environmental barriers and facilitators to a student's inclusion and participation in the school setting.
Type of Client	• Originally developed for school-aged children with motor dysfunction from 9 to 19 years of age. Can also be used with children with developmental and psychosocial disabilities
Test Format	• Semi-structured client-centered interview with student; contains 16 items with suggested follow-up questions to explore the student's functioning and need for adjustments to physical and/or social environment at school. • Manual is available for a fee of only $40 USD.
Procedures	• Semi-structured interview to first provide a context with which to understand the student's experience of school. Questionnaire—Needs for Adjustments (16 items): The therapist addresses each item as a discussion with student. If the student has recently changed schools, teachers, or classes, he or she will be asked questions about these past experiences. The therapist also asks about present and future situations at school. The therapist, together with student, rates each item on a 4-step scale, ranging from 1 (unfit—needs new adjustments) to 4 (perfect fit—no need for adjustments). • Summary Sheet: provides an overview of the student-environment fit • Planning Intervention form: used to plan the occupational therapy intervention. The therapist works collaboratively with the student to plan and implement adjustments in the school setting for items where there is poor student-environment fit. They identify environmental adjustments to make (both physical and social), team members to be involved, and steps for implementation (who, when, where, and how). • Training (about 1.5 hours) is recommended.
Time Required	• To administer and score: 40 minutes
Standardization	• User manual and score sheets available in English, Swedish, and Spanish. Has been translated into Icelandic and has undergone psychometric testing in that language
Reliability	
Test-Retest	• Reported as 90% agreement for total score; range of 76% to 100% across content areas[132]
Internal Consistency	• Not reported
Inter-Rater	• Kappa ranged between 0.76 to 1.0

(continued)

Table 16-11 (continued)

School Setting Interview (SSI) Version 3.0 (2005)

Validity	
Content	• Was designed according to the Model of Human Occupation conceptualization of the environment[4] and principles of client-centered practice. An examination with occupational therapists and content experts showed that items included were adequate for the intended purpose of the assessment. However, studies have suggested that additional items concerning physical accessibility and social interaction should be incorporated.
Construct	• All items demonstrated acceptable goodness-of-fit to the Rasch measurement model when used to evaluate a heterogeneous group of students with physical disabilities (n=87).[131] The items form a unidimensional construct and congruence with the theoretical basis for item development.
Criterion	• Not addressed.
Utility	
Research Programs	• This tool can and has been used in research to evaluate and compare the student-environment fit across various school settings (eg, integrated and segregated setting) and groups of students (eg, students in primary and in secondary schools, and students with various types of physical and psychosocial disabilities). • It can be used to describe school settings and, although it was not developed as an outcome measure, it has the potential to evaluate school setting interventions. • It also has been used as an interview guide for qualitative research. • Research findings can influence policy regarding removing barriers and providing resources to improve student participation and inclusion.
Practice Settings	• This tool supports client-centered practice and can guide therapists to identify areas of the school setting that require adjustments based on the student's needs, and examine the goodness of student-environment fit. It allows the therapist and the student to collaboratively create goals to increase student's occupational performance and participation in school. • Information obtained through the assessment can be shared with parents and teachers to support student's needs. The assessment also can be used as an evaluative measure to examine the effects of the intervention plan.
Strengths	• Relatively easy to administer and score; low cost to purchase tool. • Addresses student-environment relationships in relation to various school activities providing a profile of not only student-environment fit, but also PEO fit. • Is a client-centered assessment; student provides input directly, enabling student's involvement in the assessment and intervention planning process. • Assessment findings can help a team to tailor services and resources for individuals and groups of students.
Complexities	• Relies on input from child; this can be influenced by child's communication and/or cognitive abilities. • Not suitable for those under the age of 9 years. • Good interviewing skills and interpretation by therapist required to ensure it is used appropriately.

Table 16-12

Therapeutic Environment Screening Survey for Nursing Homes (TESS-NH)

Source	Contact: Philip D. Sloane, MD MPH or Sheryl Zimmerman, PhD, Sheps Center for Health Services Research; E-mail: psloane@med.unc.edu; sheryl_zimmerman@unc.edu http://www.unc.edu/depts/tessnh/ Cost: Free
Key References	Bicket et al[36]; Sloane et al[35,133,134]
Purpose	• To evaluate the physical aspects of long-term care facilities by gathering data on the physical environment of a long-term care facility and providing a quantitative measure of the quality of the environment in long-term care facilities
Type of Client	• Individuals with Alzheimer's disease and related disorders, occupying long-term care facilities
Test Format	• 84 items cover 13 domains reflecting 6 goals of the physical environment in caring for persons with dementia • 83 categorical items and 1 global measure of the physical environment (ordinal response format): ¤ Safety/security/health (exit control, maintenance, cleanliness, safety) ¤ Orientation (orientation/cueing) ¤ Privacy/control/autonomy (privacy, unit autonomy, outdoor access, lighting, noise, visual/tactile stimulation) ¤ Social milieu (space/seating) • Of the 84 items, 18 items form the Special Care Unit Environmental Quality Scale summary scale (SCUEQS). It is computed by adding the observed value for each item; items reflect measures of maintenance, cleanliness, safety, lighting, physical appearance/homelikeness, orientation/cueing, and noise.
Procedures	• Manual describes test procedures; guiding definitions associated with each item; modest level of training and experience in person–environment concepts are highly recommended[35]
Time Required	• Approximately 30 to 45 minutes to administer
Standardization	• Administration should follow a recommended series of steps; deviations from recommendations are not addressed. No norms identified
Reliability	
Test-Retest	• Kappa statistics above 0.60 (74% of items); where Kappa values could be calculated, percentage agreement above 80% (n = 21)[35]; SCUEQS Kappa statistic of 0.88
Internal Consistency	• Cronbach's α (SCUEQS) = 0.81 to 0.83[35]
Inter-Rater	• Percentage of agreement (average = 86.7) and kappa statistic range (0.13 to 1.0) from data collected by 2 research assistants (n = 12 SCUs) for TESS-NH items[35]; SCUEQS inter-rater reliability of 0.93[35]

(continued)

Table 16-12 (continued)

THERAPEUTIC ENVIRONMENT SCREENING SURVEY FOR NURSING HOMES (TESS-NH)	
Validity	
Content	• TESS-NH replaces 2 previous versions, Therapeutic Environment Screening Scale (TESS) and TESS2+[133] • TESS-NH grew from collaborative efforts of 10 investigative teams studying dementia special care units (SCU) • Instrument development consisted of literature review and field-testing.[35] Field testing involved 10 special care unit (SCU) study sites (204 SCU, 59 non-SCU, 10 states). On the basis of distribution of responses from field data, items were eliminated or simplified • Development of the SCUEQS items was aided by principal components and factor analysis (oblique rotation, $n = 204$ SCU)[35]
Construct	• Theoretical conceptualization structured from social ecological models (ie, the environment in terms of interactions between a physical space and the persons within it)[133]
Criterion	• Concurrent validation reported with Professional Environmental Assessment Protocol (PEAP) (reported as a standardized method of expert evaluation of the physical environment of dementia SCUs)[35]; SCUEQS significant global correlations with global PEAP ratings ($r = 0.52$, $p < 0.01$) • Reported as gold standard in recent studies
Responsiveness	• Not established
Utility	
Research Programs	• The SCUEQS can be used as a single measure of the overall environmental quality; feasible for use with comparative outcome studies of long-term care settings[35] • Future development to consider cultural and international long-term care facility standards would enrich instrument validity • Therapeutic Environment Screening Survey for Residential Care (TESS-NH/RC) has also been introduced into the research setting; developed from the TESS-NH; instrument specifically evaluates assisted living facilities[36]
Practice Settings	• Noninvasive; observation-based instrument. • TESS-NH is suitable for assessment of specialized long-term care facilities; however, instrument has been introduced into non-specialized long-term care facilities. • Provides an objective assessment of the physical/institutional environment that can be used to guide intervention and advocacy efforts at both the institutional level and the government policy level.
Strengths	• Rigorous instrument development and promising psychometric properties. • Uniquely assesses discrete elements of the physical and social environment with a specific focus on long-term care facilities. • Available through up-to-date website.
Complexities	• Care should be taken in interpretation of scores. • Promising initial psychometric properties; however, caution should be considered due to limited number of studies, small sample sizes (eg, small sample of raters were used to established inter-rater reliability).

Table 16-13

WESTMEAD HOME SAFETY ASSESSMENT (WEHSA)

Source	Co-ordinates Therapy Services, Australia http://www.therapybookshop.com/coordinates.html Cost: Approximately $118.00 USD
Key References	Clemson[29]; Clemson et al[135-137]; Pighills et al[138]
Purpose	• To identify hazards in the physical home environments of older adults at risk of falling.
Type of Client	• Older adults, 65 years and older; all diagnoses. Respondents include clients, caregivers, and service providers
Test Format	• Instrument items divided into 13 sections pertaining to places and components in the home (eg, external/internal traffic ways, bedroom, seating) and 72 hazard categories (eg, internal traffic ways includes floor mats, doorways)
Procedures	• Completed during or immediately after a home visit • Manual provides training and operationalization of terms. For example, each item is first rated as "relevant" or "not relevant"; each relevant item is then rated as a "hazard" or "not hazard"; identified hazards are categorized by type and summarized on the front page of the form to facilitate action plan development
Time Required	• Approximately 60 minutes for administration (can vary based on environment context); semistructured interview, observation of task performance, and naturalistic observation in the home environment • Scoring is dichotomous; no summary score obtained
Standardization	• The instrument is not standardized. The manual states that, "the tool is an observational aid to assist therapists in systematically identifying hazards."[29(p 48)] The manual provides operational definitions for a number of hazards
Reliability	
Test-Retest	• Not established
Internal Consistency	• Not established
Inter-Rater	• Kappa values of >0.75 for 34 items (n=21); and 0.40 to 0.75 for 31 items (n=21); Kappa could not be calculated for some items[137]
Validity	
Content	• Instrument development consisted of the following[136]: ¤ Content analysis of the falls literature ¤ 2-stage expert review consultation involving the following: – Generation of instrument specifications – WeHSA review including review of congruence of instrument specifications and relevance of items
Construct	• The WeHSA approach guided intervention practices in a qualitative study that explored challenges underlying implementation of fall prevention intervention[135]; the thematic analysis revealed support for some aspects of the WeHSA approach (eg, reported as "comprehensive," "thought provoking")
Criterion	• Not established
Responsiveness	• Not established

(continued)

Table 16-13 (continued)

Westmead Home Safety Assessment (WEHSA)

Utility	
Research Programs	• Focused tool; helpful in assisting falls prevention research programs • May be promising as a comprehensive instrument to explore a focused investigation of home hazards specific to falls risk in a multi-national setting; thus allowing for the exploration of cultural and language factors in relation person-environment relationships within the context of home hazards falls risk
Practice Settings	• Noninvasive to administer; manual guides administration and scoring • WeHSA items can be used to guide intervention planning[138] • Instrument considered to provide "a good grounding in work with clients and hazard prevention"[135(p 6)] and may be particularly beneficial in guiding novice practitioners
Strengths	• Comprehensive evaluation of home hazards specific to falls in older adults • Promising psychometric properties • Published manual supports the utility of the instrument in clinical practice
Complexities	• Instrument has a falls-specific focus with respect to home hazards identification; important to consider the clinical context in relation to the purpose and limits of the instrument • Initial psychometric properties show promise; however, responsiveness to change would be helpful to establish credibility as an outcome measure for falls prevention intervention.

Table 16-14

Work Environment Impact Scale (WEIS) V2.0

Source	Moore-Corner RA, Kielhofner G, Olsen L. Model of Human Occupation Clearinghouse, University of Illinois at Chicago; 1998; www.moho.uic.edu/ Order form available from http://www.cade.uic.edu/moho/products.aspx Cost: $40.00 USD + tax and shipping
Key References	Corner et al[139,140]
Purpose	• To describe how individuals with physical or psychosocial disabilities experience and perceive their physical and social work environment. It addresses the impact of these factors on one's ability to return to work or continue with employment after an injury/illness
Type of Client	• Individuals with physical or psychosocial disabilities who are employed and are experiencing difficulty on the job or who have had their work interrupted by an injury or illness
Test Format	• Semistructured interview and rating scale used. Requires active participation of client but no equipment
Procedures	• Examiner qualifications not addressed but typically done by an occupational therapist. Good interviewing skills and interpretation required by a professional (eg, occupational therapist). Hand scored on paper or online. Optional summary sheet available, which can be used to communicate results to other professionals

(continued)

Table 16-14 (continued)

Work Environment Impact Scale (WEIS) V2.0

Type of Client	
Time Required	• Scoring: 17 items using 4-point ordinal scales. How strongly the factor supports or interferes with return to work is identified • 30 minutes to conduct interview depending on skill level and client; 15 minutes to complete scoring • Scoring done on paper or online through anonymous numeric client ID for each client. MOHOWeb stores the assessment results and notes
Standardization	• Published manual.[140] www.moho.uic.edu/ with directions for administration, scoring, interpretation, evidence of reliability and validity. Printable and online versions available • Clear, comprehensive instructions with manual for administration and scoring • Translated into Chinese, Danish, Dutch, Finnish, French, German, Icelandic, Japanese, Korean, Norwegian, Portuguese, Slovenian, Spanish, and Swedish. Translation services available for a fee on request • Valid tool across North American and Swedish cultures
Reliability	
Test-Retest	• Calculated by weighted kappa
Internal Consistency	• 100% fit with expected response patterns of Rasch model[139]; Rasch analysis: item separation statistic=2.77 (reliability of 0.88)[139,141]
Inter-Rater	• Minimal rater bias[142]; Swedish version tested between 3 raters demonstrated differences in rater severity. Swedish version requires further study[143]
Validity	
Content	• No specific method described
Construct	• Theoretical formulations confirmed. Valid for workers with psychiatric disabilities: those with greater satisfaction, performance, and health had a higher degree of match with their occupational environment[144] • Measured a single construct (all 17 items fit criteria)[139,141] • Infit Mean Square Statistics: Acceptable in fit MnSq=1.56, Zstd: 3.7[143] • Perceptions of individuals with mental illness participation with Swedish Version, WEIS-S[145]
Criterion	• Not applicable
Responsiveness	• Not applicable
Utility	
Research Programs	• Assessment findings, notes can be stored online, can run longitudinal summary reports, can download data for research purposes • Further research that identifies the characteristics of the working environment that support individuals with mental health issues to remain on their jobs is required • The development of principles for healthy workplaces could be developed[146] of which occupational therapists can play a significant role
Practice Settings	• Can be a useful and effective instrument in a variety of settings with workers with physical or psychosocial disabilities • Workplace support is crucial for individuals with mental illnesses in order to achieve their occupational goals and well-being. Occupational therapists are well positioned to assess workplace support in order to maximize their clients' occupational performance

(continued)

Table 16-14 (continued)

Work Environment Impact Scale (WEIS) V2.0

Strengths	• Very good psychometric properties, readily available • Guiding questions and an outline are available to help structure the interview • Promotes discussion with client and employer and identifies client's views on a variety of attributes • The construct of work environment impact is well identified • English and Swedish language versions of the WEIS are validated • Available in multiple languages
Complexities	• Fairly complex to administer, score and interpret. Scoring should be done immediately after the assessment to avoid misinterpretation • Good interviewing skills and interpretation by a professional are required to ensure appropriate use • Some clients may have difficulties recalling questions with the semi-structured interview

Table 16-15

Work Environment Scale (WES), Version 4

Source	Mind Garden Inc; 855 Oak Grove Avenue, Suite 215, Menlo Park, CA 94025 http://www.mindgarden.com/products/wes.htm#data
Key References	Moos[147-149]
Purpose	• Measure workers' perceptions of the social environment including productivity, employee satisfaction, and employees' expectations of the work environment
Type of Client	• Adults, all diagnoses who work or participate in vocational rehabilitation settings • Individuals, groups, or organizations with social-ecological interventions. Employers and service providers can also complete scales
Test Format	• Self-report. Booklet of 90 statements about the work environment with items related to 10 subscales (9 items each): a) relationships (subset includes worker involvement, coworker cohesion, supervisor support); b) personal growth or goal orientation (subset includes autonomy, task orientation, work pressure); and c) the system maintenance and system change (subset includes: clarity, managerial control, innovation, physical comfort) • The answer sheet includes 2-point (true/false) answer format • 3 versions or forms that can be used together or individually. On the Real Form (Form R) respondents indicate how they view the current workplace environment • Ideal Form (Form I) respondents rate the ideal workplace goals and values. Expected Form (Form E) respondents rate work environment expectations • Manual 4th edition = $40.00 USD, which includes the scoring key. License to use options are available. Paper by mail and digital PDF downloads range from $100 to $360 USD. The online survey, which includes data collection and scoring, ranges from $120 to $400 USD; Personal Reports that interpret the score range from $15 for 1 individual report to $11/each for 51 to 100 reports. Group reports can be purchased and with consent can be shared with client/management. These reports are professionally created with colored graphics

(continued)

Table 16-15 (continued)

Work Environment Scale (WES), Version 4

Type of Client	
Procedures	• Can be hand scored or submitted online. Interpretation of personal/group reports is available • The subscales are grouped by theoretical dimensions for interpretation.[149] Interpretation by a professional with clinical training (eg, occupational therapist) recommended • Can supplement the assessment with an interview • Patterns and trends are discussed with respondents, including perceptions and their stability over time, contrasting perceptions of worker and employer/service provider, or between worker's real, ideal, or expected scores, and comparisons of different work settings
Time Required	• 15 to 20 minutes to complete and 5 to 10 minutes to score; reporting unlimited
Standardization	• Published manual[149] with directions for administration, scoring, and interpretation • Norms available
Reliability	
Test-Retest	• Intraclass coefficient >0.70
Internal Consistency	• Cronbach's $\alpha = 0.85$ when measuring workers' responses to work stressors and 0.86 for intrusion[147]; 0.90 for avoidance.[150] Cronbach's α for subscales 0.69 to 0.83 at 1 month; 0.51 to 0.63 at 12 months[148]
Inter-Rater	• N/A
Validity	
Content	• Original items were selected from a large group of Social Climate Scales[148] and underwent multiple revisions and factor analysis; items relate to the tool's purpose.
Construct	• Able to measure changes in workplaces over time during organizational change in several independent studies[151-153] • Discriminates between workplace environments in nursing units[154]; military hospitals[155]; hospital and community environments[156]; and work practice models[157]; head, staff & agency nurses[155]; midwives & nurses[158,159] • Subscales are predictive of work satisfaction, quality of life, coping strategies, staff burnout, and emotional health in several independent studies[160-164] • Confirms theoretical formulations of peer and supervisory support moderating anxiety about burnout[165]; of cultural differences in perceptions of rules and pressures[166]
Criterion	• Not applicable
Responsiveness	• Not applicable
Utility	
Translation	• Translation: With the purchase of the English version, a free translation is available for 1 of the following: Arabic, Chinese (simplified), Dutch, Estonian, French, German, Hindi, Indonesian, Italian, Japanese, Portuguese, or Spanish. You can request permission for translation into desired language at http://www. mindgarden.com/products/wes.htm#data
Research Programs	• Much of the research has been studied with nurses and doctors assessing stress related to traumatic events.[164] There is no evidence of this research with occupational therapists
Practice Settings	• Could be used to study the correlation between staff well-being and employee retention[164] • Used extensively for research purposes, but can be an effective instrument used in a variety of physical and psychosocial practice settings

(continued)

Table 16-15 (continued)

WORK ENVIRONMENT SCALE (WES), VERSION 4

Strengths	• Used extensively for research purposes but can be an effective instrument used in a variety of physical and psychosocial practice settings
Complexities	• May not reveal complete perceptions of the work environment and may require a follow-up interview with the client • Cultural implications are not fully known • The impact of the work environment for a variety of diagnoses and populations is not known • Concerns of client anonymity exist with online reports

REFERENCES

1. World Health Organization. *International Classification of Functioning, Disability and Health.* Geneva: WHO. http://www.who.int/ classification/icf/. Accessed June 19, 2016.
2. Rigby P, Letts L. Environment and occupational performance: theoretical considerations. In: Letts L, Rigby P, Stewart D, eds. *Using Environments to Enable Occupational Performance.* Thorofare NJ: SLACK Incorporated; 2003:17-32.
3. American Occupational Therapy Association (AOTA). Occupational therapy practice framework: domain and process, second edition. *Am J Occup Ther.* 2008;62:625-683.
4. Kielhofner G. *Model of Human Occupation: Theory and Application.* Philadelphia: Lippincott, Williams & Wilkins; 2008.
5. Law M, Cooper B, Strong S, Stewart D, Rigby P, Letts, L. The Person-Environment-Occupation model: a transactive approach to occupational performance. *Can J Occup Ther.* 1996;63(1):9-23.
6. Townsend EA, Polatajko HJ. *Enabling Occupation II: Advancing an Occupational Therapy Vision for Health, Well-Being and Justice Through Occupation.* Ottawa ON: Canadian Association of Occupational Therapists; 2007.
7. Baum CM, Christiansen CH. Person-environment-occupation-performance: an occupation-based framework for practice. In Christiansen CH, Baum CM, Bass-Haugen J, eds. *Occupational Therapy: Performance, Participation, and Well-Being.* 3rd ed. Thorofare, NJ: SLACK Incorporated; 2005:242-266.
8. Christiansen C, Baum CM, Bass J. The Person-Environment-Occupational Performance Model. In Duncan EAS, ed. *Foundations for Practice in Occupational Therapy.* 5th ed. London: Elsevier; 2011:93-104.
9. Hemmingsson H, Jonsson H. The issue is—an occupational perspective on the concept of participation in the international classification of functioning, disability and health—some critical remarks. *Am J Occup Ther.* 2005;59:569–576.
10. Law M, Di Rezze B, Bradley L. Environmental change to improve outcomes. In: Law M, McColl MA, eds. *Interventions, Effects and Outcomes in Occupational Therapy: Adults and Older Adults.* Thorofare, NJ: SLACK Incorporated; 2010:155-182.
11. World Health Organization. *ICF Checklist, Version 2.1a, Clinician Form for International Classification of Functioning, Disability and Health.* Geneva, Switzerland: Author; 2003. http://www.who.int/classifications/icf/training/icfchecklist.pdf. Accessed September 17, 2016.
12. Stark S, Hollingsworth H, Morgan K, Chang M, Gray DB. The interrater reliability of the community health environment checklist. *Arch Phys Med Rehabil.* 2008;89:2218-2219.
13. Ringaert L. Universal design of the built environment to enable occupational performance. In: Letts L, Rigby P, Stewart D, eds. *Using Environments to Enable Occupational Performance.* Thorofare, NJ: SLACK Incorporated; 2003:97-115.
14. Gray DB, Hollingsworth HH, Stark S, Morgan KA. A subjective measure of environmental facilitators and barriers to participation for people with mobility limitations. *Disabil Rehabil.* 2008;30:435-457.
15. Iwarsson S, Slaug B. *Housing Enabler: An Instrument for Assessing and Analyzing Accessibility Problem in Housing. User Manual.* Studentlitteratur, Lund; 2001.
16. Bedell GM, Khetani MA, Cousins M, Coster WJ, Law M. Parent perspectives to inform development of measures of children's participation and environment. *Arch Phys Med Rehabil.* 2011;92: 765-773.
17. Gillespie LD, Robertson MC, Gillespie WJ, et al. Interventions for preventing falls in older people living in the community. Cochrane Database *Syst Rev.* 2009;2:CD007146.
18. O'Brien P, Dyck I, Caron S, Mortenson P. Environmental analysis: insights from sociological and geographical perspectives. *Can J Occup Ther.* 2002;64:229-238.
19. Egilson S, Traustadottir R. Participation of students with disabilities in the school environment. *Am J Occup Ther.* 2010;63(3):264-272.
20. Stark S. Removing environmental barriers in the homes of older adults with disabilities improves occupational performance. *OTJR.* 2004;24(1):32-39.
21. Velligan DI, Mueller J, Wang M, et al. Use of environmental supports among patients with schizophrenia. *Psychiatr Serv.* 2006;57(2):219-224.
22. Clemson L, Mackenzie L, Ballinger C, Close JCT, Cumming RG. Environmental interventions to prevent falls in community-dwelling older people: a meta-analysis of randomized trials. *J Aging Health.* 2008;20:954-971.

23. Lysack C, Komanecky M, Kabel A, Cross K, Neufeld S. Environmental factors and their role in community integration after spinal cord injury. *Can J Occup Ther.* 2007;74(2):243-254.
24. Ward K, Mitchell J, Price P. Occupation-based practice and its relationship to social and occupational participation in adults with spinal cord injury. *OTJR.* 2007;27(4):149-156.
25. Chow K, Healey M. Place attachment and place identity: first-year undergraduates making the transition from home to university. *J Environ Psychol.* 2008;28:362-372.
26. Rowles GD. Beyond performance: being in place as a component of occupational therapy. *Am J Occup Ther.* 1991;45(3):265-271.
27. Proshansky H, Fabian AK, Kaminoff, R. Place identity: physical world socialization of the self. *J Environ Psychol.* 1983;3:57-83.
28. Giuliani MV. Theory of attachment and place attachment. In Bonnes M, Lee T, Bonaiuto M, eds. *Psychological Theories for Environmental Issues.* Hants: Ashgate; 2003:137-170.
29. Clemson L. *Home Fall Hazards: A Guide to Identifying Fall Hazards in the Homes of Elderly People and an Accompaniment to the Assessment Tool. The Westmead Home Safety Assessment.* West Brunswick, Australia: Coordinates Publication; 1997.
30. Hemmingsson H, Egilson ST, Hoffman O, Kielhofner G. *The School Setting Interview (SSI).* 3rd ed. Nacka: Swedish Association of Occupational Therapists; 2005.
31. Dickinson HO, Colver A. Quantifying the physical, social and attitudinal environment of children with cerebral palsy. *Disabil Rehabil.* 2011;33:36-50.
32. Colver A, Thyen U, Arnaud C, et al. Association between participation in life situations of children with cerebral palsy and their physical, social and attitudinal environment: a cross-sectional multicenter European study. *Arch Phys Med Rehabil.* 2012;93:2154-2164.
33. King G, Rigby P, Batorowicz B, et al. Development of a direct observation measure of environmental qualities of activity settings (MEQAS). *Dev Med Child Neurol.* 2014;56(8):763-769.
34. King G, Batorowicz B, Rigby P, McMain-Klein M, Thompson L, Pinto M. Development of a measure to assess youth self-reported experiences of activity settings (SEAS). *Intl J Disabil Dev Educ.* 2014;61(1):44-66.
35. Sloane P, Mitchell C, Weisman G, et al. The Therapeutic Environment Screening Survey for Nursing Homes (TESS-NH): an observational instrument for assessing the physical environment of institutional settings for persons with dementia. *J Gerontol B Psychol Sci Soc Sci.* 2002;57(2):S69–S78.
36. Bicket MC, Samus QM, McNabney M, et al. The physical environment influences neuropsychiatric symptoms and other outcomes in assisted living residents. *Int J Geriatr Psychiatry.* 2010;25:1044-1054.
37. Fleming R. An environmental audit tool suitable for use in homelike facilities for people with dementia. *Australias J Ageing.* 2011;30(3):108-112.
38. Moos RH, Lemke S. *Evaluating Residential Facilities.* Thousand Oaks, CA: Sage Publications; 1996.
39. Fougeyrollas P, Noreau L, St. Michel G, Boschen K. *Measure of the Quality of the Environment, Version 2.* Quebec: INDCP; 2008.
40. Noreau L, Fougeyrollas P, Boschen K. Perceived influence of the environment on social participation among individuals with spinal cord injury. *Topics SCI Rehabil.* 2002;7:56-72.
41. Canadian Mortgage and Housing Corporation. *Maintaining Seniors' Independence: A Guide to Home Adaptations.* Ottawa: Canadian Mortgage and Housing Corporation; 1989. http://www.cmhc-schl.gc.ca/odpub/pdf/61042.pdf. Accessed June 19, 2016.
42. Teel C, Dunn W, Jackson S, Duncan P. The role of the environment in fostering independence: conceptual and methodological issues in developing an instrument. *Topics Stroke Rehabil.* 1997;4(1):28-40.
43. Bundy AC. Play and playfulness: what to look for. In Parnham LD, Fazio LS, eds. *Play in Occupational Therapy for Children.* St. Louis, MO: Mosby; 1997:56-62.
44. Bronson M, Bundy AC. A correlational study of the Test of Playfulness and the Test of Environmental Supportiveness. *Occup Ther J Res.* 2001;21:223-240.
45. Coster W, Law M, Bedell G, Khetani M, Cousins M, Teplicky R. Development of the participation and environment measure for children and youth: conceptual basis. *Disabil Rehabil.* 2012;34(3):238-246.
46. Harms T, Cryer D, Clifford RM. *Infant-Toddler Environment Rating Scale.* Rev ed. New York: Teachers College Press; 2006.
47. Harms T, Clifford RM, Cryer D. *Early Childhood Environment Rating Scale.* Rev ed. New York: Teachers College Press; 2005.
48. Harms T, Cryer D, Clifford RM. *Family Child Care Rating Scale.* Rev ed. New York: Teachers College Press; 2007.
49. Harms T, Jacobs EV, White DR. *School-Age Care Environment Rating Scale.* Updated ed. New York: Teachers College Press; 2013.
50. Bradley RH, Caldwell BM, Corwyn RF. The Child Care HOME Inventories: assessing the quality of family child care homes. *Early Child Res Q.* 2003;18(3):294-309.
51. Brownson RC, Hoehner CM, Day K, Forsyth A, Sallis JF. Measuring the built environment for physical activity. *Am J Prev Med.* 2009;36(4 Suppl):S99-S123.
52. Whiteneck G, Harrison-Felix CL, Mellick D, Brookes CA, Charlifue, S, Gerhart KA. Quantifying environmental factors: a measure of physical, attitudinal, service, productivity and policy barriers. *Arch Phys Med Rehabil.* 2004;55:1324-1335.
53. Dijkers MP, Yavuzer G, Ergin S, Weitzenkamp D, Whiteneck G. A tale of two countries: environmental impact on social participation after spinal cord injury. *Spinal Cord.* 2002;40:351-362.
54. Fougeyrollas P. Documenting environmental factors for preventing the handicap creation process: Quebec contributions relating to ICIDH and social participation of people with functional differences. *Disabil Rehabil.* 1995;17:145-153.

55. Whiteneck GG, Fougeyrolles P, Gerhart KA. Elaborating the Model of Disablement. In Fuhrer M, ed. *Assessing Medical Rehabilitation Practices: The Promise of Outcome Research.* Baltimore, MD: Paul H. Brooks Publishing; 1997.
56. Fleming J, Nalder E, Alves-Stein S, Cornwell P. The effect of environmental barriers on community integration for individuals with moderate to severe traumatic brain injury. *J Head Trauma Rehabil.* 2014;29(2):125-135.
57. Furtado S, Sampaio R, Vaz D, et al. Brazilian version of the instrument of environmental assessment Craig Hospital Inventory of Environmental Factors (CHIEF): translation, cross-cultural adaptation and reliability. *Braz J Phys Ther.* 2014;18(3):259-267.
58. Liao L, Lau R, Pang M. Measuring environmental barriers faced by individuals living with stroke: development and validation of the Chinese version of the Craig Hospital Inventory of Environmental Factors. *J Rehabil Med.* 2012;44:740-746.
59. McCauley D, Gorter JW, Russel DJ, Rosenbaum P, Law M, Kertoy M. Assessment of environmental factors in disabled children 2-12 years: development and reliability of the Craig Hospital Inventory of Environmental Factors (CHIEF) for Children-Parent Version. *Child Care Health Dev.* 2012;39(3):337-344.
60. Nobakht Z, Rassafiani M, Rezasoltani P. Validiity and reliability of Persian version of Craig Hospital Inventory of Environmental Factors (CHIEF) in children with cerebral palsy. *Iranian Rehabil J.* 2011;9(13):3-10.
61. Whiteneck GG, Gerhart KA, Cusick CP. Identifying environmental factors that influence the outcomes of people with traumatic brain injury. *J Head Trauma Rehabil.* 2004;19:191-204.
62. Leff M, Stallones L, Xiang H, Whiteneck G. Disability, environmental factors and non-fatal injury. *Inj Prev.* 2010;16:411-415.
63. Lien W, Guo N, Lin Y, Kaun T. Relationship of perceived environmental barriers and disability in community-dwelling elderly in Taiwan—a population-based study. *BMC Geriatr.* 2014;14:59.
64. Law M, Hanna S, Anaby D, Kertoy M, King G, Xu L. Health-related quality of life of children with physical disabilities: a longitudinal study. *BMC Pediatr.* 2014;14:26.
65. Vogts N, Mackey A, Ameratunga S, Stott S. Parent-perceived barriers to participation in children and adolescents with cerebral palsy. *J Pediatr Child Health.* 2010;46:680-685.
66. Gray DB, Hollingsworth HH, Stark S, Morgan KA. A subjective measure of environmental facilitators and barriers to participation for people with mobility limitations. *Disabil Rehabil.* 2008;30:435-457.
67. Keysor J, Jette A, Haley M. Development of the Home and Community Environment (HACE) instrument. *J Rehabil Med.* 2005;37:37-44.
68. Caldwell BM, Bradley RH. *Home Observation for Measurement of the Environment: Administration Manual.* Tempe, AZ: Family & Human Dynamics Research Institute, Arizona State University; 2003.
69. Bradley RH, Caldwell BM. Using the home inventory to assess the family environment. *Pediatr Nurs.* 1988;14(2):97.
70. Bradley RH, Corwyn RF, Caldwell BM, Whiteside-Mansell L, Wasserman GA, Mink IT. Measuring the home environments of children in early adolescence. *J Res Adolescence.* 2000;10(3):247-288.
71. Bradley RH, Corwyn RF, Whiteside-Mansell L. Life at home: same time, different places—an examination of the HOME inventory in different cultures. *Early Dev Parent.* 1996;5(4):251-269.
72. Totsika V, Sylva K. The home observation for measurement of the environment revisited. *Child Adolescent Mental Health.* 2004;9(1): 25-35.
73. Bradley RH, Corwyn RF. Caring for children around the world: a view from HOME. *Int J Behav Dev.* 2005;26:468-478.
74. Bradley RH. Uses of the HOME Inventory for families with handicapped children. *Am J Ment Retard.* 1989;94(3):313-330.
75. Bradley RH. Children's home environments, health, behavior and intervention efforts: a review using the HOME Inventory as a marker measure. *Genet Soc Gen Psychol Monogr.* 1993;119:439-490.
76. Burston A, Puckering C, Kearney E. At HOME in Scotland: validation of the home observation for measurement of the environment inventory. *Child Care Health Dev.* 2005;31(5):533-538.
77. Elardo R, Bradley RH. The Home Observation for Measurement of the Environment (HOME) Scale: a review of research. *Dev Rev.* 1981;1(2):113-145.
78. Mackenzie L, Byles J, Higginbotham N. Designing the Home Falls and Accidents Screening Tool (HOME FAST): selecting the items. *Br J Occup Ther.* 2000;63:260-269.
79. Mackenzie L, Byles J, Higginbotham N. Professional perceptions about home safety: cross-national validation of the Home Falls and Accidents Screening Tool (HOME FAST). *J Allied Health.* 2002;31:22-28.
80. Mackenzie L, Byles J, Higginbotham N. Reliability of the Home Falls and Accidents Screening Tool (HOME FAST) for identifying older people at increased risk of falls. *Disabil Rehabil.* 2002;24:266-274.
81. Mackenzie L, Byles J, D'Este C. Longitudinal study of the Home Falls and Accidents Screening Tool in identifying older people at increased risk of falls. *Australas J Ageing.* 2009;28(2):64-69.
82. Mehraban A, Mackenzie L, Byles J. A self-report home environment screening tool identified older women at risk of falls. *J Clin Epidemiol.* 2011;64:191-199.
83. Carlsson G, Schilling O, Slaug B, et al. Towards a screening tool for housing accessibility problems: a reduced version of the Housing Enabler. *J Appl Gerontol.* 2009;28(1):59-80.
84. Fänge A, Iwarsson S. Accessibility and usability in housing: construct validity and implications for research and practice. *Disabil Rehabil.* 2003;25:1316-1325.
85. Iwarsson S, Isacsson A. Development of a novel instrument for occupational therapy assessment of the physical environment in the home methodological study on The Enabler. *OTJR.* 1996;16(4):227-244.
86. Iwarsson S, Nygren C, Slaug B. Cross-national and multi-professional interrater reliability of the Housing Enabler. *Scand J Occup Ther.* 2005;12(1):29-39.

87. Iwarsson S, Isacsson A. Quality of Life in the elderly population: an example exploring interrelationships among subjective well-being, ADL dependence, and housing accessibility. *Arch Gerontol Geriatr Suppl.* 1997;26(1):71-83.
88. Iwarsson S, Isacsson A, Lanke J. ADL dependence in the elderly: the influence of functional limitations and physical environmental demand. *Occup Ther Int.* 1998;5(3):1173-1193.
89. Iwarsson S, Horstmann V, Carlsson G, Oswald F, Wahl H. Person-environment fit predicts falls in older adults better than the consideration of environmental hazards only. *Clin Rehabil.* 2009;23:558-567.
90. Iwarsson S. A long-term perspective on person-environment fit and ADL dependence among older Swedish adults. *Gerontologist.* 2005;45(3):327-336.
91. Rantakokko M, Tormakangas T, Rantanen T, Haak M, Iwarsson S. Environmental barriers, person-environment fit and mortality among community-dwelling very old people. *BMC Public Health.* 2013;13:1-8.
92. Moos RH. *Life Stressors and Social Resources Inventory, and Coping Responses Inventory Annotated Bibliography.* 2nd ed. Odessa, FL: Psychological Assessment Resources; 2010.
93. Moos R, Brennan P, Schutte K, Moos B. Social and financial resources and high-risk alcohol consumption among older adults. *Alcohol Clin Exp Res.* 2010;34(4):646-654.
94. Moos R, Fenn C, Billings A, Moos B. Assessing life stressors and social resources: applications to alcoholic patients. *J Subst Abuse.* 1989;1:135-152.
95. Holanah C, Schutte K, Brennan P, Holahan C, Moos R. Episodic heavy drinking and 20-year total mortality among late-life moderate drinkers. *Alcohol Clin Exp Res.* 2014;38(5):1432-1438.
96. Stancin T, Wade S, Walz N, Yeates KO, Taylor G. Family adaptation 18 months after traumatic brain injury in early childhood. *J Dev Behav Pediatr.* 2010;31(4):317-325.
97. Humphreys K, Finney J, Moos R. Applying a stress and coping framework to research on mutual help organizations. *J Community Psychol.* 1994;22:312-327.
98. Moos RH, Finney JW, Moos BS. Inpatient substance abuse care and the outcome of subsequent community residential and outpatient care. *Addiction.* 2000;95(6):833-846.
99. Bull R, Espy K, Wiebe S, Sheffield T, Nelson J. Using confirmatory factor analysis to understand executive control in preschool children: sources of variation in emergent mathematic achievement. *Dev Sci.* 2011;14(4):679-692.
100. Peterson J, Burant C, Drotar D, et al. Predicting family burden following childhood traumatic brain injury: a cumulative risk approach. *J Head Trauma Rehabil.* 2008;23(6):357-368.
101. Zimet GD, Dahlem NW, Zimet SG, Farley GK. The Multidimensional Scale of Perceived Social Support. *J Pers Assess.* 1988;52(1):30-41.
102. Stanley MA, Beck JG, Zebb BJ. Psychometric properties of the MSPSS in older adults. *Aging Mental Health.* 1998;2(3):186-193.
103. Zimet GD, Powell SS, Farley GK, Werkman S, Berkoff KA. Psychometric characteristics of the Multidimensional Scale of Perceived Social Support. *J Pers Assess.* 1990;55:610-617.
104. Canty-Mitchell J, Zimet G. Psychometric properties of the multidimensional scale of perceived social support in urban adolescents. *Am J Comm Psychol.* 2000;28(3):391-400.
105. Dahlem N, Zimet G, Walker R. The multidimensional scale of perceived social support: a confirmation study. *J Clin Psychol.* 1991;47(6):756-761.
106. Prezza M, Costantini S. Sense of community and life satisfaction: investigation in three different territorial contexts. *J Community Appl Soc Psychol.* 1998;8(3):181-194.
107. Prezza M, Giuseppina Pacilli M. Perceived social support from significant others, family and friends and several socio-demographic characteristics. *J Community Appl Soc Psychol.* 2002;12(6):422-429.
108. Zhang J, Norvilitis J. Measuring Chinese psychological well-being with western developed instruments. *J Pers Assess.* 2002;79(3):492-511.
109. Eker D, Arkar H, Yaldiz H. Generality of support sources and psychometric properties of a scale of perceived social support in Turkey. *Soc Psychiatry Psychiatr Epidemiol.* 2000;35(5):228-233.
110. Chou KL. Assessing Chinese adolescents' social support: the multidimensional scale of perceived social support. *Personal Individ Differ.* 2000;28(2):299-307.
111. Cecil H, Stanley M, Carrion P, Swann A. Psychometric properties of the MSPSS and NOS in psychiatric outpatients. *J Clin Psychol.* 1995;51(5):593-602.
112. Hann DM, Oxman TE, Ahles TA, Furstenberg CT, Stuke TA. Social support adequacy and depression in older patients with metastatic cancer. *Psycho-Oncology.* 1995;4(3):213-221.
113. Oxman TE, Hull JG. Social support, depression, and activities of daily living in older heart surgery patients. *J Gerontol B Psychol Sci Soc Sci.* 1997;52(1):P1-P14.
114. Oxman TE, Freeman DH, Manheimer ED, Stukel T. Social support and depression after cardiac surgery in elderly patients. *Am J Geriatr Psychiatry.* 1994;2(4):309-323.
115. Ng CG, Sulaiman AR, Seng LH, Ann AYH, Wahab S, Pillai SK. Factorial validity and reliability of the Tamil version of Multidimensional Scale of Perceived Social Support among a group of participants in University Malaya Medical Centre, Malaysia. *Indian J Psychol Med.* 2013;35(4):385-388.
116. Rothan C, Stansfeld S, Matthews C, et al. Reliability of self-report questionnaires for epidemiological investigations of adolescent mental health in Cape Town, South Africa. *J Child Adolesc Ment Health.* 2011;23(2):119-128.
117. Vaingankara J, Abdina E, Chong S. Exploratory and confirmatory factor analyses of the Multidimensional Scale of Perceived Social Support in patients with schizophrenia. *Compr Psychology.* 2012;53:286-291.
118. Ng C, Amer Siddiq A, Aida S, Zainal N, Koh O. Validation of the Malay version of the Multidimensional Scale of Perceived Social Support (MSPSS-M) among a group of medical students in Faculty of Medicine, University of Malaya. *Asian J Psychiatr.* 2010;3:3-10.
119. Ahkter A, Rahman A, Husain M, Chaudhry I, Duddu V, Husain N. Multidimensional scale of perceived social support: psychometric properties in a South Asian population. *J Obstet Gynaecol Res.* 2010;36(4):845-851.

120. Clara I, Cox B, Enns M, Murray L, Torgrudc L. Confirmatory factor analysis of The Multidimensional Scale of Perceived Social Support in clinically distressed and student samples. *J Pers Assess.* 2003;81(3):265-270.
121. Kane M, DiBartolo M. Complex physical and mental health needs of rural incarcerated women. *Issues Ment Health Nurs.* 2002;23:209-229.
122. Prezza M, Sgarro M. Stress-buffering factors related to adolescents coping: a path analysis. *Adolescence.* 1992;34:715-736.
123. Wongpakaran T, Wongpakaran N, Ruktraku R. Reliability and validity of the Multidimensional Scale of Perceived Social Support (MSPSS): Thai version. *Clin Pract Epidemiol Ment Health.* 2011;7:161-166.
124. Patel SS, Shah VS, Peterson RA, Kimmel PL. Psychosocial variables, quality of life, and religious beliefs in ESRD patients treated with hemodialysis. *Am J Kidney Dis.* 2002;40(5):1013-1022.
125. Letts L, Marshall L. Evaluating the validity and consistency of the SAFER Tool. *Phys Occup Ther Geriatr.* 1995;13:49-66.
126. Chui T, Oliver R, Ascott P, et al. *Safety Assessment of Function and the Environment for Rehabilitation: Health Outcome Measurement and Evaluation (SAFER-HOME) Version 3 Manual.* Toronto, ON: VHA Rehab Solutions; 2006.
127. Letts L, Scott S, Burtney J, Marshall L, McKean M. The reliability and validity of the Safety Assessment of Function and the Environment for Rehabilitation (SAFER) Tool. *Br J Occup Ther.* 1998;61:127-132.
128. Chui T, Oliver R. Factor analysis and construct validity of the SAFER-HOME. *OTJR (Thorofare NJ)*, 2006;26:132-142.
129. Egilson S, Hemmingsson H. School participation of pupils with physical and psychosocial limitations: a comparison. *Br J Occup Ther.* 2009;72(4):144-152.
130. Hemmingsson H, Borell L. Environmental barriers in mainstream schools. *Child Care Health Dev.* 2002;28(1):57-63.
131. Hemmingsson H, Kottorp A, Bernspang B. Validity of the School Setting Interview: an assessment of the student-environment fit. *Scand J Occup.* 2004;11(4):171-178.
132. Hemmingsson H, Borell L. The development of an assessment of adjustment needs in the school setting for use with physically disabled students. *Scand J Occup Ther.* 1996;3:156-162.
133. Sloane PD, Mathew LJ. The Therapeutic Environment Screening Scale. *Am J Alzheimer's Care.* 1990;5:22-26.
134. Sloane PD, Mitchell CM, Long K, Lynn M. *TESS 2+ Instrument B: Unit Observation Checklist—Physical Environment: A Report on the Psychometric Properties of Individual Items, and Initial Recommendations on Scaling.* Chapel Hill: University of North Carolina; 1995.
135. Clemson L, Donaldson A, Hill K, Day L. Implementing person–environment approaches to prevent falls: a qualitative inquiry in applying the Westmead approach to occupational therapy home visits. *Aust Occup Ther J.* 2014;61(5):325-34.
136. Clemson L, Fitzgerald MH, Heard R. Content validity of an assessment tool to identify home fall hazards: the Westmead Home Safety Assessment. *Br J Occup Ther.* 1999;62:171-179.
137. Clemson L, Fitzgerald MH, Heard R, Cumming RG. Interrater reliability of a home fall hazards assessment tool. *OTJR.* 1999;19:83-100.
138. Pighills A, Torgerson D, Sheldon T, Drummond A, Bland M. Environmental assessment and modification to prevent falls in older people. *J Am Geriatr Soc.* 2011;59(1):26-33.
139. Corner R, Kielhofner G, Lin FL. Construct validity of a work environment impact scale. *Work.* 1997;9:21-34.
140. Corner R, Kielhofner G, Olsen L. *A User's Guide to Work Environment Impact Scale (WEIS), Version 2.* Chicago, IL: University of Illinois at Chicago; 1998.
141. Moore-Corner RA, Kielhofner G, Olson L. *User's Guide to Work Environment Impact Scale.* Chicago, IL: Model of Human Occupation Clearinghouse; 1998.
142. Kielhofner G. *Model of Human Occupation: Theory and Application.* Philadelphia, PA: Lippincott, Wilkins & Williams; 2008.
143. Ekbladh E, Fan C, Sandqvista J, Hemmingsson H, Taylor R. Work environment impact scale: testing the psychometric properties of the Swedish version. *IOS Press.* 2014;47:213-219.
144. Kielhofner G, Lai JS, Olson L, Haglund L, Ekbadh E, Hedlund M. Psychometric properties of the work environment impact scale: a cross-cultural study. *Work.* 1999;12(1):71-77.
145. Lexen A, Hofgren C, Bejerholm U. Reclaiming the worker role: perceptions of people with mental illness participating in IPS. *Scand J Occup Ther.* 2013;50:54-63.
146. Williams A, Fossey E, Harvey C. Social firms: sustainable employment for people with mental illness. *IOS Press.* 2013;43:53-62.
147. Moos R. Work as a human context. In: Pallack MS, Perloff RO, eds. *Psychology and Work: Productivity, Change and Employment (Vol. 5). Master Lecture Series.* Washington, DC: American Psychological Association; 1986:9-52.
148. Moos R. *Work Environment Scale Manual.* 3rd ed. Palo Alto, CA: Consulting Psychologists Press; 1994.
149. Moos R, Insel P. *Work Environment Scale Manual.* 4th ed. 2008. http://www.mindgarden.com/products/wes.htm#ms
150. Fischer J, Corcoran K. *Measures for Clinical Practice: A Source-Book.* London: Free Press; 1994.
151. Tommasini NR. The impact of a staff support group on the work environment of a specialty unit. *Arch Psychiatr Nurs.* 1992;6(1):40-47.
152. Maloney JP, Bartz C, Allanach BC. Staff perceptions of their work environment before and six months after an organizational change. *Mil Med.* 1991;156(2):86-92.
153. Koran LM, Moos RH, Zasslow M. Changing hospital work environments: an example of a burn unit. *Gen Hosp Psychiatry.* 1983;5(1):7-13.
154. Avallone I, Gibbon B. Nurses' perceptions of their work environment in a nursing development unit. *J Adv Nurs.* 1998;27(6):1193-1201.
155. Maloney JP, Anderson FD, Gladd DL, Brown DL, Hardy MA. Evaluation and comparison of health-care Work Environment Scale in military settings. *Mil Med.* 1996;161(5):284-289.
156. Fielding J, Weaver S. A comparison of hospital and community-based mental health nurses: perceptions of their work environment and psychological health. *J Adv Nurs.* 1994;19:1196-1204.

157. Thomas LH. Qualified nurse and nursing auxiliary perceptions of their work environment in primary, team and functional nursing wards. *J Adv Nurs.* 1992;17(3):373-382.
158. Carlisle C, Baker GA, Riley M, Dewey M. Stress in midwifery: a comparison of midwives and nurses using the Work Environment Scale. *Int J Nurs Stud.* 1994;31(1):13-22.
159. Beyer S, Brown T, Akandi R, Rapley M. A comparison of quality of life outcomes for people with intellectual disabilities in supported employment, day services and employment enterprises. *J Appl Res Intellect Disabil.* 2010;23(3):290-295.
160. Trief PM, Aquilino C, Paradies K, Weinstock RS. Impact of the work environment on glycemic control and adaptation to diabetes. *Diabetes Care.* 1999;22(4):569-574.
161. Brown T, Pranger T. Predictors of burnout for psychiatric occupational therapy personnel. *Can J Occup Ther.* 1992;59(5)258-267.
162. Chan A, Huak CY. Influence of work environment on emotional health in a health care setting. *Occup Med.* 2004;54(3):207-212.
163. Ostermann T, Bertram M, Büssing A. A pilot study on the effects of a team building process on the perception of work environment in an integrative hospital for neurological rehabilitation. *BMC Complement Altern Med.* 2010;10:10.
164. Wallbank S, Robertson N. Predictors of staff distress in response to professionally experienced miscarriage, stillbirth and neonatal loss: a questionnaire survey. *Int J Nurs Stud.* 2013;50:1090-1097.
165. Turnipseed DL. Anxiety and burnout in the healthcare work environment. *Psychol Rep.* 1998;82(2):627-642.
166. Staten DR, Mangalindan MA, Saylor C, Stuenkel DL. Staff nurse perceptions of the work environment: a comparison among ethnic backgrounds. *J Nurs Care Qual.* 2003;18(3):202-208.

Mine the Gold

Information on measures of social factors that support occupational performance is readily available in the social science and public health literature. As you explore these resources, you will learn the key words that may be used to access measures on social factors.

Become Systematic

Because most measures of social factors have been developed in other disciplines, an awareness of key resources is essential for identifying and selecting current outcomes of interest and tracking new developments in measurement of social factors.

Use Evidence in Practice

There is growing evidence about the relationships between social factors and health. Outcome measurements that demonstrate the links between social factors, health, occupational performance, and participation will build support for occupational therapy programs.

Make Occupational Therapy Contributions Explicit

Measurement of social factors along with other occupational therapy outcomes is central to efforts designed to advance health equity and well-being of all persons needing our services.

Engage in Occupation-Based, Client-Centered Practice

Occupation-based, client-centered practice requires a comprehensive understanding of the social factors that serve as enablers or barriers to occupational performance, participation, and health.

CHAPTER 17

Measuring Social Factors

Julie D. Bass, PhD, OTR/L, FAOTA and Kathryn M. B. Haugen, REHS/RS

We are all dependent on one another, every soul of us on earth. ~ George Bernard Shaw, Pygmalion, 1912

What images come to mind when you think of measuring the social factors that relate to occupational performance? Do you focus on personal characteristics such as social cognition and social anxiety? Do you attend to occupation or occupational performance characteristics such as social behavior and social functioning? Do you emphasize environmental factors such as social support and social capital? It is clear that social factors are complex and influence occupational performance in numerous ways. By the word *social*, we mean any of the factors relating to society and its organization, relationships, and networks among people and communities. The social factors of importance in practice and research vary by age and health condition. For example, social competence is commonly measured in studies of children and adolescents, while social reintegration is an important domain in rehabilitation research.

Social factors of the environment serve as enablers or barriers to occupational performance and are the focus of this chapter. That is, we will identify and examine measures that help us understand how social factors provide contextual, extrinsic support for occupational performance. There is growing evidence of the importance of these social factors to health and well-being for individuals, organizations, communities, and populations.

Before we examine concepts in more detail, consider the role of social factors in the following scenarios for an individual, organization, and population. What are the social factors that serve as enablers or barriers to occupational performance? Why would it be important to have measures of the social environment factors in each of these situations?

- *Maya*: Maya is a 43-year-old single woman who is a licensed social worker at a nonprofit organization. Her work is very important to her and she has received numerous recognitions for her contributions to the community. Maya has a chronic health condition that has resulted in physical limitations and fatigue when performing activities that require strength and endurance. She is eligible for 10 hours of support per week by a personal care attendant (PCA). To optimize her performance at work, Maya has a PCA come to her home every weekday morning and evening to assist with dressing, bathing, and household chores. Her neighbor helps her on weekends with some household chores. The social support that Maya receives from her PCA and neighbor enables her to have optimal performance in meaningful life activities.
- *Special Olympics*: Special Olympics is an organization that uses sports to help people with intellectual disabilities discover their full potential and experience success. The mission of Special Olympics could not be realized without the involvement of volunteers. Volunteers promote social inclusion of participants, break down stereotypes about intellectual disabilities, provide athletes with assistance and support, and offer their expertise in specialized areas of need. Volunteers also receive enormous benefits from their involvement in the organization by virtue of the rewards that come from knowing their contributions are making the world a better place. Special Olympics has designed a webpage that describes the community of people who are involved in Special Olympics and the ways they support each other.
- *Refugee community*: A group of leaders from a newer refugee population are concerned about the prevalence of developmental disabilities in their community's children. They worry about the fear and

Law M, Baum C, Dunn W, eds. *Measuring Occupational Performance: Supporting Best Practice in Occupational Therapy, Third Edition (pp 393-412).*

Structural and Social Determinants		*Intermediary Determinants*
Socioeconomic/Political Context	*Structural Indicators*	*Individual Context*
Social Policies	Social Capital	
Culture and Societal Values	Social Cohesion	
Public Policies	Socioeconomic	Social Support/Psychosocial Factors
Microeconomic Policies	Social class	Behaviors/Biological Factors
Governance	Gender/Ethnicity	Material Circumstances
	Education	Health System
	Occupation	
	Income	

Figure 17-1. Adapted from the World Health Organization's Commission on the Social Determinants of Health (CSDH) Conceptual Framework.[1]

myths that are circulating regarding the causes of developmental disabilities and the limited access that community members have to accurate information. This leadership group strives to help the refugee community by developing broad partnerships and outreach initiatives to improve health and quality of life. For this particular issue, the leaders take an inventory of potential partners, including state and local health departments, university faculty, health professionals, volunteers, and other community leaders. They also identify the optimal communication strategies for providing information and support to the community (public awareness campaign, call center, information sessions, town hall meetings, email, text messages, social media).

In each of these scenarios, it is clear that people make a difference in the everyday life of an individual, an organization's capacity to realize its mission, and a community's efforts to improve quality of life. Social factors such as these are critical to occupational performance, participation, and health.

Overview of Social Factors

Key Concepts

Three different social factors related to occupational performance, health, and participation are examined in this chapter: social determinants of health, social support, and social capital. *Social determinants of health* is an umbrella term for a variety of social factors that are associated with the health of populations. Social support and social capital are important social factors with applications in both practice and research.

Social Determinants of Health

The term *social determinants of health* is used to describe the many complex person and environment factors that influence health along with performance, participation, and well-being. Some of these factors are clearly social in nature (eg, social support, social capital). Other factors focus on the sociocultural or system-level characteristics (eg, public policies, income) of individuals and populations.

Conceptual models and frameworks for the social determinants of health continue to evolve. The World Health Organization's Commission on the Social Determinants of Health proposed a conceptual framework that makes distinctions between structural and social determinants and intermediary determinants (Figure 17-1).[1] Structural and social determinants consist of the key institutions and systems related to the socioeconomic and political context and the indicators that measure individuals' positions within society. These determinants are the main factors associated with health inequities. Intermediary determinants of health are the individual and life circumstances that are distributed unequally in populations and also contribute to health inequalities. Thus, social determinants of health include not only specific social factors, but also other system and individual factors that occur unequally in populations. Social support and social capital, 2 primary concepts discussed in this chapter, are evident in this framework. Social support is an intermediary determinant of health while social capital is placed along both the structural and intermediary dimensions.

Social Support

Social support is a complex and multidimensional construct that is a critical social determinant of health for individuals. Three dimensions are important in the measurement of social support: structure, function, and perception.[2] Structure and function are sometimes identified as received social support as compared with perception or perceived social support. The structural dimension focuses on the quantity and characteristics of one's social network. Functional aspects of social support emphasize the behaviors and exchanges between people that may enable occupational performance. The perceptual dimension examines subjective perspectives (eg, confidence, adequacy, satisfaction) with the quality of relationships and social network.

Functional social support is central to individuals as they engage in everyday life. Four types of functional social support may be evident in a specific situation.[3,4] Emotional support (ie, social support in the form of comfort and caring) is especially critical in a crisis stage. Informational support becomes more important when advice and guidance on issues is needed, especially when recovering from or adapting to a new life circumstance. Tangible support includes the provision of materials or services (eg, loan, transportation, housing) and is needed over the long term. Being a part of something or a sense of belonging is important at every stage.

Social Capital

Social capital is a multidisciplinary term that has been studied in 2 primary ways.[5] Burt described social capital in terms of one's access to informational and supportive resources (eg, knowledge, support) because of relationships with other people and social networks.[5] Putnam summarized social capital in terms of the level of involvement one has in social networks and organizations.[5] The phrase, "the glue that holds people together," illustrates the main idea in social capital. A more formal definition of social capital is the "institutions, relationships, attitudes, and values that govern interactions among people and contribute to economic and social development."[6(p 2)]

There are 2 forms and 3 scopes of social capital that are important to consider in measurement.[6,7] The forms of social capital include both structural and cognitive components. Structural social capital is the objective and observable connectedness one has with different networks, associations, and institutions. Cognitive social capital is the subjective perceptions one has regarding reciprocity, support, sharing, and trust in relationships. Social capital may also be examined and understood for its scope that expands from individual to the community level. Social capital may be examined at the micro level (networks of individuals or households), meso level (networks of groups), and macro level (networks of institutional relationships and structures). The relationship between form (structural, cognitive) and scope (micro, meso, macro) has been depicted in a 2-dimensional drawing to illustrate specific avenues for measurement.[6] The nature of the social network may also be explored through measures of social capital. Distinctions have been made between social capital that is available through horizontal social connections with people having similar demographic characteristics (bonding) or different characteristics (bridging) and vertical social connections with people having greater stature and authority (linking).[5]

There has been growing interest in the role of social capital on the health and vitality of individuals and communities. Studies have examined the social capital characteristics of at-risk and developing communities. Health and economic initiatives have included objectives to build social capital as a means to address health and social inequalities.

Other Social Factors

There are other social factors that support occupational performance and may be important to measure in specific areas of practice. Concepts such as social connectedness, cohesion, cognition, inclusion, anxiety, behavior, functioning, competence, participation, and reintegration may be found in the literature on social factors. Measures for these social factors are readily available and may be appropriate for research and practice.

Importance of Measurement in Social Factors

A comprehensive understanding of occupational performance, participation, and well-being requires measurement of the social factors that are supports and barriers for an individual or community. In some occupational therapy roles, measurement of social factors may be part of the occupational profile or overall evaluation plan. In other roles, occupational therapy practitioners may draw on the outcomes of social factor measurement conducted by other professionals or organizations. Measurement may focus on the social characteristics of a given individual or may examine what is known about a specific community or population.

Why is it necessary for occupational therapists to examine social factors within the context of an individual's occupational performance? There is growing evidence that social factors are associated with health outcomes. Two examples are highlighted here. Social support has been shown to have substantial effects on adherence to recommended intervention programs; a meta-analysis of over 50 years of research found that social support that is practical or functional in nature may enable better health because an individual is more likely to carry out prescribed programs.[8] Social support has also been linked to physiological status. An extensive review of the literature indicated that positive structural and functional social support is beneficial for the cardiovascular, neuroendocrine, and immune systems and so social support may provide a pathway to better physical health.[9] Thus, an occupational therapy practitioner may use social factor measures to evaluate a client's social network and the type of support they can provide. Then, a client's family and friends may be enlisted to assist in an intervention program with a byproduct of improved health along with occupational performance and participation.

Why is it necessary to incorporate population- or community-based measures of social factors in occupational therapy practice? National and global population health agendas provide occupational therapy with ample opportunity to contribute to societal goals of improved health for all. Healthy People 2020 (https://www.healthypeople.gov/), Health Canada (http://www.hc-sc.gc.ca/ahc-asc/index-eng.php), European Union Health Strategy (http://ec.europa.eu/health/index_en.htm), Australian Government Department of Health (http://www.health.gov.au/internet/publications/publishing.nsf/Content/corporate-plan-2016-17-toc), United Nations Millennium Development Goals (http://www.un.org/millenniumgoals/), and World Health Organization Health Promotion Programme (http://www.who.int/healthpromotion/about/goals/en/) have similar goals for population health. In direct and indirect ways, these plans recognize that social factors are a key to improving overall health and well-being. Thus, governmental (local, regional, national) and nongovernmental organizations have made strategic investments in measuring the social factors that are known or believed to influence health. Social factors are particularly important in addressing goals related to health equity and health disparities and in community development. In developing effective and efficient occupational therapy programs, it makes sense that knowledge of the social context (social determinants, social support, social capital) would be factored into the design, implementation, monitoring, and evaluation of programs. For example, the occupational therapy services that would be developed for a community that has documented problems of social isolation, social deterioration, and structural racism would be different from that of a community with strong social cohesion in neighborhoods, an array of social service organizations, and intergenerational social networks.

Factors to Remember

There are several issues that must be considered when measuring the social factors that influence occupational performance, participation, and well-being. Occupational therapy practitioners should be aware of ongoing development of measures of social factors, the interdisciplinary nature of knowledge on social factors, the secondary sources of data from social factor measures in practice, and the reliance on self-report in most social factor measures.

The theoretical frameworks, concepts, and corresponding measures of specific social factors continue to evolve in the literature. Occupational therapy practitioners must keep abreast of new developments and advances in knowledge regarding how social factors support health and occupational performance. Tracking psychometric studies is particularly important because new measures of social factors and improved measurement characteristics for existing measures are introduced in peer-reviewed literature.

Occupational therapy practitioners are also challenged when exploring the breadth of literature on social factors. Most of the relevant research and practice information is interdisciplinary and so is not readily available in many occupational therapy journals and textbooks. The measures used to evaluate the social factors related to occupational performance also require some ability to translate discipline-specific occupational therapy terminology into interdisciplinary terminology that is used in the health and social sciences. For example, the term *health behaviors* may be used as a key word in studies of social support rather than health management and maintenance, an instrumental activity of daily living (IADL) term in the Occupational Therapy Practice Framework.[10]

Occupational therapy practitioners also need to determine the optimal sources of data on social factor measures. In occupational therapy, narratives and occupational profiles may provide direct information on the social factors that influence occupational performance. When working on interdisciplinary or interprofessional teams to provide services for an individual client, other professionals may have primary responsibility for administering and interpreting the formal social factors measures. When working with organizations, communities, and populations to improve occupational performance, measures of social factors may be conducted by designated agencies with a specific mission and expertise to evaluate aggregate data. Thus, a challenge for occupational therapy practitioners is to focus their professional development on eliciting pertinent social factors information through interview and observation and becoming effective users of data from formal measures that have been collected by others.

The final issue to remember when measuring social factors is that most of these measures are based on self-report. Although the measurement of social factors requires the perspective and perceptions of the individual, it is challenging to establish the accuracy of information from self-reports. For example, a meta-analysis of the relationship between received and perceived social support in 23 studies showed only a moderate correlation ($r=.32$-$.35$) and thus, there are clearly other factors at play in perceptions of social factors.[11] These limitations in measures of social factors must be considered in the evaluation process.

Strategies for Selecting Measures for Social Factors

Selecting measures for social factors requires consideration of the target client population, the identified construct and purpose of the measure, relevant psychometric properties, practical information and characteristics, and the credibility of the sponsoring individual or organization. Finding the best match between available measures and a specific need for measurement in practice entails review of all of these characteristics.

Target Client Population

Defining the target client population is important when exploring available measures. A clear description of client characteristics in terms of gender, age, medical conditions or social circumstances, primary language and culture, practice setting, and geographic residence will be helpful in searching for measures that were developed for the client population. The types of measures selected will also depend on the definition of the client as an individual or family, organization, community, or population.

Construct and Purpose

Three social factor constructs were introduced in this chapter in more detail: social determinants, social support, and social capital. Additional social factor constructs are described in the literature and may be relevant to a particular area of practice. The identified purpose of measuring a specific construct must also be examined. For example, some measures may be extensively used in research but have not been fully developed for use in practice. Similarly, some measures may be extremely valuable as a means to understand trends in populations but have limited applicability to evaluate individual clients in clinical settings.

Relevant Psychometric Properties

All measures undergo some degree of development. The care that was taken in the development stage and the description of the development process provides valuable evidence regarding the quality of a measure. An examination of the publication manual (if available) and/or initial journal article(s) provides important clues on the psychometric properties of a measure. Later psychometric studies on a measure may extend the recommended applications for a measure and further support its overall quality. Even older measures may continue to have relevance if there is supporting evidence and currency of use. It is also important to identify the relevant psychometric properties for a given type of measure. For example, a measure based on item response theory as compared to classical test theory has different measurement assumptions and will demonstrate the quality of the measure in different ways.

Practical Information and Characteristics

A variety of practical considerations may also be important when selecting measures of social factors. The answers to the following types of questions may be helpful in narrowing the options among similar measures. What are the required qualifications and expertise of the user of the measure? How much time is required to administer, score, and interpret the measure? Is the measure readily available and how much does it cost?

Credibility of the Sponsoring Individual or Organization

There are countless measures of social factors available in print and on the Internet. A first step in selecting measures for further review is to answer a few questions regarding the credibility of the author or sponsoring organization. Has the measure been described and reviewed in peer-reviewed journal articles? Is the author associated with an academic institution, governmental agency, practice setting, or foundation that provides oversight for research? Is the measure recommended for use by an organization that is committed to ethical and trustworthy information (eg, HONcode)? How widespread is the adoption and use of a measure? What summary and research information is available on the measure?

Strategies for Reporting About Social Factors

Occupational therapy is still developing its capacity to contribute to reports on social factors. As we increase our focus on the occupational performance needs of communities and populations and national and international initiatives to support health equity, we will find growing opportunities to contribute to evaluations of and interventions for social factors. The types of reporting methods to use when reporting in team meetings, to families, and as part of research protocols will depend on the setting, the roles of other professionals, and the client as individual, family, organization, community, or population.

Individual or Family

When the client is an individual or family, the occupational therapy practitioner may report on the outcomes of social factors measures that relate to occupational performance and participation. The measures may be administered and interpreted by an occupational therapist or, at times, another professional may have primary responsibility. For example, one client might need physical assistance or cueing to complete ADL upon discharge. The occupational therapy practitioner's team may report on the availability of tangible support to meet needs in ADL.

Community or Population

There is a growing emphasis on initiatives that address the health of communities and populations outside the medical system. In this context, reporting is consistent with standards of practice in public and population health. For practitioners who are interested in expanding the role of occupational therapy in community and population health, several strategies may be useful to prepare for giving reports on social factors. Become familiar with the literature in international development, public and population health, public policy and affairs, sociology and psychology, social work, economics, and governmental and international agencies. Use published exemplars to learn interdisciplinary terminology that is associated with occupational therapy concepts and how measures of social factors are summarized. For example, some components of structural social capital are aligned with the areas of occupation in the Occupational Therapy Practice Framework.[10] When reporting on the outcomes of social factors measures related to occupational performance, use messages that resonate with the common terms used by the target audience.

Organization

The strategies to develop skills in reporting to organizations are similar to those recommended for populations and communities. In addition, occupational therapy practitioners are encouraged to review the organization's mission and vision and other documents that may be helpful in "translating" occupational therapy reports to standard reports used by a specific organization. For example, a nonprofit organization that serves individuals who are homeless will use a different reporting system than a large corporation that is addressing the needs of its employees.

Future Directions for Practice and Research in Measures of Social Factors

Although there have been considerable advances in the development of social factor measures, additional work is needed. Several recommendations are identified in the interdisciplinary literature on social factor measurement.[12] Many measures need further conceptual and operational development and psychometric studies. The factor structure of existing social support instruments also needs to be examined in specific populations. Finally, additional studies are needed to understand the role of social support in supporting health and addressing the needs of people with health conditions.

As occupational therapy practitioners develop their knowledge of the contributions of social factors to occupational performance and participation, increased involvement on interdisciplinary research and practice teams will be important to build stronger linkages between social factor concepts and occupational therapy. The role of occupational therapy in social factor measurement needs to be explicated as it relates to person, environment, and occupational performance. Some occupational performance measures may be improved by adding social factor components. Occupational therapy outcome studies should examine the relationship between social factors and occupational performance. Occupational therapy must commit to addressing the social determinants of health that relate to inequities in performance, participation, and health.

Overview of Measures of Social Factors

A comprehensive review of the literature was conducted to identify and select the social factor measures that are included in this chapter. Measures that are discussed in detail as well as those included in the summary tables were selected based on their stage of development, conceptual framework and completed psychometric studies, usage and currency in research and practice, availability, breadth of target populations, credibility of the author or sponsoring organization, longevity of applications in research and practice, and quantity and quality of peer-reviewed research studies. Other measures were omitted from this chapter because of limited information, availability, and usage. Because social factors have growing relevance to our understanding of occupational performance and participation, readers are invited to expand this list to include other measures of social determinants of health, social support, and social capital and measures of other social factors as well (eg, social connectedness, social functioning).

Social Determinants of Health

Measures of social determinants of health are important in understanding patterns of health and health inequities in populations. Social determinants of health are routinely measured as part of large population surveys and used to establish health priorities. Data from these measures are collected and analyzed by local, state, and national government agencies or from foundations with a mission that is focused on this area. In this chapter, a brief overview of measures of social determinants of health is provided rather than in full detail (see Table 17-1) because occupational therapy practitioners need to be effective users of data from sources but typically will not have primary responsibility for administering and interpreting these measures.

Social Support

Many measures of social support have been developed since the 1980s. Table 17-2 provides a brief summary of an array of interdisciplinary social support measures that have been described in the literature. Four measures have been selected for a more detailed review: The Inventory of Socially Supportive Behaviors (ISSB); Medical Outcomes Study: Social Support Survey (MOS-SS or MOS-SSS) and Modified Medical Outcomes Study: Social Support Survey (mMOS-SS); Multidimensional Scale of Perceived Social Support (MSPSS); and Patient Reported Outcomes Measurement System (PROMIS). These measures have been used extensively and have published information on the conceptual framework and psychometric properties.

The Inventory of Socially Supportive Behaviors (ISSB) was initially developed in the 1980s to measure the frequency of received support in the last month[13,14] (see Table 17-3). The original measure has 40 items that yielded 4 subscales in a confirmatory factor analysis: directive guidance, nondirective support, positive social exchange, and tangible assistance.[15] The short version of the ISSB has 19 items. Each item is scored on a 5-point Likert scale according to frequency of occurrence during the last month (not at all, once or twice, about once per week, several times per week, about every day). The leading question for all items is, "During the past 4 weeks, how often did other people do these activities for you, to you, or with you?" Examples of questions that are on both the original and short version of the measure are as follows:

- Gave you some information on how to do something
- Did some activity together to help you get your mind off things

The ISSB has been used in studies of children, adolescents, college students, older adults, employees, mental health issues, stroke, cardiac conditions, and developmental disabilities.

The Medical Outcomes Study: Social Support Survey (MOS-SS or MOS-SSS) and Modified Medical Outcomes Study: Social Support Survey (mMOS-SS) is a multidimensional self-report measure of the functional dimensions of social support (see Table 17-4). The original MOS-SS consists of 19 items resulting in 4 factors (emotional/informational, tangible, affectionate, and positive social interaction)[16] and the modified mMOS-SS has 8 items yielding 2 factors (instrumental and emotional). Respondents identify the frequency of social support for each item on a 5-point Likert scale (none of the time, a little of the time, some of the time, most of the time, all of the time) in response to the following leading question, "People sometimes look to others for companionship, assistance, or other types of support. How often is each of the following kinds of support available to you if you need it?" Examples of items that are on both the original and modified version of the measure are as follows:

- To help you if you were confined to bed?
- To have a good time with?

The MOS-SS or mMOS-SS is part of the large scale Medical Outcomes Study by the Rand Corporation and has been used in studies of chronic conditions, cancer, cardiac conditions, caregivers, hospice, and older adults and has been adopted as a social support measure in international studies that include Taiwan, Mozambique, and Australia.

The Multidimensional Scale of Perceived Social Support (MSPSS) is a brief (12 items) self-report measure of perceptions of social support received from family, friends, and significant others[17,18] (see Table 17-5). Respondents identify their level of agreement with each item on a 7-point Likert scale (very strongly agree/disagree, strongly agree/disagree, mildly agree/disagree, neutral). Scoring results in a total social support score and scores for each source of support. Examples of items include the following:

- There is a special person who is around when I am in need.
- My family really tries to help me.

Although the MSPSS does not have the conceptual framework of other measures, it continues to be a common measure of social support. The MSPSS has been used in studies across the lifespan, in various countries and cultures, and for many medical and mental health conditions.

The Patient Reported Outcomes Measurement System (PROMIS) is a comprehensive measure of physical, mental, and social health for adults and children[19] (see Table 17-6). The PROMIS initiative began in 2004 as a means to expand the assessment of self-reported health in both practice and research. For adults, social health includes the domains of ability to participate in social roles and activities, satisfaction with social roles and activities, social support, social isolation, and companionship. Although the social support domain is still under development, many of the other social health domains include items that may be associated with received or perceived social support. For example, an item in the companionship domain asks respondents to indicate on a 5-point Likert scale (never, rarely, sometimes, usually, always) their response to the question, "Do you have someone with whom to have fun?"

For children, social health includes the domains of peer relationships, family belongingness, and family involvement. For example, the peer relationships domain asks respondents (or a parent surrogate) to identify their response on the same 5-point Likert scale to the statement, "In the past 7 days, I was able to count on my friends."

PROMIS measures are available in either a computerized adaptive test (CAT) format based on item response theory or as static short forms. Most PROMIS measures are also available in Spanish. The PROMIS Assessment Center (http://www.nihpromis.org) provides a free, online data collection tool for researchers and resources to enable practitioners to incorporate patient-reported outcomes in their assessment process.

Social Capital

There are a growing number of measures of social capital described in the literature. It has been recommended that social capital be examined along 6 dimensions within the context of specific topics and using a variety of key sources.[20] Six dimensions should be included in evaluation of social capital: groups and networks, trust and solidarity, collective action and cooperation, social cohesion and inclusion, information and communication, and empowerment and political action.. Social capital may be examined within the context of topics such as crime/violence, economics/finance/trade, education, environment/water/sanitation, health/nutrition, information technology, poverty reduction/economic development, and rural and urban development. Families, communities, firms, civic groups, public sector, ethnic, and gender groups are key sources for social capital. Because there is not a single measure of social capital, determination of the relevant dimensions is necessary in selecting measures. Table 17-7 provides a brief summary of interdisciplinary social capital measures that have good documentation. Three measures have been selected for a more detailed review: Personal Social Capital Scale (PSCS), Integrated Questionnaire for the Measurement of Social Capital (SC-IQ) (and Social Capital Integrated Questionnaire [SOCAP IQ] for developing countries), and Social Capital Assessment Tool (SOCAT). These measures have been used extensively and have information on the conceptual framework and psychometric properties.

The Personal Social Capital Scale (PSCS) is a self-report measure of an individual's (rather than community's) bonding (horizontal similar) and bridging (horizontal different) social networks (see Table 17-8). The original version of the measure consists of 10 items with 32 bonding subitems and 10 bridging subitems.[21] Preliminary psychometric studies indicate adequate internal consistency, reliability, construct validity, and predictive validity. Respondents identify the characteristics of their social capital using a forced choice scale. Examples of items and subitems include the following:

- Do you participate in activities for how many of each of these 2 types of groups and organizations?
  - Governmental, political, economic, and social groups/organizations
  - Cultural, recreational, and leisure groups/organizations
- When all groups and organizations in the 2 categories are considered, how many possess the following assets/resources?
  - Significant power for decision making
  - Solid financial basis
  - Broad social connections
  - Great social influence

Two shorter versions of the PSCS (16 sub-item, 8 subitem) have recently been described in the literature.[22] Because the PSCS is relatively new, there is little information or recommendations regarding applications in practice and research settings.

The Integrated Questionnaire for the Measurement of Social Capital (SC-IQ) (and Social Capital Integrated Questionnaire [SOCAP IQ] for developing countries) is a self-report measure of social capital at micro (household or individual) level (see Table 17-9). The measure consists of 7 areas with 6 to 33 questions per area and is available through the World Bank.[23] Areas include groups and networks (structural), trust and solidarity (cognitive), collective action and cooperation (output), information and communication, social cohesion and inclusion, empowerment and political action, and CORE questions across 6 dimensions. It is intended for use in larger household surveys and for understanding social capital in developing countries. Reliability and validity have not been reported. Respondents answered questions that were either open-ended or on a Likert scale. Examples of questions include the following:

- How well do people in your village/neighborhood help each other out these days?
  - Always helping
  - Helping most of the time
  - Helping sometime
  - Rarely helping
  - Never helping
- In the last month, how many times have you gotten together with people to play games, sports, or other recreational activities?

This measure is especially useful in developing countries. There is little information or recommendation regarding applications in practice and research settings.[23]

The Social Capital Assessment Tool (SOCAT) is a self-report measure that measures multidimensional aspects of social capital, including both structural and cognitive forms and macro, meso, and micro scopes (see Table 17-10). This measure is a multi-stage assessment involving 3 instruments for measuring the community profile, a household survey, and the organizational profile, and is available through the World Bank Group.[6,24] The community profile includes open-ended community discussions and a structured questionnaire. The household survey includes 5 sections, including an introduction, household characteristics, genogram/family tree, structural dimensions, and cognitive dimensions. Lastly, the organizational profile involves semi-structured interviews or focus groups with leaders, members, and key informants. The reliability of this measure has not been reported, but empirical validity is reported. Question formats included open-ended, multiple choice, and Likert scale. Examples of questions include the following:

- What are the groups, organizations, or associations that function in this village/neighborhood? Which groups play the most active role in helping improve the well-being of community members?
- What is the organization's capacity to carry out its specialized tasks?
  - Excellent
  - Good
  - Adequate
  - Deficient

This measure is useful in providing baseline and monitoring data for programs, measuring social capital at the household, community, and organizational levels and the structural and cognitive dimensions.[6,24]

Summary

Measures of social factors provide occupational therapy practitioners with new avenues for understanding the enablers and barriers of occupational performance that are influenced by societal characteristics, relationships, and networks among people and communities. This chapter provided an introduction to commonly used measures of social determinants of health, social support, and social capital. As occupational therapy has broadened its scope of practice to address health equities, participation, and community engagement, inclusion of social factors in the evaluation process has become critical to research on occupational performance and the development of effective occupational therapy interventions.

Table 17-1

ASSESSMENTS FOR SOCIAL FACTORS

Title of Assessment	*Construct or Factor Assessed*	*Description*
Social Determinants of Health		
American Community Survey[25]	*Population*: Basic, social, economic *Housing*: financial, physical economic	Annual US survey; sampling of about 1 in 38 US households each year
Behavioral Risk Factor Surveillance System (BRFSS)[26]	Risk behaviors and events, chronic health conditions, use of preventive services (national and state level data)	Annual US health-related interviews; sample of more than 400,000 adults
ENACT, THRIVE (Prevention Institute)[27]	Community-level characteristics that have been found to be important for strong communities	Community-level inventories of social determinants of health and related strategies to address barriers
Kids Count Data Center (Annie E. Casey Foundation)[28]	Well-being of children in the United States (national and state level data)	Provides population-based data for the US and by state for demographics, economic well-being, education, family and community, health, safety and risky behaviors
Health Inequality		
CHANGE: Community Health Assessment and Group Evaluation[29]	Assets and limitations of community institutions/organizations, health care, schools, and worksite sectors as they relate to an assessment of community health at large.	Data may be collected using observation, survey, focus groups, walkability audits, and photovoice.
Disability Adjusted Life Year (DALY)[30]	Population measure of the burden of disease	DALY = YLL + YLD where YLL is years of life lost due to premature death and YLD is years of life lost due to disability.
Gini Index[31]	Individual or group measure of inequality (eg, income, premature mortality)	Relative difference in individuals or groups on a theoretical scale from 1 to 0 (1 = perfect or maximum inequality, 0 = perfect equality)
HALex[31]	Individual measure of health-related quality of life	Measures self-rated health and activity limitation in national surveys on a theoretical scale from 0 to 1 (1 = no activity limitation; excellent health, 0.10 = limited in activities and health)
Healthy days[31]	Group measure of the number of healthy days (physical and mental health) in last 30 days	Estimated by the BRFSS; comparisons by state, income levels, and other population groups

Table 17-2

ASSESSMENTS FOR SOCIAL SUPPORT FACTORS

Title of Assessment	*Construct or Factor Assessed*	*Description*
Berkman-Syme Social Network Index (SNI)[32,33]	Type, size, closeness, and frequency of contacts in the current social network	11 items; self-reported questionnaire; published predictive validity Modified versions
Interpersonal Support Evaluation list (ISEL)[34]	Perceived availability of potential social resources	20-item scale; 4 support subscales: tangible, belonging, self-esteem, appraisal

(continued)

Table 17-2 (continued)

Assessments for Social Support Factors

Title of Assessment	*Construct or Factor Assessed*	*Description*
The Inventory of Socially Supportive Behaviors (ISSB)[2,13,14]	Frequency of received social support in the last month	Original version: 40 items; 5-point Likert scale Dimensions: tangible and intangible forms of support Short Version: 19 items
Medical Outcomes Study Social Support Survey (MOS-SS)[16,35,36] http://www.rand.org/health/surveys_tools/mos/social-support.html	Multidimensional, self-administered measure of functional dimensions of social support	Original: 4-factor model Modified: 2-factor model
Multidimensional Scale of Perceived Social Support (MSPSS)[17,18] http://gzimet.wix.com/mspss	Measures perceptions of social support from family, friends, and significant other	Three factors: family, friends, significant others 12-item scale 7-point Likert scale Versions: multiple languages including Spanish, Swedish, Portuguese, Chinese, Farsi; applications in developing countries
Patient Reported Outcomes Measurement System (PROMIS)[19,37] http://www.nihpromis.org/	Patient-reported outcomes on social health and other domains	Versions: adult (5 domains), pediatric (3 domains) Short form (4 to 10 items) or computerized adaptive testing (3 to 7 items)
Social Relationship Scale[38]	Extent of a network of social relationships and perceived helpfulness of these relationships on the life stresses and health	Six items representing work, money and finances, home and family, personal health, personal and social, and society in general
Social Support Questionnaire (SSQ)[39-41]	Availability and satisfaction with social support	27-item self-administered scale; 6-point rating scale; overall support score (SSQN) calculated; established criterion validity, inter-item correlation, internal consistency, test-retest reliability

Table 17-3

The Inventory of Socially Supportive Behaviors (ISSB)

Source	Measurement Instrument Database for the Social Sciences (MIDSS): http://www.midss.org/content/inventory-socially-supportive-behaviors-issb-long-and-short-form
Key References	Barrera et al[35]; Stokes and Wilson[36]; Chronister et al[37]
Purpose	• Measures amount of social support an individual is receiving from others. • The instrument conceptualizes social support as including tangible forms of assistance, such as the provision of goods and services, and intangible forms of assistance, such as guidance and expressions of esteem.

(continued)

Table 17-3 (continued)

The Inventory of Socially Supportive Behaviors (ISSB)

Type of Client	• Self-report measure.
Test Format	• 40-item self-report measure that assesses frequency of assistance during the preceding month using 5-point Likert scales (1 = not at all, 2 = once or twice, 3 = about once per week, 4 = several times per week, and 5 = about every day). • 19-item short version is available.
Procedures	• Brief instructions for completing and scoring the survey are provided.
Time Required	• Brief measure
Standardization	• A total frequency score or average frequency score may be obtained from the 5-point ratings of each item. The average frequency score permits calculation of a global score.
Reliability	
Test-Retest	• Over a 2-day interval (.88), over a 1-month interval (.63 to .80) for undergraduates.
Internal Consistency	• > .9
Inter-Rater	• N/A
Validity	
Factor Structure	• 3 clusters: Guidance, Emotional Support, and Tangible Support
Utility	• Primary purpose is research
Strengths	• Available in the public domain, no charge for use. May be reproduced and modified. It is a global measure of a unidimensional construct.
Complexities	• Limited information available on administration, scoring, interpretation, and application to practice settings.

Table 17-4

Medical Outcomes Study: Social Support Survey (MOS-SS or MOS-SSS) and Modified Medical Outcomes Study: Social Support Survey (mMOS-SS)

Source	Rand Health: http://www.rand.org/health/surveys_tools/mos/mos_socialsupport.html
Key References	Sherbourne and Stewart[16]; Gjesfjeld et al[35]; Moser et al[36]
Purpose	• Measures multiple dimensions of functional social support • Original: emotional/informational, tangible, affectionate, and positive social interaction • Modified: instrumental, emotional
Type of Client	• Self-report survey.
Test Format	• Self-administered survey in paper format, 5-point Likert scale • Original: 19 items for 4 dimensions • Modified: 8 items for 2 dimensions
Procedures	• Short self-explanatory instructions provided on survey.
Time Required	• Brief amount of time.
Standardization	• Subscale scores and overall index of social support available.

(continued)

Table 17-4 (continued)

Medical Outcomes Study: Social Support Survey (MOS-SS or MOS-SSS) and Modified Medical Outcomes Study: Social Support Survey (mMOS-SS)

Reliability	
Internal Consistency	• MOS-SS: Chronbach's alpha >.5 • mMOS-SS: Chronbach's alpha .67 to .97
Validity	
Factor Structure	• MOS-SS: original scale had 5 subscales; emotional and informational subscales were combined because of overlap in items • mMOS-SS: factorial analysis resulted in 2-factor solution
Construct	• MOS-SS: significant correlations with health and other social factors • mMOS-SS: moderate significant correlations with population characteristics
Discriminant	• MOS-SS: dimensions were supported in an analyses • mMOS-SS: significant differences between demographic groups
Utility	• Original: Longitudinal research studies for patients with chronic conditions • Application to many populations
Strengths	• Widely used, global applications, multiple languages, public documents and available without charge, part of the large scale Medical Outcomes Study by the Rand Corporation that includes other measures
Complexities	• Limited information available on administration, scoring, interpretation, and application to practice settings

Table 17-5

Multidimensional Scale of Perceived Social Support (MSPSS)

Source	Zimet; Multidimensional Scale of Perceived Social Support (MSPSS); http://gzimet.wix.com/mspss
Key References	Zimet et al[17,18]; Stanley et al[42]; Bruwer et al[43]; Cecil et al[44]
Purpose	• Measure perceptions of support from 3 sources: family, friends, and significant other
Type of Client	• Self-report survey
Test Format	• 12 items, with 4 items each for family, friends, and significant other • 7-point Likert scale • Paper version
Procedures	• Limited information available • Self-explanatory
Time Required	• Very brief survey
Standardization	• No established population norms • Mean scores for 3 subscales and total scale
Reliability	
Test-Retest	• Coefficient: .72 to .85
Internal Consistency	• Chronabach's coefficient alphas for subscales and total scale: (.81 to .98)

(continued)

Table 17-5 (continued)

MULTIDIMENSIONAL SCALE OF PERCEIVED SOCIAL SUPPORT (MSPSS)

Validity	
Confirmatory factor analysis	• 3 factors
Construct	• Positive social support was inversely related to 1) depression and anxiety for family ($p < 0.01$), 2) depression for friends ($p < 0.01$) and significant other ($p < 0.05$)
Utility	• Research and Clinical Studies • Self-Management Programs • Populations: youth, older adults, mental illness, various mental conditions, immigration, developing countries, at-risk populations
Strengths	• Translated into over 20 languages • Applications to many populations, including youth, older adults, psychiatric conditions, and populations in developing countries
Complexities	• Wide application but limited recent review articles and no available guidelines for administration and interpretation of results

Table 17-6

PATIENT-REPORTED OUTCOMES MEASUREMENT SYSTEM (PROMIS)

Source	PROMIS: Dynamic Tools to Measure Health Outcomes from the Patient Perspective: http://www.nihpromis.org/ Webinars: https://www.youtube.com/playlist?list=PLn4-TLdSKwaRrNYt14Ipw4WVdBarSo8Yx
Key References	Cella et al[19]; Hahn et al[37]; Heinemann[45]
Purpose	• Obtain patient reported outcomes on social health and other domains • Adult Self-Report Domains: ¤ Ability to participate in social roles and activities ¤ Satisfaction with social roles and activities ¤ Social support ¤ Social isolation ¤ Companionship • Pediatric Self-Report and Proxy Domains ¤ Peer Relationships ¤ Family Belongingness ¤ Family involvement
Type of Client	• Adult: Self-Report • Pediatric: Self-Report and Proxy
Test Format	• Short forms (4 to 10 items) or computerized adaptive testing (3 to 7 items) • Each question/statement has 5 response options • 7-day recall period for most items
Procedures	• Website has extensive training materials and manuals. • There is free access to the computerized and paper versions of the assessment

(continued)

Table 17-6 (continued)

Patient-Reported Outcomes Measurement System (PROMIS)

Type of Client	
Procedures	• Assessment may be administered in computerized or paper format • 50 is the average score in the reference population with a standard deviation of 10
Time Required	• Very short. Actual time is dependent on the chosen domains.
Standardization	• Calibration studies testing included representative sample from 2000 Census demographic data, including individuals with chronic conditions
Reliability	• Reference population: US general population • Precision: Good precision across the broad domain especially when using computerized adaptive testing (CAT) with 10 items
Validity	
Concurrent	• Scores on PROMIS correlate with scores on similar measures
Responsiveness	• PROMIS effect size changes as people experience clinical benefit or change
Utility	• Can be used across chronic conditions and with both children and adults. • Is available in multiple languages • Free computerized adaptive testing is available and includes scoring
Strengths	• NIH supported development of PROMIS to provide practitioners and researchers with PROs that can be used with a variety of populations and have strong psychometric properties.
Complexities	• An introduction to Item Response Theory and Computerized Adaptive Testing is necessary to understand the measurement theory used in PROMIS. Written materials and videos are readily available on the website.

Table 17-7

Measures for Social Capital Factors

Title of Assessment	*Construct or Factor Assessed*	*Brief Description*
Individual		
Personal Social Capital Scale (PSCS)[21,22]	Individual network connections, the links a person has to society. Includes bonding and bridging social capital	Original version: 10 items with 32 bonding sub-items: 5 sub-item areas 10 bridging sub-items: 5 sub-item areas 5-point Likert scale Short versions: 16 sub-items, 8 sub-items Utility: behavioral and health research
Resource Generator[46]	Individual social capital measures	3 theoretical classifications Item response theory 33 social resource items Dichotomous scale Utility: cross-sectional, prospective research

(continued)

Table 17-7 (continued)

MEASURES FOR SOCIAL CAPITAL FACTORS

Title of Assessment	*Construct or Factor Assessed*	*Brief Description*
Community		
Adapted Social Capital Assessment Tool (A-SCAT)[7]	Social capital for 2 domains: structural (connectedness) and cognitive (reciprocity, sharing, trust)	Quantitative; 7 questions for structural social capital and 11 questions for cognitive social capital
Integrated Questionnaire for the Measurement of Social Capital (SC-IQ) and Social Capital Integrated Questionnaire (SOCAP IQ)[20,24]	Social capital for 6 dimensions: groups and networks, trust and solidarity, collective action and cooperation, information and communication, social cohesion and inclusion, empowerment and political action.	Quantitative; part of a larger household survey; SOCAP-IQ is an extension of the SC-IQ for developing countries
Our Community U of MN[47]	Social capital in rural communities. Includes bonding, bridging, and linking social capital.	34 items 7 conceptual domains: bonding (trust, engagement), bridging (trust, engagement), linking (trust, engagement), efficacy Utility: research on social capital, resource for education, community assessment tool
Social Capital Assessment Tool (SOCAT)[6,20]	Social capital data on households, communities, and organizations Forms: structural, cognitive Scope: macro (community), meso, micro (individual)	Qualitative/quantitative. Includes both structural and cognitive components Three instruments: community, household, organizational
Social Capital Community Benchmark Survey http://www.hks.harvard.edu/saguaro/communitysurvey/	Widespread, systematic measure of social capital in communities. Allows comparisons across communities	Versions: 2000, 2006, short 11 dimensions Utility: research database, tool for communities, program development and evaluation
Social Capital Questionnaire for Adolescent Students (SCQ-AS)[48]	Social capital for adolescents for 3 subscales: social network/cohesion/sense of belonging, trust, autonomy and control	Quantitative; 12 items; 3-point Likert scale

Table 17-8

PERSONAL SOCIAL CAPITAL SCALE (PSCS)

Source	Chen et al[21]
Key References	Wang et al[22]
Purpose	• Measure individual network connections, links a person has to society. Includes bonding and bridging
Type of Client	• Self-report survey
Test Format	• Forced choice survey, 5-point Likert scale • Original version: 10 items with 32 bonding sub-items and 10 bridging sub-items.

(continued)

Table 17-8 (continued)

Personal Social Capital Scale (PSCS)

Type of Client	
Test Format	• Bonding sub items areas: ◦ (a) perceived network size ◦ (b) frequency of contact with network members ◦ (c) the number of network members who are perceived as trustful ◦ (d) the number of network members possessing resources (education, professional job, position, social influence, and political power) ◦ (e) the number of network members who are reciprocal • Bridging sub-items areas: ◦ (a) perceived group size ◦ (b) participation in group activities ◦ (c) if the groups represent personal rights and interests ◦ (d) resources possessed by these groups ◦ (e) the likelihood to receive help from the groups upon request • Short versions: 16 sub-items or 8 sub-items
Procedures	• Manual and guidelines are not readily available • One participant per household • Paper and pencil or computer-based questionnaire
Time Required	• 30 to 45 minutes
Standardization	• 10 item scores • Two-factor model: bonding and bridging • Total score
Reliability	• Psychometric studies are still in progress
Internal Consistency	• Positive correlations between all item scores and total scale score. • Total scale score: Correlations between item cores and total scale score (.37 to .77), Cronbach alpha=.87 • Bonding capital subscale: Correlations between items and subscale (53 to .77), Cronbach alpha=.85 • Bridging capital subscale: Correlations between items and subscale (.42 to .74). Cronbach alpha=.84 • Short versions also have adequate reliability.
Validity	• Psychometric studies are still in progress
Construct	• Two-factor model established from confirmatory factor analysis • Construct validity was supported for known group differences on gender, education, age, residence
Predictive	• Regression was used in predictive validity studies, positive associations were demonstrated between PSCS scores and informational, instrumental, and emotional support, and perceived collective efficacy using regression • Short versions preserved 2-factor model and had high correlations with original PSCS
Utility	• An instrument for health and behavioral research
Strengths	• Available in English and Chinese
Complexities	• Length of original version

Table 17-9

Integrated Questionnaire for the Measurement of Social Capital (SC-IQ) and Social Capital Integrated Questionnaire (SOCAP IQ) for Developing Countries

Source	World Bank Group
Key References	Grootaert[23]
Purpose	• Measure social capital at the household or individual level (micro): ◦ Groups and networks (structural)—33 questions ◦ Trust and solidarity (cognitive)—6 questions ◦ Collective action and cooperation (output)—7 questions ◦ Information and communication—11 questions ◦ Social cohesion and inclusion—23 questions ◦ Empowerment and political action—15 questions ◦ CORE questions across 6 dimensions—27 questions
Type of Client	• Self-report
Test Format	• Likert scale • Open-ended questions
Procedures	• Questionnaire may be conducted in telephone interview
Time Required	• 30 to 60 minutes
Standardization	• Script and standard questions • Response options for forced choice questions
Reliability	• Not reported
Validity	• Not reported
Utility	• Intended use in larger household surveys
Strengths	• Intended application to understand social capital in developing countries • May be used as part of a larger household survey
Complexities	• Length of survey and time to complete • Emphasis on recall of past events on some questions

Table 17-10

Social Capital Assessment Tool (SOCAT)

Source	World Bank Group
Key References	Grootaert and Van Bastelaer[6,24]
Purpose	• Measures multidimensional aspects of social capital • Forms: structural and cognitive • Scope: macro, meso, micro
Type of Client	• Self-report • Quantitative and qualitative

(continued)

Table 17-10 (continued)

Social Capital Assessment Tool (SOCAT)

Type of Client	
Test Format	• Three instruments: 1. Community profile: 1) open-ended community discussions based on participatory interview guide, 2) standardized structured questionnaire 2. Household survey: quantitative 1) introduction, 2) household characteristics, 3) genogram/family tree, 4) structural dimensions, 5) cognitive dimensions 3. Organizational profile: semi-structured key informant or focus groups interviews with leaders, members, nonmembers
Procedures	• Multi-stage assessment
Time Required	• Community profile: one-half to 1 day • Household surveys: 15 to 120 minutes, depending on household characteristics • Organizational profile: 45 to 60 minutes for key informant interviews, 15 to 30 minutes for focus groups interviews; 3 to 4 hours total time
Standardization	• Guidelines for community and organizational profiles. • Script and standard questions for household surveys
Reliability	• Not reported
Validity	• Empirical validity reported, but details on analyses not provided
Utility	• Provides baseline and monitoring data for programs
Strengths	• Integrated quantitative/qualitative tool • Measures social capital at household, community, and organizational levels • Provides detailed information about structural and cognitive dimensions
Complexities	• Length of survey and time to complete • Interpretation

References

1. Solar O, Irwin A. *A Conceptual Framework for Action on the Social Determinants of Health: Social Determinants of Health Discussion Paper 2 (Policy and Practice).* Geneva, Switzerland: World Health Organization Press; 2007.
2. Chronister JA, Johnson EK, Berven NL. Measuring social support in rehabilitation. *Disabil Rehabil.* 2006;28(2):75-84.
3. Bowlby J. *Attachment and Loss: Loss, Sadness and Depression.* Vol 3. New York: Basic Books; 1980.
4. Thoits PA. Conceptual, methodological, and theoretical problems in studying social support as a buffer against life stress. *J Health Soc Behav.* 1982;23:145-159.
5. Grootaert C, Narayan D, Jones VN, Woolcock M. *Measuring Social Capital: An Integrated Questionnaire.* The World Bank Working Paper. No 18. Washington, DC: World Bank Publications; 2004. https://openknowledge.worldbank.org/bitstream/handle/10986/15033/281100PAPER0Measuring0social0capital.pdf. Accessed September 12, 2016.
6. Grootaert C, Van Bastelaer T, eds. *Understanding and Measuring Social Capital: A Multidisciplinary Tool for Practitioners.* Vol 1. Washington DC: World Bank Publications; 2002. http://www-wds.worldbank.org/external/default/WDSContentServer/WDSP/IB/2002/07/31/000094946_02071104014990/Rendered/PDF/multi0page.pdf. Accessed June 16, 2016.
7. Harpham T, Grant E, Thomas E. Measuring social capital within health surveys: key issues. *Health Policy Plan.* 2002;17(1):106-111.
8. DiMatteo MR. Social support and patient adherence to medical treatment: a meta-analysis. *Health Psychol.* 2004;23(2):207.
9. Uchino BN. Social support and health: a review of physiological processes potentially underlying links to disease outcomes. *J Behav Med.* 2006;29(4):377-387.
10. American Occupational Therapy Association. Occupational therapy practice framework: domain and process. 3rd ed. *Am J Occup Ther.* 2014;68(Suppl 1):S1-S48.

11. Haber MG, Cohen JL, Lucas T, Baltes BB. The relationship between self-reported received and perceived social support: a meta-analytic review. *Am J Community Psychol.* 2007;39(1-2):133-144.
12. Lindsey AM, Yates BC. Social support: conceptualization and measurement instruments. In: Stromborg FM, Olsen SJ, eds. *Instruments for Clinical Health-Care Research.* Sudbury, MA: Jones & Bartlett Learning; 2004:164-199.
13. Barrera M, Sandler IN, Ramsay TB. Preliminary development of a scale of social support: studies on college students. *Am J Community Psychol.* 1981;9(4):435-447.
14. Stokes JP, Wilson DG. The inventory of socially supportive behaviors: dimensionality, prediction, and gender differences. *Am J Community Psychol.* 1984;12(1):53-69.
15. Finch JF, Barrera M Jr, Okun MA, Bryant WHM, Pool GJ, Snow-Turek AL. Factor structure of received social support: dimensionality and the prediction of depression and life satisfaction. *J Soc Clin Psychol.* 1997;16:323-342.
16. Sherbourne CD, Stewart AL. The MOS social support survey. *Soc Sci Med.* 1991;32(6):705-714.
17. Zimet GD, Dahlem NW, Zimet SG, Farley GK. The Multidimensional Scale of Perceived Social Support. *J Pers Assess.* 1988;52(1):30-41.
18. Zimet GD, Powell SS, Farley GK, Werkman S, Berkoff KA. Psychometric characteristics of the Multidimensional Scale of Perceived Social Support. *J Pers Assess.* 1990;55(3-4):610-617.
19. Cella D, Riley W, Stone A, et al. The Patient-Reported Outcomes Measurement Information System (PROMIS) developed and tested its first wave of adult self-reported health outcome item banks: 2005–2008. *J Clin Epidemiol.* 2010;63(11):1179-1194.
20. Dudwick N, Kuehnast K, Nyhan Jones V, Woolcock M. *Analyzing Social Capital in Context: A Guide to Using Qualitative Methods and Data.* Washington, DC: World Bank Publications, 2006. http://documents.worldbank.org/curated/en/601831468338476652/pdf/389170Analyzin11in1Context01PUBLIC1.pdf. Accessed September 12, 2016.
21. Chen X, Stanton B, Gong J, Fang X, Li X. Personal Social Capital Scale: an instrument for health and behavioral research. *Health Educ Res.* 2009;24(2):306-317.
22. Wang P, Chen X, Gong J, Jacques-Tiura AJ. Reliability and validity of the Personal Social Capital Scale 16 and Personal Social Capital Scale 8: two short instruments for survey studies. *Soc Indicators Res.* 2014;119:1133-1148.
23. Grootaert C. *Measuring Social Capital: An Integrated Questionnaire.* No. 18. Washington, DC: World Bank Publications; 2004.
24. Grootaert C, Van Bastelaer T. Understanding and measuring social capital: a synthesis of findings and recommendations from the social capital initiative. *The World Bank Social Capital Initiative Working Paper.* No 24. Washington DC: World Bank Publications; 2001. http://siteresources.worldbank.org/INTSOCIALCAPITAL/Resources/Social-Capital-Initiative-Working-Paper-Series/SCI-WPS-24.pdf. Accessed June 16, 2016.
25. US Department of Commerce, US Census Bureau. American Community Survey. http://www.census.gov/acs/www/. Published 2012. Accessed June 22, 2016.
26. US Centers for Disease Control and Prevention. Behavioral Risk Factor Surveillance System (BRFSS). http://www.cdc.gov/brfss/. Published 2013. Accessed June 22, 2016.
27. Prevention Institute. Tools. http://preventioninstitute.org/tools.html. Published 2014. Accessed June 22, 2016.
28. The Annie E. Casey Foundation. KIDS COUNT data center. http://datacenter.kidscount.org/. Published 2014. Accessed June 22, 2106.
29. US Centers for Disease Control and Prevention. Community Health Assessment and Group Evaluation (CHANGE) Action Guide: building a foundation of knowledge to prioritize community needs. http://www.cdc.gov/nccdphp/dch/programs/healthycommunitiesprogram/tools/change/pdf/changeactionguide.pdf. Published 2010. Accessed June 22, 2016.
30. World Health Organization. Metrics: disability-adjusted life year (DALY). http://www.who.int/healthinfo/global_burden_disease/metrics_daly/en/. Published 2014. Accessed June 22, 2016
31. Truman BI, Smith CK, Roy K, et al. Rationale for regular reporting on health disparities and inequalities—United States. *MMWR Suppl.* 2011;60(1):3-10.
32. Berkman LF, Syme SL. Social networks, host resistance, and mortality: a nine-year follow-up study of Alameda County residents. *Am J Epidemiol.* 1979;109(2):186-204.
33. House JS, Umberson D, Landis KR. Structures and processes of social support. *Ann Rev Sociol.* 1988;14:293-318.
34. Cohen S, Hoberman HM. Positive events and social supports as buffers of life change stress. *J Appl Soc Psychol.* 1983;13(2):99-125.
35. Gjesfjeld CD, Greeno CG, Kim KH. A confirmatory factor analysis of an abbreviated social support instrument—The MOSS-SSS. *Res Soc Work Pract.* 2008;18(3):231-237.
36. Moser A, Stuck AE, Silliman RA, Ganz PA, Clough-Gorr KM. The eight-item modified Medical Outcomes Study Social Support Survey: psychometric evaluation showed excellent performance. *J Clin Epidemiol.* 2012;65(10):1107-1116.
37. Hahn EA, DeVellis RF, Bode RK, et al. Measuring social health in the patient-reported outcomes measurement information system (PROMIS): item bank development and testing. *Qual Life Res.* 2010;19(7):1035-1044.
38. McFarlane AH, Neale KA, Norman GR, Roy RG, Streiner DL. Methodological issues in developing a scale to measure social support. *Schizophr Bull.* 1981;7(1):90-100.
39. Sarason IG, Levine HM, Basham RB, Sarason BR. Assessing social support: the social support questionnaire. *J Pers Soc Psychol.* 1983;44(1):127.
40. Sarason IG, Sarason BR. Social support: mapping the construct. *J Soc Pers Relat.* 2009;26(1):113-120.
41. Sarason IG, Sarason BR, Shearin EN, Pierce GR. A brief measure of social support: practical and theoretical implications. *J Soc Pers Relat.* 1987;4(4):497-510.
42. Stanley MA, Beck JG, Zebb BJ. Psychometric properties of the MSPSS in older adults. *Aging Ment Health.* 1998;2(3):186-193.
43. Bruwer B, Emsley R, Kidd M, Lochner C, Seedat S. Psychometric properties of the Multidimensional Scale of Perceived Social Support in youth. *Compr Psychiatry.* 2008;49(2):195-201.

44. Cecil H, Stanley MA, Carrion PG, Swann A. Psychometric properties of the MSPSS and NOS in psychiatric outpatients. *J Clin Psychol.* 1995;51(5):593-602.
45. Heinemann AW. Measurement of participation in rehabilitation research. *Arch Phys Med Rehabil.* 2010;91(9):S1-S4.
46. Van Der Gaag M, Snijders TA. The Resource Generator: social capital quantification with concrete items. *Soc Networks.* 2005;27(1):1-29.
47. Chazdon S, Allen R, Horntvedt J, Scheffert DR. Developing and validating University of Minnesota Extension's social capital model and survey. University of Minnesota Extension Center for Community Vitality. http://www.extension.umn.edu/community/civic-engagement/social-capital/. Published 2013. Accessed June 22, 2016.
48. Paiva PCP, de Paiva HN, de Oliveira Filho PM, et al. Development and validation of a Social Capital Questionnaire for Adolescent Students (SCQ-AS). *PloS One.* 2014;9(8):e103785.

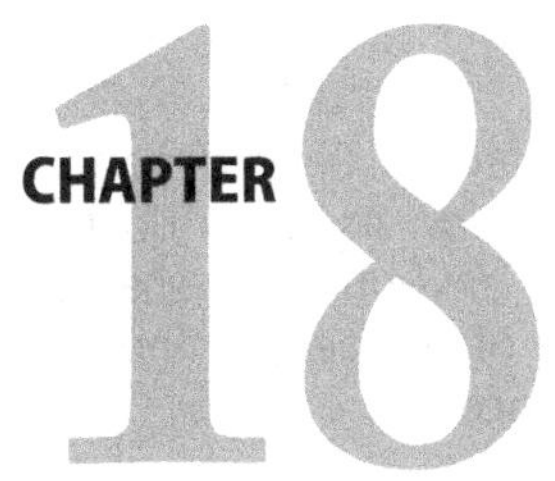

Applying an Occupational Performance Measurement Approach

Challenges and Strategies in Implementation

Mary Law, PhD, FCAOT; Carolyn Baum, PhD, OTR/L, FAOTA; and Winnie Dunn, PhD, OTR, FAOTA

The purpose of this book has been to help the reader understand the importance of using an occupational performance measurement approach and have ready access to occupational performance assessment tools for occupational therapy practice. Occupational performance represents the unique contribution that occupational therapy contributes to health and the changing health system. Using and reporting on people's occupational performance capacities and needs is the greatest asset professionals bring to the patients or clients they serve because it puts the emphasis on the client's needs, activities, and goals.

Incorporating outcome measurement into every occupational therapy practice is no longer a choice made by individual therapists. With increased pressure for fiscal accountability, changing accreditation and regulatory standards, increased responsibility to ensure competent practice, and increased expectations from consumers, occupational therapists must have reliable and valid methods to document the effects of their practice. Because participation is our desired outcome with the persons we serve, valid and reliable outcome measurement of participation is the way to provide this documentation.

It is our hope that this book will help student occupational therapists and occupational therapists in practice to develop measurement strategies that are efficient and inform both their practice and their colleagues and consumers about the practice of occupational therapy. Let us conclude our dialogue by examining questions about measurement, its implementation, and the challenges inherent in the effective use of measurement that more clearly represents the core philosophy of occupational therapy.

Why Do We Need to Ensure That Measurement Is Integral to Our Practice?

Identity

From the earliest time in the history of occupational therapy, occupational therapists have placed value on supporting persons to engage in occupations that are important to them within their daily lives. The profession of occupational therapy began with recognition that there is an important and significant relationship between occupation, health, and well-being. Unfortunately, these early values were displaced during the middle of the 20th century when occupational therapists began to focus their treatment on changing impairments such as mood, range of motion, and strength, rather than enabling engagement in occupation. Because of this shift in focus, the outcomes that were measured during therapy emphasized changes in impairment or performance components rather than measuring the impact of these component changes on participation outcomes. Beginning in the 1970s, occupational therapy shifted back to its roots with a renewed emphasis on interventions designed to facilitate clients to perform chosen occupations in the environments in which they live, work, and play.

However, this shift back to our roots has not been complete. Even today, in many practice locations, occupational therapy practice remains in conflict between the core values of the profession (ie, a focus on enabling and providing opportunities for improved occupational performance and more satisfaction with living) and the demands of

Law M, Baum C, Dunn W, eds. *Measuring Occupational Performance: Supporting Best Practice in Occupational Therapy, Third Edition (pp 413-420).*

some settings that compel therapists to remain focused on addressing the impairments of individuals.

The entire health system is now focusing on function, well-being, and quality of life. The World Health Organization (WHO) International Classifications of Functioning, Disability and Health (ICF)[1] emphasizes activity and participation as critical features of a comprehensive view of healthy living. This expansion of the traditional medical model view from "fixing impairments" or "cure" toward function, well-being, and quality of life requires occupational therapy to take a leadership role in identifying what a person needs and wants to do and the environmental supports that make that doing possible. Our unique contribution goes beyond impairment at the activity and participation level that provides and supports performance and removes the barriers that limit an individual's participation in life activities. It is this uniqueness that gives us our identity. Charles Christiansen, in his 1999 Eleanor Clarke Slagle Lecture, reminds us that what we do shapes our identities of ourselves and what others perceive us to be.[2] Our measurement approach has everything to do with that identity.

Furthermore, with a new focus on participation, more and more occupational therapists will have the opportunity to provide services in community settings not previously served by occupational therapy. Our ability to contribute to and provide leadership within these new systems will be possible by establishing a strong identity that is associated with performance and participation. Conducting measurement that addresses performance in context will make that expertise clear to everyone.

Uniqueness

A shift is occurring toward a focus on function as one of the primary indicators of intervention effectiveness.[3,4] What, then, is the unique contribution of occupational therapy in service systems? A careful review of the Institute of Medicine report *Enabling America*[5] identifies nursing, physical therapy, engineering, and occupational therapy as disciplines that focus on improving the function of the person with a disability. The goal of promoting function is shared by occupational therapy, physical therapy, nursing, social work, psychology, and medicine, among others.[6]

It is the occupational therapy perspective that makes our contribution unique. Occupational therapists understand and analyze the relationship between persons, the occupations they choose to do, and the environments in which persons carry out these occupations. Occupational therapists identify the supports and barriers to a person's chosen occupation and can collaborate with that person and his or her family to ensure successful participation in these occupations. Unlike other disciplines, we are making our best contribution when we stand at the intersection between the person and his or her desired participation. Occupational therapists are the only discipline whose focus is on activity as distinct from the environment. Other disciplines are more likely to focus on the person's ways of handling participation or on the environment's characteristics related to desired performance. Occupational therapy, through its focus on the interaction between persons and environment, enables the team to use the best aspects of the person and the environment to support performance.

Core Knowledge

At the core of what we do is what we know—our specialty is occupational performance. Our subspecialty may be in working with children, older adults, persons with mental illness, or individuals with hand injuries or spinal cord injuries. Our core knowledge is not who or what we treat—it is how our knowledge will empower our clients to achieve their objectives in performing occupations of their choice.

Therefore, it is impossible to address a person's engagement in daily occupations without a strong understanding of what the person wants and needs to do and knowledge of how performance components and environmental factors influence that person's performance. Occupational therapists often describe themselves as taking a holistic approach to care. This approach comes from having knowledge of the factors that contribute to the occupational performance of the individual or community that we are serving. We must use measurement tools to gather the information to support our unique contribution to the health and well-being of those we serve. Hopefully, this text has provided knowledge and strategies to enable the practitioner to employ the type of measurement in his or her daily practice with clients of different diagnoses, cultures, and social situations that reflect our interest and expertise in the person's ability to perform, the environment's capacity to support desired performance, and the task's characteristics to enable successful performance. It is only in creating congruence between what we say is our expertise and what others observe in our measurement and intervention strategies that we inform others about ourselves.

Evidence of Making a Difference

Occupational therapy clients come to receive intervention that will enable them to conduct their lives in a successful and satisfying way. They expect that our interventions are effective, appropriate to their needs, and cost efficient. In addition to our clients' expectations, there is a need for increased accountability in all service systems and from regulatory bodies. Just as others expect it, occupational therapists must expect themselves to employ best practices. As described earlier in this book, best practice combines research evidence with clinical reasoning and client's values and preferences to provide effective occupational therapy intervention. In such an evidence-based practice, therapists use research knowledge while collaborating with clients to identify occupational performance needs, analyze the reasons for participation difficulties, and provide intervention to improve occupational performance.

Knowledge of the effectiveness of interventions is drawn from the research literature and from an active outcome measurement protocol within each occupational therapist's practice. It is important for every therapist to employ outcome measurement strategies that will enable him or her to acquire evidence of whether occupational therapy intervention is effective as it is happening. Every occupational therapist needs to know whether his or her intervention has made a difference overall for his or her clients. Our more traditional strategies of measuring performance components will not provide this evidence because the relationship between improved component skills and participation has not been demonstrated. Occupational therapists will serve themselves better to make the direct link between the measurement of performance in context and the intervention process.

Focus on Societal Needs: Quality of Life, Well-Being

About 50 million Americans (20%) and 3.4 million Canadians (14.6%)[7] have a physical or mental impairment that interferes with their daily activities; 41% of them are so severe that they cannot work or participate in their communities. Disability is a public health problem that affects not only individuals and their immediate families, but also society.[5,8]

There are a number of issues facing society that occupational therapists can address. Persons with chronic disease, illness, and neurological or mental health conditions need the resources and skills to lead productive lives and participate with family as they live and work in their communities. Children present another challenge. Those with chronic disease and disability need the support to grow into adulthood with the skills to achieve independence in their lives. Technology has made independence possible for those who previously were not physically capable of independent living. Workers continue to have injuries, and more and more are suffering needless injuries from the movements required in their jobs. Providing workers with the skills to avoid injuries is becoming basic to employee education programs in many industries. Not only do people miss work because of injury, more and more are finding it difficult to manage aging parents on a day-to-day basis. This creates important opportunities for occupational therapists who focus on occupational performance and employ measurement strategies focused on what people need and want to do.

Hospitals have joined into health care networks and, as the funding systems approach payment based on covered lives, they are building programming to ensure that the communities they serve are healthy. Health costs less than illness. Occupational therapists can play key roles in supporting healthy communities by helping their clients attain the knowledge to prevent secondary conditions. This often means building community follow-up programs and linking clients to community resources and independent living centers to help them gain the confidence and skills to perform the activities and roles that are meaningful to them. Occupational therapists play a role in facilitating community independence and can provide important contributions to a population-based approach to health.

Occupational therapists have traditionally played a role in the school systems based on legal mandates, but with an occupational performance perspective, occupational therapy personnel can have an expanded role. Society is looking for ways to prepare children with the skills and behaviors for life. For example, occupational therapists can play a role with children who have behavior disorders by helping them achieve satisfaction in meaningful tasks that provide an outlet for their frustration and a forum to highlight their strengths, rather than continuing to expect them (and their teachers) to struggle within a context that amplifies limitations in performance. Within the context of schools, occupational therapists are also sources of knowledge to improve classroom organization, teaching modifications and building planning in service to all the students and teachers within the school. Expanding our roles beyond the traditional service to persons with specific disabilities provides opportunities for occupational therapy knowledge to support a more successful and satisfying experience for everyone.

Our towns and cities are facing a crisis with the increase in older adults who need housing and supportive services to live independently. Occupational therapists are a natural resource to support the health, fitness, and social needs of older adults who are at risk of losing their independence. Occupational therapists are also important resources for families as they struggle to make good decisions about support mechanisms for their older family members. Occupational performance must be the focus of identifying problems that limit full participation in community life.

Society is progressively developing a universal environment that makes the disabilities we identify today transparent; this means that the barriers that prohibit successful participation are being removed for everyone. For example, although curb cuts have been installed to comply with the Americans with Disabilities Act (ADA), they are used by many more citizens without traditional "disabilities" (eg, parents with strollers, or adults who wish to avoid joint trauma from stepping off the curb). Occupational therapists have the expertise to work with architects, engineers, and city planners to remove barriers that place unnecessary restraints on individuals. The measurement models we are recommending in this text provide an entry into community planning. Occupational therapists who employ an occupational performance approach will demonstrate immediate relevance for this societal evolution. At the center of all of these issues is occupation. Society's problems become exaggerated when its citizens cannot work, cannot care for themselves, and cannot care for others.

Occupational therapists can influence the health of their communities by taking knowledge of occupational performance into new arenas of health care. It is the occupational therapist's responsibility to help policy makers understand how occupational therapy's unique contribution to occupational performance reduces health care costs, as it directs its services to help individuals with or at risk for disabilities to live independently. These functions can be achieved in many ways, from challenging insurance denials, encouraging professional direction, and stimulating laws and regulations, to becoming involved in consumer groups and advocacy-oriented organizations that share the same concerns for persons with disabilities.

All public policy initiatives require the practitioner to become involved in the communities in which they live and work and educate people about the benefits of occupational therapy as they interact with people whose job or interest it is to improve the health and lives of the people in that community. This is possible when data regarding the performance needs of persons with disabilities have been collected and summarized at a level that policy makers can understand.

A Profession's Responsibility

Occupational therapy (as reflected in us as professionals) has the professional responsibility to address the needs of our societies as it struggles with issues of chronic disease, disability, and handicapping situations. To societies, these issues mean lost productivity and costly services; to individuals, they mean poorer health and compromised well-being. A brief review of the health issues of Canada and the United States will set a context to examine what occupational therapists can do to highlight our contribution to helping both society and the individuals who can benefit from our interventions.

The problems associated with chronic disease and disability are so prevalent that, in 2010, the US Department of Health and Human Services published the Healthy People 2020 Objectives,[9] with priorities to challenge communities and health professionals to promote prevention strategies for their citizens. A number of the objectives should be of interest to occupational therapists. Of particular interest should be the objectives for activity and participation.

Activities and Participation

- DH-13 (Developmental) Increase the proportion of people with disabilities who participate in social, spiritual, recreational, community, and civic activities to the degree that they wish
- DH-14 Increase the proportion of children and youth with disabilities who spend at least 80% of their time in regular education programs
- DH-15 Reduce unemployment among people with disabilities
- DH-16 Increase employment among people with disabilities
- DH-17 Increase the proportion of adults with disabilities who report sufficient social and emotional support
- DH-18 (Developmental) Reduce the proportion of people with disabilities who report serious psychological distress
- DH-19 (Developmental) Reduce the proportion of people with disabilities who experience nonfatal, unintentional injuries that require medical care
- DH-20 Increase the proportion of children with disabilities, birth through age 2 years, who receive early intervention services in home- or community-based settings

In Canada, the federal government has worked to improve the health and participation of Canadians through health-promotion strategies.[10,11] Health is viewed as much more than the absence of disease, and many provinces in the country have set health goals for their populations. One example is the province of Ontario, where the health goals include an emphasis on health promotion and disease prevention; building healthy, supportive communities; reducing illness, disability, and death; improving the physical environment; and ensuring accessible and affordable health services for all.[12]

Raising Issues in Public Forums

As society builds strategies to manage its needs, occupational therapists must be able to answer some important questions that will place occupational therapy in a key position in the new health system. Most importantly, we need to be able to address key issues in public forums to educate the policy makers who make decisions about the allocations of resources that pay for occupational therapy services. The following are offered as examples; each question is related to an area where occupational therapists currently work and must have the data to retain our positions:

- What occupational performance measures document the activity participation, instrumental activity levels, and effectiveness of environmental modifications that will allow older adults to retain their independence in their communities?
- Do people who receive occupational therapy services demonstrate productive work behaviors, are they able to problem solve, or manage multiple tasks, and can they sustain productivity with environmental or job modifications?
- Do those who receive occupational therapy service, and engage in community life, experience fewer secondary health conditions?
- What impact does assistive technology have on community participation?
- Does occupational therapy improve the child's participation in the classroom, in the family, and in community activities?

It is through public policy that support is garnered for community living, that children with disabilities gain access to services, that the mentally ill have access to programs that give them the skills for living, and that individuals with disabilities gain access to the services that will help them learn to live and work as productive individuals. Governments provide funding for all of these programs.

Because occupational therapy is so closely linked to the legislative process, it is important for therapists to be informed and involved. The therapists' responsibilities go beyond their relationship with their clients and beyond their role as health care professionals. As citizens in a democracy, they also have a responsibility to propose policy and raise the issues that affect necessary legislation. To become vitally involved in the political system, each therapist must take the responsibility of gaining the skills necessary to influence policy. Such skills are acquired by mobilizing resources and learning the workings of the system in which the policy will be changed.

Major Challenges of Incorporating Measures Into Occupational Therapy Practice

Where to Start

What if you have not been exposed to the measures that answer the questions about how persons engage in occupations of their choice within many different environments in their community? Start by thinking about the type of outcome measure you need to evaluate occupational performance outcomes. What occupations do your clients want or need to perform? There is a need to move beyond impairment-level measures and exert our uniqueness in helping people achieve their occupational objectives.

We suggest that you start by developing an understanding of the principles of measurement and how measurement is used in occupational therapy. Review Chapter 3 in this text and the decision-making process for measurement outlined in the chapter. Get together with colleagues and focus on one area of your practice to determine an outcome measure that you could use. Do not try to do everything at once. Choose an instrument that you think will strengthen your understanding of your client's issues and use it. Discuss with your colleagues how you might implement a measurement model that will illustrate the unique contribution of occupational therapy to your institution's program. If you start identifying one measure to incorporate into your practice and then try others, outcome measurement will soon become an integral part of what you do every day as an occupational therapist.

In these discussions, you will also want to identify measures or data collection procedures that you can stop using so that your assessment does not become unmanageable. For example, if you begin with a performance in context measure, this may inform you about a narrower focus for further assessment, thus reducing what you have to use as follow-up assessment. You might also have data from other sources (eg, observation, referral, other discipline's tests) that give you what you need without duplicating effort.

What If I Do not Have Time?

Measurement tools must have clinical utility in order to be incorporated into occupational therapy assessment and to be useful for intervention planning. Review the measures identified in this book to determine which are most efficient for your practice. Many assessments included in this text are self-reports and can be completed and brought to the occupational therapy session for the therapist and clients to review together. The caregiver instruments provide a way to engage the caregiver in the planning process and help the therapist to ensure that intervention addresses true occupational performance issues. Remember this—although some measures take time to do, the information from occupational performance measures can save time during occupational therapy intervention. For example, use of the Canadian Occupational Performance Measure to identify a client's occupational performance issues leads to more focused assessment strategies and intervention, which increases client motivation and saves time in the long run.

The Protocols Used in Our Facility Do Not Include Measurement

People establish protocols to find the most effective and efficient way to serve a particular group. The occupational therapist and other health care professionals must be vigilant in adapting protocols to include measurement strategies and data that facilitate life planning, such as discharge decisions, transitions from school to work, and other factors that address the client's participation. Because we have to generate data about the cost-effectiveness of our interventions, such as reduced health care usage overall, outcome measurement contributes to both positive intervention planning and documentation for effectiveness. Other health professionals want to add measures to answer their specific questions; occupational therapists can join with colleagues to be sure the right measures are being used to document the effectiveness of the interventions.

My Team Expects Certain Information From Me

Over time, team members come to expect certain roles from their colleagues. Changing these roles can be difficult. To address this, you can meet with the team to explicitly discuss the occupational therapist's role. Such a discussion is an opportunity for you to highlight the focus that occupational therapist's place on occupational performance and how measurement of this concept can provide information to the team about clients' functioning. The occupational therapist also needs to highlight expectations for the other team members. Physical therapists contribute knowledge of movement, speech-language pathologists contribute knowledge of communication, and occupational therapists contribute knowledge of occupational performance.

Another strategy is to find ways to incorporate information from other disciplines into your reporting mechanisms. Sometimes more than one team member comes to the meeting with similar data; although this is validating, it can also be wasteful. Team members must have trust in each other's ability to gather information, and we demonstrate our trust by using data collected by others in our characterization of the person's status and our interpretation of the meaning of that data for performance needs.

Third, occupational therapists can use a transition strategy. We can report on performance in context with our "new" measures and include comments on the "expected" data from our observations. This strategy makes the link between component function and performance. For example, if you begin to incorporate the School Function Assessment into your measurement strategy, you can comment on the functional range of motion the child demonstrates in the same tasks from your observations of that task. With the new and more expansive participation information added to the expected information, the team can learn about the broader possibilities for effecting change.

Most Outcome Measures Do Not Apply to My Clients

Although it is true that there are some low-incidence populations that are not well represented in assessment samples, this issue is not as critical for measures that focus on performance in context. Some of the measures in this book emphasize the characteristics of the environment, thus making them relevant to whatever environment the person exists within. Others focus on the performance itself; again, systematic ways of recording performance can be helpful to any therapist serving any population. Some of the measures require significant others, including family and other service providers, to complete the information about the individual you are serving; in these cases, applicability is related to the informant's interest and ability to complete the forms with or without the therapist's assistance. Traditional standardized measures of the person's skills and abilities does limit applicability when your client doesn't match the sample in the measure. However, with performance in context, these same restrictions are not relevant; contexts are what they are, regardless of the person's characteristics. Additionally, making whatever the person does relevant for the assessment process sets therapists free from former restraints. The measurement strategies we are recommending in this book set therapists free from former restraints.

One other comment is critical here. The central focus of occupational therapy practice is performance in daily life; everything we do must support this focus. Therefore, when we drift very far from this goal, we must ask ourselves whether we are still providing occupational therapy. There are many things an occupational therapist might know how to do from specialized training. It does not make it occupational therapy just because an occupational therapist performs the task. It is only occupational therapy when the focus is performance of occupations within daily life.

What Measure Do I Use?

The most appropriate outcome measure in each client's situation depends on what information you need to build a client-centered care plan. By reading through the book, we are sure that you have found a number of instruments that would help you help your clients. The reviews we have prepared will help you to have confidence in the measures that you choose. We also have reviewed several individualized measurement strategies that can be used in almost all intervention encounters. You will have to try some to find the ones that are congruent with your team's style; that is a great way to get others committed to this transition because they will "own" the process with you.

What Happens to All of My Other Knowledge?

Some therapists worry that they will lose the skills that they have developed in testing specific performance components. In fact, you will still need these skills but may use them at different points in the therapeutic process. As outlined in Chapter 3, the first step in the measurement process is to use an assessment to enable clients to identify occupational performance issues for intervention. After that has been completed, the therapist needs to gather information about performance components and environmental factors that are either helping or hindering the client's occupational performance. It is at this stage that other knowledge, such as testing performance components and environmental assessment, is required. You may also find that you will have a more focused performance component assessment because you will see that only certain aspects will be relevant to particular performance. For example, the family might provide cues and supports during the personal hygiene rituals that make testing perceptual and memory skills irrelevant to getting teeth brushed and hands washed (eg, including a game or song in the morning ritual, which the parents enjoy). Although occupational therapy knowledge is holistic, you do need to know how the person's impairment is limiting his or her occupational performance, and then you can focus energy appropriately.

We Have No Money to Buy Assessments

This is a common dilemma in occupational therapy practice today. One of the ways to address this issue is to ensure that you use the assessments that you purchase often. If this is the case, you can justify the purchase because it provides the outcome information you need. It is important to review the measurement carefully, as there may be assessments that are similar but less costly. Many of the assessments we have discussed are in the public domain and do not need to be purchased. Others cost less than $100.

The Focus on Occupational Performance Outcomes in Occupational Therapy—Is This Just a Trend That Will Go Away Soon?

Occupational performance has been the focus of the profession since it began in 1918. The person-environment perspective is implicit in occupational therapy values and is reflected now in the way in which all outcomes of health are measured in well-being, satisfaction, and quality of life. This is an expertise for which we are recognized.

What Do I Write in My Reports and How Do I Ensure Reimbursement?

National health policies within the United States such as Medicare and most payment systems recognize individuals' progress to the level that they were achieving prior to their illness or injury. Documentation must focus on how the person is making progress and achieving function to overcome the impairments caused by the illness or injury. One strategy involves measuring and documenting the occupations that the person can now perform in light of the impairments that were causing difficulty in performance. However, some systems such as HMOs and some Medicare systems are offering a lump sum for the person's care. In these systems, there is currently less concern for specific outcomes by the reimbursement agent; the service agencies have the responsibility to decide which interventions will yield the most efficient and effective way of releasing the person from care because less time in care means better use of the money available. Balancing between efficient use of resources on a person's behalf and providing quality care will be the challenge for these systems. Your documentation needs to reflect both a respectfulness for efficient use of resources and your concern for the person's performance. For example, in discussing cooking as a desired outcome, you can write about the home instructions for practice, include information about safety in the home to "reduce the chances for accidents," thereby reducing re-hospitalization, and discuss the changes in other status due to the person's increased participation. You must tailor your documentation to the particular system without losing track of the occupational therapy focus.

These situations make the need for evidence about our contributions to efficiency and effectiveness even more critical. Your documentation of each case can provide portions of the evidence that can develop into a convincing argument. In addition, these situations make it even more critical for occupational therapists to illustrate their unique contributions explicitly. It is no wonder that some rehabilitation endeavors are viewing occupational therapy and physical therapy as duplication of service when they both document measurement of the same person-variable data. We must be willing to take the risk to shine the light on our differences in perspective through documentation and to contribute to databases that can show reduction in use of health care dollars across time with increased independence. Emphasize the person's ability to care for him- or herself, which requires less home care follow-up and fewer readmissions and reoccurrences.

When documenting for children and families, we must be better about projecting outcomes across time, even toward adulthood. Supporting the team to make these projections provides a yardstick for prioritizing how to spend the child's time at various stages in development. It is very easy to get caught up in reaching milestones without continuing to consider whether these skills are contributing to long-term planning.

Another pitfall to avoid when serving children and families is measuring only to determine the child's eligibility for services. We primarily use status measures of the child's skills to establish a discrepancy between capacity and performance. However, these measures do not guide practice. The measures we have included in this text provide information for intervention planning, and many of them provide a means for including the family in the data collection process. When families have something explicit to contribute, they become full members of the team as the law intended.

Teaching the Next Generation of Occupational Therapists

One of the biggest challenges for our profession is to determine the best strategies for passing along best practices to our developing colleagues and, at the same time, provide information to our practicing colleagues. Educators must take a leadership role in making best practice information available to both groups. This book is a great resource for students and their teachers because it guides you through the rationale and application of best practices in measurement (ie, to make sure that our measurement approaches clearly reflect the core concepts of occupational therapy). For faculty, we urge you to use this book as your resource for exploring occupation-centered practice. Students can complete many of the measures on their own families and friends and discuss what insights they gained from using them. You can work with the students on groups of measures that might become a packet for fieldwork placements. If you have meetings with your supervising therapists, you can make the measures available for them to review and discuss.

For new graduates, using this book to build your initial repertoire of measures will prepare you to implement these best practices on fieldwork and in your work. The student's biggest challenge after learning these best practices is how to handle fieldwork and initial job situations that are using more traditional performance component measurements. First and foremost, students and new graduates must feel empowered to effect change in these systems by having studied and practiced the appropriate measures and by preparing a rationale for why the alternatives you offer are worth a try. We recommend that students use this topic as one of their teaching/inservice opportunities for the staff; your supervisors take students because they want to keep current, so take advantage of this. We also recommend that you include some of these measures along with others traditionally used and prepare to point out the utility of the additional information to your supervisor and the team. These strategies both inform the therapist of new information and invite the systems to try a new way.

References

1. World Health Organization. *International Classification of Functioning, Disability, and Health (ICF)*. Geneva, Switzerland: WHO; 2001.
2. Christiansen C. The 1999 Eleanor Clarke Slagle Lecture. Defining lives: occupation as identity – an essay on relationships, competence and the creation of meaning. *Am J Occup Ther.* 1999;53(6):547-548.
3. Ware JE. Measures for a new era of health assessment. In: Steward AL, Ware JE, eds. *Measuring Functioning and Well-Being.* Durham, NC: Duke University Press; 1993:3-12.
4. Ware JE. Conceptualization and measurement of health-related quality of life: comments on an evolving field. *Arch Phys Med Rehabil.* 2003;84(4 Suppl 2):43-51.
5. Brandt EN Jr, Pope AM. *Enabling America: Assessing the Role of Rehabilitation Science and Engineering.* Washington, DC: National Academy Press; 1997.
6. Fisher AG. The foundation—functional measures, part 1: what is function, what should we measure, and how should we measure it? *Am J Occup Ther.* 1992;46(2):183-185.
7. Statistics Canada. *A Profile of Disability in Canada, 2001.* Ottawa, ON: Statistics Canada; 2002.
8. Pope AM, Tarloff AR. *Disability in America: Toward a National Agenda for Prevention.* Washington, DC: National Academy Press; 1991.
9. US Department of Health and Human Services. Healthy People 2020 Objectives. https://www.healthypeople.gov/2020/topics-objectives. Accessed June 20, 2016.
10. Health and Welfare Canada. *Achieving Health for All: A Framework for Health Promotion.* Ottawa, Ont: Government of Canada; 1986.
11. Health and Welfare Canada. *Active Health Report.* Ottawa, Ont: Government of Canada; 1987.
12. Premier's Council on Health, Well-Being and Social Justice. *Our Environment, Our Health.* Toronto, Ont: Province of Ontario; 1993.

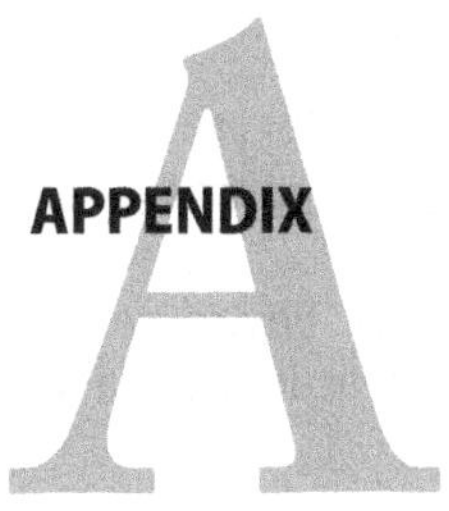

APPENDIX

LIST OF MEASURES (ALPHABETICAL)

Activities Scale for Kids (ASK)
Activity Card Sort (ACS)
ADL Situational Test
Adolescent Role Assessment
Arnadottir OT-ADL Neurobehavioral Evaluation (A-ONE)
Arthritis Impact Measurement Scales (AIMS)
Assessment of Ludic Behaviors (ALB)
Assessment of Motor and Process Skills (AMPS)
Assessment of Occupational Functioning—Collaborative Version
Barthel Index (BI)
Canadian Occupational Performance Measure (COPM)
Caregiver Assessment of Functional Dependence and Upset (CAFU)
Child Behaviors Inventory of Playfulness (CBIP)
Child Health Questionnaire (CHQ)
Child-Initiated Pretend Play Assessment (ChIPPA)
Children's Assessment of Participation and Enjoyment (CAPE)
Children's Health Assessment Questionnaire (CHAQ)
Community Integration Measure
Community Integration Questionnaire
Coping Inventory for Children
Craig Handicap Assessment and Reporting Technique (CHART)
Craig Hospital Inventory of Environmental Factors (CHIEF) and CHIEF Short Form
Direct Assessment of Functional Abilities (DAFA)
Direct Assessment of Functional Status (DAFS)
Early Coping Inventory
Experience Sampling Method (ESM)
Extended Activities of Daily Living Scale (EADLS)
Feasibility Evaluation Checklist
Functional Autonomy Measurement System (SMAF)
Functional Behavior Profile (FBP)
Functional Independence Measure (FIM) & WeeFIM
Health Assessment Questionnaire (HAQ)
Home and Community Environments: Measure of Processes of Care (MPOC)
Home Environment
Home Environment: Home Observation for Measurement of the Environment, Revised Edition (HOME)
Home Falls and Accidents Screening Tools
Home Observation for Measurement of the Environment (HOME)
Interest Checklist and Activity Checklist
Interpersonal Support Evaluation List
Interview Schedule for Social Interaction (ISSI)
Job Content Questionnaire (JCQ)
Juvenile Arthritis Functional Assessment Report (JAFAR)
Juvenile Arthritis Functional Assessment Scale (JAFAS)
Juvenile Arthritis Self-Report Index (JASI)
Katz Index of Activities of Daily Living
Kitchen Task Assessment (KTA)
Leisure Activity Profile (LAP)
Leisure Boredom Scale
Leisure Competence Measure (LCM)
Leisure Diagnostic Battery (LDB)
Leisure Satisfaction Questionnaire/Leisure Satisfaction Scale (LSS)
Lifease Software: Ease 3.2 Basic and Ease 3.2 Deluxe
Life Habits Assessment (LIFE-H)
Life Role Salience Scale
Life Stressors and Social Resources Inventory—Adult Form (LISRES-A)
London Handicap Scale
Measure of Quality of the Environment
Melville Nelson Self-Care Assessment
Memory and Behavior Problems Checklist: Revised
Multidimensional Scale of Perceived Social Support (MSPSS)
National Institutes of Health Activity Record (ACTRE)

Law M, Baum C, Dunn W, eds. *Measuring Occupational Performance: Supporting Best Practice in Occupational Therapy, Third Edition (pp 421-422).*

Occupational Circumstances Assessment-Interview and Rating Scale (OCAIRS)
Occupational Performance History Interview II
Occupational Questionnaire (OQ)
Occupational Role History
Occupational Self-Assessment
Parenting Stress Index (PSI)
Patient Specific Function Scale (PSFS)
Pediatric Activity Card Sort (PACS)
Pediatric Evaluation of Disability Inventory (PEDI)
Pediatric Interest Profiles: Survey of Play for Children and Adolescents
Perceived Efficacy and Goal Setting System (PEGS)
Performance Assessment of Self-Care Skills (PASS)
Person in Environment System
Personal Care Participation Assessment and Resource Tool (PC- PART)
Personal Projects Analysis (PPA)
Physical Self-Maintenance Scale (PSMS)
Play History
Preferences for Activities of Children (PAC)
Reintegration to Normal Living Index
Revised Knox Preschool Play Scale (PPS-R)
Role Checklist
Safety Assessment of Function and the Environment for Rehabilitation (SAFER)
Safety Assessment of Function and the Environment for Rehabilitation—Home Outcome Measurement and Evaluation (SAFER-HOME)
School Function Assessment (SFA)
Social Problem Questionnaire
Social Support Inventory for People with Disabilities (SSIDP)
Spinal Function Sort
Structured Assessment of Independent Living Skills (SAILS)
Structured Observation and Report Technique (SORT)
Test of Environmental Supportiveness (TOES)
Test of Grocery Shopping Skills
Test of Playfulness (ToP) Version 4
Transdisciplinary Play-Based Assessment (TPBA) 2nd Ed
Valpar Component Work Samples (VCWS)
Vineland Adaptive Behavior Scales (VABS)
Westmead Home Safety Assessment
Work Environment Scale (WES)
Worker Role Interview
Workplace Environment: Work Environment Impact Scale
World Health Organization—Disability Schedule II (WHO-DAS II)

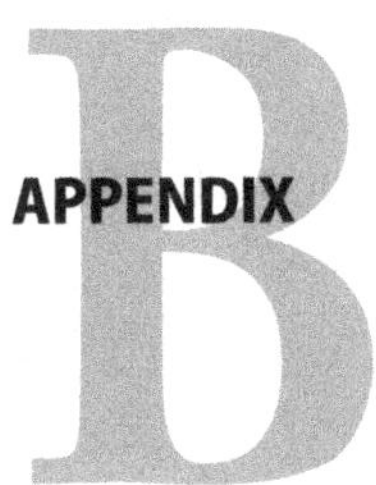

APPENDIX B

List of Measures by Occupational Performance Area

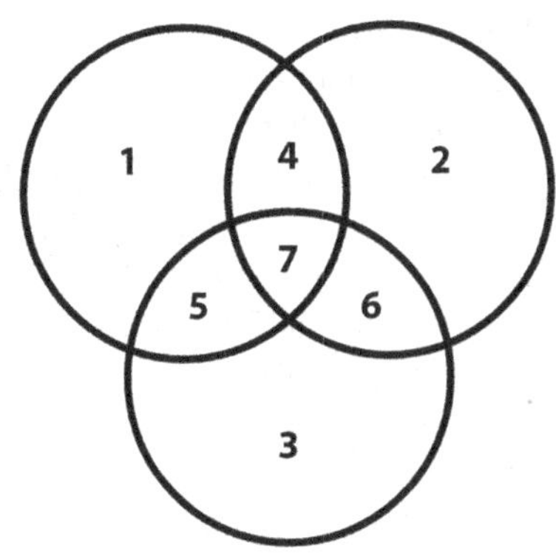

PEO Diagrams Linked to Outcome Measures

Space 1 illustrates the person variables alone. Measures of performance components would fit here.

Space 2 illustrates the environmental variables alone. This would include measures of the features of the environment, such as those included in Chapter 17.

Space 3 illustrates the occupation variables alone. There are no measures of this type in this book.

Space 4 represents the intersection of person and environment. Measures in this category will inform you about how the person fits into or responds to environmental conditions. Various chapters include measures of this type.

Space 5 represents the intersection of person and occupation. Measures in this category will inform you about the person's interests and needs for occupational performance. Various chapters will introduce these measures to you.

Space 6 represents the intersection of occupation and the environment. Measures in this category address the capacity of environments to support particular tasks and the match between tasks and environments. This classification is not used in this book.

Space 7 represents the intersection of all 3 variables, occupational performance. Many of the measures in this section capture this relationship, and therefore are very useful tools for intervention planning in natural environments.

Space 1

Child Behaviors Inventory of Playfulness (CBIP)
Child Health Questionnaire (CHQ)
Leisure Boredom Scale
Memory and Behavior Problems Checklist: Revised

Space 2

Home and Community Environments: Measure of Processes of Care (MPOC)
Home Falls and Accidents Screening Tool (HOME FAST)
Life Stressors and Social Resources Inventory—Adult Form (LIS- RES-A)
Measure of Quality of the Environment (MQE)
Safety Assessment of Function and the Environment for Rehabilitation (SAFER)
Safety Assessment of Function and the Environment for Rehabilitation—Health Outcome Measurement and Evaluation (SAFER-HOME)
Westmead Home Safety Assessment
Workplace Environment: Work Environment Impact Scale

Space 4

Coping Inventory for Children
Early Coping Inventory
Home Environment
Home Observation for Measurement of the Environment (HOME)

Law M, Baum C, Dunn W, eds. *Measuring Occupational Performance: Supporting Best Practice in Occupational Therapy, Third Edition (pp 423-424).*

Interpersonal Support Evaluation List
Interview Schedule for Social Interaction (ISSI)
Lifease Software: Ease 3.2 Basic and Ease 3.2 Deluxe
Multidimensional Scale of Perceived Social Support (MSPSS)
Parenting Stress Index (PSI)
Post-Occupancy Evaluation (POE)
Social Support Inventory for People with Disabilities (SSIDP)
Test of Environmental Supportiveness (TOES)
Work Environment Scale (WES)

Space 5

Activities Scale for Kids (ASK)
Activity Card Sort (ACS)
ADL Situational Test
Adolescent Role Assessment
Arnadottir OT-ADL Neurobehavioral Evaluation (A-ONE)
Arthritis Impact Measurement Scales (AIMS)
Barthel Index (BI)
Caregiver Assessment of Functional Dependence and Upset (CAFU)
Child-Initiated Pretend Play Assessment (ChIPPA)
Community Integration Measure
Community Integration Questionnaire
Craig Handicap Assessment and Reporting Technique (CHART)
Direct Assessment of Functional Status (DAFS)
Experience Sampling Method (ESM)
Extended Activities of Daily Living Scale (EADLS)
Functional Behavior Profile (FBP)
Interest Checklist and Activity Checklist
Juvenile Arthritis Functional Assessment Report (JAFAR)
Juvenile Arthritis Functional Assessment Scale (JAFAS)
Juvenile Arthritis Self-Report Index (JASI)
Leisure Diagnostic Battery (LDB)
Leisure Satisfaction Questionnaire/Leisure Satisfaction Scale (LSS)
Life Role Salience Scale
London Handicap Scale
National Institutes of Health Activity Record (ACTRE)
Occupational Questionnaire (OQ)
Patient Specific Function Scale (PSFS)
Pediatric Activity Card Sort (PACS)
Pediatric Interest Profiles: Survey of Play for Children and Adolescents
Personal Projects Analysis (PPA)
Preferences for Activities of Children (PAC)
Reintegration to Normal Living Index
Role Checklist
Spinal Function Sort
Structured Assessment of Independent Living Skills (SAILS)
Test of Grocery Shopping Skills
Test of Playfulness (ToP) Version 4
Valpar Component Work Samples (VCWS)
Vineland Adaptive Behavior Scales (VABS)

Space 7

Assessment of Ludic Behaviors (ALB)
Assessment of Motor and Process Skills (AMPS)
Assessment of Occupational Functioning—Collaborative Version
Canadian Occupational Performance Measure (COPM)
Children's Assessment of Participation and Enjoyment (CAPE)
Children's Health Assessment Questionnaire (CHAQ)
Craig Hospital Inventory of Environmental Factors (CHIEF) and CHIEF Short Form
Direct Assessment of Functional Abilities (DAFA)
Feasibility Evaluation Checklist
Functional Autonomy Measurement System (SMAF)
Functional Independence Measure (FIM) & WeeFIM
Health Assessment Questionnaire (HAQ)
Job Content Questionnaire (JCQ)
Katz Index of Activities of Daily Living
Kitchen Task Assessment (KTA)
Leisure Activity Profile (LAP)
Leisure Competence Measure (LCM)
Leisure Diagnostic Battery (LDB)
Life Habits Assessment (LIFE-H)
Melville Nelson Self-Care Assessment
Occupational Circumstances Assessment-Interview and Rating Scale (OCAIRS)
Occupational Performance History Interview II
Occupational Role History
Occupational Self-Assessment
Pediatric Evaluation of Disability Inventory (PEDI)
Perceived Efficacy and Goal Setting System (PEGS)
Performance Assessment of Self-Care Skills (PASS)
Person in Environment System
Personal Care Participation Assessment and Resource Tool (PC- PART)
Physical Self-Maintenance Scale (PSMS)
Play History
Revised Knox Preschool Play Scale (PPS-R)
School Function Assessment (SFA)
Structured Observation and Report Technique (SORT)
Transdisciplinary Play-Based Assessment (TPBA) 2nd Ed.
Worker Role Interview
World Health Organization-Disability Schedule II (WHO-DAS II)

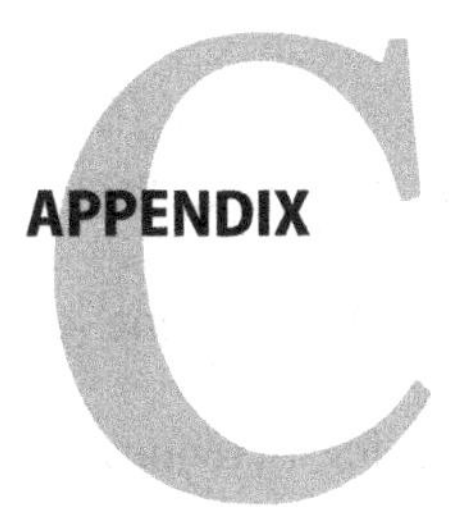

APPENDIX C

LIST OF MEASURES BY SOURCE/AUTHOR

Amatea ES, Cross EG, Clark JE, Bobby CL, Life Role Saliance Scale

American Guidance Service Inc, Vineland Adaptive Behavior Scales (VABS)

Arnadottir G, Arnadottir OT-ADL Neurobehavioral Evaluation (A-ONE)

Baron K, Kielhofner G, Ienger A, Goldhammer V, Wolenski J, Occupational Self-Assessment

Baum C, Activity Card Sort (ACS)

Baum C, Functional Behavior Profile (FBP)

Baum C, Edwards DF, Kitchen Task Assessment (KTA)

Behnke C, Fetkovich MM, Play History

Black MM, Adolescent Role Assessment

Bosche K, Measure of Quality of the Environment (MQE)

Bradley R, Caldwell BM, Home Observation for Measurement of the Environment (HOME)

Bryze K, Play History

Bundy A, Test of Environmental Supportiveness (TOES)

Bundy A, Test of Playfulness (ToP) Version 4

Caldwell BM, Bradley RH, Home Environment: Home Observation for Measurement of the Environment (HOME) (Revised Edition)

Canadian Occupational Therapy Association, Pediatric Activity Card Sort (PACS)

Canadian Occupational Therapy Association Comprehensive Rehabilitation and Mental Health Services, Safety Assessment of Function and the Environment for Rehabilitation (SAFER Tool)

Canadian Occupational Therapy Association Comprehensive Rehabilitation and Mental Health Services, Safety Assessment of Function and the Environment for Rehabilitation—Health Outcome Measurement and Evaluation (SAFER-HOME)

Career/Lifeskills Resources, Work Environment Scale (WES)

Center for Rehabilitation Effectiveness, Pediatric Evaluation of Disability Inventory (PEDI)

Centre d'expertise, Functional Autonomy Measurement System (SMAF)

Centre for Outcome Measurement in Brain Injury at Craig Hospital, Craig Hospital Inventory of Environmental Factors (CHIEF), and CHIEF Short Form

Centre interdisciplinaire de recherche en réadaptation et intégration sociale, Life Habits Assessment (LIFE-H)

Cohen S, Mermelstein R, Kamarck T, Hoberman HM, Interpersonal Support Evaluation List

Coordinates Publications, Westmead Home Safety Assessment

Corney RH, Clare AW, Social Problem Questionnaire

Csikszentmihalyi M, Larson R, Experience Sampling Method (ESM)

Data System (Marita Kloseck), Leisure Competence Measure (LCM)

Deshpande S, Kielhofner G, Henriksson C, et al, Occupational Circumstances Assessment-Interview and Rating Scale (OCAIRS)

Dickerson AE, Role Checklist

Employment Potential Improvement Corporation, Spinal Function Sort

Ferland F, Assessment of Ludic Behaviors (ALB)

Fisher AG, Assessment of Motor and Process Skills (AMPS)

Florey LL, Michelman SM, Occupational Role History

Fries JF, Health Assessment Questionnaire (HAQ)

Furst G, National Institutes of Health Activity Record (ACTRE)

Gitlin LN, Roth DL, Burgio L, et al, Caregiver Assessment of Functional Dependence and Upset (CAFU)

Hamera E, Brown C, Test of Grocery Shopping Skills

Health Act, Child Health Questionnaire (CHQ)

Henderson S, Duncan-Jones P, Byrne DG, Scott R, Interview Schedule for Social Interaction (ISSI)

Holm MB, Rogers JC, Performance Assessment of Self-Care Skills (PASS)

Howe S, Levinson J, Shear E, et al, Juvenile Arthritis Functional Assessment Report (JAFAR)

Idyll Arbor Inc, Leisure Satisfaction Questionnaire/Leisure Satisfaction Scale (LSS)

Law M, Baum C, Dunn W, eds. *Measuring Occupational Performance: Supporting Best Practice in Occupational Therapy, Third Edition (pp 425-426).*

Iso-Ahola SE, Weissinger E, Leisure Boredom Scale
Iwarsson S, Isacsson A, Home Environment
Karagiozis H, Gray S, Sacco J, Shapiro M, Kawas C, Direct Assessment of Functional Abilities (DAFA)
Karasek RA, Job Content Questionnaire (JCQ)
Katz S, Ford AB, Moskowitz RW, Jackson BA, Jaffe MW, Katz Index of Activities of Daily Living
Kielhofner G, Mallinson T, Crawford C, et al, Occupational Performance History Interview II
King S, Rosenbaum P, King G, Home and Community Environments: Measure of Processes of Care (MPOC)
Knox S, Revised Knox Preschool Play Scale (PPS-R)
Law M, Baptiste S, Carswell A, McColl MA, Polatajko H, Pollock N, Canadian Occupational Performance Measure
Lawton MP, Brody EM, Physical Self-Maintenance Scale (PSMS)
Lifease Corporation, Lifease Software: Ease 3.2 Basic and 3.2 Deluxe
Linder TW, Transdisciplinary Play-Based Assessment (TPBA) 2nd Ed
Little BR, Personal Projects Analysis (PPA)
Loewenstein D, Amigo E, Duara R, et al, Direct Assessment of Functional Status (DAFS)
Lovell DJ, Howe S, Shear E, et al, Juvenile Arthritis Functional Assessment Scale (JAFAS)
Mackenzie L, Byles J, Higginbotham N, Home Falls and Accidents Screening Tools
Mahoney SI, Barthel DW, Barthel Index (BI)
Mahurin RK, DeBittignies BH, Pirozzolo FJ, Structured Assessment of Independent Living Skills (SAILS)
Mann WC, Talty P, Leisure Activity Profile (LAP)
McColl MA, Davies D, Community Integration Measure
McColl MA, Friedland J, Social Support Inventory for People with Disabilities (SSIDP)
Medical Outcomes Trust, London Handicap Scale
Meenan RF, Arthritis Impact Measurement Scales (AIMS2)
Mellnick D, Craig Handicap Assessment and Reporting Technique (CHART)
Melville DL, Nelson LL, Melville Nelson Self-Care Assessment
Missiuna C, Pollock N, Law M, Perceived Efficacy and Goal Setting System (PEGS)
Moore-Corner RA, Keilhofner G, Olsen L, Workplace Environment: Work Environment Impact Scale
No author, Interest Checklist & Activity Checklist
Nouri FM, Lincoln NB, Extended Activities of Daily Living Scale (EADLS)
Oakley F, Kielhofner G, Barris R, Reichler R, Role Checklist
PART Group, Personal Care Participation Assessment and Resource Tool (PC-PART)
Preiser WFE, Rabinowitz HZ, White ET, Post-Occupancy Evaluation (POE)
Program in Occupational Therapy, Feasibility Evaluation Checklist
Psychological Assessment Resources, Life Stressors and Social Resources Inventory—Adult Form (LISRES-A)
Psychological Assessment Resources, Parenting Stress Index (PSI)
Psychological Corporation, Children's Assessment of Participation and Enjoyment (CAPE)
Psychological Corporation, Preferences for Activities of Children (PAC)
Psychological Corporation, School Function Assessment (SFA)
Rintala DH, Uttermohlen DM, Buck EL, et al., Structured Observation and Report Technique (SORT)
Rogers CS, Impara JC, Frary RB, et al, Child Behaviors Inventory of Playfulness (CBIP)
Rogers JC, Holm MB, Performance Assessment of Self-Care Skills (PASS)
Rogers JC, Holm M, Goldstein G, McCue M, Nussbaum P, Performance Assessment of Self-Care Skills (PASS)
Scholastic Testing Service, Inc, Coping Inventory for Children
Scholastic Testing Service, Inc, Early Coping Inventory
Singh G, Athreya BH, Fries JF, Goldsmith DP, Children's Health Assessment Questionnaire (CHAQ)
Skurla E, Rogers JC, Sunderland T, ADL Situational Test
Smith NR, Kielhofner G, Watts JH, Occupational Questionnaire (OQ)
Stagnitti, K, Child-Initiated Pretend Play Assessment (ChIPPA)
Stratford P, Gill C, Westaway M, Binkley J, Patient Specific Function Scale (PSFS)
Takata N, Play History
Teri L, Truax P, Logsdon R, Uomoto J, Zarit S, Vitaliano PP, Memory and Behavior Problems Checklist: Revised
Therapy Skill Builders, Pediatric Interest Profiles: Survey of Play for Children and Adolescents
Uniform Data System for Medical Rehabilitation, Functional Independence Measure (FIM) & WeeFIM
Valpar International Corporation, Valpar Component Work Samples (VCWS)
Velozo CA, Kielhofner G, Fisher G, Worker Role Interview
Watts JH, Madigan JM, Assessment of Occupational Functioning-Collaborative Version
Whiteneck G, Charlifue S, Gerhart K, Overholser D, Richardson G, Craig Handicap Assessment and Reporting Technique (CHART)
Willer B, Rosenthal M, Kreutzer JS, Gordon WA, Rempel R, Community Integration Questionnaire
Williams JBW, Karls JM, Wandrei K, Person in Environment System
Witt P, Ellis G, Leisure Diagnostic Battery (LDB)
Wood-Dauphinee S, Opzoomer A, Williams JI, Marchand B, Spitzer WO, Reintegration to Normal Living Index
World Health Organization, Disability Schedule II (WHO-DAS II)
Wright FV, Law M, Crombie V, Goldsmith C, Dent P, Shore A, Juvenile Arthritis Self-Report Index (JASI)
Young NL, Activities Scale for Kids (ASK)
Zimet GD, Dahlem NW, Zimet SG, Farley GK, Multi-dimensional Scale of Perceived Social Support (MSPSS)

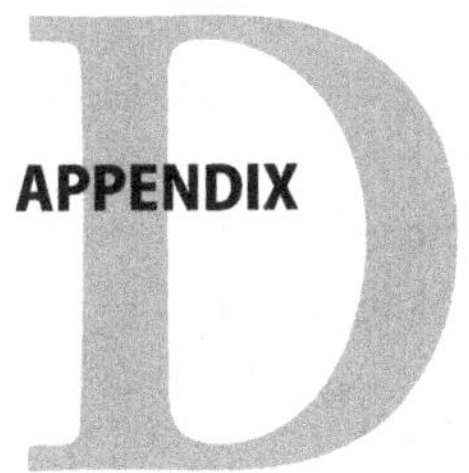

APPENDIX D

LIST OF MEASURES MAPPED TO THE INTERNATIONAL CLASSIFICATION OF FUNCTIONING

GENERAL TASKS AND DEMANDS

Activities Scale for Kids (ASK)
Activity Card Sort (ACS)
Adolescent Role Assessment
Arnadottir OT-ADL Neurobehavioral Evaluation (A-ONE)
Arthritis Impact Measurement Scales (AIMS)
Assessment of Ludic Behaviors (ALB)
Assessment of Motor and Process Skills (AMPS)
Assessment of Occupational Functioning—Collaborative Version
Barthel Index (BI)
Canadian Occupational Performance Measure (COPM)
Caregiver Assessment of Functional Dependence and Upset (CAFU)
Child Behaviors Inventory of Playfulness (CBIP)
Child Health Questionnaire (CHQ)
Child-Initiated Pretend Play Assessment (ChIPPA)
Children's Assessment of Participation and Enjoyment (CAPE)
Children's Health Assessment Questionnaire (CHAQ)
Community Integration Measure
Community Integration Questionnaire
Coping Inventory for Children
Craig Handicap Assessment and Reporting Technique (CHART)
Direct Assessment of Functional Abilities (DAFA)
Direct Assessment of Functional Status (DAFS)
Early Coping Inventory
Experience Sampling Method (ESM)
Extended Activities of Daily Living Scale (EADLS)
Feasibility Evaluation Checklist
Functional Autonomy Measurement System (SMAF)
Functional Behavior Profile (FBP)
Health Assessment Questionnaire (HAQ)
Home Observation for Measurement of the Environment (HOME)
Interest Checklist & Activity Checklist
Interpersonal Support Evaluation List
Interview Schedule for Social Interaction (ISSI)
Job Content Questionnaire (JCQ)
Juvenile Arthritis Functional Assessment Report (JAFAR)
Juvenile Arthritis Functional Assessment Scale (JAFAS)
Juvenile Arthritis Self-Report Index (JASI)
Katz Index of Activities of Daily Living
Kitchen Task Assessment
Leisure Activity Profile (LAP)
Leisure Boredom Scale
Leisure Competence Measure (LCM)
Leisure Diagnostic Battery (LDB)
Leisure Satisfaction Questionnaire/Leisure Satisfaction Scale (LSS)
Life Habits Assessment (LIFE-H)
London Handicap Scale
Melville Nelson Self-Care Assessment
Memory and Behavior Problems Checklist: Revised
National Institutes of Health Activity Record (ACTRE)
Occupational Circumstances Assessment-Interview and Rating Scale (OCAIRS)
Occupational Performance History Interview II
Occupational Questionnaire (OQ)
Occupational Role History
Occupational Self-Assessment
Parenting Stress Index (PSI)
Patient Specific Function Scale (PSFS)
Pediatric Activity Card Sort (PACS)

Law M, Baum C, Dunn W, eds. *Measuring Occupational Performance: Supporting Best Practice in Occupational Therapy, Third Edition (pp 427-432).*

Pediatric Evaluation of Disability Inventory (PEDI)
Pediatric Interest Profiles: Survey of Play for Children and Adolescents
Perceived Efficacy and Goal Setting System (PEGS)
Performance Assessment of Self Care Skills (PASS)
Person in Environment System
Personal Projects Analysis (PPA)
Physical Self-Maintenance Scale (PSMS)
Play History
Preferences for Activities of Children (PAC)
Reintegration to Normal Living Index
Revised Knox Preschool Play Scale (PPS-R)
Role Checklist
School Function Assessment (SFA)
Social Problem Questionnaire
Social Support Inventory for People with Disabilities (SSIDP)
Spinal Function Sort
Structured Assessment of Independent Living Skills (SAILS)
Structured Observation and Report Technique (SORT)
Test of Grocery Shopping Skills
Test of Playfulness (ToP) Version 4
Transdisciplinary Play-Based Assessment (TPBA) 2nd Ed.
Valpar Component Work Samples (VCWS)
Vineland Adaptive Behavior Scales (VABS)
Worker Role Interview
World Health Organization-Disability Schedule II (WHO-DAS II)

Communication

ADL Situational Test
Arnadottir OT-ADL Neurobehavioral Evaluation (A-ONE)
Assessment of Ludic Behaviors (ALB)
Assessment of Occupational Functioning—Collaborative Version
Canadian Occupational Performance Measure (COPM)
Caregiver Assessment of Functional Dependence and Upset (CAFU)
Child-Initiated Pretend Play Assessment (ChIPPA)
Children's Assessment of Participation and Enjoyment (CAPE)
Coping Inventory for Children
Direct Assessment of Functional Abilities (DAFA)
Direct Assessment of Functional Status (DAFS)
Experience Sampling Method (ESM)
Functional Autonomy Measurement System (SMAF)
Functional Independence Measure (FIM) & WeeFIM
Home Observation for Measurement of the Environment (HOME)
Life Habits Assessment (LIFE-H)
National Institutes of Health Activity Record (ACTRE)
Occupational Questionnaire (OQ)
Patient Specific Function Scale (PSFS)
Pediatric Evaluation of Disability Inventory (PEDI)
Performance Assessment of Self Care Skills (PASS)
Personal Projects Analysis (PPA)
Preferences for Activities of Children (PAC)
Revised Knox Preschool Play Scale (PPS-R)
School Function Assessment (SFA)
Structured Assessment of Independent Living Skills (SAILS)
Structured Observation and Report Technique (SORT)
Test of Playfulness (ToP) Version 4
Transdisciplinary Play-Based Assessment (TPBA) 2nd Ed.
Valpar Component Work Samples (VCWS)
Vineland Adaptive Behavior Scales (VABS)
World Health Organization—Disability Schedule II (WHO-DAS II)

Mobility

Activities Scale for Kids (ASK)
Activity Card Sort (ACS)
ADL Situational Test
Arnadottir OT-ADL Neurobehavioral Evaluation (A-ONE)
Arthritis Impact Measurement Scales (AIMS)
Assessment of Ludic Behaviors (ALB)
Assessment of Motor and Process Skills (AMPS)
Assessment of Occupational Functioning—Collaborative Version
Barthel Index (BI)
Canadian Occupational Performance Measure (COPM)
Child Health Questionnaire (CHQ)
Children's Assessment of Participation and Enjoyment (CAPE)
Children's Health Assessment Questionnaire (CHAQ)
Craig Handicap Assessment and Reporting Technique (CHART)
Early Coping Inventory
Experience Sampling Method (ESM)
Extended Activities of Daily Living Scale (EADLS)
Functional Autonomy Measurement System (SMAF)
Health Assessment Questionnaire (HAQ)
Interest Checklist and Activity Checklist
Job Content Questionnaire (JCQ)
Juvenile Arthritis Functional Assessment Report (JAFAR)
Juvenile Arthritis Functional Assessment Scale (JAFAS)
Juvenile Arthritis Self-Report Index (JASI)
Katz Index of Activities of Daily Living
Leisure Activity Profile (LAP)
Leisure Competence Measure (LCM)
Leisure Diagnostic Battery (LDB)
Life Habits Assessment (LIFE-H)
London Handicap Scale
National Institutes of Health Activity Record (ACTRE)
Occupational Questionnaire (OQ)

Patient Specific Function Scale (PSFS)
Pediatric Activity Card Sort (PACS)
Pediatric Evaluation of Disability Inventory (PEDI)
Perceived Efficacy and Goal Setting System (PEGS)
Performance Assessment of Self Care Skills (PASS)
Personal Care Participation Assessment and Resource Tool (PC- PART)
Personal Projects Analysis (PPA)
Physical Self-Maintenance Scale (PSMS)
Preferences for Activities of Children (PAC)
Revised Knox Preschool Play Scale (PPS-R)
School Function Assessment (SFA)
Spinal Function Sort
Structured Assessment of Independent Living Skills (SAILS)
Structured Observation and Report Technique (SORT)
Transdisciplinary Play-Based Assessment (TPBA) 2nd Ed.
Valpar Component Work Samples (VCWS)
Vineland Adaptive Behavior Scales (VABS)
Worker Role Interview
World Health Organization—Disability Schedule II (WHO-DAS II)

Self-Care

Activities Scale for Kids (ASK)
Activity Card Sort (ACS)
ADL Situational Test
Arnadottir OT-ADL Neurobehavioral Evaluation (A-ONE)
Arthritis Impact Measurement Scales (AIMS)
Assessment of Motor and Process Skills (AMPS)
Assessment of Occupational Functioning—Collaborative Version
Barthel Index (BI)
Canadian Occupational Performance Measure (COPM)
Caregiver Assessment of Functional Dependence and Upset (CAFU)
Child Health Questionnaire (CHQ)
Children's Health Assessment Questionnaire (CHAQ)
Craig Handicap Assessment and Reporting Technique (CHART)
Direct Assessment of Functional Abilities (DAFA)
Direct Assessment of Functional Status (DAFS)
Experience Sampling Method (ESM)
Extended Activities of Daily Living Scale (EADLS)
Functional Autonomy Measurement System (SMAF)
Functional Independence Measure (FIM) & WeeFIM
Health Assessment Questionnaire (HAQ)
Interest Checklist and Activity Checklist
Juvenile Arthritis Functional Assessment Report (JAFAR)
Juvenile Arthritis Functional Assessment Scale (JAFAS)
Juvenile Arthritis Self-Report Index (JASI)
Katz Index of Activities of Daily Living
Kitchen Task Assessment
Life Habits Assessment (LIFE-H)
London Handicap Scale
Melville Nelson Self-Care Assessment
Memory and Behavior Problems Checklist: Revised
National Institutes of Health Activity Record (ACTRE)
Occupational Performance History Interview II
Occupational Questionnaire (OQ)
Occupational Self-Assessment
Patient Specific Function Scale (PSFS)
Pediatric Activity Card Sort (PACS)
Pediatric Evaluation of Disability Inventory (PEDI)
Performance Assessment of Self Care Skills (PASS)
Personal Care Participation Assessment and Resource Tool (PC- PART)
Personal Projects Analysis (PPA)
Physical Self-Maintenance Scale (PSMS)
Reintegration to Normal Living Index
School Function Assessment (SFA)
Structured Assessment of Independent Living Skills (SAILS)
Structured Observation and Report Technique (SORT)
Vineland Adaptive Behavior Scales (VABS)
World Health Organization—Disability Schedule II (WHO-DAS II)

Domestic Life

Activity Card Sort (ACS)
Adolescent Role Assessment
Arthritis Impact Measurement Scales (AIMS)
Assessment of Motor and Process Skills (AMPS)
Assessment of Occupational Functioning—Collaborative Version
Canadian Occupational Performance Measure (COPM)
Caregiver Assessment of Functional Dependence and Upset (CAFU)
Children's Assessment of Participation and Enjoyment (CAPE)
Community Integration Questionnaire
Direct Assessment of Functional Abilities (DAFA)
Direct Assessment of Functional Status (DAFS)
Experience Sampling Method (ESM)
Extended Activities of Daily Living Scale (EADLS)
Functional Autonomy Measurement System (SMAF)
Functional Independence Measure (FIM) & WeeFIM
Interest Checklist & Activity Checklist
Juvenile Arthritis Functional Assessment Report (JAFAR)
Juvenile Arthritis Functional Assessment Scale (JAFAS)
Juvenile Arthritis Self-Report Index (JASI)
Katz Index of Activities of Daily Living
Life Habits Assessment (LIFE-H)
London Handicap Scale
National Institutes of Health Activity Record (ACTRE)
Occupational Performance History Interview II

Occupational Questionnaire (OQ)
Occupational Self-Assessment
Parenting Stress Index (PSI)
Patient Specific Function Scale (PSFS)
Personal Care Participation Assessment and Resource Tool (PC- PART)
Personal Projects Analysis (PPA)
Preferences for Activities of Children (PAC)
Role Checklist
Structured Observation and Report Technique (SORT)
Test of Grocery Shopping Skills
World Health Organization—Disability Schedule II (WHO-DAS II)

Interpersonal Interactions and Relationships

Activity Card Sort (ACS)
Adolescent Role Assessment
Assessment of Occupational Functioning—Collaborative Version
Canadian Occupational Performance Measure (COPM)
Child Behaviors Inventory of Playfulness (CBIP)
Child Health Questionnaire (CHQ)
Child-Initiated Pretend Play Assessment (ChIPPA)
Children's Assessment of Participation and Enjoyment (CAPE)
Community Integration Questionnaire
Coping Inventory for Children
Craig Handicap Assessment and Reporting Technique (CHART)
Direct Assessment of Functional Abilities (DAFA)
Early Coping Inventory
Experience Sampling Method (ESM)
Extended Activities of Daily Living Scale (EADLS)
Functional Behavior Profile (FBP)
Home Observation for Measurement of the Environment (HOME)
Interpersonal Support Evaluation List
Interview Schedule for Social Interaction (ISSI)
Job Content Questionnaire (JCQ)
Leisure Activity Profile (LAP)
Leisure Competence Measure (LCM)
Leisure Diagnostic Battery (LDB)
Leisure Satisfaction Questionnaire/Leisure Satisfaction Scale (LSS)
Life Habits Assessment (LIFE-H)
London Handicap Scale
Memory and Behavior Problems Checklist: Revised
National Institutes of Health Activity Record (ACTRE)
Occupational Questionnaire (OQ)
Parenting Stress Index (PSI)
Patient Specific Function Scale (PSFS)
Pediatric Evaluation of Disability Inventory (PEDI)
Pediatric Interest Profiles: Survey of Play for Children and Adolescents
Perceived Efficacy and Goal Setting System (PEGS)
Person in Environment System
Personal Projects Analysis (PPA)
Play History
Preferences for Activities of Children (PAC)
Reintegration to Normal Living Index
Revised Knox Preschool Play Scale (PPS-R)
Role Checklist
School Function Assessment (SFA)
Social Problem Questionnaire
Social Support Inventory for People with Disabilities (SSIDP)
Structured Assessment of Independent Living Skills (SAILS)
Structured Observation and Report Technique (SORT)
Test of Grocery Shopping Skills
Test of Playfulness (ToP) Version 4
Transdisciplinary Play-Based Assessment (TPBA) 2nd Ed.
Valpar Component Work Samples (VCWS)
Vineland Adaptive Behavior Scales (VABS)
World Health Organization—Disability Schedule II (WHO-DAS II)

Learning and Applying Knowledge

Activity Card Sort (ACS)
Adolescent Role Assessment
Assessment of Ludic Behaviors (ALB)
Assessment of Motor and Process Skills (AMPS)
Assessment of Occupational Functioning—Collaborative Version
Canadian Occupational Performance Measure (COPM)
Child-Initiated Pretend Play Assessment (ChIPPA)
Children's Assessment of Participation and Enjoyment (CAPE)
Coping Inventory for Children
Direct Assessment of Functional Abilities (DAFA)
Early Coping Inventory
Experience Sampling Method (ESM)
Functional Autonomy Measurement System (SMAF)
Functional Behavior Profile (FBP)
Interest Checklist and Activity Checklist
Interpersonal Support Evaluation List
Job Content Questionnaire (JCQ)
Kitchen Task Assessment
Leisure Activity Profile (LAP)
Leisure Boredom Scale
Leisure Competence Measure (LCM)
Leisure Diagnostic Battery (LDB)
Leisure Satisfaction Questionnaire/Leisure Satisfaction Scale (LSS)

Life Habits Assessment (LIFE-H)
London Handicap Scale
Memory and Behavior Problems Checklist: Revised
National Institutes of Health Activity Record (ACTRE)
Occupational Questionnaire (OQ)
Occupational Role History
Patient Specific Function Scale (PSFS)
Pediatric Activity Card Sort (PACS)
Perceived Efficacy and Goal Setting System (PEGS)
Performance Assessment of Self Care Skills (PASS)
Personal Projects Analysis (PPA)
Play History
Preferences for Activities of Children (PAC)
Reintegration to Normal Living Index
Revised Knox Preschool Play Scale (PPS-R)
School Function Assessment (SFA)
Structured Assessment of Independent Living Skills (SAILS)
Structured Observation and Report Technique (SORT)
Test of Grocery Shopping Skills
Transdisciplinary Play-Based Assessment (TPBA) 2nd Ed
Valpar Component Work Samples (VCWS)
Vineland Adaptive Behavior Scales (VABS)
Worker Role Interview

Major Life Areas

Activity Card Sort (ACS)
Adolescent Role Assessment
Arthritis Impact Measurement Scales (AIMS)
Assessment of Occupational Functioning—Collaborative Version
Canadian Occupational Performance Measure (COPM)
Caregiver Assessment of Functional Dependence and Upset (CAFU)
Children's Assessment of Participation and Enjoyment (CAPE)
Community Integration Questionnaire
Craig Handicap Assessment and Reporting Technique (CHART)
Direct Assessment of Functional Abilities (DAFA)
Direct Assessment of Functional Status (DAFS)
Early Coping Inventory
Experience Sampling Method (ESM)
Feasibility Evaluation Checklist
Interpersonal Support Evaluation List
Job Content Questionnaire (JCQ)
Juvenile Arthritis Functional Assessment Report (JAFAR)
Juvenile Arthritis Functional Assessment Scale (JAFAS)
Juvenile Arthritis Self-Report Index (JASI)
Leisure Activity Profile (LAP)
Life Habits Assessment (LIFE-H)
Life Role Salience Scale
Life Stressors and Social Resources Inventory—Adult Form (LISRES-A)
London Handicap Scale
National Institutes of Health Activity Record (ACTRE)
Occupational Performance History Interview II
Occupational Questionnaire (OQ)
Occupational Role History
Occupational Self-Assessment
Patient Specific Function Scale (PSFS)
Pediatric Activity Card Sort (PACS)
Perceived Efficacy and Goal Setting System (PEGS)
Performance Assessment of Self Care Skills (PASS)
Personal Projects Analysis (PPA)
Preferences for Activities of Children (PAC)
Reintegration to Normal Living Index
Role Checklist
Social Problem Questionnaire
Spinal Function Sort
Structured Assessment of Independent Living Skills (SAILS)
Structured Observation and Report Technique (SORT)
Valpar Component Work Samples (VCWS)
Vineland Adaptive Behavior Scales (VABS)
Worker Role Interview

Community, Social, and Civic Life

Activity Card Sort (ACS)
ADL Situational Test
Adolescent Role Assessment
Arthritis Impact Measurement Scales (AIMS)
Assessment of Occupational Functioning—Collaborative Version
Canadian Occupational Performance Measure (COPM)
Caregiver Assessment of Functional Dependence and Upset (CAFU)
Children's Assessment of Participation and Enjoyment (CAPE)
Community Integration Measure
Community Integration Questionnaire
Coping Inventory for Children
Craig Handicap Assessment and Reporting Technique (CHART)
Direct Assessment of Functional Abilities (DAFA)
Direct Assessment of Functional Status (DAFS)
Early Coping Inventory
Experience Sampling Method (ESM)
Functional Autonomy Measurement System (SMAF)
Functional Behavior Profile (FBP)
Home Observation for Measurement of the Environment (HOME)
Interest Checklist and Activity Checklist
Interpersonal Support Evaluation List
Interview Schedule for Social Interaction (ISSI)

Juvenile Arthritis Functional Assessment Report (JAFAR)
Juvenile Arthritis Functional Assessment Scale (JAFAS)
Juvenile Arthritis Self-Report Index (JASI)
Katz Index of Activities of Daily Living
Leisure Activity Profile (LAP)
Leisure Competence Measure (LCM)
Leisure Diagnostic Battery (LDB)
Leisure Satisfaction Questionnaire/Leisure Satisfaction Scale (LSS)
Life Habits Assessment (LIFE-H)
Life Role Salience Scale
Life Stressors and Social Resources Inventory—Adult Form (LISRES-A)
London Handicap Scale
Memory and Behavior Problems Checklist: Revised
Multidimensional Scale of Perceived Social Support (MSPSS)
National Institutes of Health Activity Record (ACTRE)
Occupational Questionnaire (OQ)
Patient Specific Function Scale (PSFS)
Pediatric Activity Card Sort (PACS)
Pediatric Evaluation of Disability Inventory (PEDI)
Perceived Efficacy and Goal Setting System (PEGS)
Person in Environment System
Personal Projects Analysis (PPA)
Play History
Preferences for Activities of Children (PAC)
Role Checklist
Structured Observation and Report Technique (SORT)
Vineland Adaptive Behavior Scales (VABS)
World Health Organization—Disability Schedule II (WHO-DAS II)

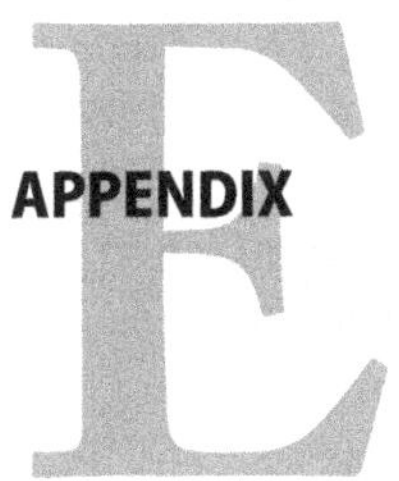

APPENDIX

Outcome Measures Rating Forms and Guidelines

OUTCOME MEASURES RATING FORM

CanChild Centre for Childhood Disability Research
Institute of Applied Health Sciences, McMaster University
1400 Main Street West. Room 408
Hamilton, Canada L8S 1C7
Fax (905) 522-6095
lawm@mcmaster.ca

To be used with: Outcome Measures Rating Form Guidelines (CanChild, 2004)

Name and initials of measure: ____________________
Author(s): ____________________
____
Source and year published: ____________________
____
Date of review: ____________________
Name of reviewer: ____________________

1. Focus

A. Focus of measurement—Using the ICF framework

- ☐ Body functions..........................Are the physiological functions of body systems (includes psychological functions).
- ☐ Body structures.........................Are anatomical parts of the body such as organs, limbs, and their components.
- ☐ Activities and participation....Activity is the execution of a task or action by an individual. Participation is involvement in a life situation.
- ☐ Environmental factors.............Make up the physical, social and attitudinal environment in which people live and conduct their lives.

B. Attribute(s) being measured—Check as many as apply.

This list is based on attributes cited in the ICF, 2001: WHO.

Body Functions

Global mental functions

- ☐ Consciousness
- ☐ Orientation
- ☐ Sleep
- ☐ Intellectual
- ☐ Global psychosocial
- ☐ Temperament and personality
- ☐ Energy and drive

Law M, Baum C, Dunn W, eds. *Measuring Occupational Performance: Supporting Best Practice in Occupational Therapy, Third Edition (pp 433-444).*

Specific mental functions

- ☐ Attention
- ☐ Memory
- ☐ Psychomotor
- ☐ Mental function of sequencing complex measurements
- ☐ Thought
- ☐ Higher level cognitive
- ☐ Calculation
- ☐ Mental functions of language
- ☐ Experience of self and time
- ☐ Perceptual

Sensory functions and pain

- ☐ Seeing and related
- ☐ Hearing and vestibular

Voice and speech functions

- ☐ Voice
- ☐ Articulation
- ☐ Fluency and rhythm of speech
- ☐ Alternative vocalization

Functions of the cardiovascular, hematological, immunological, and respiratory systems

- ☐ Cardiovascular
- ☐ Hematological and immunological systems
- ☐ Respiratory system
- ☐ Additional functions and sensations of the cardiovascular and respiratory systems

Functions of the digestive, metabolic, and endocrine systems

- ☐ Related to the digestive system
- ☐ Related to metabolism and the endocrine system

Genitourinary and reproductive functions

- ☐ Urinary
- ☐ Genital and reproductive

Neuromuscular and movement-related functions

Joints and Bones

- ☐ Mobility of joint
- ☐ Stability of joint
- ☐ Mobility of bone

Muscle

- ☐ Muscle power
- ☐ Muscle tone
- ☐ Muscle endurance

Movement

- ☐ Motor reflex
- ☐ Involuntary movement reaction
- ☐ Control of voluntary movement
- ☐ Involuntary movement
- ☐ Sensations related to muscle and movement
- ☐ Gait patterns

Functions of the skin and related structures

Skin

- ☐ Protection
- ☐ Repair
- ☐ Other functions
- ☐ Sensations

Hair

- ☐ Function of the hair

Nails

- ☐ Function of nails

Body Structures

Structures of the nervous system

- ☐ Brain
- ☐ Sympathetic nervous system
- ☐ Spinal cord and related structures
- ☐ Parasympathetic nervous system
- ☐ Meninges

Eye, ear, and related structures

- ☐ Eye socket
- ☐ Eyeball
- ☐ Around eye
- ☐ External ear
- ☐ Middle ear
- ☐ Inner ear

Structures involved in voice and speech

- ☐ Nose
- ☐ Mouth
- ☐ Pharynx
- ☐ Larynx

Structures of the cardiovascular, immunological, and respiratory systems

Cardiovascular system	☐ Heart	☐ Veins
	☐ Arteries	☐ Capillaries
Immune system	☐ Lymphatic vessels	☐ Lymphatic nodes
	☐ Thymus	☐ Spleen
	☐ Bone marrow	
Respiratory system	☐ Trachea	☐ Lungs
	☐ Thoracic cage	☐ Muscles of respiration

Structures related to the digestive, metabolic, and endocrine systems

- ☐ Salivary glands
- ☐ Oesophagus
- ☐ Stomach
- ☐ Pancreas
- ☐ Liver
- ☐ Gall bladder
- ☐ Intestines
- ☐ Endocrine glands

Structures related to the genitourinary and reproductive systems

- ☐ Urinary system
- ☐ Pelvic floor
- ☐ Reproductive system

Structures related to movement

- ☐ Head and neck
- ☐ Upper extremity
- ☐ Shoulder region
- ☐ Trunk
- ☐ Lower extremity
- ☐ Pelvic region
- ☐ Additional musculoskeletal structures related to movement

Skin and related structures

- ☐ Skin
- ☐ Nails
- ☐ Skin and glands
- ☐ Hair

Activities and Participation

Learning and applying knowledge

Purposeful sensory	☐ Watching	☐ Other purposeful sensing
	☐ Experiences	☐ Listening
Basic learning	☐ Copying	☐ Rehearsing
	☐ Learning to read	☐ Learning to write
	☐ Learning to calculate	☐ Acquiring skills
Applying knowledge	☐ Focusing attention	☐ Calculating
	☐ Thinking	☐ Solving problems
	☐ Reading	☐ Making decisions
	☐ Writing	

General tasks and demand

- ☐ Undertaking a single task
- ☐ Carrying out daily routine
- ☐ Undertaking multiple tasks
- ☐ Handling stress and other psychological demands

Communication

- ☐ Receiving (verbal, nonverbal, written, formal sign language)
- ☐ Producing (verbal, nonverbal, written, formal sign language)
- ☐ Conversation and use of communication devices and techniques

Mobility

- ☐ Changing and maintaining body position
- ☐ Walking and moving
- ☐ Carrying, moving, and handling objects
- ☐ Moving around using transportation

Self-care

- ☐ Washing oneself
- ☐ Caring for body parts
- ☐ Toileting
- ☐ Dressing
- ☐ Eating
- ☐ Drinking

Looking after one's health

☐ Ensuring oneself physical	☐ Maintaining one's health comfort	☐ Managing diet and fitness

Domestic life

Acquisition of necessities	☐ Acquiring a place to live	☐ Acquisition of goods and services
Household tasks	☐ Preparing meals	☐ Doing housework
	☐ Caring for household objects and assisting others	

Interpersonal interactions and relationships

General	☐ General interpersonal interactions (basic and complex)	
Particular interpersonal	☐ Informal social relationships	☐ Relating with strangers
Relationships	☐ Family relationships	☐ Formal relationships
	☐ Intimate relationships	

Major life areas

Education	☐ Informal	☐ Preschool
	☐ School	
Work and employment	☐ Apprenticeship	☐ Acquiring, keeping, and terminating a job
	☐ Renumerative employment	☐ Non-renumerative employment
Economic life	☐ Basic economic transactions	☐ Complex economic transactions
	☐ Economic self-sufficiency	

Community, social, and civic life

Community	☐ Community life	
Recreation and leisure	☐ Play	☐ Crafts
	☐ Sports	☐ Hobbies
	☐ Arts and culture	☐ Socializing
Civic	☐ Religion and spirituality	☐ Political life and citizenship
	☐ Human rights	

<u>Environmental Factors</u>

Products and technology

☐ Communication	☐ Education	☐ Employment
☐ Culture, recreation, and sport	☐ Products or substances for personal consumption	☐ Products and technology for personal use in daily living
☐ Design, construction, and buildings for public use	☐ Design, construction, and buildings for private use	☐ For personal indoor and outdoor mobility and transportation
☐ Religion and spirituality	☐ Land development	☐ Assets

Natural environment and human-made changes to environment

☐ Physical geography	☐ Sound	☐ Human events
☐ Flora and fauna	☐ Air quality	☐ Time-related changes
☐ Natural events	☐ Population	☐ Vibration
☐ Light	☐ Climate	

Support and relationships

☐ Immediate family	☐ Extended family	☐ Friends
☐ Health professionals	☐ Other professionals	☐ Strangers
☐ People in positions of authority	☐ People in subordinate positions	☐ Domesticated animals
☐ Acquaintances, peers, colleagues, neighbors, and community members		☐ Personal care providers and personal assistants

Attitudes

- ☐ Of immediate family
- ☐ Of strangers
- ☐ Of people in positions of authority
- ☐ Of acquaintances, peers, colleagues, neighbors, and community members
- ☐ Of extended family
- ☐ Of health professionals
- ☐ Of people in subordinate positions
- ☐ Of personal care providers and personal assistants
- ☐ Of friends
- ☐ Of health-related professionals
- ☐ Societal attitudes
- ☐ Social norms, practices, and ideologies

Services, systems, and policies

- ☐ Production of consumer goods
- ☐ Open space planning
- ☐ Utilities
- ☐ Transportation
- ☐ Legal
- ☐ Media
- ☐ Architecture and construction
- ☐ Social security
- ☐ Health
- ☐ Labor and employment
- ☐ Housing
- ☐ Communication
- ☐ Associations and organizations
- ☐ Civil protection
- ☐ Economic
- ☐ General social support
- ☐ Education and training
- ☐ Political

C. Does this measure assess a single attribute or multiple attributes?

- ☐ Single
- ☐ Multiple

D. Check purposes that apply and indicate (*) primary purpose of the measure

- ☐ To describe or discriminate
- ☐ To predict
- ☐ To evaluative

Comments: ______________________________

____

E. Perspective—Indicate possible respondents

- ☐ Client
- ☐ Caregiver/parent
- ☐ Service provider
- ☐ Other professional
- ☐ Other

F. Population measure designed for:

Age: Please specify all applicable ages if stated in the manual

- ☐ Infant (birth to < 1 year)
- ☐ Adult (> 18 years to < 65 years)
- ☐ Child (1 year to < 13 years)
- ☐ Senior (> 65 years)
- ☐ Adolescent (13 to < 18 years)
- ☐ Age not specified

Diagnosis: ______________________________

List the diagnostic group(s) for which this measure is designed to be used: ______________________________

____

G. Evaluation context—Indicate suggested/possible environments for this assessment

- ☐ Home
- ☐ Workplace
- ☐ Other ______________________________
- ☐ Education setting
- ☐ Community agency
- ☐ Community
- ☐ Rehabilitation center/health care setting

2. Clinical Utility

A. Clarity of Instructions (Check one of the ratings)

- ☐ Excellent: Clear, comprehensive, concise, and available
- ☐ Adequate: Clear, concise, but lacks some information
- ☐ Poor: Not clear and concise or not available

Comments: ______________________________

____

B. Format (check applicable items)

☐ Interview
☐ Naturalistic observation
☐ Task performance
☐ Questionnaire: ☐ Self completed ☐ Interview administered ☐ Caregiver completed
☐ Other ______

Physically invasive:	☐ Yes	☐ No
Active participation of client:	☐ Yes	☐ No
Special equipment required:	☐ Yes	☐ No

C. Time to complete assessment: ____ minutes

Administration:	☐ Easy	☐ More complex
Scoring:	☐ Easy	☐ More complex
Interpretation:	☐ Easy	☐ More complex

(Consider time, amount of training, and ease)

D. Examiner qualifications: Is formal training required for administering and/or interpreting?

☐ Required ☐ Recommended ☐ Not required
☐ Not addressed

E. Cost (Canadian Funds)

Manual: $ ______

Score sheets: $ ______ for ______ sheets

Indicate year of cost information: ______

Source of cost information: ______

F. Manual (check one of the ratings)

☐ Excellent: Published manual which outlines specific procedures for administration, scoring and interpretation, evidence of reliability and validity
☐ Adequate: Manual available and generally complete but some information is lacking or unclear regarding administration, scoring and interpretation, evidence of reliability and validity
☐ Poor: No manual available or manual with unclear administration, scoring and interpretation, no evidence of reliability and validity

G. Overall Clinical Utility

☐ Excellent: Excellent manual or published document, acceptable to client, feasible to purchase, administer, score, and interpret
☐ Adequate: Adequate to excellent manual or published document; some area of concern in terms of feasibility recost, time, complexity, acceptability
☐ Poor: Poor/no manual or not feasible due to major concerns of cost, time, complexity, or acceptability

3. Scale Construction

A. Which specific domain does this measure assess?

☐ Physical ☐ Psychological ☐ Social
☐ School functioning ☐ Environmental ☐ Personal care
☐ Other

B. Item Selection (check one of the ratings)

- ☐ Excellent: Included all relevant characteristics of attribute based on comprehensive literature review and survey of experts
- ☐ Adequate: Included most relevant characteristics of attribute
- ☐ Poor: Convenient sample of characteristics of attribute

Comments: ____

____

C. Weighting

Are the items weighted in the calculation of total score?	☐ Yes	☐ No
If yes, are the items weighted?	☐ Implicitly	☐ Explicitly

D. Level of Measurement

☐ Nominal	☐ Ordinal
☐ Interval	☐ Ratio

Scaling method (Likert, Guttman, etc.): ______________________

Number of items: ______________________

Indicate if subscale scores are obtained:	☐ Yes	☐ No
If yes, can the subscale scores be used alone?		
Administered:	☐ Yes	☐ No
Interpreted:	☐ Yes	☐ No

List subscales:	Number of items:
__________	__________
__________	__________
__________	__________

4. Standardization

A. Norms available (N/A for instrument whose purpose is only evaluative)

☐ Yes ☐ No ☐ N/A

Age: Please specify all applicable ages for which norms are available

☐ Infant (birth to < 1 year)	☐ Child (1 year to < 13 years)	☐ Adolescent (13 to < 18 years)
☐ Adult (> 18 years to < 65 years)	☐ Senior (> 65 years)	

Populations for which it is normed: ____

____

Size of sample: n = _____

5. Reliability

A. Rigor of standardization studies for reliability (check one of the ratings)

- ☐ Excellent: More than 2 well-designed reliability studies completed with adequate to excellent reliability values
- ☐ Adequate: 1 to 2 well-designed reliability studies completed with adequate to excellent reliability values
- ☐ Poor: Reliability studies poorly completed, or reliability studies showing poor levels of reliability
- ☐ No evidence available

Comments: ____

____

B. Reliability Information

Type of reliability	Statistic used	Value	Rating (excellent, adequate, poor)
________	________	________	________
________	________	________	________
________	________	________	________

*Guidelines for levels of reliability coefficient (see instructions)

Excellent: >0.80   Adequate: 0.60 to 0.79   Poor: <0.60

6. Validity

A. Rigor of standardization studies for validity (check one of the ratings)

- ☐ Excellent: More than 2 well-designed validity studies supporting the measure's validity
- ☐ Adequate: 1 to 2 well-designed validity studies supporting the measure's validity
- ☐ Poor: Validity studies poorly completed or did not support the measure's validity
- ☐ No evidence available

Comments: ____

____

B. Content validity (Check one of the ratings)

- ☐ Excellent: Judgmental or statistical method (eg, factor analysis) was used and the measure is comprehensive and includes items suited to the measurement purpose
  Method: ☐ Judgmental ☐ Statistical
- ☐ Adequate: Has content validity but no specific method was used
- ☐ Poor: Instrument is not comprehensive
- ☐ No evidence available

C. Construct validity (Check one of the ratings)

- ☐ Excellent: More than 2 well-designed studies have shown that the instrument conforms to prior theoretical relationships among characteristics or individuals
- ☐ Adequate: 1 to 2 studies demonstrate confirmation of theoretical formulations
- ☐ Poor: Construct validation poorly completed, or did not support measure's construct validity
- ☐ No evidence available

Strength of association: ____

____

D. Criterion validity (Check ratings that apply)

- ☐ Concurrent ☐ Predictive
- ☐ Excellent: More than 2 well-designed studies have shown adequate agreement with a criterion or gold standard
- ☐ Adequate: 1 to 2 studies demonstrate adequate agreement with a criterion or gold standard measure
- ☐ Poor: Criterion validation poorly completed or did not support measure's criterion validity
- ☐ No evidence available

Criterion measure(s) used: ____

____

Strength of association: ____

____

E. Responsiveness (Check one of the ratings)

- ☐ Excellent: More than 2 well-designed studies showing strong hypothesized relationships between changes on the measure and other measures of change on the same attribute.
- ☐ Adequate: 1 to 2 studies of responsiveness
- ☐ Poor: Studies of responsiveness poorly completed or did not support the measure's responsiveness
- ☐ N/A
- ☐ No evidence available

Comments: ____

____

7. Overall Utility
(Based on an Overall Assessment of the Quality of This Measure)

- ☐ Excellent: Adequate to excellent clinical utility, easily available, excellent reliability, and validity
- ☐ Adequate: Adequate to excellent clinical utility, easily available, adequate to excellent reliability, and adequate to excellent validity
- ☐ Poor: Poor clinical utility, not easily available, poor reliability and validity

Comments/notes/explanations: ____

____

____

____

Materials Used for Review/Rating

Please indicate the sources of information used for this review/rating:

- ☐ Manual
- ☐ Journal articles (attach or indicate location)
    - ☐ By author of measure
    - ☐ By other authors

List sources: ____

____

____

____

- ☐ Books: Provide reference
- ☐ Correspondence with author (attach)
- ☐ Other sources: ____

____

____

____

OUTCOME MEASURES RATING FORM

CanChild Centre for Childhood Disability Research
Institute of Applied Health Sciences, McMaster University
1400 Main Street West. Room 408
Hamilton, Canada L8S 1C7
Fax (905) 522-6095
lawm@mcmaster.ca
Prepared by: Mary Law, Ph.D. O.T.(C)

For further discussion of issues: Law M. Measurement in occupational therapy: scientific criteria for evaluation. *Can J Occup Ther.* 1987;54:133-138.

General information: Name of Measure, Authors, Source and Year.

1. Focus

A. *Focus of measurement.* Use the ICF framework to indicate the focus of the measurement instrument that is being reviewed. The definitions are as follows:
   - Body Functions: Are the physiological functions of body systems (including psychological functions).
   - Body Structures: Are anatomical parts of the body such as organs, limbs, and their components.
   - Activities and Participation: Activity is the execution of a task or action by an individual. Participation is involvement in a life situation.
   - Environmental Factors: Make up the physical, social and attitudinal environment in which people live and conduct their lives.

B. *Attributes being measured.* The rating form lists attributes organized using the ICF framework. Check as many attributes as apply to indicate what is being measured by this instrument.

C. *Single or multiple attribute.* Check the appropriate box to indicate whether this measure assesses a single attribute only or multiple attributes.

D. *List the primary purpose for which the scale has been designed.* Secondary purposes can also be listed but the instrument should be evaluated according to its primary purpose (ie, discriminative, predictive, evaluative).
   - *Discriminative.* A discriminative index is used to distinguish between individuals or groups on an underlying dimension when no external criterion or gold standard is available for validating these measures.
   - *Predictive.* A predictive index is used to classify individuals into a set of predefined measurement categories, either concurrently or prospectively, to determine whether individuals have been classified correctly.
   - *Evaluative.* An evaluative index is used to measure the magnitude of longitudinal change in an individual or group on the dimension of interest. (Kirshner B, Guyatt G. A methodological framework for assessing health indices. *J Chronic Dis.* 1985;38:27-36.)

E. *Perspective.* Indicate the possible respondents.

F. *Population for which it is designed (AGE).* If no age is stated, mark as age unspecified. List the diagnostic groups for which the measure is used.

G. *Evaluation context.* Refers to the environment in which the assessment is completed. Check all possible environments in which this assessment can be completed.

2. Clinical Utility

A. *Clarity of instructions.* Check one of the ratings. Excellent: clear, comprehensive, concise and available; Adequate: clear, concise but lacks some information; Poor: not clear and concise or not available.

B. *Format.* Check all applicable items to indicate the format of data collection for the instrument. Possible items include naturalistic observation, interview, a questionnaire (self-completed, interview administered or caregiver-completed) and task performance.
   - *Physically invasive.* Indicates whether administration of the measure requires procedures that may be perceived as invasive by the client. Examples of invasiveness include any procedure that requires insertion of needles or taping of electrodes, or procedures that require clients to take clothing on or off.
   - *Active participation of client.* Indicate whether completion of the measure requires the client to participate verbally or physically.
   - *Special equipment required.* Indicate whether the measurement process requires objects that are not part of the test kit and are not everyday objects. Examples of this include stopwatches, a balance board, or other special equipment.

C. *Time to complete the assessment.* Record in minutes. For Administration, Scoring, and Interpretation, consider the time and the amount of training and the ease with which a test is administered, scored, and interpreted, and indicate whether these issues are easy or more complex. For Administration, Scoring, and Interpretation to be rated as easy, each part of the task should be completed in under 1 hour with minimal amount of training and be easy for the average service provider to complete.

D. *Examiner qualifications.* Indicate whether formal training is required for administering and interpreting this measure.

E. *Cost.* In Canadian funds, indicate the cost of the measurement manual and score sheets. For score sheets, indicate the number of sheets obtainable for that cost. List the source and the year of the cost information so readers will know whether the information is up to date.

3. Scale Construction

A. *Item selection.* Check one of the ratings. Excellent: included all relevant characteristics of the attribute based on comprehensive literature review and survey of experts—a comprehensive review of the literature only is enough for an excellent rating, but a survey of experts alone is not enough; Adequate: included most relevant characteristics of the attribute; Poor: convenient sample of characteristics of the attribute.

B. *Weighting.* Indicate whether the items in the tool are weighted in the calculation of the total score. If items are weighted, indicate whether the authors have weighted these items implicitly or explicitly. Implicit weighting occurs when there are a number of scales and each have a different number of items and the score is obtained by simply adding the scores for each item together. Explicit weighting occurs when each item or score is multiplied by a factor to weight its importance.

C. *Level of measurement.* State whether the scale used is nominal (descriptive categories), ordinal (ordered categories), or interval or ratio (numerical) for single and for summary scores. Indicate the scaling method that was used and the number of items in the measure. Indicate if subscale scores are obtained. Indicate whether the subscales can be administered alone and the scores interpreted alone. In some cases, the scores can be interpreted alone, but the whole measure must be administered first. List the subscales with the number of items and indicate whether there is evidence of reliability and validity for the subscales so that the scores can be used on their own. Standardization is the process of administering a test under uniform conditions.

4. Standardization

A. *Manual.* Check one of the ratings. Excellent: published manual which outlines specific procedures for administration; scoring and interpretation; evidence of reliability and validity. Adequate: manual available and generally complete but some information is lacking or unclear regarding administration; scoring and interpretation; evidence of reliability and validity. Poor: no manual available or manual with unclear administration; scoring and interpretation; no evidence of reliability and validity.

B. *Norms.* Indicate whether norms are available for the instrument. Please note that instruments that are only meant to be evaluative do not require norms. Indicate all ages for which norms are available, the populations for which the measure has been normed (eg, children with cerebral palsy, people with spinal cord injuries), and indicate the size of the sample that was used in the normative studies.

5. Reliability

Reliability is the process of determining that the test or measure is measuring something in a reproducible and consistent fashion.

A. *Rigour of standardization studies for reliability.* Excellent: More than 2 well-designed reliability studies completed with adequate to excellent reliability values; Adequate: 1 to 2 well-designed reliability studies completed with adequate to excellent reliability values; Poor: No reliability studies or poorly completed, or reliability studies showing poor levels of reliability.

B. *Reliability information.* Internal Consistency: the degree of homogeneity of test items to the attribute being measured. Measured at one point in time. Observer: 1) Intraobserver—Measures variation that occurs within an observer as a result of multiple exposures to the same stimulus, 2) Interobserver—Measures variation between 2 or more observers. Test-Retest: Measures variation in the test over a period of time.

Complete the table and reliability information by filling in the type of reliability that was tested (internal consistency, observer, test-retest); the statistic that was used (eg, Cronbach's coefficient alpha, kappa coefficient, Pearson correlation, intra-class correlation); the value of the statistic that was found in the study; and the rating of the reliability. Guidelines for levels of the reliability coefficient indicate that it will be rated excellent if the coefficient is greater than 0.80, adequate if it is from 0.60 to 0.79, and poor if the coefficient is less than 0.60.

6. Validity

A. *Rigour of standardization studies for validity.* Excellent: More than 2 well designed validity studies supporting the measure's validity; Adequate: 1 to 2 well designed validity studies supporting the measure's validity; Poor: No validity studies completed, studies were poorly completed or did not support the measure's validity.

B. *Content validity.* Check one of the ratings. Content validity: the instrument is comprehensive and fully represents the domain of the characteristics it claims to measure. (Nunnally JC. *Psychometric Theory.* New York: McGraw-Hill; 1978.) Excellent: Judgmental or statistical method (eg, factor analysis) was used and the measure is comprehensive and includes items suited to the measurement purpose; Adequate: Has content validity, but no specific method was used; Poor: Instrument is not comprehensive. Method: Note whether a judgmental (eg, consensus methods) or statistical method (eg, factor analysis) of establishing content validity was used.

C. *Construct validity.* The measurements of the attribute conform to prior theoretical formulations or relationships among characteristics or individuals. (Nunnally JC. *Psychometric Theory.* New York: McGraw-Hill; 1978.) Excellent: More than 2 well-designed studies have shown that the instrument conforms to prior theoretical relationships among characteristics or individuals; Adequate: 1 to 2 studies demonstrate confirmation of theoretical formulations; Poor: No construct validation completed. Indicate the strength of association of the findings for construct validity by listing the value of the correlation coefficients found.

D. *Criterion validity.* Check one of the ratings. Criterion validity: The measurements obtained by the instrument agree with another more accurate measure of the same characteristic, that is, a criterion or gold standard measure. (Nunnally, J. C. (1978). Psychometric theory. New York: McGraw-Hill.) Indicate whether the type of criterion validity that was investigated is concurrent, predictive, or both. Excellent: More than 2 well-designed studies have shown adequate agreement with a criterion or gold standard; Adequate: 1 to 2 studies demonstrate adequate agreement with a criterion or gold standard measure; Poor: No criterion validation completed. Indicate the strength of association of the evidence for criterion validity by listing the values of the correlation coefficients that were found in the criterion validity studies. Using the information from the assessment that has been completed on this measure, check the appropriate rating to give an overall assessment of the quality of the measure.

E. *Responsiveness.* Check one of the ratings (applicable only to evaluative measures). Responsiveness: The ability of the measure to detect minimal clinically important change over time. (Guyatt G, Walter SD, Norman GR. Measuring change over time: assessing the usefulness of evaluative instruments. *J Chronic Dis.* 1987;40:171-178.) Excellent: More than 2 well-designed studies showing strong hypothesized relationships between changes on the measure and other measures of change on the same attribute; Adequate: 1 to 2 studies of responsiveness; Poor: No studies of responsiveness; N/A: Check if the measure is not designed to evaluate change over time.

7. Overall Utility

Excellent: Adequate to excellent clinical utility, easily available, and excellent reliability and validity. Adequate: Adequate to excellent clinical utility, easily available, adequate to excellent reliability, and adequate to excellent validity. Poor: Poor clinical utility, not easily available, poor reliability, and validity.

8. Materials Used

Please indicate and list the sources of information that were used for this review. By listing sources of information and attaching appropriate journal articles or correspondence with authors, it will be easier to find further information about this measure if it is required.

Financial Disclosures

Dr. Catherine Backman has no financial or proprietary interest in the materials presented herein.

Dr. Julie D. Bass has no financial or proprietary interest in the materials presented herein.

Dr. Carolyn Baum receives royalties from sale of the *Activity Card Sort* from AOTA Press.

Dr. Jackie Bosch has no financial or proprietary interest in the materials presented herein.

Mark Burghart has no financial or proprietary interest in the materials presented herein.

Dr. Mary A. Corcoran has no financial or proprietary interest in the materials presented herein.

Oana Craciunoiu has no financial or proprietary interest in the materials presented herein.

Dr. Winnie Dunn is the author of the Sensory Profiles. Pearson Publishing owns the copyright, and Dr. Dunn receives a royalty for their sale.

Dr. Mary Forhan has no financial or proprietary interest in the materials presented herein.

Dr. Lauren Foster has no financial or proprietary interest in the materials presented herein.

Apeksha Gohil has no financial or proprietary interest in the materials presented herein.

Dr. Meredith P. Gronski has no financial or proprietary interest in the materials presented herein.

Dr. Joy Hammel has no financial or proprietary interest in the materials presented herein.

Kathryn M. B. Haugen has no financial or proprietary interest in the materials presented herein.

Dr. Jenna Heffron has no financial or proprietary interest in the materials presented herein.

Dr. Margo B. Holm has no financial or proprietary interest in the materials presented herein.

Dr. Vicki Kaskutas has no financial or proprietary interest in the materials presented herein.

Dr. Mary Law is an author of the Canadian Occupational Performance Measure (COPM) and receives a royalty for its sale and income from an online learning module and COPM translations.

Dr. Danbi Lee has no financial or proprietary interest in the materials presented herein.

Dr. Lori Letts has no financial or proprietary interest in the materials presented herein.

Dr. Joy MacDermid has received payment from Elsevier for the *Journal of Hand Therapy.*

Dr. Susan Magasi has no financial or proprietary interest in the materials presented herein.

Dr. Mary Ann McColl is an author of the COPM and a director and shareholder in COPM Inc.

Dr. Kira Meskin has no financial or proprietary interest in the materials presented herein.

Dr. Laura Miller has no financial or proprietary interest in the materials presented herein.

Dr. Becky Nicholson has no financial or proprietary interest in the materials presented herein.

Dr. Monica S. Perlmutter has no financial or proprietary interest in the materials presented herein.

Nancy Pollock is an author of the COPM and a director and shareholder in COPM Inc.

Dr. Anne A. Poulsen has no financial or proprietary interest in the materials presented herein.

Dr. Patricia Rigby has no financial or proprietary interest in the materials presented herein.

Dr. Joan C. Rogers has no financial or proprietary interest in the materials presented herein.

Jill Stier has no financial or proprietary interest in the materials presented herein.

Dr. Linda Tickle-Degnen has no financial or proprietary interest in the materials presented herein.

Anna Wallisch has no financial or proprietary interest in the materials presented herein.

Dr. Jenny Ziviani has no financial or proprietary interest in the materials presented herein.

INDEX

Printed in the United States
by Baker & Taylor Publisher Services